Manual of Allergy and Immunology

Fourth Edition

Manual of Allergy and Immunology
Fourth Edition

Edited by

Daniel C. Adelman, M.D.
Associate Adjunct Professor of Medicine
Division of Allergy and Immunology
University of California, San Francisco
San Francisco, California

Thomas B. Casale, M.D.
Director of Clinical Research, School of Medicine
Professor and Assistant Chair, Department of Medicine
Chief, Allergy and Immunology
Creighton University
Omaha, Nebraska

Jonathan Corren, M.D.
Associate Clinical Professor
Department of Medicine
University of California, Los Angeles;
Medical Director
Allergy Research Foundation
Los Angeles, California

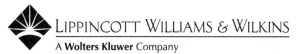

LIPPINCOTT WILLIAMS & WILKINS
A **Wolters Kluwer** Company
Philadelphia · Baltimore · New York · London
Buenos Aires · Hong Kong · Sydney · Tokyo

Acquisitions Editor: Jonathan W. Pine
Developmental Editor: Selina M. Bush
Production Editor: Melanie Bennitt
Manufacturing Manager: Timothy Reynolds
Cover Designer: Mark Lerner
Compositor: Circle Graphics
Printer: Vicks Lithograph

© **2002 by LIPPINCOTT WILLIAMS & WILKINS**
530 Walnut Street
Philadelphia, PA 19106 USA
LWW.com

Printed in the USA
Previous Editions: 1995, 1988, 1981

Library of Congress Cataloging-in-Publication Data

Manual of allergy and immunology.—4th ed. / [edited by] Daniel C. Adelman, Thomas B.
  Casale, Jonathan Corren.
    p. ; cm.
  Includes bibliographical references and index.
  ISBN 0-7817-3052-X
    1. Allergy—Handbooks, manuals, etc. 2. Immunology—Handbooks, manuals, etc. I.
  Adelman, Daniel C. II. Casale, Thomas B. III. Corren, Jonathan.
    [DNLM: 1. Immunologic Diseases—Handbooks. 2. Hypersensitivity—Handbooks. WD
  301 M294 2002]
    RC584 .M36 2002
  616.97—dc21

                                                                          2001050543

---

10 9 8 7 6 5 4 3 2 1

To my wife, Deborah, and children, Arielle, Nathan, and Gabriel, for their patience, tolerance, and understanding; and to my parents, Barnet and Beverly, for the years of support and encouragement.

Daniel C. Adelman, M.D.

To the memory of my father, William J. Casale, Sr.; to my mother, Nancy; my wife, Jean; and my son, Jeffrey, for their loving support and encouragement.

Thomas B. Casale, M.D.

To the memory of my father, Herman Corren, M.D., for his inspiration and encouragement, and to my mother, Mildred, my wife, Martha, and children Jeremy and Rachel, for their loving support.

Jonathan Corren, M.D.

CONTENTS

CONTRIBUTING AUTHORS

Julian L. Ambrus, Jr., M.D.
Associate Professor, Department of Medicine, State University of New York at Buffalo; Director, Autoimmune Disease Research Center, Department of Medicine, Buffalo General Hospital–Kaleida Health, Buffalo, New York

Robert Ausdenmoore, M.D.
Volunteer Professor of Pediatrics, Division of Allergy and Immunology, Children's Hospital Medical Center, Cincinnati, Ohio

Alan N. Baer, M.D.
Associate Professor, Department of Medicine, State University of New York at Buffalo; Chief, Division of Rheumatology, Erie County Medical Center, Buffalo, New York

Vincent S. Beltrani, M.D.
Associate Clinical Professor of Dermatology, Columbia University College of Physicians and Surgeons, New York, New York; Associate Visiting Professor, Allergy and Rheumatology, UMDNJ Asthma and Allergy Research Center, Newark, New Jersey

Leonard Bielory, M.D.
Associate Professor, Departments of Medicine, Pediatrics, and Ophthalmology, UMDNJ, New Jersey Medical School; Director, UMDNJ Asthma and Allergy Research Center, and UMDNJ University Hospital, Newark, New Jersey

Jack J. H. Bleesing, M.D.
Assistant Professor, Department of Pediatrics, University of Arkansas for Medical Sciences; Pediatric Faculty, Department of Pediatrics, Arkansas Children's Hospital, Little Rock, Arkansas

Bruce S. Bochner, M.D.
Professor, Department of Medicine, Division of Clinical Immunology, Johns Hopkins University School of Medicine, Johns Hopkins Asthma and Allergy Center, Baltimore, Maryland

John M. Boggs, M.D.
Consultant, Infectious Diseases, Department of Internal Medicine, Palo Alto Medical Foundation, Palo Alto, California; Assistant Clinical Professor, Department of Medicine, Stanford University Medical Center, Stanford, California

Mark Boguniewicz, M.D.
Professor, Department of Pediatrics, University of Colorado School of Medicine; Senior Faculty Member, National Jewish Medical and Research Center, Denver, Colorado

A. Wesley Burks, M.D.
Professor, Department of Pediatrics, University of Arkansas for Medical Sciences, and Arkansas Children's Hospital, Little Rock, Arkansas

Robert K. Bush, M.D.
Professor, Department of Medicine, University of Wisconsin at Madison; Chief of Allergy, William S. Middleton VA Hospital, Madison, Wisconsin

Ernest N. Charlesworth, M.D.
Department of Dermatology, Shannon Clinic, San Angelo, Texas

Beth W. Colombe, M.D.
Associate Professor and Director, Immunogenetics and Tissue Typing Laboratory, Thomas Jefferson University, Philadelphia, Pennsylvania

Jonathan Corren, M.D.
Associate Clinical Professor, Department of Medicine, University of California at Los Angeles, Los Angeles, California

Charlotte Cunningham-Rundles, M.D.
Mount Sinai Medical Center, New York, New York

Lloyd E. Damon, M.D.
Professor, Department of Medicine, University of California at San Francisco, San Francisco, California

Mark S. Dykewicz, M.D.
Associate Professor of Internal Medicine, Division of Allergy and Immunology, Director, Training Program in Allergy and Immunology, Saint Louis University Medical School; Attending Physician, Department of Internal Medicine, Saint Louis University Hospital, St. Louis, Missouri

Thomas A. Fleisher, M.D.
Chief, Department of Laboratory Medicine, National Institute of Health, Bethesda, Maryland

David B. K. Golden, M.D.
Associate Professor, Department of Medicine, Johns Hopkins University; Director of Allergy, Department of Medicine, Sinai Hospital, Baltimore, Maryland

Paul A. Greenberger, M.D.
Professor of Medicine, Division of Allergy Immunology, Northwestern University Medical School; Attending Physician, Department of Medicine, Northwestern Memorial Hospital, Chicago, Illinois

Alfredo A. Jalowayski, M.D.
Respiratory Physiologist Specialist, Department of Pediatrics and Surgery, University of California at San Diego, La Jolla, California

Susann Kircher, M.D.
Fellow, Department of Allergy and Immunology, University of California at San Diego; Fellow, VA Hospital, San Diego, California

Eric C. Kleerup, M.D.
Assistant Professor, Department of Medicine, Division of Pulmonary and Critical Care, University of California, Los Angeles, School of Medicine, Los Angeles, California

Michelle Lierl, M.D.
Adjunct Associate Professor, Department of Clinical Pediatrics, Children's Hospital Medical Center, Cincinnati, Ohio

Eric Macy, M.D.
Assistant Clinical Professor, Department of Medicine, University of California, San Diego, School of Medicine; Partner Physician, Department of Allergy, Kaiser Permanente Medical Center, San Diego, California

Diana Marquardt, M.D.
Associate Professor, Department of Medicine, University of California at San Diego, San Diego, California

Joseph L. McGerity, M.D.
Director of Allergy Service, Student Health Service, San Francisco State University; Clinical Professor of Medicine, Allergy-Immunology Division, University of California at San Francisco, San Francisco, California

Michael H. Mellon, M.D.
Associate Clinical Professor, Department of Pediatrics, University of California at San Diego School of Medicine, La Jolla, California; Staff Physician, Department of Allergy, Kaiser Permanente Medical Center, San Diego, California

Edina Moylett, M.D.
Fellow in Allergy and Immunology, Department of Pediatrics, Baylor College of Medicine; Department of Pediatrics, Texas Children's Hospital, Houston, Texas

Ali I. Musani, M.D.
Fellow, Department of Medicine, Division of Critical Care, Pulmonary, Allergic, and Immunologic Diseases, Jefferson Medical College, Thomas Jefferson University, and Thomas Jefferson University Hospital, Philadelphia, Pennsylvania

William Neaville, M.D.
Fellow, Allergy and Immunology Training Program, University of Wisconsin at Madison, Madison, Wisconsin

Kathleen M. O'Neil, M.D.
Clinical Associate Professor, Department of Pediatrics, State University of New York at Buffalo School of Medicine and Biomedical Sciences; Director, Department of Allergy, Immunology, and Rheumatology, Children's Hospital of Buffalo, Buffalo, New York

Rodolfo M. Pascual, M.D.
Fellow, Department of Medicine, Division of Critical Care, Pulmonary, Allergic, and Immunologic Diseases, Jefferson Medical College, Thomas Jefferson University, and Thomas Jefferson University Hospital, Philadelphia, Pennsylvania

Roy Patterson, M.D.
Professor of Medicine, Department of Allergy-Immunology, Northwestern University Medical School, Chicago, Illinois

Stephen P. Peters, M.D.
Jefferson Medical College, Philadelphia, Pennsylvania

Michael D. Roth, M.D.
Division of Pulmonary Disease and Critical Care Medicine, University of California at Los Angeles, Los Angeles, California

Sarbjit S. Saini
Johns Hopkins Asthma and Allergy Center, Baltimore, Maryland

Alvin M. Sanico, M.D.
Assistant Professor, Department of Medicine, Division of Clinical Immunology, Johns Hopkins Asthma and Allergy Center, Baltimore, Maryland

Michael Schatz, M.D.
Chief, Department of Allergy, Kaiser Permanente Medical Center; Clinical Professor, Department of Medicine, University of California at San Diego School of Medicine, San Diego, California

William T. Shearer, M.D., Ph.D.
*Professor and Section Head, Department of Pediatrics, Baylor College of Medicine;
Chief of Service, Department of Allergy and Immunology, Texas Children's Hospital,
Houston, Texas*

Michelle Zeidler, M.D.
*Senior Fellow, Department of Medicine, Division of Pulmonary and
Critical Care, University of California at Los Angeles School of Medicine,
Los Angeles, California*

Robert S. Zeiger, M.D., Ph.D.
*Clinical Professor, Department of Pediatrics, University of California at San Diego,
La Jolla, California; Director of Allergy Research, Department of Allergy, Kaiser
Permanente Medical Center, San Diego, California*

PREFACE

The fourth edition of the *Manual of Allergy and Immunology* is designed to serve health care professionals in the diagnosis and management of allergic and other immunological disorders. Our goals have been to present the basic and essential material clearly and to provide specific information to assist in clinical decision-making and treatment planning.

We selected contributors to this edition for their specific expertise. Only currently accepted therapeutic regimens and dosages are recommended; all material that is considered investigative is so identified. We have attempted to minimize didactic material; what is included has been carefully edited to allow a basic understanding of each subject. More extensive discussions of each subject are referenced in each chapter under Selected Readings. In addition, useful addresses on the World Wide Web have been referenced when such sites are available.

Our overall goal is to have the *Manual* contain the basic information, collected in a single source, that is required for the practice of allergy and clinical immunology. The specialist will find this manual a convenient reference handbook, while the generalist will be able to use the *Manual* as a helpful guide in formulating a diagnostic and therapeutic approach to patients suspected of having an allergic or immunologic disorder, or in choosing immunologic diagnostic studies generally available for the evaluation of patients with such conditions as infectious diseases, hematologic disorders, or rheumatic disease. We hope that students, house officers, and other health care professionals will find the *Manual* a useful guide to the clinical practice of allergy and immunology.

Our heartfelt thanks to all of our contributors, for unselfishly giving their time and considerable effort preparing their respective chapters. We also thank Lippincott Williams & Wilkins for giving us the opportunity to publish the *Manual*; and our editors, Jonathan Pine and Selina Bush, for patiently giving encouragement and editorial assistance throughout the preparation of this edition.

Daniel C. Adelman
Thomas B. Casale
Jonathan Corren

1. INTRODUCTION TO THE IMMUNE SYSTEM

Susann Kircher and Diana Marquardt

The function of the immune system is to distinguish self from nonself and to protect the organism from the latter. Such a system is necessary for survival in all animals. In humans, a functioning immune system is required to prevent attack by endogenous factors, such as tumors or autoimmune phenomena, as well as external factors, such as microorganisms or toxins. Dysfunction or deficiency of the immune system leads to clinical diseases of varying expression and severity, ranging from mild atopic disease to severe rheumatoid arthritis, combined immunodeficiency, or cancer. This chapter serves as a brief introduction to the complexities of the immune system. In the subsequent chapters and the suggested reading lists are additional explanations.

I. Cells of the immune system

A. Lymphocytes are responsible for the initial specific recognition of an antigen. Lymphocytes comprise approximately 40% of the total number of white blood cells. They are principally divided into **B lymphocytes** and **T lymphocytes** on the basis of their phenotypic expression of cell surface molecules (see Chapter 19) as well as their functional differences. Structurally, B and T cells cannot be distinguished from each other under the microscope, although about 10% to 15% are B cells, and 70% to 80% of circulating blood lymphocytes are T cells; the remainder of lymphocytes are neither B nor T cells, and are often referred to as **null cells**.

1. **Phenotypic identification** of B and T lymphocytes is accomplished by immunofluorescence staining using monoclonal antibodies reactive with individual cell surface molecules or antigens. **Monoclonal antibodies** are produced by antibody-producing hybridoma cell lines, which are capable of forming an antibody that is highly specific and always identical. Fusing a nonsecreting myeloma cell and the antibody-forming cell creates this hybrid cell, which results in an immortalized cell line that produces antibody recognizing a specific antigen. The hybridoma cells can be stored and retrieved to obtain the same antibody whenever needed. The display of many cell surface antigens not only differs by cell type, but also by the particular stage of differentiation and maturation of the cell; thus, the phenotypic expression of these developmentally regulated cell-surface molecules enables distinction between resting and activated cells. Dozens of monoclonal antibodies have been produced that react with cell surface antigens, enabling identification of B- and T-cell subsets and even distinction of cells by their stages of differentiation. Cell surface molecules identified by monoclonal antibodies and subsequently cloned are known as **clusters of differentiation (CD)** and are numbered sequentially. For example, CD19 is associated with mature B cells, whereas CD3 signifies activated T cells. These molecules are discussed more extensively in Chapter 19.

2. **Lymphocyte subtypes and function.** Collectively, the functions of the T and B cells encompass an entity termed the **adaptive immune system**. B lymphocytes are coated with surface membrane-bound immunoglobulin and a wide variety of other molecules; functionally, B lymphocytes produce antibody. Minor populations of B cells develop in the bone marrow, are polyreactive, and express the CD5 marker, an adhesion and cell surface molecule. These are referred to as **B1 cells**. The B1 cells express immunoglobulin M (IgM), are polyreactive, and often have a relatively low receptor binding affinity. Other B cells develop lacking the CD5 molecule and are known as B2 cells. Prior to encountering antigen, mature B2 cells coexpress IgM and IgD antibodies on their surface. However,

1

once B2 cells encounter antigen, they usually switch their antigen receptors to IgG, IgA, or IgE. Within secondary lymphoid tissues, complexes of antigen, antibody, and complement are localized in follicular dendritic cells. When these complexes encounter one another, **germinal centers** are formed, which can be seen on histologic examination as discrete areas in the spleen and lymph nodes. It is within these germinal centers that B2 cells encounter antigen and undergo immunoglobulin class switching via the interaction of CD40 and its ligand, CD40L (also known as CD154). CD40 is a surface marker constitutively expressed on B cells, and CD40L is expressed on an appropriately activated subset of CD4 T cells, known as T helper 2 (Th2) cells. It is the interaction of these two molecules that allows immunoglobulin class switching. It is during immunoglobulin class switching that somatic hypermutation of the antigen receptor genes occurs and high-affinity, antigen-specific IgG, IgA, or IgE are produced. The final stages of B-cell differentiation into antibody-secreting plasma cells continues to occur in secondary lymphoid tissues, but outside the germinal centers. Memory cells and plasma cell precursors are also formed in the germinal centers.

3. **T lymphocytes** mediate a number of functions, notably the **cell-mediated immune responses**, such as delayed hypersensitivity, graft rejection, and immune surveillance of neoplastic cells. Quantitative and functional differences distinguish the principal T-cell subsets. CD4 cells predominate over CD8 cells in blood by a ratio of 2 : 1. CD4 cells provide helper and "inducer" signals for B and T lymphocytes (through various cytokines). CD4 cells also help to mediate CD8 cell cytotoxic actions. In addition, CD4 cells provide inducer signals for macrophages that help to augment the cytotoxic capabilities of macrophages. The CD4 cells are made up of two predominant cell types: **Th1 and Th2 cells**. These T-cell subsets differentiate from the Th0 cell following antigenic stimulation. A Th1 cell is a helper cell that produces a specific phenotypic profile of cytokines such as interleukin-2 (IL-2) and interferon-γ (IFN-γ). These cytokines generally inhibit the growth and growth and differentiation of Th2 cells. Th1 cells are primarily involved in cell-mediated immunity, in that they activate macrophages and cytotoxic T cells. A Th2 cell is a helper cell that produces such cytokines as IL-4, 5, 6, 10, and 13. These cells likewise inhibit Th1 responses and are involved primarily in humoral immunity and allergic inflammation. The paradigm of the Th1/Th2 subsets will be discussed in further detail in **section III, Immune system functional components**. CD8 cells, when influenced by CD4 cells, suppress B lymphocyte immunoglobulin production and T lymphocyte responses to major histocompatibility antigens, and enhance cytotoxicity and natural killing. The **CD8⁺ cells** are known as cytotoxic T cells and can function as both suppressor cells and mediate delayed-type hypersensitivity (DTH) reactions. CD8 molecules interact with major histocompatibility complex (MHC) class I molecules. The peptides presented by CD8 cells are derived from endogenous proteins, tumor cells, and viruses found within the antigen presenting cell (APC). Cytotoxic T cells and their relation to the Th1/Th2 paradigm will be discussed in section III.B.

4. **Null cells**, a part of the innate immune system, include a number of different cell types, including **natural killer (NK) cells**, which express the markers CD16 and CD56. These cells do not possess the typical appearance of a lymphocyte; they are slightly larger with a kidney-shaped nucleolus and have a granular appearance (**large granular lymphocytes [LGL]**). NK cells are capable of binding IgG because they have a membrane receptor for the IgG molecule. When a cell is coated with an antibody and destroyed by an NK cell, this phenomenon is called **antibody-dependent cell-mediated cytotoxicity (ADCC)**. Alternatively, NK cells can destroy cells without involvement of antibody (e.g., virally infected cells or tumor cells). Other characteristics of NK cells include recognition of antigens without major histocompatibility restric-

tions, lack of immunologic memory, and regulation of activity by cytokines and arachidonic acid metabolites.

B. **Phagocytic cells** are a part of the innate immune system, and consist of **monocyte–macrophages**, **polymorphonuclear leukocytes**, and **eosinophils**. These cells mature in the bone marrow, circulate in the blood for a short time as mature cells, and enter the tissue spaces by diapedesis through capillary walls, in response to cytokines and chemotactic factors.

1. **Macrophages** play a central role in the innate immune response. Derived from the blood monocytes, they circulate for a few days in the blood and then leave the vascular compartment to become active tissue macrophages. Macrophages possess receptors for carbohydrates, such as mannose, that are not normally found on the cells of vertebrates. This allows the macrophages to discriminate self from nonself. Receptors for antibodies and complement are found on both neutrophils and macrophages. This adaptation allows for enhanced phagocytosis of foreign organisms coated with antibody or complement. Macrophages have the following important functions: chemotaxis (cell movement), phagocytosis (antigen engulfment), and most important of all, processing and presentation of antigen in an immunogenic form recognizable to T lymphocytes. Microorganisms engulfed by macrophages can be destroyed when they encounter a wide range of toxic intracellular molecules produced by macrophages. Some of these molecules include superoxide anion, hydroxyl radicals, hypochlorous acid, nitric oxide, plasma proteins and peptides, lysozyme, arachidonic acid metabolites, nucleotide metabolites (cyclic adenosine monophosphate), and cytokines (IL-1, IL-6, and tumor necrosis factor [TNF]). Many tissue-specific cells are of macrophage lineage and function to process and present antigen (e.g., Langerhan cells and oligodendrocytes).

2. **Polymorphonuclear leukocytes** originate from pluripotent bone marrow stem cells. These cells circulate in the blood and tissue, and their primary function is phagocytosis and destruction of foreign antigens. These cells function in an antigen-nonspecific fashion, and have receptors for antibodies as well as for complement, so that if microorganisms are coated with either of these components, phagocytosis will be enhanced.

3. **Eosinophils**, often found in inflammatory sites or at sites of immune reactivity, play a role in host defense against parasites and other large metazoan pathogens. Although eosinophils show certain functional characteristics similar to those of neutrophils, they are only weakly phagocytic. One proposed mechanism for their ability to kill parasites is via the release of cationic proteins and reactive oxygen metabolites into extracellular fluid. In addition to releasing mediators, eosinophils also possess the ability to synthesize and secrete prostaglandins, leukotrienes, and various cytokines. Eosinophils appear to have a modulatory or regulatory function in various types of inflammation. However, in the airway inflammatory response in asthma, eosinophil-derived mediators of inflammation—including major basic protein (MBP), eosinophil-derived neurotoxin (EDN), eosinophil cationic protein (ECP), and lysophospholipase (LPL)—are toxic to respiratory epithelium. Therefore, in certain instances, eosinophils promote tissue injury, and in this particular example, contribute to the pathogenesis of allergen-triggered inflammation in diseases such as asthma. The exact mechanism by which eosinophils cause oxidative damage is not known. Bromide ion is thought to be a substrate for eosinophil peroxidase, and eosinophil oxidative damage may occur via bromination of tyrosine residues.

C. **Basophils and mast cells** release the mediators of immediate hypersensitivity (e.g., histamine, leukotrienes, prostaglandins, and platelet-activating factor [PAF]) (see Chapter 2), which have significant effects on the vasculature and on smooth muscle. Basophils circulate, whereas mast cells are present only in tissue, and in much larger numbers. These cells have high-affinity receptors for IgE (FcεRI) and are involved in immediate and late-phase allergic reactions.

II. Development of the immune system

A. Phylogenetic development. Evolutionarily, the innate immune system evolved or developed before the adaptive immune response and appears to be inherent in all multicellular organisms. One feature that differentiates the innate and adaptive immune systems is the possession of germ-line-encoded receptors found within the innate immune system. These germ-line-encoded receptors mediate innate immune recognition. These receptors are predetermined genetically and thus have evolved through natural selection to possess specificity against infectious microorganisms. The immune system in higher animals and humans evolved with increasing complexity in terms of its specific antibody and cell-mediated immune response capacity, i.e., the adaptive immune response. Despite the complexity of the human immune system, host defense is still highly dependent on surface barriers and phagocytic mechanisms. The absence of phagocytic functions (as in severe neutropenia or in neutrophil function disorders, such as chronic granulomatous disease) or the loss of physical barriers (as with extensive cutaneous burns) can present a risk of fulminant, life-threatening invasion by microorganisms that normally are not pathogenic.

B. Ontogenetic development

  1. **In mature mammals, the primary lymphoid organs are the thymus and bone marrow**. During fetal development the liver is one of the primary organs of lymphoid development. In early fetal development, lymphocyte precursors are derived from the fetal yolk sac. By the fourth or fifth week of gestation, lymphocytes originate from the liver and thereafter from the bone marrow. In the bone marrow, pluripotent stem cells differentiate into lymphocytes, granulocytes, monocytes, erythrocytes, and megakaryocytes. B cells undergo early growth in the bone marrow and finally emerge with membrane-bound surface IgM or both IgM and IgD, although they have not yet encountered antigen. This growth that takes place in the bone marrow is antigen-independent B-lymphocyte maturation. B cells also proliferate in response to antigen-dependent signals and eventually differentiate into antibody-secreting cells or plasma cells. This proliferation is dependent on antigen binding to the B-cell receptor. This receptor comprises membrane-bound immunoglobulin and two additional chains required for its stable expression, Ig-α and Ig-β. There are two such heterodimers that flank the membrane-bound immunoglobulin and help to mediate signal transduction. B-cell activation also requires costimulation in the form of T cell help in two ways. The first is stimulation with IL-4, produced by the CD4+ T cell, which is an important B-cell growth factor. The second is T- and B-cell interaction via the molecules CD40 and CD40L (CD154); CD40 is expressed on the B cell, and CD40L is found on CD4 T cells. The interaction of these molecules facilitates class switching to IgA, IgG, and IgE. In a rare clinical immunodeficiency state, patients with X-linked hyper-IgM syndrome lack CD40L and are unable to produce antibodies of the IgA, IgG, and IgE classes. B cells also possess a cell surface molecule, B7 (CD80), which is up-regulated after ligation of CD40. B7 is a counterreceptor for CD28, a costimulatory molecule expressed on T cells. This costimulatory molecular interaction optimizes cytokine secretion and the T–B cell interaction.

     A human fetus is capable of synthesizing IgM antibody by 10.5 weeks of gestation, IgG by 12 weeks, and IgA antibody by 30 weeks. The immunocompetent human infant, typically born without antigen stimulation (unless infected in utero), has little circulating IgA and IgM. IgG antibody in the newborn is almost completely derived from the mother by active and selective transport across the placenta. Adult serum levels of IgG, IgM, and IgA are attained at different developmental stages (Fig. 1.1). See Appendix V for serum immunoglobulin levels by age.

     From 6 to 8 weeks of gestation, T-lymphocyte precursors migrate through the thymus, which is derived from the third and fourth embryonic pharyngeal pouches and is located in the mediastinum. The thymus func-

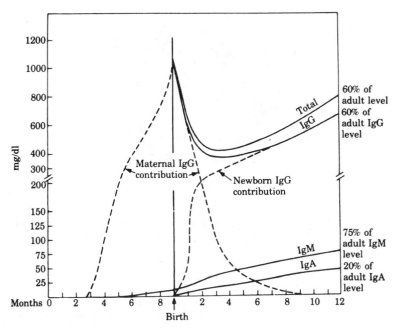

FIG. 1.1. Immunoglobulin (IgG, IgM, IgA) serum levels in the fetus and infant in the first year of life. IgG in the fetus and newborn infant is solely of maternal origin. The maternal IgG disappears by the age of 9 months, at which time endogenous synthesis of IgG by the infant is well established. The IgM and IgG at birth are entirely neonatal in origin (no placental transfer). (From Stiehm ER. Immunoglobulins and antibodies. In: Stiehm ER, Fulginiti VA, eds. *Immunologic disorders in infants and children.* Philadelphia: Saunders, 1973, with permission.)

tions to produce T lymphocytes and is the site of initiation of T-lymphocyte differentiation. A large number of T cells migrate to the thymus and become fully immunocompetent T cells. In addition, a number of T cells that are autoreactive die in the thymus. Under the influence of various cytokines (such as thymosin), T cells in the thymus undergo growth and differentiation and deletion of autoreactive clones. Functional development of cellular responses progressively matures as the fetus develops through parturition and infancy into adulthood.

2. **Phagocytic cells** are seen in the human fetus at 2 months of gestation as a few myelocytes and histiocytes present in the early yolk sac stage of hematopoiesis. Monocytes first appear in the spleen and lymph nodes at 4 to 5 months of gestation, with gradual maturation of macrophage function with advanced fetal age. The spleen, lymph nodes, and gut-associated lymphoid tissue are considered secondary lymphoid organs. Lymph nodes are peripherally dispersed throughout the body and function to localize the spread of infection. Lymph nodes are arranged in a reticular pattern with a cortex and medulla. B-lymphocytes are found in the cortex (follicles and germinal centers) as well as in the medulla, whereas T lymphocytes are primarily found in the medullary and cortical areas of the lymph nodes (see Fig. 1.2). The spleen is also divided into T- and B-cell areas similar to that of the lymph node. The spleen functions primarily to filter and process antigens from the blood.

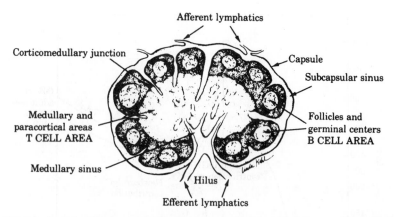

FIG. 1.2. Lymph node structure indicating primary T-cell and B-cell areas. (From Thaler MS, Klausner RD, Cohen HJ. Foundations of the immune response. In: *Medical immunology*. Philadelphia: Lippincott, 1977, with permission.)

3. **Complement components** are synthesized by the fetus early in gestation, either at the same time as or just before the beginning of immunoglobulin synthesis. There is almost no placental transfer of complement components C1q, C2, C4, C3, and C5, and the total hemolytic complement in the newborn is low. Such deficiency and dysfunction may be responsible for the relative opsonic deficiency in newborns. Complement plays a very important role in both innate and adaptive immunity. In the humoral immune response, complement opsonizes antigen as well as immune complexes for uptake by the complement receptor type 2 (CR2, CD21), is a coreceptor for B-cell activation, and is expressed primarily on B cells, follicular dendritic cells (FDC), and some T cells. Many different mechanisms are responsible for the complement-mediated promotion of the humoral immune response. These include:
   a. Enhancing antigen uptake and processing by both antigen-specific and nonspecific B cells for presentation to specific T cells.
   b. Activating a CD21/CD19 complex-mediated signaling pathway in B cells (this stimulus is synergistic to that induced by antigen interaction with the B-cell receptor).
   c. Promoting the interaction between B cells and follicular dendritic cells, in which C3d-bearing immune complexes participate in intracellular bridging. C3d is the ligand for CR2 on B cells, and is instrumental in B cell activation.
      CR2 can play a role in the development of autoimmune disease by determining B cell tolerance toward self-antigens. CR2 may be a key factor in the observed correlation between autoimmune disease and deficiency of the early complement components.

III. **Immune system functional components**
   The immune system consists of specific and nonspecific components that have distinct, yet overlapping functions. These two entities are known as the adaptive and the innate immune systems. The antibody-mediated and cell-mediated immune systems (parts of the adaptive immune system) provide specificity and a memory of previously encountered antigens. Phagocytic cells and complement proteins (parts of the innate immune system) are nonspecific cellular mechanisms and nonspecific plasma factors, respectively. Despite their lack of specificity, these components are essential because they are responsible for the natural immunity to a vast array of environmental microorganisms.

A. Antibody-mediated immunity. Antigen-specific activation of B cells occurs following the binding of antigen to membrane-bound immunoglobulin. Under the influences of a variety of cytokines released from monocytes and T cells (see Development of the immune system, section II.B. on page 4), B cells undergo clonal expansion and finally, differentiation into plasma cells capable of secreting large quantities of antibody. Small subsets of mature B cells become **memory B cells**, which are responsible for the recall responses after reexposure to antigen. When an individual first encounters a foreign antigen, an antibody response is mounted. There are typically four stages that characterize the **primary immune response**. During the first stage, no antibody is detected for the first 4 to 5 days. During the second phase, IgM antibodies form in high titers, followed several days later (typically 10 to 14 days after antigen exposure) by the production of IgG antibodies directed toward the same antigen. In the third stage, the antibody titer stabilizes, and during the fourth stage, there is a decline in antibody titer over a period of months to years, as the antibody is either cleared or catabolized. The **secondary antibody response** occurs upon reexposure to the same antigen; antibody, primarily IgG, appears more rapidly, persists longer, and reaches a higher titer.

    1. **Immunoglobulin structure.** Immunoglobulins are glycoproteins composed of four polypeptide chains (two light and two heavy chains), linked by disulfide bonds that allow the chains to form a bilaterally symmetric immunoglobulin molecule (Fig. 1.3). The N terminus of each chain possesses a variable domain, which, through the use of the hypervariable complementarity-determining regions, binds antigen. Both the heavy and light chains have C-terminal regions. These regions form the constant regions and further define the class and subclass of the antibody. This region also determines if the antibody light chain will be kappa (κ) or lambda (λ). There are five classes of immunoglobulins, called IgA, IgG, IgM, IgD, and IgE, based on the structure of their heavy chains (see Table 1.1). There are two subclasses of IgA and four subclasses of IgG. All immunoglobulins are glycoproteins and contain between 3% and 13% carbohydrate. The carbohydrate portion essentially maintains the structure of the immunoglobulin. Each antibody can exist as two forms: as a circulating molecule or as a stationary molecule attached to the B-cell surface which functions as the B-cell receptor. The stationary form has a hydrophobic transmembrane portion that functions as an anchor. There are only two classes of light chains: kappa and lambda. Each immunoglobulin molecule has only one class of light chain and only one class of heavy chain, although each class of immunoglobulin can have either kappa or lambda light chains. A monomeric antibody, such as IgG, consists of a single immunoglobulin molecule. Polymeric antibodies, such as IgM and IgA, consist of multiple basic units (e.g., IgM antibody consists of 10 light chains and 10 heavy chains). In addition to the polypeptide chains, other structures can be incorporated into the immunoglobulin molecule, including the **J chain**, also known as the joining chain, which is associated with all polymeric forms of antibody and is a polypeptide that stabilizes the polymer and the secretory piece of IgA. The **secretory component** of IgA can help to protect the IgA molecule from proteases within the gastrointestinal tract. This secretory component is only found on the secretory form of IgA.

    2. **Antibody diversity.** To respond to the enormous variety of antigens that humans and other animals encounter, the immune system must be capable of producing approximately 10^{15} antigen-specific antibodies. The source of antibody diversity lies in the structure and arrangement of the immunoglobulin genes and the ability of B cells to modify these genes by chromosomal rearrangement. There are three genetic components that encode immunoglobulin. These three components are found

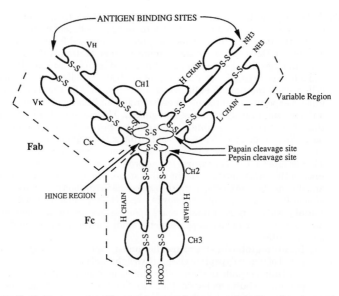

FIG. 1.3. Basic immunoglobulin structure with immunoglobulin subunits produced by enzyme. Interchain disulfide bonds are shown (large S–S), but intrachain bonds have been omitted for clarity. The number of H–H disulfide bonds varies with each class and subgroup of immunoglobulin. V_H and V_κ indicate the variable regions of the heavy and light (kappa) chains, respectively; C_H1–3 and C_κ indicate constant regions of the heavy and light (kappa) chains, respectively. H and L indicate heavy and light, respectively. Fab indicates the antibody-binding portion of the antibody molecule; Fc indicates the crystallizable receptor and complement-binding portion of the antibody molecule. Polymeric forms of immunoglobulin M (IgM) and IgA are not shown but are joined at the Fc region of the carboxy terminus.

on three separate chromosomes and are named as follows: (i) the IGH cluster (named for the heavy chain and located on chromosome 14), (ii) the IGK cluster (named for the kappa light chain and located on chromosome 2), and (iii) the IGL cluster (named for the lambda light chain and located on chromosome 22).

The antigen specificity of an antibody molecule depends upon the amino acid sequences in the antigen-binding portions of the heavy and light chain variable domains (Fig. 1.3). The information needed for an immunoglobulin molecule to be produced is coded for in the DNA. The chromosomal light and heavy chain DNA is separated into multiple gene segments that code for the variable (V), joining (J), and constant (C) regions of the light and heavy chains of the antibody molecule and the diversity (D) region of the immunoglobulin heavy chain. The IGK and IGL clusters lack the D segment. Rearrangement of these genes—with one V gene (of which there are approximately 50 functional V segments) recombining with one J gene and one D gene, and together recombining with a C gene—allows for the generation of virtually unlimited antibody diversity from a relatively small pool of chromosomal DNA. In addition, the fully recombined VDJ (heavy chain) and VJ (light chain) genes undergo point mutations (**somatic mutation**), which can alter the specificity or the affinity of the antibody for the antigen. The process of somatic mutation takes place in the germinal centers of secondary lymphoid tissue, during B-cell proliferation.

Table 1.1. Characteristic features of the five classes of immunoglobulins

Immuno-globulin	Heavy chains	Light chains	Molecular weight (daltons)	Serum concen-tration (mg/dL)	Locali-zation in secre-tions	Presence of other structures	Serum half-life (days)	Pla-cental trans-fer	Classic comple-ment activa-tion	Alter-nate comple-ment activation	Biologic activity (function)
IgG	Gamma (γ_1) (γ_2) (γ_3) (γ_4)	Kappa or lambda	150,000	1200 [a]	–	–	23	+ + + + +	+ + + +	–	Neutralization, opson-ization, bacteriolysis, agglutination, hemolysis
IgM	Mu (μ)	Kappa or lambda	900,000	150	±	J chain	5	–	+	–	Neutralization, hemoly-sis, agglutination, bac-teriolysis, opsonization, first detectable anti-body, receptor on B lymphocyte
IgA	Alpha (α_1) (α_2)	Kappa or lambda	160,000 (secre-tory IgA, 370,000)	300	+	J chain and secretory component for secre-tory IgA	6	–	–	+	Neutralization, present in body secretions
IgD	Delta (δ)	Kappa or lambda	180,000	3	–	–	3	–	–	+	Receptor on B lymphocyte
IgE	Epsilon (ε)	Kappa or lambda	200,000	0.03	±	–	2	–	–	+	Mast-cell binding and increased vascular permeability on anti-gen exposure

Ig, immunoglobulin; +, present; –, absent; ±, possibly present.
[a] IgG1 is the most abundant.

3. **Structural–functional correlates.** Study of the immunoglobulin subunits can help to localize and specify the function of biologically active sites.
    a. Enzymes such as papain and pepsin, dilute acids, or wetting agents such as urea can be used to cleave the immunoglobulin molecule into its component fragments. Papain breaks the molecule into two Fab fragments and one Fc fragment, and pepsin breaks the molecule into a single F(ab)2 fragment and multiple Fc fragments (Fig. 1.3).
        (1) The **Fab** end of an immunoglobulin molecule is called the amino-terminal end, which, with the presence of both light and heavy chains, is the antigen-binding site. The amino-terminal end possesses marked variability in the amino acid sequence. This **hypervariability** enables the immunoglobulin molecule to combine with a variety of antigens.
        (2) The **Fc** end is the carboxy-terminal end, and contains only heavy chain components. The Fc, or constant region, has a fixed amino acid sequence and is responsible for conferring biologic activity on the immunoglobulin molecule, such as placental transfer, complement fixation, and binding to skin and effector cells (e.g., macrophages, platelets, granulocytes, and mast cells). In addition, the Fc portion of the immunoglobulin molecule plays a critical role in the rate of synthesis and catabolism of the molecule. The Fc fragment is not involved in antigen recognition.
    b. Various genetic markers are localized on the constant region of the light and heavy chains. Genetic variation in light chains produces certain amino acid sequences, creating genetic allotypes. Light chain allotypes are called **Km** and **Oz** markers; heavy chain allotypes are called **Gm**, **Am**, and **Mm** markers. These are inherited in mendelian fashion.
4. **Immunoglobulin classes.** Immunoglobulins are divided into five major classes, or isotypes. The characteristic features of the immunoglobulin isotypes and subclasses are summarized in Table 1.1.
    a. **Immunoglobulin G** is primarily involved in the secondary or recall immune response. IgG antibodies are composed of two light chains and two heavy chains. The ability of IgG to diffuse into body tissue facilitates the combination and efficient elimination of antigens. This molecule is further divided into four different subclasses, **IgG1**, **IgG2**, **IgG3**, and **IgG4**, based on structural differences in the γ-heavy chain. These subclasses also have functional variations in terms of complement fixation, alternative complement pathway activation, macrophage adherence, and ease of placental transfer. All of the subclasses are transferred across the placenta and all of the subclasses partake in antibody-dependent cellular cytotoxicity. IgG1 and IgG3 are the subclasses with the most potent complement fixation abilities. IgG2 also fixes complement, but to a lesser degree, and IgG4 does not activate the classical complement pathway. IgG1 is the most abundant of the subclasses, is the primary subclass responsible for immunity to tetanus/diphtheria, and is also very important in the primary immune response against viral respiratory agents. IgG2 is of primary importance in the body's ability to respond to polysaccharide antigens, such as pneumococcal and meningococcal bacteria. IgG3, along with IgG1, is involved in the primary immune response against viral respiratory agents; IgG3 is the IgG subclass that fixes complement most efficiently. In addition, IgG3 appears to be the primary subclass involved in the antibody response against *Moraxella catarrhalis*. There is much controversy over the clinical significance of IgG subclass deficiency, but some studies suggest that patients with subclass deficiency are prone to develop sinus and respiratory tract infections. Furthermore, it appears that IgG2 and IgG3 are decreased in 15% to 20% of IgA-deficient individuals. IgG3 is the most commonly deficient subclass

in adults, whereas IgG2 deficiency is the most commonly deficient subclass in children.

b. Immunoglobulin M is the major part of the early antibody response, especially in response to nonprotein bacterial antigens. The IgM molecule consists of five subunits that are linked by disulfide bonds and J chains. The antibody is not transferred across the placenta, and its polymeric structure makes for efficient agglutination. IgM readily fixes complement, allowing for the efficient lysis of antigen by primarily activating the classical complement pathway.

c. Immunoglobulin A is the primary immunoglobulin of all mucosal surfaces and exocrine secretions. It exists either as a monomer, dimer, or even a trimer of the basic four-chain structure. IgA can be found in the serum or in exocrine secretions. **Secretory IgA** is equipped with a polypeptide secretory piece that permits secretion of the IgA molecule across mucous membranes, providing initial protection against pathogens at the mucosal level. Selective IgA deficiency is the most common primary immunodeficiency in humans, affecting between 1 in 500 and 1 in 700 individuals.

d. Immunoglobulin D is present in very small quantities in the serum. Although its structure is similar to that of the other immunoglobulins, its functional role is not well characterized. Notably, there is a rare syndrome, hyper-IgD, characterized by periodic fevers, flushing, gastrointestinal complaints, and arthralgias.

e. Immunoglobulin E (reaginic antibody) is normally present in very low concentrations, although elevated levels are seen in atopic disease and in a number of other disorders (see Chapter 2). IgE antibody is made up of the basic four-chain structure. Mast cells and basophils have high-affinity receptors for the Fc region of IgE (FcεRI). IL-4 is primarily responsible for the promotion of IgE isotype switching. The bridging of two IgE molecules by antigen results in the release of inflammatory mediators that characterize the immediate hypersensitivity response (see Chapter 2). A new therapy for allergic disease and asthma consists of an anti-IgE antibody. This antibody has been engineered to bind only to the free, circulating IgE, not receptor-bound IgE. Thus, it does not initiate mast cell activation or degranulation by IgE receptor cross-linking.

B. Cell-mediated immunity consists of a set of immune phenomena distinct from antibody-mediated immunity. As seen in Table 1.2, several features distinguish the humoral and cellular arms of the immune system. Specifically, cell-mediated immunity is mediated by T cells and monocytic cells and requires either intact cells to carry out their immune functions by direct cell-to-cell contact or acts through production of soluble factors, or **cytokines** that control and/or regulate specific immunologic functions (see Table 1.3).

1. The T helper 1/T helper 2 paradigm. T-cell elaboration of cytokines contributes to both the regulation of immunoglobulin synthesis and

(text continues on page 14)

Table 1.2. Differences between humoral and cell-mediated immunity

Humoral-mediated immunity	Cell-mediated immunity
Antibody mediated	Cell mediated
Responsible cell: B lymphocyte	Responsible cell: T lymphocyte or cell products required for transfer of immunity
Transfer of immunity with serum	
Primary defense against bacterial infection	Responsible for host defense against viruses, fungi, intracellular organisms, tumor antigens, allograft rejection

Table 1.3. Selected cytokines and their major sources and activities

Cytokine	Primary sources	Primary biologic effects
Granulocyte colony stimulating factor (G-CSF)	Monocytes, fibroblasts, epithelial cells	Maturation and differentiation
Granulocyte macrophage colony-stimulating factor (GM-CSF)	Activated macrophages and T cells	Proliferation, differentiation, activation and prolonged survival of eosinophils, neutrophils, and macrophages; enhanced cytokine production; eosinophil degranulation; platelet production
Interferon-alpha (IFN-α)	Monocytes/macrophages and to a lesser extent B cells and NK cells	Inhibits viral replication
Interferon-beta (IFN-β)	Monocytes/macrophages	Similar to IFN-α
Interferon-gamma (IFN-γ)	CD4$^+$ Th1, lymphocytes, NK cells, and some CD8$^+$ lymphocytes	Differentiation; activation to express FcγR, MHC class I and II, nitric oxide synthase, IL-1, and TNF in macrophages; shift of Th2 to Th1; growth and expression of IL-2R; increased cytotoxicity; activation of CD8$^+$ cells and NK cells
Interleukin-1 (IL-1)	Monocytes/macrophages	Cytokine production; cellular cytotoxicity, cytokine production; differentiation, proliferation, and immunoglobulin production; acute phase reactant
Interleukin-2 (IL-2)	CD4$^+$ lymphocytes	Clonal expansion of Ag-specific cells; differentiation and cytokine expression; maturation of CD8$^+$ cells; promotes T cell maturation and growth
Interleukin-3 (IL-3)	T-lymphocytes	Proliferation and differentiation of hematopoietic stem cells
Interleukin-4 (IL-4)	CD4$^+$ lymphocytes (Th2 cells)	Growth and activation of T and B lymphocytes; production of MHC class II, IL-6, TNF, CD23, CD72; switch factor for IgE, enhances IgE, IgG1, and IgG4 and inhibits IgM, IgG2, and IgG3 production; inhibits IFN-γ production; enhances IL-5 production
Interleukin-5 (IL-5)	CD4$^+$ and CD8$^+$ lymphocytes	Proliferation, chemoattraction, adhesion, activation, enhanced survival, and degranulation of eosinophils

Table 1.3. *Continued*

Cytokine	Primary sources	Primary biologic effects
Interleukin-6 (IL-6)	Monocytes/macrophages	Acute phase reactant; activates B cells to mature into plasma cells; switch factor for IgG1 and IgA; inhibits LPS stimulates IL-1 and TNFα production
Interleukin-7 (IL-7)	Bone marrow stromal cells and thymic stromal cells	Proliferation of progenitor B cells; proliferation of activated T cells
Interleukin-8 (IL-8)	Macrophages	Neutrophil chemotactic factor and histamine releasing regulatory factor
Interleukin-9 (IL-9)	Enhances response of B cells to IL-4	Enhances responses of B cells to IL-4
Interleukin-10 (IL-10)	Murine CD4$^+$ Th2; human CD4$^+$ Th10, Th1, Th2, and CD8$^+$ lymphocytes (inhibited by IL-4 and IFN-γ)	Differentiation of monocytes to macrophages; inhibits expression of MHC class II and many adhesion molecules; inhibits IFN-γ and TNF-production, resulting in switch of T cell differentiation from Th1 to Th2
Interleukin-11 (IL-11)	Bone marrow stromal cell	Similar to IL-6
Interleukin-12 (IL-12)	Monocytes/macrophages	Activates NK cells; stimulates IFN-γ and TNF-α production by Th-1 cells; inhibits IL-4, IL-5, and IL-10 production by Th2 cells
Interleukin-13 (IL-13)	CD4$^+$ Th2 lymphocytes	Similar to IL-4; enhances production of MHC class II and integrins; reduced production of IL-1 and TNF
Interleukin-14 (IL-14)	Activated T lymphocytes	Expands clones of B cells and suppresses immunoglobulin secretion
Interleukin-15 (IL-15)	Monocytes/macrophages	Proliferation; increased cytotoxicity; expression of ICAM-3; acts on T cells and NK cells
Interleukin-16 (IL-16)	CD8$^+$ lymphocytes	Chemoattractant, growth factor of CD4$^+$ lymphocytes
Interleukin-17 (IL-17)	CD4$^+$ memory cells	Autocrine proliferation and activation of CD4$^+$ cells
Interleukin-18 (IL-18; IFN-γ-inducing factor)	Macrophages, Kupffer cells	Similar to IL-12; inhibits IgE production by increasing IFN-γ
Platelet-derived growth factor (PDGF)	Platelet α granule; monocytes/ macrophages	Proliferation; chemoattractant for fibroblasts; active in wound healing, atherogenesis, and airway remodeling

continued

Table 1.3. *Continued*

Cytokine	Primary sources	Primary biologic effects
Stem cell factor (SCF) (c-kit ligand, mast cell growth factor)	Bone marrow stroma; fibroblasts	Chemoattractant for mast cells, with IL-3 stimulates growth; also has histamine-releasing activity
Transforming growth factor-beta (TGF-β)	Platelets and to a lesser extent T and B cells	Inhibits IL-2-stimulated growth; switch factor for IgA but inhibits IgM and IgG production; counteracts IL-4 stimulation of IgE; inhibits cytotoxicity
Tumor necrosis factor-alpha (TNF-α) (also called cachectin)	Monocytes/macrophages	Enhanced apoptosis through DNA fragmentation; enhanced cytokine MHC classes I and II, and adhesion molecule expression; cytotoxicity; effects are similar to IL-1

Ag, antigen; NK, natural killer; CD, clusters of differentiation; Th, T helper; LPS, lipopolysaccharide; MHC, major histocompatibility complex; ICAM, intracellular adhesion molecule; TNF, tumor necrosis factor; IgG, immunoglobulin G.

secretion, and cell-mediated immunity. Subsets of CD4$^+$ T lymphocytes are characterized on the basis of patterns of cytokine release: Th1 cells differ from Th2 cells in that Th1 cells produce IL-2 and IFN-γ, whereas Th2 cells produce IL-4, IL-5, IL-9, IL-10, and IL-13, among other cytokines. Th2 cells promote preferential production of some immunoglobulin isotypes, whereas Th1 cells mediate delayed hypersensitivity responses and inhibit the proliferation of the Th2 cells. Table 1.3 summarizes the actions of many of the cytokines. Unlike B cells, T cells must migrate to the sites within the body where antigen is found, because T-cell responses to pathogens are dependent on the T cell being in direct contact with the pathogenic antigen. In adults, there are approximately 25 million to 100 million distinct "naïve" T cell clones that have never encountered antigen. In contrast, there are only several thousand T cells bearing receptors that recognize individual antigen. **Naïve T cells** are first given the task of determining whether or not antigen is present, and second, whether or not this antigen is a threat to the body. Dendritic cells are instrumental in presenting antigen to T cells and are found in secondary lymphoid organs. These organs collect and trap antigen that is present in other parts of the body. Naïve T cells begin to migrate to these lymphoid organs in a process known as "homing." When a T cell encounters an antigen, a cascade is initiated that results in an approximate thousand-fold clonal expansion of T cells with identical antigen specificity. In time, the activated T cells acquire effector function and once again home a second time to areas of inflammation. At these sites of inflammation, the T cells interact with eosinophils, basophils, mast cells, and antigen-presenting cells. There is another set of effector cells that contact activated B cells in lymphoid tissue and facilitate humoral immune responses. Although most effector T cells die after the antigen is cleared, a few remain and become memory cells and are able to mount rapid immune responses when specific antigen returns.

In humans, Th1 cells produce IL-2, IFN-γ, lymphotoxin, and possibly small amounts of IL-6, IL-10, and IL-13. Th2 cells produce IL-4, IL-5, IL-6, IL-9, IL-10, and IL-13. Both Th1 and Th2 cells produce TNF-α, granulocyte macrophage colony-stimulating factor (GM-CSF), and chemokines. In reality, there is significant overlap in the types of cytokines produced by these cell populations. A third subset of T helper cells exists and is termed Th0. **Th0 cells express cytokines inherent to both Th1 and Th2 cells.**

2. **T helper 1 and T helper 2 cells exhibit functionally distinct characteristics.** For example, Th1 cells primarily are involved in cell-mediated inflammatory reactions and thus the cytokines they produce activate cytotoxic and inflammatory reactions. IFN-γ, a Th1 cytokine, is often found at sites of delayed-type hypersensitivity reactions. Th1 cells mediate these reactions; likewise, Th2 cytokines augment antibody production, particularly IgE responses, and enhance eosinophil production. Therefore, the Th2 cytokines are often found in association with allergic and antibody-driven immune responses.

3. **T helper 1 and T helper 2 cells regulate cellular function.** Specific Th1 cytokines promote Th1 proliferation and differentiation, but these cytokines act to inhibit the differentiation and effector function of Th2 cells and cytokines. For example, IFN-γ selectively inhibits Th2 proliferation, whereas IL-10 (a Th2 cytokine) inhibits Th1 cytokine production. Likewise, throughout the entire body, Th1 and Th2 cells interact to suppress each other. Pregnancy is a special condition in which there is systemic "immune tolerance" partly mediated through a shifting of the Th1/Th2 balance. During pregnancy, the Th1 system is suppressed while the Th2 system is enhanced. This facilitates fetal survival because Th1 cytokines can be harmful to the placenta, whereas IL-10 is protective against fetal loss.

4. Phagocyte-dependent host responses are partially controlled by Th1 cells, whereas phagocyte-independent immune responses are controlled by Th2 cells. Specifically, Th1 cells promote the production of opsonizing and complement-fixing antibodies, macrophage activation, antibody-dependent cell cytotoxicity, and delayed-type hypersensitivity. Th2 cells primarily provide help for humoral immune responses such as IgE- and IgG1-isotype switching and mucosal immunity. Th2 cells also provide signals that induce mast cell and eosinophil growth and differentiation and facilitate IgA synthesis. Moreover, some Th2-derived cytokines (such as IL-4, IL-10, and IL-13) inhibit certain macrophage functions. Recently, two activation markers have been identified that are associated with the two primary subsets of T helper cells. **Lymphocyte activation gene-3 (LAG-3)** is an activation marker associated with Th1 cells and is a member of the immunoglobulin superfamily. **CD30** is an activation marker associated with Th2 cells, and is a member of the TNF receptor family.

5. **Both** CD4+ and CD8+ cells participate in the T helper1/T helper 2 paradigm. There is increasing evidence that Th2-like CD8+ cells exist in both humans and mice, and can be derived under similar conditions. IL-12 and IFN-γ facilitate differentiation of Th1 or cytotoxic type 1 (Tc1) CD8+ T cells, whereas IL-4 facilitates differentiation into Th2 or cytotoxic type 2 (Tc2) CD8+ T cells. However, in order for these CD8+ Tc2 cells to become IL-4 secreting, they need to be exposed to require higher levels of IL-4 during the initial priming than do CD4+ Th2 cells. Once committed to a Tc2 lineage, these CD8+ cells secrete the Th2 cytokines IL-4, 5, 9, 10, and 13. Different types of infectious organisms can affect which subsets of CD8+ cells will predominate during an immune response to that infection. Tc2-like cells have been isolated from patients with lepromatous leprosy, human immunodeficiency virus (HIV), and Job syndrome. In contrast, Tc1-like cells have been isolated from patients with tuberculoid leprosy. Although the Tc2 cells function in a "helper" manner, by secreting the appropriate cytokines, they can be just as cytotoxic as Tc1 cells. Both cell subsets kill via Ca^{2+}/perforin-dependent mechanisms and by activation of Fas. Although Tc2 cells can help B cells, they do not do

so in a cognate manner. Cognate help by Tc2 cells is unlikely because these cells do not recognize antigen processed and presented by MHC class II cells, as Tc2 cells are restricted to recognizing MHC class I. However, it is possible that Tc2 cells can help B cells via bystander, or non-cognate mechanisms.

6. **Histocompatibility.** T lymphocytes do not recognize antigens directly, but do so after the antigen is processed and presented on the surface of an antigen-presenting cell associated with a cell surface glycoprotein, which is coded for by the MHC. This glycoprotein is termed the MHC class II molecule. Histocompatibility molecules are classified into two major groups: class I molecules (which regulate interactions between CD8+ cells and target cells), and class II molecules (which regulate interactions between CD4+ cells and antigen-presenting cells). The function of both class I and II MHC molecules is to present antigen to T cells, thus initiating the adaptive immune response. T cells are able to interact with the histocompatibility molecules only if they are genetically identical; this phenomenon is known as **MHC restriction**.

   a. In humans, the MHC is located on chromosome 6. It is divided into four major regions: A, B, C, and D. The A, B, and C regions code for class I molecules, and the D region codes for class II molecules. The histocompatibility leukocyte antigen (HLA) complex comprises more than 200 genes. The class I genes code for the α-polypeptide chain of the class I molecule, whereas the beta$_2$-microglobulin gene, on chromosome 15, encodes for the β-chain of the class I molecule, and is the light chain of the class I molecule. The α-chain has four domains: two peptide-binding domains (α_1 and α_2); one immunoglobulin-like domain (α_3), and the last domain is the cytoplasmic tail. The class II molecules contain α and β polypeptide chains, which are encoded by the class II genes. The class II genes are also found on chromosome 6 and have a special system used for designation and nomenclature of their loci. Specifically, three letters are used. The three letters signify **class, family**, and **chain**. The first letter is always a D and indicates the class. The second letter is an M, O, P, Q, or R and represents the family. The third letter in the series is an A or B and represents the α or β chain, respectively.

   In addition, each of the class II α and II β chains has four domains: the peptide-binding domain (α_1 or β_1), the immunoglobulin-like domain (α_2 or β_2), the transmembrane region, and the cytoplasmic tail.

   With rare exception, class I genes are expressed on all cells of the body, whereas class II genes are primarily expressed by antigen-presenting cells, such as B cells, dendritic cells, macrophages, some activated T cells, and thymic epithelial cells. Class I and II molecules process antigen differently. Class I molecules process intracellular proteins that are marked by **ubiquitin**. The proteins unfold and enter proteosomes, where they are processed and degraded into peptides. Next, they enter the endoplasmic reticulum. The peptide is then transported to the outer surface of the cell and bound to the HLA I molecule. Class II molecules degrade extracellular proteins via a different pathway. These are taken into the cell via invaginations, which pinch off and form endocytic vesicles. These vesicles join with lysosomes and at this point, the peptides are exposed to proteolytic enzymes. The lysosome–endocytic vesicle complex becomes known as an endosome. Once digested, the peptides are placed on the outer surface of the cell and are bound to the HLA class II molecules.

   MHC class II molecules lacking the peptide ligands are unstable and disassemble at low pH. MHC class II molecules require a ligand to occupy the peptide-binding groove in order to remain stable. Therefore, a peptide can be regarded as the "third subunit" of a mature MHC class II molecule. HLA-DM has been shown to bind the empty class II dimers and thus stabilize the groove in the absence of peptides.

T-cell receptors discriminate between MHC class I and II molecules. In general, **CD8 cells bind HLA class I** and down-regulate the expression of CD4 molecules, whereas **CD4 cells bind class II** and down-regulate the expression of CD8 molecules. Generally, CD4$^+$ T lymphocytes become helper T cells and CD8$^+$ T lymphocytes become cytotoxic T cells. As thymocytes enter the thymic cortex, they attempt to match their receptors with HLA peptide complexes on the cortical epithelial cells. If the receptors and ligands do not match up, which happens in the majority of cases, the thymocytes die via apoptosis mechanisms. A minority of thymocytes undergoes positive selection, in which these cells engage HLA peptide complexes and bind with low affinity. This low-affinity binding is sufficient to block apoptosis. Next, at the corticomedullary junction, the thymocytes are given the opportunity to undergo negative selection. At this point, they encounter antigen-presenting cells that express costimulatory molecules and proteases (cathepsins). This expression allows for a high-affinity interaction between the T-cell receptor and the HLA peptide. This interaction creates a signal instructing the thymocyte to undergo apoptosis. This process is termed negative selection and takes place so that self-reacting (or autoreactive) T cells, which can cause autoimmune disease, can be destroyed. Of all the progenitor cells that enter the thymus and proliferate in it, fewer than 1% mature into T cells.

The MHC gene products have important roles in clinical immunology. For example, transplanted tissues are rejected if transplants are performed across MHC barriers (see Chapter 16).

   b. The majority of cellular immunity is mediated by the CD4$^+$ cell, which is responsible for the following immune phenomena:

   (1) Delayed hypersensitivity reactions (e.g., tuberculin skin test response).

   (2) Contact sensitivity (e.g., poison ivy dermatitis).

   (3) Immunity to intracellular organisms.

   (4) Immunity to viral and fungal antigens.

   (5) Tissue graft rejection.

   (6) Elimination of tumor cells bearing foreign antigens.

   (7) Formation of chronic granulomas.

IV. Phagocytic immunity

The phagocytic arm of the immune system can be divided into two major groups: the **circulating** and **fixed** components. Circulating cells with phagocytic capacity include all of the granulocytes (including eosinophils) and the monocytes. The fixed tissue phagocytes include cells of the monocyte/macrophage lineage, specifically Kupffer cells of the liver, splenic macrophages, pulmonary alveolar macrophages, lymph node macrophages, and the microglial cells of the brain. Together, the fixed-tissue phagocytes are referred to as the **reticuloendothelial system**. The ability of the granulocytes, monocytes, and macrophages to destroy foreign antigen by phagocytosis is crucial for host defense. Failure of either of these systems invariably results in an increased susceptibility to infection.

The following steps are necessary for adequate phagocytosis and destruction of foreign antigen: (i) **random movement**; (ii) **neutrophil adherence** to vascular endothelium; (iii) **transmembrane migration (diapedesis)**; (iv) **chemotaxis**; (v) **opsonization** and **fixation** of the bacteria or foreign material; (vi) **ingestion** of the antigen; (vii) **metabolic activation** of the phagocytes to destroy the foreign material; and (viii) **destruction** of the organism. Specific features of this system are as follows.

   A. Phagocytic cells migrate either in a random manner or in response to biochemical signals. This directed movement is called **chemotaxis**. Known chemoattractants include the activated complement components C3a, C4a, C5a, bacterial products, various leukotrienes, and other arachidonic acid metabolites.

B. Opsonization is the process by which antibody coats a bacterial cell wall or foreign material and increases its susceptibility to phagocytosis.

C. Phagocytosis is the process of engulfing foreign material into the phagocytic cell. After an intracellular phagocytic vacuole, or **phagosome**, is formed around the foreign material, lysosomal enzymes are released into this vacuole, resulting in the degradation of the foreign material. Neutrophil-generated, oxygen free radicals also play an important role in the destruction of phagocytosed microbes. Stimulated neutrophils can use the enzyme nicotinamide adenine dinucleotide phosphate (NADPH) oxidase directly to generate superoxide anion radicals, which are rapidly converted to hydrogen peroxide and hydroxyl radicals. The latter two metabolic products provide the majority of the microbicidal activity in the phagosome. When halides and myeloperoxidase are present in the phagosome, hypochlorous acid and free halides are generated. During this process an increased burst of metabolic activity, with increased oxygen consumption, can be measured and used to assess neutrophil-killing capacity.

V. The complement system

The complement system is made up of more than 25 plasma and cell membrane proteins, which are activated sequentially, and play important roles in immunologic effector mechanisms and host defense. Complement promotes bacterial, viral, and cellular lysis. Complement also acts to promote phagocytosis by the process of opsonization involving the deposition of specific complement fragments onto the surface of foreign microbes or cells. Receptors for these complement fragments are on phagocytic cells, leading to enhanced recognition and binding of the cell membrane to the phagocyte. Complement regulates inflammatory and immune responses, and has also been shown to play a role in acquired immunity because it helps to ensure the retention of antigen by follicular dendritic cells (FDC) in germinal centers, thereby providing a constant source of antigenic stimulus to activated, antigen-specific B cells.

Complement proteins can be grouped into four functional divisions according to their interaction with the third component (C3): (i) classic pathway activation, (ii) alternative pathway activation, (iii) the amplification mechanism, and (iv) the effector mechanism (Fig. 1.4). An additional pathway of complement activation is the lectin pathway. Activation of this pathway is mediated by **mannose binding lectin (MBL)**. The structure of MBL is similar to the C1q molecule of the classical complement pathway and is a pattern recognition receptor specific for mannose carbohydrates found only in bacteria and yeasts. **MBL** associates with two serine proteases (mannin binding lectin associated proteases 1 and 2 [**MASP-1 and -2**]). This entire complex cleaves downstream components of complement.

A. The classic activation pathway depends on the interaction of three complement proteins (C1, C4, and C2) with antigen-bound antibody to activate the initial cleavage of C3. C1, the first complement component, consists of three subcomponents, C1q, C1r, and C1s, which form a complex in the presence of calcium. Antigen–antibody complexes (containing IgG1, IgG2, IgG3, or IgM) can activate C1 to its enzymatically active form. Activated C1 then cleaves its two complement substrates, C4 and C2, to form a bimolecular complex, C4b2ba. This complex, known as **C3 convertase**, is capable of cleaving C3 to initiate activation of the effector sequence. Once C3 is activated, there is subsequent activation of the terminal components of the pathway. Complement enhances the immune response. The attachment of C3 to an antigen has been demonstrated to affect various phases of the acquired immune response. C3 is involved in (i) the promotion of antigen uptake, processing, and presentation by B cells to antigen-specific T cells; (ii) direct activation of B cells; and (iii) facilitation of B cell interactions.

B. Alternative pathway activation. Microbial and mammalian cell surfaces can activate the alternative pathway in the absence of specific antigen–antibody complexes. This nonspecific activation offers a major physiologic advantage, because host protection can be generated before the induction of an antibody-mediated immune response. Factors capable of activating the alternative pathway include inulin, zymosan, bacterial polysaccharides, and

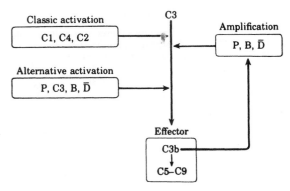

FIG. 1.4. Overview of four-compartment complement system. (P, properdin; D, activated factor D.) (From Fearon DT, Austen KF. Immunochemistry of the classical and alternative pathways of complement. In: Glynn LE, Steward MW, eds. *Immunochemistry: an advanced textbook*. New York: Wiley, 1977, with permission.)

aggregated immunoglobulins IgG4, IgA, and IgE. Proteins involved in this reaction include properdin, factor D, factor B, and C3.

C. **Amplification.** Constituent proteins of the amplification pathway include **C3b, factors B and D, and properdin**. Under normal circumstances, an alternative pathway convertase, which amplifies the activation of this pathway, is quite unstable and rapidly decays. Properdin binds to this alternative pathway convertase, stabilizing and retarding its decay and allowing it to perpetuate the complement cascade (Fig. 1.5).

D. **Effector mechanism.** The classic and alternative C3 pathways generate C3b, which serves a number of functions, including interaction of C4b2a (the classic C3 convertase) and C3bBb (the alternative pathway C3 convertase) to allow further activity on C5 and subsequent activation of the terminal sequence (Fig. 1.5). In the final steps, formation of membrane-bound C5b67 permits binding of C8 to the C5 fragment to cause a partial membrane lesion resulting in slow cell lysis. By complexing with C9, the cytolytic reaction is accelerated.

E. **The membrane attack complex** (MAC). After activated C5 binds to C6, C7 and C8 subsequently bind, forming the complex C5b678, which is then capable of binding multiple molecules of C9. This forms a cylindrical structure, C5b6789, termed the MAC. This structure is inserted through the cell membrane, breaching the osmotic barrier of the cell wall, ultimately resulting in death of the cell.

Type I: Immediate hypersensitivity
(IgE-mediated)
Antigen
Preformed intragranular mediators
Histamine
Proteinases
   Chymases
   Tryptases
   Carboxypeptidases
   Cathepsin G-like proteinases
Acid hydrolases
   β-Hexosaminidase
   β-Glucuronidase
   β-D-Galactosidase
   Arylsulfatase A

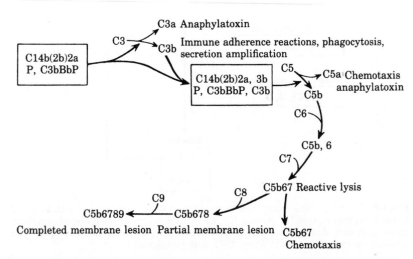

FIG. 1.5. Terminal complement sequence. (From Soter NA, Austen KF. Effector systems of inflammation. In: Fitzgerald TB, et al., eds. *Dermatology in general medicine*. New York: McGraw-Hill, with permission.)

Proteoglycans
  Heparin
  Chondroitin sulfate E
Chemotactic factors
Newly formed mediators
  Arachidonic acid metabolites
  Prostaglandins
  Thromboxanes
  5-, 12-Hydroxyeicosatetraenoic (HETEs)
  Leukotrienes
  Platelet activating factor
Free radicals
  Nitric oxide
  Superoxide anion
  Hydrogen peroxide
  Hydroxyl radicals
Cytokines
  TNF-α and TNF-β
  IL-1, 2, 3, 4, 5, 6, 8
  IFN-γ GM-CSF
  Macrophage inflammatory protein (MIP)-2
  Basic fibroblast growth factor (bFGF)
  Leukemia inhibitory factor (LIF)
Mast cell

Antigen–Antibody Interactions

An antigen is a substance that can stimulate an immune response and react with an antibody or a sensitized T cell. The capacity of an antigen to elicit an immune response is termed its **immunogenicity**; its ability to react with an antibody is termed its **antigenicity**. Low molecular weight substances (e.g., drugs) are not immunogenic by themselves unless combined with a carrier protein. These small molecules are called **haptens**. Although they cannot evoke an antibody response when injected alone, they can by themselves react with antibody. Immunogenicity is a complex phenomenon that depends not only on the physical properties of the antigen, but also on the biologic system, route of administration, and method of immunization.

Classification of Immunologic Reactions

Although the function of the immune system is protection of the host from foreign antigens, abnormal immune responses can lead to tissue injury and disease. Gell and Coombs classified the mechanisms of immune tissue injury into four distinct types of reactions, which allows for a better understanding of the immunopathogenesis of disease (Fig. 1.6).

I. **Type I: anaphylactic or immediate hypersensitivity.** Antigen binding to preformed IgE antibodies attached to the surface of the mast cell or basophil causes release of inflammatory mediators, e.g., histamine, leukotrienes, cytokines, proteases, arachidonic acid metabolites, and enzymatic mediators (see Chapter 2), which produce the clinical manifestations. Examples of type I diseases include anaphylactic shock, allergic rhinitis, allergic asthma, and acute drug allergic reactions.

II. **Type II: cytotoxic reactions.** Cytotoxic reactions involve the binding of either IgG or IgM antibody to cell-bound antigens. Antigen–antibody binding results in activation of the complement cascade and the destruction of the cell to which the antigen is bound. Examples of tissue injury by this mechanism include immune hemolytic anemia and Rh hemolytic disease in the newborn. Diseases such as autoimmune hyperthyroidism in which thyroid-stimulating antibodies stimulate the thyroid tissue, or thyroid-stimulating hormone (TSH)-binding inhibitory antibodies inhibit the binding of TSH to its receptor; or myasthenia gravis in which antibodies are directed to the acetylcholine receptor blocking this neuromediator from interacting with its receptor are also type II reactions. In this latter group of diseases, cytolysis is not a component of these reactions.

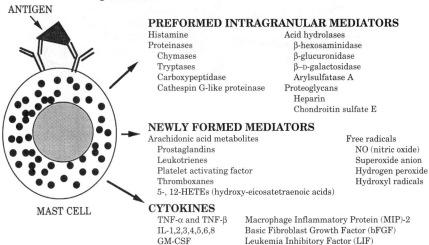

FIG. 1.6. Classification of allergic reactions (Gell and Coombs).

TYPE II: CYTOTOXIC

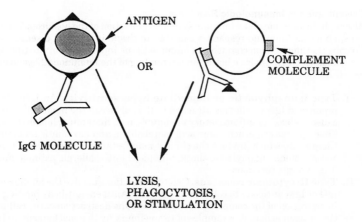

B

TYPE III: IMMUNE COMPLEX MEDIATED REACTIONS

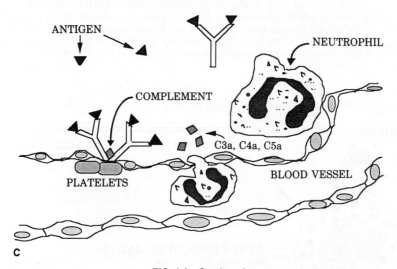

C

FIG. 1.6. *Continued*

III. **Type III: immune-complex-mediated reactions.** Immune complexes are
   formed when antigens bind to antibodies. They are usually cleared from the circulation by the phagocytic system. However, deposition of these complexes in
   tissues or in vascular endothelium can produce immune complex-mediated tissue
   injury. Two important factors leading to injury by this mechanism include increased quantity of circulating complexes and the presence of vasoactive amines,
   which increase vascular permeability and favor tissue deposition of immune complexes. Immune complex deposition leads to complement activation, anaphyla-

TYPE IV: CELL-MEDIATED DELAYED HYPERSENSITIVITY

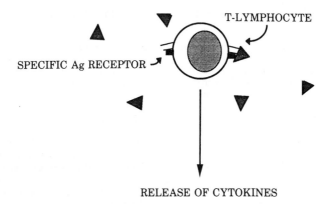

D   RELEASE OF CYTOKINES

FIG. 1.6. *Continued*

toxin generation, chemotaxis of polymorphonuclear leukocytes, phagocytosis, and tissue injury. Clinical examples are serum sickness, certain types of nephritis, and certain features of bacterial endocarditis.

IV. Type IV: delayed hypersensitivity. Unlike the other types of hypersensitivity reactions, type IV reactions are not mediated by antibody. Delayed hypersensitivity reactions are mediated primarily by T lymphocytes (cell-mediated immunity). The classic examples are the tuberculin skin test reactions and contact dermatitis.

Selected Readings

Adelman DC. Functional assessment of mononuclear cells. *Immunol Allergy Clin North Am* 1994;14:241–263.

Delves PJ, Roitt IM. The immune system. First of two parts. *N Engl J Med* 2000; 343:37–49.

Klein J, Sato A. The HLA system. First of two parts. *N Engl J Med* 2000;343:702–709.

Klein J, Sato A. The HLA system. Second of two parts. *N Engl J Med* 2000;343:782–786.

Medzhitov R, Janeway C Jr. Innate immunity. *N Engl J Med* 2000;343:338–344.

Mosmann TR, Sad S. The expanding universe of T-cell subsets: Th1, Th2 and more. *Immunol Today* 1996;17:138–146.

Nielsen CH, Fisher EM, Leslie RG. The role of complement in the acquired immune response. *Immunology* 2000;100:4–12.

Presta LG, Lahr SJ, Shields RL, et al. Humanization of an antibody directed against IgE. *J Immunol* 1993;151:2623–2632.

Romagnani S. Short analytic review: Th1 and Th2 in human diseases. *Clin Immunol Immunopathol* 1996;80:225–235.

Shearer WT, Huston DP. The immune system. An overview. In: Middleton E, Reed CE, Ellis EF, et al., eds. *Allergy principles and practice.* St. Louis: Mosby, 1993:3–21.

Von Andrian UH, Mackay CR. T-cell function and migration. Two sides of the same coin. *N Engl J Med* 2000;343:1020–1033.

2. IMMEDIATE HYPERSENSITIVITY: APPROACH TO DIAGNOSIS

Alvin M. Sanico, Bruce S. Bochner, and Sarbjit S. Saini

I. Background: historical perspective of immunoglobulin E

Nearly a century ago, Portier and Richet reported a paradoxical immunological effect when trying to enhance the resistance of dogs to sea anemone toxin by injecting the dogs with the toxin. Rather than conferring the expected protection, when reinjected weeks later with minute amounts of the same toxin, several animals died within minutes of cardiorespiratory collapse. To describe this phenomenon, they coined the term **anaphylaxis** (meaning antiprotection). Subsequent studies determined that these reactions required prior exposure to the foreign substance and a period of weeks to manifest the response. It was also found that anaphylactic sensitivity could be transferred from one animal to another by injecting or infusing a serum-derived factor, initially referred to as **reagin**. Soon thereafter, studies in humans revealed that injection of serum from an anaphylactically sensitive individual into a nonsensitive individual (**passive transfer**) led to local sensitization (transfer of a wheal and flare reaction) in the recipient at the cutaneous site. The passive transfer experiment, sometimes referred to as the PK test or reaction (named after Prausnitz and Kustner, who performed the early experiments), gave the first indication that allergic hypersensitivity resulted from a serum protein. This type of response became known as **immediate hypersensitivity** due to the rapidity of the response. However, the composition of reagin remained a mystery until the 1960s, when Ishizaka and Ishizaka purified and identified **immunoglobulin E (IgE)**, establishing that reagin was an antibody molecule. It is now clear that the presence of specific IgE antibodies represents the single most important determinant of allergic sensitivity. Synthesis or passive transfer of IgE antibodies sensitizes the recipient for both the immediate allergic response and any subsequent reactions. Today, the term **allergen** refers to a protein, typically a common innocuous antigen that elicits IgE antibody production. **Allergy** refers to the clinical manifestations of IgE-dependent immunological reactions, whereas **atopy** is used to describe the genetic tendency to generate IgE responses.

II. Antigen characteristics

Antigens. For a substance to generate an immune response, it must be presented to the immune system in an appropriate fashion. Characteristics of the antigen can determine whether the immune system develops an antibody response of a particular class or whether an antibody response is generated at all. For example, so-called T-cell-independent antigens such as polysaccharides do not typically give rise to IgE antibodies. Thus, the nature of the antigen is an important determinant of the host response. Although a complete understanding of what makes an antigen an allergen has not been achieved, several general principles can be stated. Most common allergens (e.g., pollen, dust mites, animal dander) that cause airway symptoms in humans are proteins with a molecular weight of 10 to 20 kD, are highly water-soluble, and can act as complete allergens. Repeated, low-level exposure to these proteins (typically in the submicrogram range) diffusing across mucosal surfaces is particularly efficient at inducing an IgE response. Host characteristics are also key in generating IgE responses, given that about 20% of the exposed population, that is, those with the atopic trait, will generate IgE antibodies. Some of the most prevalent aeroallergens, such as dust mites (*Der p 1,* a cysteine protease) have enzymatic functions in their natural state. A clear association between the functional properties of an allergen and its **immunogenicity**, that is, the ability to generate immunologic responses in susceptible subjects, is lacking. It has also been difficult to identify common structural features among known allergenic proteins to allow predictions of the immunogenicity of novel peptides. However, the cross-reactivity of a protein with preexisting IgE antibodies to another allergen has been shown to be based on structural similarities and presents clinically, for example, in the **oral allergy syndrome**. Here, the ingestion of labile proteins found in, for instance, fresh apples, can cross-react with an individual's existing birch–pollen-specific IgE, leading to the occurrence of itching of the oral mucosa.

A. **Complete protein allergens.** By definition, proteins that are complete allergens have (i) the property to induce the production of IgE antibodies; (ii) the ability to elicit an allergic reaction or trigger symptoms in a sensitive host; and (iii) the property to bind IgE antibodies with sufficient numbers of antigenic determinants.

B. **Incomplete protein allergens.** An incomplete allergen is one that is able to elicit symptoms in a sensitive host, but cannot independently generate an IgE antibody response. Commonly, these are low molecular weight drugs such as the β-lactam family of antibiotics. On the basis of studies with penicillin, the β-lactam molecule generates reactive metabolites in vivo that covalently bind to a number of the host's normal proteins, such as albumin. These reactive compounds are termed **haptens**, and by definition they must bind to other proteins (haptenate) in vivo to elicit an IgE response. Penicillin hapten–protein complexed allergens, also called major and minor determinants, have been identified and used for diagnostic skin testing. However, it has been difficult to establish standard skin testing reagents for the evaluation of other incomplete drug allergens given the multiple pathways to generate drug intermediates and their potential for haptenization.

III. **Production of immunoglobulin E**

If many individuals are exposed to the same antigen by the same route, only a few develop IgE antibodies, and therefore only a few of these people are at risk for allergic reactions upon reexposure. Why only a minority of people make antigen-specific IgE and become allergic remains unknown. If such events are to occur, however, a distinct series of immunological events must happen (Fig. 2.1). These include internalization of the antigen by antigen-presenting cells, such as dendritic cells, and its processing and presentation to T lymphocytes. If an IgE antibody response is to occur, these events must take place in the presence of specific cytokines, the most important of which is interleukin (IL)-4 released by T lymphocytes and other cells. IL-4 is critical for the generation of the T lymphocytes (Th2 cells) themselves and for subsequent stimulation by these cells of B lymphocytes. If this stimulation occurs in the presence of IL-4, the B cells undergo immunoglobulin gene class switching, leading to their terminal differentiation into plasma cells that produce antigen-specific IgE antibodies. Generation of IgE-producing plasma cells is also facilitated by binding of CD40 ligand on the Th2 cell to CD40 on the B cell. Once plasma cells undergo these steps, they release the exact same antigen-specific IgE for the rest of their lives. This IgE secretion by plasma cells typically takes place at mucosal sites, but it can also occur in lymph nodes and other lymphoid organs. Among immunoglobulins, IgE has several unique features. For example, unlike IgG, IgE cannot cross the placenta. IgE contains an additional region in its heavy chain that makes the molecule uniquely capable of binding to specific IgE receptors. IgE is also heavily glycosylated, although the biological significance of this is uncertain. Finally, although the presence of IgE correlates with allergic diseases, high levels of IgE are seen in other disorders, such as helminthic parasite infections.

IV. **High-affinity immunoglobulin E receptor**

Secreted IgE produced by allergen-specific B cells binds to specialized Fc receptors on the surface of mast cells and basophils throughout the body. Although free IgE has a short serum half-life (2 to 3 days compared to 21 days for IgG), IgE bound to the surface of mast cells can persist for several months. The high-affinity IgE receptor (FcεRI) expressed by human mast cells and basophils is a tetramer composed of one alpha, one beta, and two gamma chains. Despite the low serum concentration of IgE (typically in the nanogram per milliliter range), most surface FcεRI receptors are occupied, given that the dissociation constant is 1×10^{-10}M. The alpha chain binds to IgE at its third heavy chain constant

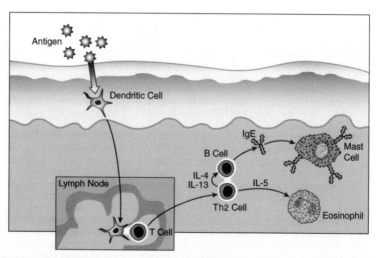

FIG. 2.1. Allergen sensitization. Activation of the immune system by an antigen requires exposure such as may occur when allergen breaches a mucosal surface. Antigen-presenting cells such as dendritic cells can ingest antigens in the tissue and present digested peptide fragments via their major histocompatibility complex (MHC) immune recognition system. Activated antigen-presenting cells travel via the lymphatics to local lymph nodes and make contact with T cells whose specific antigen receptors recognize one of the peptides in their MHC class II. A productive interaction occurs and the antigen-specific T lymphocyte is activated. Antigen-specific T cells are then capable of activating antigen-specific B cells to produce immunoglobulin E (IgE) antibodies either in primary or secondary lymphoid tissue or within the local tissue site. If the T cells are a subset referred to as Th2, i.e., those associated with allergic inflammation, then the B cells will shift the isotype of immunoglobulin produced to the IgE isotype under the influence of unique cell–cell attachment (via clusters of differentiation 40 [CD40] and CD40 ligand) and cytokines, such as interleukin-4 (IL-4) or IL-13, produced by T cells. Once released by plasma cells, antigen specific IgE binds to high-affinity IgE receptors on mast cells and basophils, leading to sensitization of these cell types. When mast cells and basophils with such IgE on their surface come in contact with native protein antigen, they are induced to degranulate, releasing granule contents such as histamine, proteoglycans, and some enzymes. Th2 cells also secrete the cytokine IL-5, which can activate eosinophils and prolong their survival in tissues. (From Dr. Robert Schleimer and Jacqueline Schaffer, with permission)

domain, whereas the β and γ subunits of the receptor are involved in transducing signals generated by activation of the receptor complex (Fig. 2.2). The therapeutic anti-IgE antibody being developed for clinical use takes advantage of this fact by binding to the third heavy chain of free IgE, preventing the IgE from binding to the alpha chain of FcεRI. The overall number of high-affinity receptor complexes on basophils ranges from a few thousand to 1 million molecules per cell and is related to the level of circulating free IgE as well as to levels of expression of the beta subunit. Both IgE and IL-4 are believed to enhance mast cell FcεRI expression. An alternate, trimeric high-affinity IgE receptor (composed of one α and two γ chains) occurs on monocytes, dendritic cells, and Langerhans cells, especially in allergic hosts, and may assist in antigen presentation by these cells to T cells.

Another receptor for IgE, termed FcεRII, is of low affinity with a single transmembrane chain that is unrelated to FcεRI. The FcεRIIα isoform is found on

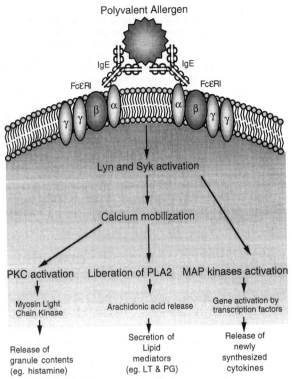

FIG. 2.2. Cross-linking of immunoglobulin E (IgE) activates intracellular biochemical pathways. Once mast cells or basophils are sensitized by IgE binding to the FcεRI alpha chain, they can be activated by polyvalent allergen that cross-links adjacent receptors. See V.D. on pages 30, 31 for details.

resting B cells and acts as an adhesion molecule as well as a regulator of IgE synthesis. The FcεRIIβ (CD23) isoform is inducible on B cells, monocytes, and some T cells by IL-4 or IL-13 stimulation.

V. Mast cells and basophils

A. Origin and distribution. Mast cells and basophils can be identified microscopically by the presence of cytoplasmic granules that contain acidic molecules that take up basic dyes and stain metachromatically. Both cell types also bear high-affinity IgE receptors. They both originate from CD34+ hematopoietic, pluripotent stem cells residing in the bone marrow, but differ in their developmental stages. Undifferentiated mast cells migrate from the bone marrow to the connective tissues of mucosal and epithelial surfaces of the body. They subsequently mature and take up residence in close proximity to blood vessels and body surfaces in contact with the external environment. Mast cells (and some basophils) also uniquely express c-kit, a receptor that binds the important growth factor, stem cell factor (SCF). The local tissue environment can provide SCF as well as influence mast cell mediator content, granule ultrastructure, and functionality, thus contributing to heterogeneity among mast cell populations. In contrast, basophils mature in the bone marrow under the influence of IL-3 and reside in the circulation as mature, nondividing cells. In the past, basophils were thought to be a form of circulating mast cell, but are now considered closer in lineage to eosinophils. Basophils can migrate to tissue sites in response to inflammatory stimuli, such as those generated during the late phase of an allergic response. Seasonal allergen exposure can cause an increase in the number of circulating basophils and tissue mast cells. Local application of steroids, such as in the nose of rhinitis patients, will blunt the increase in mast cells that is normally observed during the pollen season.

B. Pathways of mast cell and basophil mediator release. The major consequences of allergen cross-linking IgE bound to the surface of mast cells and basophils are cellular activation, degranulation, and inflammatory mediator release. The complex of symptoms associated with **immediate hypersensitivity** begins minutes after allergen exposure and has been linked to release of preformed and rapidly generated mediators from mast cells and basophils. Depending on the site and circumstances of allergen exposure, symptoms can range in severity from sneezing and rhinorrhea following pollen inhalation, to anaphylaxis following systemic allergen exposure (e.g., drug, insect sting, or food) leading to possible death. The implicated mediators are typically classified based on their pattern of release and include those that are preformed in granules and released by exocytosis (e.g., histamine), those that are rapidly synthesized from membrane lipids (e.g., prostaglandins), and lastly, cytokines that are synthesized and released over several hours. The nature of each mediator, its cellular source, and main action are summarized in Table 2.1.

One classic manifestation of immediate hypersensitivity is the wheal and flare response to allergen in the skin. The diagnostic skin test is based on the

Table 2.1. Mast cell and basophil mediators released by IgE cross-linking

Mediator	Cell	Actions
PREFORMED		
Histamine	MC, B	Vasodilatation, increased vascular permeability, smooth muscle contraction, bronchospasm, mucous secretion, P-selectin induction, fibroblast proliferation
Proteoglycans		
Heparin	MC	Anticoagulant, storage matrix
Chondroitin sulfate	MC, B	Storage matrix
Neutral proteases		
Tryptase	MC_T, MC_{CT}, B*	Generate C3a and bradykinin, degrades neuropeptides such as VIP, induces epithelial IL-8 production
Chymase	MC_{CT}, B*	Bronchial mucus secretion (animals)
Carboxypeptidase A	MC_{CT}	Undefined
Enzymes		
Superoxide dismutase	MC	Actions in human allergic disease unknown
Peroxidase		
Lysosomal acid hydrolases		
β-Hexosamidase	MC	Function unclear
β-Glucuronidase	MC	Cleaves tissue matrix
Preformed cytokines		
TNF-α, IL-16	MC	*See* CYTOKINES *next page*

Table 2.1. *Continued*

Mediator	Cell	Actions
NEWLY FORMED		
Arachidonic acid metabolites		
LTB_4	MC	Neutrophil chemoattractant
LTC_4	MC, B	Bronchoconstriction, mucus secretion, increased vascular permeability, eosinophil chemoattractant (formerly SRS-A)
PGD_2, PGF_2	MC	Bronchoconstriction, mucus secretion, edema, vasodilation, neutrophil chemoattractant
PAF	MC	Chemoattractant for eosinophils, neutrophils, platelet aggregation
CYTOKINES		
IL-6	MC	Increased IgE synthesis
IL-8	MC, B	Neutrophil chemoattractant
IL-4	B, MC	Induction of endothelial VCAM-1, IgE production by B cells, differentiation of Th2 cells, increased FcεRI and CD23, epithelial eotaxin
IL-13	B, MC	Induction of endothelial VCAM-1, IgE production, mucus secretion, epithelial eotaxin
IL-16	MC	Lymphocyte chemoattractant
GM-CSF, IL-5	MC	Eosinophil growth, activation, survival
TNF-α	MC	Induction of endothelial adhesion molecules, epithelial chemokines, mucus secretion, leukocyte cytokine secretion
CHEMOKINES		
MCP-1	MC	Monocyte and T-cell chemotaxis
MIP-1 alpha	MC, B	Macrophage differentiation, neutrophil chemotaxis and cytotoxicity
MIP-1 beta	MC‡	Chemotaxis of monocytes
RANTES	MC‡	Chemotaxis of eosinophils, basophils, lymphocytes

MC_{CT}, Chymase tryptase-containing mast cell, found in skin, blood vessels, and intestinal submucosa; MC_T, tryptase-containing mast cell, typically found in lung, nasal cavity, intestinal mucosa; B*, extremely low levels of this mediator have been found in basophils (<1% of that in mast cells); MC‡, HMC-1, a human mast cell leukemia cell line; IgE, immunoglobulin E; LT, leukotriene; PG, prostaglandin; PAF, platelet-activating factor; IL, interleukin; VIP, vasoactive intestinal peptide; SRS-A, slow-reacting substance of anaphylaxis; VCAM-1, vascular cell adhesion molecule-1; Th2, T helper 2; CD, clusters of differentiation; GM-CSF, granulocyte macrophage colony-stimulating factor; TNF, tumor necrosis factor; MCP, monocyte chemotactic protein; MIP, macrophage inflammatory protein; RANTES, regulated upon activation, normal T cell expressed and secreted.

ability of IgE-sensitized skin mast cells to respond to specific allergen exposure within minutes by releasing vasoactive mediators at the site of allergen application, a so-called immediate or **early-phase response**. Approximately 50% of subjects challenged with allergen in the skin, nose, or lungs also develop a reaction 4 to 12 hours after allergen exposure. This **late response** is characterized by recurrence of clinical symptoms as well as the local influx of circulating leukocytes such as eosinophils, lymphocytes, and basophils to the tissue in response to the mediators released during the early phase. Many features of the late-phase reaction are similar to those observed in chronic human allergic disease.

In addition to allergen, experimental antibodies and autoantibodies (present in some patients with chronic urticaria) that can cross-link cell-bound IgE or FcεRI receptors can also activate mast cells and basophils. In either case (allergen or cross-linking antibodies), bridging of as few as 1% of the total surface FcεRI (about 300 to 500 receptors) can be sufficient to activate the cells. In the case of a nonatopic individual, the surface-expressed IgE may be directed against several antigens without a single antigen-specific IgE expressed in sufficient quantity to trigger release.

A number of IgE-independent and FcεRI-independent pathways for activation of mast cells and basophils also exist. Most of these depend on the influx of calcium for cellular activation. Examples of *in vivo* triggers are drugs such as opiates (for skin mast cells), aspirin and other nonsteroidal antiinflammatory drugs (NSAIDS), smooth muscle relaxants, and intravenous radiocontrast dyes. Examples of in vitro agents are calcium ionophore and compound 48/80 (the latter for mast cell activation). There are also numerous biologic inflammatory stimuli that can activate or potentiate mediator release, including histamine releasing factors, products of complement activation (C3a, C5a), nerve-related peptides (tachykinins, nerve growth factor, calcitonin gene-related peptide), adenosine triphosphate (ATP), IL-1, IL-3, and several chemokines. In addition, skin mast cells in certain subjects can be activated by a variety of physical stimuli (such as cold temperature, pressure, sunlight, heat, or exercise) to produce urticaria.

C. **Releasability.** The wide variation noted in the extent of histamine release from basophils of different individuals has been termed releasability. Factors that determine the sensitivity of basophils or mast cells to allergen activation, or the magnitude of their mediator release, are still not clear, although in about 5% to 10% of people, their basophils refuse to release any histamine after IgE receptor cross-linking. These "nonreleaser" basophils appear to have a deficiency in Syk, a tyrosine kinase necessary for proper signal transduction (see Fig 2.2 on page 27). Immunotherapy leads to a higher threshold for allergen-induced basophil mediator release and may be one of the benefits of this form of treatment. In cultured mast cell systems, the induction of greater numbers of FcεRI receptors by either IL-4 or IgE leads to increased sensitivity to allergen and increased magnitude of mediator responses. However, similar effects of increased FcεRI expression or surface-bound IgE on basophil mediator responses have not been observed.

D. **Biochemical signaling pathways triggered by multivalent allergen.** IgE-dependent FcεRI aggregation leads to the stimulation of several intracellular signaling events as well as calcium influx into the cell. Although these events have been extensively studied, there remain many missing details in the order of events and the exact molecules that participate in each cell type. Figure 2.2 depicts a possible schema for FcεRI-related signaling events. The bridging of adjacent surface-bound IgE molecules by polyvalent allergen leads to the activation of a receptor-associated src family kinase, Lyn, which phosphorylates the receptor subunits and starts the cascade. The tyrosine kinase Syk is next recruited to the receptor, and this is followed by a cascade of intermediate molecules and secondary messengers that ultimately lead to the endpoints of granule secretion, lipid metabolite generation, and synthesis of cytokines. One proposed pathway involves Syk activation of phospholipase C (PLC), which in turn hydrolyzes phosphatidylinositol bisphosphate (PIP_2, found in the plasma membrane) to inositol 1,4,5-trisphosphate (IP_3) and 1,2-diacylglycerol (DAG). IP_3 functions as a secondary messenger to mobilize internal calcium stores, leading to an increase in the cytosolic concentration of calcium, a central signaling event. Both DAG and calcium can activate the protein kinase C (PKC) family of enzymes. PKC is able to phosphorylate many substrates including myosin light chain kinase (MLCK), which may act to change the cytoskeleton to permit degranulation. A separate pathway traced to the FcεRI complex activation involves the p21 ras molecule leading to downstream activation of the mitogen-activated protein kinases (MAPKs). The p21ras pathway is common to several receptors and involved in numerous cell functions including the activation of transcription factors that can enter the nucleus to activate cytokine genes. Elevations in intracellular calcium and phosphorylation of other MAPKs can activate cytoplasmic phospholipase A_2 ($cPLA_2$). $cPLA_2$ cleaves membrane phospholipids to generate arachidonic acid and eventually leads to synthesis of prostaglandins and eicosanoids.

It is important to note that several agents can inhibit cellular degranulation, including ethylenediaminetetraacetic acid (EDTA) (by calcium chelation), cyclic adenosine monophosphate (cAMP), colchicine, cromolyn, beta-agonists, and corticosteroids (true for basophils, but not mast cells). Therapeutic drugs that can block mediator release include those that target cAMP by either increasing its levels (e.g., beta-adrenergic agonists) or preventing the breakdown of cAMP by inhibiting phosphodiesterases (e.g., theophylline). Although it is known to inhibit degranulation, the specific intracellular targets of cromolyn are not understood. Potential therapeutics that are in development may specifically inhibit events early in the signaling cascade, such as the activation of Lyn or Syk tyrosine kinases.

VI. Mediators of immediate hypersensitivity
A. Preformed, granule-based mediators
1. **Histamine.** Bioactive factors such as histamine are stored within the granules of mast cells and basophils and are essentially fully released within 30 minutes of FcεRI activation. The *in vivo* administration of histamine reproduces many of the symptoms of acute allergen exposure and, therefore, is the mediator most often identified with immediate hypersensitivity reactions. On the basis of allergen challenge studies, histamine released in the acute phase is thought to be of mast cell origin, whereas basophils are responsible for its reappearance in the late phase. Histamine is produced from histidine by histidine decarboxylase and is packaged with heparin and other proteoglycans in the granule matrix. Degradation of histamine occurs rapidly *in vivo* by two pathways, either by deamination by histaminases or methylation by *N*-methyltransferase. Histamine acts by binding to specific receptor subtypes H1, H2, and H3 (the latter located mainly in the central nervous system [CNS]), the tissue distribution of which determine the character of the response. Given the wide range of biologic responses to allergen, the use of specific histamine receptor antagonists has aided the definition of tissue responses. Histamine binding to H1-receptors is linked to contraction of airway and gastrointestinal smooth muscle, increased vascular permeability, mucus production in the nose, pruritus, and cutaneous vasodilation. H2 receptor activation leads to increased gastric acid secretion, esophageal muscle contraction, vascular permeability and dilation, airway mucus secretion, and pruritus. Furthermore, H2 receptors are on lymphocytes and are mainly inhibitory while promoting CD8+ lymphocyte activity. Also, H2 receptor activation of basophils, eosinophils, and neutrophils suppresses degranulation.

The actions of histamine in the skin lead to the classic **wheal and flare response**, which is inhibited most effectively by H1-receptor antagonists. Injection of histamine into the skin initially causes vascular leak leading to a raised area or "wheal" from local edema. This is followed by a neuronal reflex leading to increased vasodilatation and vascular permeability at the periphery of the wheal, yielding the erythema or "flare" response. The resemblance of this skin lesion to urticaria has led to the common use of antihistamines for this condition.

Histamine exerts a bronchoconstrictive effect on the smooth muscle of the lower airway, leading to bronchospasm and wheezing. In addition, edema formation and increased mucous gland secretion are seen in both the lung and nose. Experimental histamine inhalation has been used as a measure of bronchial smooth muscle hyperreactivity, a characteristic of asthma. Clinical experience with antihistamines has shown efficacy in the treatment of allergic rhinitis, but somewhat surprisingly, little therapeutic benefit in managing bronchoconstriction in asthma, indicating that the latter is primarily attributable to other mediators.

In the gastrointestinal tract, histamine secretion stimulates both gastric and mucosal cells, leading to increased gastric acid and fluid secretion as well as smooth muscle contraction, resulting in increased peristalsis, hypermotility, and diarrhea.

2. **Neutral proteases and proteoglycans.** Mast cell secretory granules vary in electron microscopic appearance (scrolls, latticed, or grating architecture) as well as in their relative content of neutral serine proteases. These granules are also filled with highly negatively charged proteoglycans such as chondroitin sulfate or heparin that are packaged with the positively charged histamine and neutral proteases. These proteoglycans influence the activity of the proteases by limiting their inactivation as well as slowing the rate of diffusion into the local tissue site. Neutral proteases are the most abundant proteins in mast cell granules and are represented by **chymase, tryptase**, and **carboxypeptidase A.** Classification of mast cells by their granule protease content has led to the identification of tryptase-predominant mast cells located in the mucosa of the lung and gastrointestinal tract, with dual chymase and tryptase-predominant mast cells located in the skin and in submucosal areas. The general actions of these proteases are not well defined, but may include digestion of the basement membrane, increased vascular permeability, and activation of proteins involved in wound healing.

The serine protease **tryptase** accounts for up to 20% of all protein produced by the mast cell and can cause bronchial hyperresponsiveness. In animals, tryptase acts as a fibroblast growth factor. It interacts with and activates thrombin as well as the protease-activated receptor-2 (PAR-2). Two forms of tryptase exist, alpha-tryptase and beta-tryptase. Serum measurements of the two types can be useful diagnostically. **Alpha tryptase** is constitutively released into the serum at low levels and therefore serves as an indirect measure of the total number of mast cells in the body. Significant elevations in alpha-tryptase are seen in disorders with mast cell hyperplasia such as **mastocytosis**. In contrast, **beta-tryptase** is released acutely during mast cell degranulation. Clinically, beta-tryptase is used as a marker of anaphylaxis, particularly given its elevated presence in the serum for about 6 hours, with a half-life of 90 minutes, in contrast to the much shorter half-life of histamine. Tryptase and histamine have been detected in fluids recovered from allergen-challenged lung, nose, and skin.

The other major mast cell protease, chymase, is prominent in skin and submucosal mast cells and is typically found with carboxypeptidase in the secretory granules. It has been reported to stimulate bronchial mucus secretion in animals and can also cleave vasoactive intestinal peptide (VIP), a mediator of smooth muscle relaxation.

B. **Newly synthesized mediators**

1. **Leukotrienes.** The arachidonic acid derivatives include members of the leukotriene (LT) and prostaglandin families generated through the lipoxygenase and cyclooxygenase (COX) pathways, respectively (Fig. 2.3).

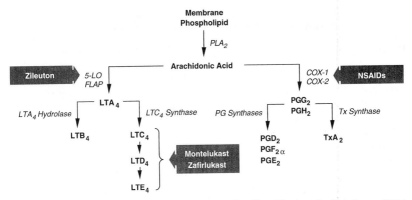

FIG. 2.3. Synthesis of leukotrienes and prostaglandins. Various leukotrienes (LTs) and prostaglandins (PGs) are generated from free arachidonic acid through the 5-lipoxygenase (5-LO) and cyclooxygenase (COX) pathways, respectively. The 5-LO and COX enzymes can be pharmacologically inhibited by zileuton and by nonsteroidal antiinflammatory drugs (NSAIDs), respectively, whereas effects of the cysteinyl LTs can be inhibited by receptor antagonists such as montelukast and zafirlukast.

LTs collectively represent what was identified in the 1940s as slow-reacting substance of anaphylaxis (SRS-A). Arachidonic acid released from membrane phospholipids by phospholipase A_2 (PLA$_2$) is translocated to the 5-lipoxygenase activating protein (FLAP) on the nuclear envelope. It is then converted by 5-lipoxygenase (5-LO) to 5-hydroperoxy-eicosatetraenoic acid (5-HPETE) and subsequently to leukotriene A_4 (LTA$_4$). LTA$_4$ is then converted to dihydroleukotriene B_4 (LTB$_4$) by LTA$_4$ hydrolase or to the cysteinyl leukotriene LTC$_4$ by LTC$_4$ synthase. LTC$_4$ is secreted and in extracellular locations, it is sequentially converted to LTD$_4$ and LTE$_4$ by enzymatic cleavage of glutamine and glycine, respectively. The LTs are synthesized and released by various cellular participants in allergic inflammation, including mast cells, basophils, and eosinophils. The levels of LTs in bronchoalveolar and nasal lavage fluids significantly increase minutes after local challenge with relevant allergen in atopic individuals. The cysteinyl LTs (LTC$_4$, LTD$_4$, and LTE$_4$) cause prolonged bronchoconstriction with up to a thousand-fold greater potency than histamine. They also induce mucus secretion, increased vascular permeability, and mucosal swelling. Cysteinyl LTs and LTB$_4$ are chemotactic for eosinophils and neutrophils, respectively. Other effects of LTs are listed in Table 2.2. The effects of LTs are mediated by two G protein-coupled receptors, CysLT1 and CysLT2, which are localized on various organs including the lungs. Pharmacological antagonists of the CysLT1 receptor (e.g., montelukast and zafirlukast) as well as an inhibitor of the 5-LO enzyme (zileuton) improve pulmonary function and ameliorate asthma symptoms. The effectiveness of this form of treatment for allergic rhinitis is presently being investigated.

2. **Prostaglandins.** The prostaglandins are generated from arachidonic acid by two forms of COX. COX-1 is constitutively expressed in a wide variety of cell types, whereas COX-2 is highly inducible in mast cells, macrophages, neutrophils, and other cells by proinflammatory factors. During the immediate phase of an allergic reaction, mast cells (but not basophils) release prostaglandin D_2 (PGD$_2$), which can serve as a marker that distinguishes these cells from basophils. PGD$_2$ causes bronchoconstriction, with

Table 2.2. Major effects of the lipoxygenase and cyclooxygenase products of arachidonic acid metabolism

Effect	LO- or COX-derived mediator
Airway hyperreactivity	LTE_4
Bronchoconstriction	LTC_4, LTD_4, LTE_4, PGD_2, $PGF_{2\alpha}$, TxA_2
Bronchodilation	PGE_2
Microvascular constriction	$PGF_{2\alpha}$, TxA_2
Microvascular dilation and plasma extravasation	LTC_4, LTD_4, LTE_4, PGD_2, PGE_2, PGI_2
Glandular secretion	LTC_4, LTD_4
Hyperalgesia	PGE_2, PGI_2, LTB_4
Leukocyte chemotaxis and adherence to endothelium	LTB_4, TxA_2, LTD_4
Enhanced platelet aggregation	TxA_2
Suppressed platelet aggregation	PGI_2

LO, lipoxygenase; COX, cyclooxygenase; LT, leukotriene; PG, prostaglandin; Tx, thromboxane.

up to a 30-fold greater potency than histamine, as well as vasodilation and resultant nasal obstruction. The other prostanoids and their actions are listed in Table 2.2. Note that $PGF_{2\alpha}$ likewise causes bronchoconstriction, but increases nasal patency because of its vasoconstrictive effect. PGE_2 has been postulated to have a protective role that counterbalances the bronchoconstrictive effects of PGD_2, $PGF_{2\alpha}$, and the cysteinyl LTs. The production of these prostaglandins is dependent on the presence of the appropriate synthase enzyme in the involved cells.

   3. **Platelet activating factor.** Platelet activating factor (PAF) is synthesized by neutrophils and eosinophils, as well as by mast cells, monocytes, macrophages, endothelial cells, and others. Intradermal injection of PAF in nonallergic subjects causes neutrophil infiltration and plasma extravasation with up to a thousand-fold greater potency than histamine; in allergic subjects, eosinophil infiltration also occurs. Nasal provocation with PAF causes congestion as well as an influx of eosinophils and neutrophils, whereas its inhalation causes bronchoconstriction that is LT-dependent. PAF was initially regarded as a potent mediator in asthma, but clinical trials of PAF antagonists have failed to demonstrate clinical efficacy.
   C. **Other mediators**
      1. **Neuropeptides and neurotrophins.** Histamine released during the immediate phase of the allergic reaction can activate sensory nerve fibers in the nasal mucosa, thus inducing the sneezing and secretory reflexes. Such activation can also induce an axon reflex whereby the tachykinins **substance P** and **neurokinin A**, as well as **calcitonin gene-related peptide**, are released from nociceptive nerve endings. These neuropeptides can cause vasodilation, increased vascular permeability, bronchoconstriction, and cell migration. **Bradykinin** can also be generated from kininogens during an allergic reaction. This mediator can induce bronchoconstriction, coughing, and plasma extravasation. **Nerve growth factor** is likewise released upon allergen provocation, putatively from epithelial cells, eosinophils, and mast cells. This neurotrophin influences the development of tachykinergic nerve fibers and might thus play a role in the development of hyperreactivity noted in allergic airway disease.
      2. **Cytokines.** The exact role of cytokines produced by mast cells and basophils in allergic responses *in vivo* remains unclear. IgE-dependent acti-

vation of cultured human mast cells and tissue-derived mast cells results in the production of a large number of cytokines, including IL-1, -2, -3, -4, -5, -6, -8, and -13 as well as granulocyte macrophage colony-stimulating factor (GM-CSF), interferon-γ (IFN-γ), and tumor necrosis factor (TNF-α). As with preformed mediators, mast cell cytokine production also appears to be heterogeneous. Activated basophils can synthesize and release sizeable quantities of IL-4 and IL-13, whereas TNF-α is released by mast cells. The relative importance of each of these cytokines can be inferred based on patterns of release and comparisons to other cellular sources of these products. In particular, the production of IL-4 and IL-13 from these cells may act to amplify allergic inflammatory events. Among the possible effects of these cytokines are enhanced IgE production from B cells, upregulation of the vascular cell adhesion molecule-1 (VCAM-1) on endothelial cells, and the differentiation of Th2 lymphocytes. Furthermore, release of TNF-α by these cells can have multiple pro-inflammatory effects, including inducing the transcription factor NFκB that can enhance expression of chemokines, adhesion molecules, and other proinflammatory genes. A limited quantity of preformed TNF-α exists in mast cells. There is also evidence that cultured mast cells or mast cell lines release chemokines such as macrophage inflammatory protein-α (MIP-1α) (also basophils), MIP-1β, monocyte chemotactic protein-1 (MCP-1), RANTES, and IL-8, which can act to recruit specific leukocyte subtypes.

Following allergen exposure of sensitive individuals, acute allergic reactions subside within minutes, but can often be followed hours later by a second inflammatory response termed the late-phase response. In the skin, the **late-phase response** manifests as reoccurrence of diffuse induration and erythema, while in the airways nasal congestion or bronchoconstriction recur. There are many similarities between late phase reactions and chronic allergic diseases, including: (i) their dependence upon IgE, (ii) the pattern of cellular infiltration (especially eosinophils, basophils, and Th2 lymphocytes), (iii) the association with reversible airways obstruction and increased airways hyperreactivity (typical characteristics of asthma), (iv) the generation of edema and mucus hypersecretion, and (v) the quantities and types of inflammatory mediators released (e.g., histamine, leukotrienes, cytokines, and chemokines). The late-phase IgE-mediated inflammatory events in humans help to explain how chronic or recurrent allergen exposure leads to enhanced allergen sensitivity ("priming") and the chronic symptoms of allergic rhinitis and asthma.

Local tissue accumulation of eosinophils is prominent in allergic diseases. This is likely due to a combination of factors, including those that mediate preferential eosinophil adhesion (e.g., IL-4, IL-13), via induction of the endothelial adhesion molecule VCAM-1, recognized by the integrin very late-activation antigen-4 (VLA-4) on the eosinophil surface. Preferential migration occurs in response to chemokines (chemotactic cytokines) of the C-C chemokine family (such as eotaxins and MCP-4) that are produced by tissue-resident cells such as the respiratory epithelium. Chemokines are recognized by specific receptors. For example, the chemokine receptor CCR3 (which selectively binds eotaxins) is prominently and selectively expressed on eosinophils, basophils, and mast cells. Together with cytokines that prolong their survival (e.g., IL-5, GM-CSF) eosinophilic inflammatory infiltrates get established. Each of these molecules is thus a possible target for the development of new drugs to combat allergic diseases.

VII. Atopic diseases

Atopic diseases are conditions related to IgE-mediated hypersensitivity. Both genetic and environmental factors appear to influence an individual's allergic disease susceptibility, and/or severity of disease. A genetic basis for asthma, rhinitis, and atopic dermatitis is supported by observations of familial clustering and of increased concordance rates in monozygotic, compared with dizygotic, twins. Several chromosomal markers (e.g., 5q23-q31, 11q13, 12q14-q24.33, 17p11.1-q11.2, and other loci) have been linked to asthma, and they appear to vary among different ethnic groups. Environmental factors that can interact with genetic susceptibility include exposure to allergens, tobacco smoke, and various pathogens. The following are brief descriptions of conditions related to atopy as well as examples of specific type I, IgE-mediated allergic reactions to allergen exposure.

A. Atopic conditions

1. **Anaphylaxis** is an immediate systemic reaction caused by IgE-mediated release of potent mediators from tissue mast cells and peripheral blood basophils. The clinical presentation of this potentially life-threatening event may include mucocutaneous changes such as pruritus and urticaria, laryngeal edema, bronchospasm, cardiovascular collapse, and/or gastrointestinal symptoms. Commonly implicated etiologic factors include certain drugs, foods, insect venoms, and latex allergens.

2. **Allergic rhinosinusitis** is the most common atopic disease, affecting up to 20% of the United States population and up to 9 of 10 asthmatic patients. The symptoms of sneezing, nasal pruritus, and rhinorrhea may be attributable to histamine, whereas nasal congestion may be attributable to cysteinyl leukotrienes, released upon aeroallergen exposure.

3. **Asthma** is a complex disease characterized by inflammation, reversible airflow obstruction, and hyperreactivity to various inhaled substances. It affects about 17 million Americans, with a prevalence that has increased over the last two decades. Like other chronic atopic diseases, asthma is associated with a high socioeconomic cost. It is the most common nonsurgical indication for hospitalization in the pediatric age group. The typical symptoms of asthma include recurrent wheezing, dyspnea, chest tightness, and/or cough.

4. **Allergic conjunctivitis** is commonly associated with rhinosinusitis, but it can also be the single manifestation of atopy, especially in children. Its signs and symptoms include recurrent lacrimation, ocular pruritus, and swelling.

5. **Atopic dermatitis** is a chronic pruritic inflammatory skin disease that affects more than 10% of children, usually during the first 5 years of life. It frequently predates the development of allergic airway disease, which occurs in up to 80% of affected patients in a progression termed the allergic march. Approximately 40% of infants and young children with moderate to severe atopic dermatitis have food allergy. Acute skin lesions include erythematous papules with serous exudate, whereas chronic changes include thickened plaques or lichenification. As in other atopic conditions, its features include an elevated serum total IgE, eosinophilia, and increased releasability of histamine from basophils.

6. **Urticaria and angioedema** are clinical manifestations of mucocutaneous vasodilation and increased vascular permeability with resultant superficial or deep tissue swelling, respectively. There are several types of urticaria and angioedema, and those specifically associated with IgE-mediated hypersensitivity are typically acute and transient. Chronic forms of these conditions are rarely related to an allergy, and in such situations the etiology may be difficult or impossible to ascertain.

B. Specific allergies

1. **Food allergy** is most common in young children, especially among those with atopic dermatitis. The manifestations of a true IgE-mediated adverse reaction to food occur within minutes to a few hours after ingestion, and generally involve the dermatologic, gastrointestinal, and/or respiratory systems. About 80% to 90% of verified allergic reactions to food in children are attributable to egg, milk, peanuts, soy, fish, tree nuts, and wheat. In adults, allergic reactions are to a more limited variety of foods, including peanuts, tree nuts, fish, and shellfish. Peanuts and tree nuts account for more than 90% of fatalities due to food allergy.

2. **Drug allergy** accounts for only a small percentage of adverse drug reactions, most of which are not associated with IgE-mediated hypersensitivity. Reactions to drugs that have an immunologic basis can range from transient urticaria to fatal anaphylaxis. They typically require a period of sensitization and can occur at doses below the therapeutic range. Penicillin and other β-lactam antibiotics constitute the most common causes of drug allergy.

3. **Insect venom allergy** causes about 40 deaths yearly in the United States, and it is likely that additional cases are undiagnosed and unreported. Most insect stings produce local reactions in nonallergic people, but systemic effects ranging from airway obstruction to hypotension can also occur in venom-sensitive individuals. Stinging insects responsible for such IgE-mediated reactions include yellow jackets, hornets, wasps, honeybees, and fire ants.

4. **Latex allergy** affects less than 1% of the general population, but certain individuals have a significantly higher risk of developing this condition. For example, it has been reported that latex allergy affects 24% to 60% of patients with spina bifida and 5% to 15% of healthcare workers.

C. **Approach to the patient**

As in other medical conditions, a complete history and physical examination is mandatory for the diagnosis and management of patients with allergic disease. The following aspects generally require particular attention.

1. **History**

a. **Onset of symptoms.** The age at onset of symptoms may suggest whether or not the condition is IgE-mediated. For example, more than 90% of patients with rhinitis symptoms that started before age 10 years have positive skin tests, whereas fewer than 40% of those whose symptoms started after age 40 have allergen sensitivity. Food allergy is much more prevalent during infancy and early childhood, although sensitivity could also manifest later in life.

b. **Character, duration, frequency and severity of symptoms.** Allergy-related changes may be localized, or may involve the respiratory, dermatologic, cardiovascular, and gastrointestinal systems. Respiratory or ocular symptoms may be due to an infectious process if they only last 1 to 2 weeks, but are likely related to allergies if they are more persistent. Urticaria has a greater probability of having an allergic etiology if it is acute rather than chronic. The frequency and severity of symptoms may help determine whether to prescribe medications to be used daily or only as needed.

c. **Temporal nature of symptoms.** The allergic condition may be intermittent, year-round, strictly seasonal, or year-round with seasonal exacerbations. Persistent respiratory symptoms during the spring, summer, or fall seasons may indicate sensitivity to tree, grass, or weed allergens, respectively (Table 2.3). Year-round symptoms may be attributable to perennial sources of aeroallergens such as dust mites, cockroaches, indoor molds, rodents, or fur-bearing pets.

d. **Topological nature of symptoms.** The patient's disease can be exacerbated at home, in school, or at work. This may indicate sensitivity to allergens or hyperreactivity to irritants that could be present in these places. Of note, cat allergens can be detected in schools even in the absence of these pets, presumably transported there on clothing. About 5% of asthma cases are believed to be related to the workplace. Certain patients could have increased work-related risks for sensitivity and exposure to latex, laboratory animals, or biochemical products.

e. **Trigger factors.** Substances in the environment can initiate or exacerbate the patient's symptoms. These can include known sources of aeroallergens as well as nonallergenic elements. Most patients with allergic airway disease develop symptoms upon exposure not only to allergens, but also to tobacco smoke and other irritants. This can be

Table 2.3. Typical seasonal pattern of selected common aeroallergens

Common name	Major allergen	Spring	Summer	Fall	Year round
Trees					
Oak	*Que a* 1	X			
Birch	*Bet v* 1	X			
Grasses					
Timothy	*Ph1 p* 5[a]		X		
Orchard	*Dac g* 5[a]		X		
Weeds					
Plantain			X	X	
Ragweed	*Amb a* 1[a]			X	
Molds					
Alternaria	*Alt a* 1			X	
Aspergillus	*Asp f* 1				X
Indoor allergens					
Cat	*Fel d* 1[a]				X
Dog	*Can f* 1[a]				X
Dust mite	*Der p* 1[a]				X
Cockroach	*Bla g* 1				X

[a] Standardized extracts available in the United States.

explained by exaggerated mucosal tissue responsiveness to sensory nerve stimulation in the presence of allergic inflammation. Environmental factors such as temperature, humidity, or barometric changes can also affect symptoms of allergic airway disease.

f. **Activity and behavioral factors.** Physical exercise may trigger asthma and, more rarely, anaphylaxis. Outdoor activities may predispose the patient to aeroallergen exposure or to insect stings. Tobacco smoking could significantly worsen allergic airway disease.

g. **Impact of disease on the patient.** Chronic allergic disease can adversely affect the patient's daily activities and performance in school or at work. For example, allergic rhinitis contributes to a total of more than 800,000 missed schooldays and a similar number of lost workdays annually. Quality of life is an important outcome that needs to be evaluated and monitored as treatment is initiated and continued.

h. **Personal history of atopy.** The occurrence of atopic dermatitis during early childhood increases the probability of subsequent allergic airway disease. Allergic rhinitis likewise often predates asthma.

i. **Family history of atopy.** A history of allergic airway disease or atopic dermatitis in one or both parents can increase the child's risk of developing the same condition. For example, the incidence of allergic rhinitis in children is 1.5 and 3 times greater if one or both of their parents, respectively, have a history of having this disease.

j. **Other comorbidities.** The patient can have a disease requiring medications such as beta-blockers that can worsen asthma, cause nasal congestion, or can interfere with the management of anaphylaxis. The presence of hypertension, narrow-angle glaucoma, or urinary retention can preclude the use of decongestants alone or in combination with antihistamines.

2. **Physical examination**

a. The entire **skin** should be examined for acute and chronic changes, including urticarial lesions, angioedema, dermatitis, and lichenification. The presence of dermatographism can confound the interpretation of skin test results.

  b. The **eyes** should be examined for conjunctival hyperemia and chemosis (edema). Giant papillae greater than 1 mm in size that give a cobblestone appearance to the conjunctivae indicate an allergic, rather than an infectious process, although these can also be found in contact lens users. Preauricular adenopathy is absent in allergic conjunctivitis and, if present, suggests viral or bacterial conjunctivitis. Changes in visual acuity also suggest a nonatopic condition. The presence of cataracts that can occasionally be associated with atopic dermatitis and, more rarely, with chronic use of high dose steroids should be assessed by funduscopy.

  c. Examination of the **tympanic membranes** with an otoscope and of the frontal and maxillary **sinuses** by palpation and percussion should be done to check for comorbidities associated with allergic airway disease, such as otitis media and sinusitis, respectively.

  d. External examination of the **nose** can reveal a transverse crease resulting from repetitive upward rubbing of the nose, known as the **allergic salute**. The interior of the nose should be assessed with adequate illumination and exposure using a headlight and nasal speculum or, alternatively, with an otoscope with a large speculum. A more extensive examination of the upper airway can be achieved using a fiberoptic nasopharyngoscope. The evaluation should note the color of the mucosa; quantity and quality of secretions; and presence and severity of swelling, nasal polyps, ulcerations, and anatomic abnormalities such as septal deviation. If severe swelling is present, topical decongestants can be applied to allow adequate examination.

  e. The **oropharynx** should be examined for the presence of erythema, edema, tonsillar hypertrophy, posterior drainage, or oral thrush, the latter being a side effect seen in patients using inhaled corticosteroids.

  f. **Chest evaluation.** The chest should be examined by visual inspection for the presence of hyperinflation or use of accessory muscles, and by auscultation for adventitious sounds such as wheezing.

3. **Clinical and laboratory tests**
   Certain tests can be performed to confirm or further characterize the allergic condition suggested by the history and physical examination, as well as to monitor the progression of disease or its response to treatment. The pretest probability of a positive result should be taken into account in determining whether the test is warranted and in interpreting the results.

Primary Tests

  a. **Skin tests**
     (1) **Indication.** Demonstrating the presence of antigen-specific IgE antibodies is important in establishing the diagnosis of atopic disease and in identifying allergens for which avoidance measures and/or immunotherapy could be effective. Recognition of a positive skin test by the patient can be useful in gaining cooperation and compliance with these measures. Validated skin testing for immediate hypersensitivity is available for aeroallergens, foods and insect venoms, as well as for penicillin.

     (2) **General guidelines and methods for skin testing.** Scratch tests initially were used to assess sensitivity to allergens, but they have now been replaced by percutaneous (also known as epicutaneous, prick, or puncture) and intracutaneous (also known as intradermal) skin tests. The following guidelines are applicable for these techniques (see Appendix II for skin testing methods).

        (a) **Quality control** should be applied to ensure the reliability and consistency of the individual tester as well as of the employed devices and allergen extracts. The composition and concentration of allergen extracts should be documented and standardized whenever possible. The potency of these extracts deteriorates over time, particularly after being diluted and/or exposed to warm temperature. Allergen solutions of 1:100 weight/volume concentration that are kept in the refrigerator at 2° to 8°C usually maintain their antigenicity for up to 1 year.

(b) **Testing with both negative and positive controls** (diluent such as phosphate-buffered saline with 0.4% phenol and histamine phosphate 0.1% or 0.01% for percutaneous or intracutaneous tests, respectively) need to be performed to allow proper interpretation of results. Note that wheal formation can occur even with the diluent negative control if the patient has dermatographism, whereas the response to the histamine positive control can be suppressed by certain medications with antihistaminic properties.

(c) **Avoid oral antihistamines to prevent suppression of skin test reactivity.** Most first-generation antihistamines should be avoided at least 72 hours before testing. Hydroxyzine should be withheld at least for the preceding 96 hours. Second-generation antihistamines must be avoided for at least 1 week before the test. Tricyclic antidepressants may also affect the test if taken within the prior 1 to 2 weeks. H2 blockers can cause mild suppression of skin test reactivity if taken less than 1 day before the test, but this usually is not a problem. Short-term use of systemic steroids does not affect skin testing, but chronic, high-dose, topical steroid therapy may partially suppress reactivity by reducing the number of tissue mast cells. Therefore, potent topical steroids should be avoided on the forearms for 2 to 3 weeks before skin testing. A diminished response to skin testing can also be observed in infants and the elderly, and possibly in patients on vasopressors.

(d) Adverse events, including fatal anaphylaxis, are extremely rare, and can occur in highly sensitive individuals following intracutaneous testing. Appropriate emergency equipment and drugs, as well as a physician, should thus be readily available for treatment of a potentially life-threatening reaction. Skin testing in symptomatic asthmatics should be deferred to avoid even the small risk of further deterioration of lung function. Because systemic reactions could include uterine contractions, pregnant patients should be skin tested only if the potential benefit outweighs the risk.

(e) Skin tests are typically performed on the volar aspect of the forearm as the preferred site, or sometimes the upper back is used. Aseptic techniques should be employed. For percutaneous testing, a drop of concentrated allergen extract is placed on the skin surface, and a superficial puncture is made through the drop using one of several metal or plastic devices manufactured for this purpose. Alternatively, there are individual or multitest applicators in which the allergen solutions can be preloaded onto the tip of the puncturing device. For intracutaneous testing, the dose of allergen used is usually 1/100 to 1/1000 of the solution used for the percutaneous test. Approximately 0.02 mL of the allergen solution is injected intradermally to create a 1- to 3-mm bleb.

(f) Percutaneous skin tests are generally less sensitive, but more specific than intracutaneous tests. Percutaneous testing correlates better with exacerbation of allergic airway disease symptoms following inhalational challenge with grass or cat allergens. Intracutaneous testing should be considered only when the percutaneous test is negative and there is a history that is strongly suggestive of allergen sensitivity and of relevant exposure. Intracutaneous testing, however, should not be done for food allergy to avoid false-positive results and anaphylactic reactions.

(g) The selection of the number and type of inhalant allergens used for skin testing should be based rationally on their geographic relevance as well as utility in disease management that includes environmental control and/or immunotherapy.

Interpretation of Results

The skin test results should be read at the peak of the reaction, usually 15 to 20 minutes after application. The average diameters of the resultant wheal and of the typically wider area of erythema are recorded. The presence of pseudopods, which are lateral extensions from the central wheal that indicate a high degree of sensitivity, should also be noted. A test is considered positive if the wheal diameter produced by the allergen is at least 3 mm greater than that produced by the diluent. It is important to keep in mind that the clinical significance of such results should be based on their correlation with the patient's history. False-negative results can arise from improper technique, loss of allergen potency, recent anaphylaxis, or drugs that suppress skin reactivity, whereas false-positive results may be caused by skin test materials used at inappropriately high concentrations that induce nonspecific histamine release or local irritation. In general, the sensitivity and negative predictive value of skin tests are higher than their specificity and positive predictive value, respectively.

    b. Radioallergosorbent tests and related *in vitro* tests for allergen-specific immunoglobulin E. Although *in vivo* skin testing is the preferred method of evaluating IgE-mediated hypersensitivity, *in vitro* measurement of allergen-specific IgE using immunoadsorption methods can be applicable in certain situations. These assays can be useful in cases involving (i) dermatographism or generalized dermatitis; (ii) ongoing treatment with long-acting antihistamines or tricyclic antidepressants that cannot be discontinued; (iii) uncooperative patients; (iv) evaluation of cross-reactivity between insect venoms; (iv) a clinical history suggesting a significant risk of systemic reaction to skin tests; (v) a situation where reliable skin test reagents are not available (e.g., latex); and (vi) postmortem evaluation of fatal anaphylaxis. Drawbacks of this method include generally lower test sensitivity, higher cost, delay in obtaining results, and lack of a universal consensus in defining what constitutes a positive test. For the assessment of children with food allergy and atopic dermatitis, however, cutoff levels of IgE antibodies with excellent predictive values are available for egg, milk, peanut, and fish.

    c. Pulmonary function testing. Spirometric evaluation of lung function and reversibility of airway obstruction, if present, should be part of the initial assessment of a patient suspected of having asthma. Follow-up pulmonary function tests may also be warranted during return visits to monitor disease progression or response to treatment. Of note, the perception of asthma severity often does not correlate with the degree of objectively measured airway obstruction. Routine spirometry provides more information than a peak expiratory flow meter, but is less convenient. Neither provides measurements of lung volume or diffusing capacity, which may need to be determined for the evaluation of other diagnostic possibilities.

Secondary Tests

    a. Provocative tests that are usually only performed in a research setting can be useful in the clinical evaluation of allergic disease. These techniques should be done only by experienced personnel with the same precautions advised for skin testing regarding the readiness to manage serious reactions. Double-blind, placebo-controlled food challenges can confirm or rule out sensitivity to food in cases wherein the skin test result does not correlate with the clinical history. This can also help to determine whether a patient previously diagnosed with food allergy during early childhood has outgrown this affliction. Bronchial challenge with a work-related allergen can assist in the diagnosis of occupational asthma. Bronchoprovocation with increasing amounts of a known spasmogen, such as methacholine, to determine the concentration that causes a 20% decrease in forced expiratory volume in 1 second (FEV_1) (PC_{20}), can demonstrate the presence of hyperresponsiveness that is compatible with asthma. Although rarely indicated, this test, if normal, is particularly useful in excluding the diagnosis of asthma. Provocative testing is not warranted in cases where the diagnosis is already clearly evidenced by the history and other examinations.

b. A **chest radiograph** can assist in evaluating differential diagnoses as well as the complications of asthma. Chest **computed tomography** (CT) scanning can demonstrate bronchiectasis compatible with allergic bronchopulmonary aspergillosis. **Limited sinus CT scans** with coronal sections, compared to radiographs, provide greater information regarding the ostiomeatal complex and other structures involved in persistent or recurrent sinus infections.

c. **Serum total immunoglobulin E** levels are of little use in the evaluation of atopic diseases because of their broad and overlapping range across affected and healthy populations. Total IgE levels could be elevated in other clinical conditions such as helminthic parasitic disease, hyper-IgE syndrome, progressive human immunodeficiency virus (HIV) infection, IgE myeloma, drug-related adverse reactions such as interstitial nephritis, graft versus host disease, and allergic bronchopulmonary aspergillosis.

d. Levels of **antigen-specific IgG** to insect venoms produced in response to immunotherapy correlate with protection from reactions to an insect sting. However, other than for experimental purposes, there is no clinical value to measuring IgG to other allergens during or after immunotherapy.

e. The peripheral blood **eosinophil count** can be normal or slightly elevated in patients with atopic disease. However, eosinophilia greater than 20% or an absolute eosinophil count greater than 1,500 per mm^3 should initiate a search for nonallergic causes. The eosinophilia can be greater during the pollen season or during asthma exacerbations among susceptible individuals, but is typically suppressed among those being treated with steroids or leukotriene modifiers. Similarly, eosinophil counts in nasal or bronchoalveolar lavage fluids, induced sputum, and nasal smears or mucosal scrapings can fluctuate with pollen exposure or medication use. However, these cytological analyses are not routinely indicated in the assessment of allergic disease.

f. The levels of histamine, leukotrienes, and other **mediators** in biological fluids obtained *in vivo* or released *in vitro* correlate with allergic disease and are useful outcomes that are measured particularly for research purposes. Measurement of serum beta-tryptase levels, which remain elevated for several hours after being released by mast cells during a systemic allergic reaction, can be clinically indicated in the assessment of possible anaphylaxis. Although histamine can sometimes also be detected in anaphylaxis, it only remains elevated for about 1 hour. In addition, plasma, rather than serum, should be assayed because unintended artifactual basophil degranulation is less likely to occur in clotted blood. Assays to determine serum levels of alpha-tryptase can also be useful to evaluate the presence of masto-cytosis.

   g. Miscellaneous tests to measure sedimentation rate, α-1-antitrypsin, complement proteins, 5-hydroxyindole acetic acid, stool ova and parasites, sweat chloride, and others can be considered to rule out differential diagnoses of, or conditions associated with, the various allergic diseases. In the setting of recurrent infections, the measurement of quantitative immunoglobulins should be considered.

4. **Controversial and unproven tests.** Several techniques have been developed for possible application in the diagnosis of allergic disease, but have been shown to be either invalid for any purpose, inapplicable for the evaluation of IgE-mediated sensitivity, or inappropriate for clinical use because of significant inherent limitations. These include so-called cytotoxic testing, provocation-neutralization testing, electrodermal diagnosis, applied kinesiology, the reaginic pulse test, and chemical analysis of body tissues.

Acknowledgement

S. S. Saini was supported by NIH grant AI01564.

Selected Readings

Bochner BS, Lichtenstein LM. Anaphylaxis. *N Engl J Med* 1991;324:1785–1790.

Busse WW, Lemanske RF. Asthma. *N Engl J Med* 2001;344:350–362.

Diagnosis and management of anaphylaxis. Joint Task Force on Practice Parameters, American Academy of Allergy, Asthma and Immunology, American College of Allergy, Asthma and Immunology, and the Joint Council of Allergy, Asthma and Immunology. *J Allergy Clin Immunol* 1998;101:S465–S528.

Grant JA, Li H. Biology of basophils. In: Middleton E, Reed CE, Ellis EF, et al., eds. *Allergy principles and practice*. St. Louis: Mosby, 1998:277–284.

Kay AB. Allergy and allergic diseases. *N Engl J Med* 2001;344:30–37.

Bernstein IL, Storms WW. Practice parameters for allergy diagnostic testing. *Ann Allergy Asthma Immunol* 1995;75:543–625.

Primer on allergic and immunologic diseases. *JAMA* 1997;278:1815–2025.

Rothenberg ME. Eosinophilia. *N Engl J Med* 1998;338:1592–1600.

Schwartz LB, Huff T. Biology of mast cells. In: Middleton E, Reed CD, Ellis EF, et al., eds. *Allergy principles and practice*. St. Louis: Mosby, 1998:261–276.

Siraganian R. Biochemical events in basophil or mast cell activation and mediator release. In: Middleton E, Reed CD, Ellis EF, et al., eds. *Allergy principles and practice*. St. Louis: Mosby, 1998:204–227.

3. AEROALLERGENS AND ENVIRONMENTAL FACTORS

William Neaville, Robert K. Bush, Robert Ausdenmoore, and Michelle Lierl

Aeroallergens

Aeroallergens are relatively large and complex particles, such as pollens, molds, insect parts, animal dander, plant fragments, and house dust mites, that are capable of eliciting allergic reactions in susceptible persons. These particles contain many molecular components, only some of which are antigenic. When specific antigenic components have been identified, they usually are proteins with some carbohydrate subunits and have a molecular weight of 10,000 to 40,000 D. The **antigenicity** of these molecules is fundamentally a property of their **size**, **spatial configuration**, and **chemical groupings**. The overall **allergic importance** of these particles is not only a function of their **antigenicity**, but also of their **availability** in the environment for contact with susceptible persons and the suitability of **particle size** for impingement on the respiratory mucosa.

I. **Sources and size of aeroallergens**
  A. **Biogenic** particulate matter commonly identifiable in air samples includes pollen grains and fungal spores. **Unidentifiable biogenic** particulate materials include insect parts, plant fragments, animal dander, and fragmented pollen and fungi. These may be identifiable by immunoassay. **Nonbiogenic** materials, such as hydrocarbons, dirt, salt crystals, or other particulate substances, especially from neighboring farm or industrial activities, may modify allergic responses, but are not aeroallergens. **Nonbiogenic, nonparticulate** gases such as chlorine, hydrogen sulfide, formaldehyde, gasoline, wood smoke, tobacco smoke, and cooking odors are also not allergens but may influence allergic reactions and act directly as irritants.
  B. Most airborne substances of allergic importance identifiable microscopically are between 2 and 60 µm in diameter. Most of these particles (particularly those greater than 15 µm diameter) strike ocular, nasal, and pharyngeal surfaces because of their linear momentum. Because the majority of allergenic particles do not reach the bronchi, it has been postulated that the bronchial pathophysiologic features in asthma result from a bronchial reflex stimulated by nasopharyngeal receptors. Alternatively, active allergenic material may be eluted from the particles in the nasopharynx and aspirated, or may reach the bronchi by a hematogenous route.
II. **Sampling techniques: volumetric methods**
  A. Particles heavier than air also exhibit inertial forces, so placing an obstruction in the flow of air causes the particles to impinge on the obstruction. Several sampling techniques take advantage of this fact, but currently these techniques are not recommended because they do not provide volumetric data and significantly underrepresent small particles.
  B. With the **rotating arm impactor**, a coated surface is rotated for specific periods of time at a fixed and known speed. Then the particles are counted and expressed as pollen grains or spores per cubic meter of sample. Such methods reduce the factors of wind velocity and direction. One adaptation, the Rotorod Sampler (Fig. 3.1), involves the use of clear acrylic collector rods coated with a thin layer of silicone grease to enhance retention of impacted particles. Other modifications provide **timed intermittent rotation** to prevent overloading and shields to cover exposed surfaces between operating intervals. The American Academy of Allergy, Asthma and Immunology currently recommends the intermittent rotoslide sampler as the standard volumetric collector for larger particles.
  C. **Inertial suction samplers.** When a given volume of air is drawn through membrane filters with defined pore sizes or is aspirated through an orifice with a defined size, particles of a given density leave the air stream and

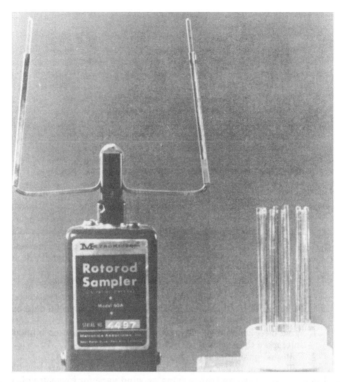

FIG. 3.1. Rotorod sampler (rotating arm impactor), which is well suited to short periods of continuous collection. Field carrier for storage of additional Lucite rods is shown at **right** (Courtesy of Air Pollution Training Institute, Research Triangle Park, NC.)

impinge on a collecting plate as the air changes direction because of the plate. One modification, the **Burkhard (Hirst) spore trap** (Fig. 3.2), contains a collecting plate (rotated at the rate of 2 mm per hour) within the trap to allow observations of the fluctuations in the count. In addition, a rudder eliminates the factor of wind direction. A more sophisticated sampler, the **AccuVol** (Fig. 3.3), allows collection of particles less than 1 μm. Spore traps are the preferred method for sampling particles over a broad particle size range. Immunochemical assay of collected material is highly specific and quantitative for specific allergens, e.g., ragweed allergen *Amb a* 1.

D. Interpretation of sampling data

  1. For most sampling procedures, volumetric samples are preferred. Manuals with identification guidelines are available for pollens and mold spores (see Selected Readings). Tabulation of their concentrations (by counting under the microscope) can help determine seasonal prevalences of common aeroallergens in given locales (see Appendix VI). Correlation of particle counts with clinical symptoms on a given day must be cautiously interpreted. There are great variations in the pollen and mold concentrations within any collection period. Allergic symptoms may be manifested in an individual because of a high peak concentration even if the total daily count is low. Allergen concentrations may be high as those measured by immunoassay in some circumstances, even though the pollen or mold concentration by visual count is low. Unfortunately, some news agencies report daily pollen or mold counts to help promote

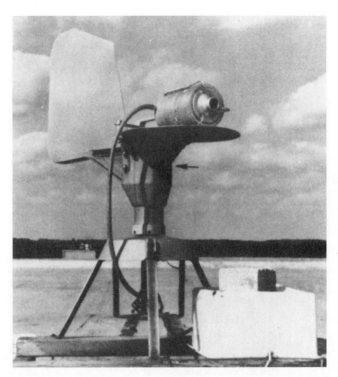

FIG. 3.2. Buckard (Hirst) spore trap serving as wind vane for exposure of Anderson sampler in free air. The intake orifice (**arrow**) of the spore trap is 2 mm × 14 mm. Particles are collected on a greased, tape-coated drum, which is advanced by a clock mechanism. (From Air Pollution Training Institute, Research Triangle Park, NC, with permission.)

medication advertisements to a lay public unaware of sampling limitations, the important aspects of personal exposure variations, the effects of multiple sensitivities, or complex allergen dose-response relationships.

2. **Immunochemical quantitation** of allergens in air samples can be made using labeled antibody toward the allergen being measured. Fractions of these allergens can be separated by size by collecting them on filters with progressively smaller pore sizes. Correlations of quantitative data derived by immunochemical means with clinical symptom scores, especially in asthma, is considerably better than the correlation with pollen or mold spore counts. Relatively few studies of this type have been carried out and, thus far, only data with respect to ragweed (*Amb a* 1), insect allergens, and *Alternaria* (*Alt a* 1) have been published. This new, more precise method of quantitating allergen in the air may not only provide better data to correlate with clinical symptoms, but also may increase the understanding of the effect of antigens not recognizable under the microscope (e.g., dander and insect fragments in dwellings and workplaces).

III. Pollen aeroallergens

Pollen grains are male reproductive structures of seed-bearing plants and function to carry the male gametes (sperm) to the female gametes (egg), which remain on the plant. Pollen transfer for plants with showy, colorful, and fragrant flowers is accomplished by insects (entomophily). In these instances, the pollen is often large, with an adhesive coating. Remarkable adaptations of some plants allow dissemination of pollen by birds, bats, mice, or even snails.

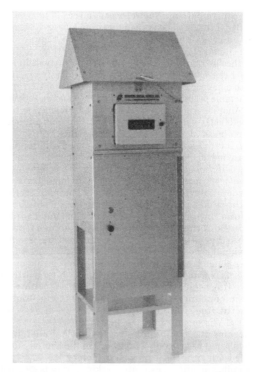

FIG. 3.3. The AccuVol volumetric air sampler draws air through a fiberglass filter at a set flow rate. Particles down to 0.3 μm in diameter are deposited on the filter. A size-selective inlet can be installed, allowing selective sampling of particles less than 10 μm in diameter. (From General Metal Works, Cleveland, OH, with permission.)

Most **pollens of allergic importance are windborne** (anemophily). Plants with windborne pollen transfers are typically drab, with small, inconspicuous, and odorless flowers. Their pollen is usually small and nonadhesive, with a smooth unsculptured surface.

Most pollen is shed in the early morning hours, but dispersal by wind currents usually produces maximal pollen concentrations in the afternoon or early evening. Although pollen grains are viable for only a few hours, nonviable pollen is still an active allergen. A gentle wind can carry pollen of anemophilous plants for many miles and produce high pollen concentrations in urban and metropolitan areas, far from their rural or suburban source. A floristic map and regional pollen guide listing the periods of prevalence and relative importance of various pollens in various regions of the United States and Canada appear in Appendix VI.

A. Weeds. Although many different classes of plants may be considered weeds, such as Polygonaceae (buckwheat family), Amaranthaceae (pigweed and waterhemp family), Chenopodiaceae (goose foot family), and Plantaginaceae (plantain family), plants from within the family Compositae are most important from an allergy perspective. Within this family, ragweed (*Ambrosia* sp) is the single most important cause, quantitatively and qualitatively, of seasonal allergic rhinitis (hay fever) in the United States. The highest concentrations of ragweed pollen occur in the central plains and eastern agricultural regions. Cultivation of soil as seen in the midwestern grain fields allows dense ragweed growth and the greatest seasonal exposure risk for the ragweed pollen-sensitive patient. Ragweed pollen season is typically considered to last 2 to 3 months, with peaks ranging from late August to early October, depending on geographic locale. Peak times for ragweed pollination in the southern United States occur considerably later than in the north. Peak dates occur at the same time for each locale—generally within a 2-week period.

Amb a 1 (formerly termed antigen E) is a highly reactive fraction of ragweed with a molecular weight of 37,800 D, representing approximately 6% of the extractable protein of ragweed. It is 200 times as active as whole ragweed extract. Another fraction, *Amb a* 2 (formerly termed antigen K) (molecular weight 38,000 D) is somewhat less potent than *Amb a* 1, but still produces reactions in almost all ragweed-sensitive patients.

B. **Grasses.** It is difficult to distinguish the pollen of different grasses solely on the basis of morphology. Consequently, the importance of individual species is largely determined on the basis of total grass-pollen counts combined with a knowledge of the regional presence of individual grass species.

    1. In general, **Bermuda grass** is the predominant species throughout the **southern** half of the United States and the **southern Pacific coast regions**. In the **northeastern** and **northern midwestern states, the bulk of the grass pollen usually comes from the blue grass, orchard grass, timothy grass, and redtop** (see Appendix VI.A for individual locales).

    2. Grass pollen is seen only during the **growing seasons**, so that seasonal patterns (spring and summer) are noted in the north, and more perennial patterns are observed in the south. As with weed pollen, **grass pollen concentrations are generally low at high altitudes, such as in the Rocky Mountain area**. They are also low in the far north regions of Wisconsin, Michigan, and Maine.

    3. Regarding the **frequency** and **severity** of allergic symptoms, grass pollen ranks second only to ragweed in the United States. In other parts of the world, it is the leading aeroallergen.

        Significant cross-sensitivity on skin testing is seen between blue, timothy, orchard, and redtop grasses, but Bermuda grass is antigenically distinct. The extensive cross-reactivity of grass pollens makes skin testing with individual grass extracts unnecessary. Studies indicate that one species is usually sufficient for in vitro diagnosis of grass pollen allergy.

C. **Trees.** The pollens of wind-pollinating (anemophilous) trees are the principal causes of respiratory allergy in this botanical group. Insect-pollinating (entomophilous) trees (e.g., ornamental and fruit trees) and the anemophilous conifers whose pollen has a thick exine or outer covering (e.g., pine trees) are of minor allergic significance.

    1. **Each tree genus produces pollen morphologically distinct from that of any other genus** and exhibits marked individual variation with respect to the duration, intensity, and seasonal pattern of pollination.

    2. **Little cross-antigenicity is noted between genera.** In addition, clustering of certain genera often occurs within the same floristic zone. As a result of these factors, an allergic patient can have selective sensitivity (frequently only to one genus or a few different genera). Pollens from the Fagales order are an important source of allergens in spring in the temperate climate zone. *Bet v* 1 from birch pollen is an important allergen from this class and has been studied fairly closely. There are common cross-sensitizations to food in birch-allergic patients. A well-known example is with raw apple. This is commonly known as the oral allergy syndrome.

    3. In general, the period of pollination within a given locality is short, with the result that tree-sensitive patients often exhibit correspondingly brief periods of discomfort.

        Pollination occurs before, during, or shortly after leaves develop in deciduous trees. In more temperate climates, tree pollination concludes by late spring when the trees are fully leaved; in warmer areas this season may be extended (see Appendix VI.A).

IV. Fungi as aeroallergens

Fungi are often considered to belong to a kingdom of multicellular eukaryotes separate from the plant and animal kingdom.

Mold is a term frequently used interchangeably with fungus, but the term fungus is correct, whereas mold more properly refers to amorphous masses of fungi not necessarily of the same type. Despite their simplicity, fungi are among the most successful organisms on earth. They exist in large numbers in almost every environment—dry areas virtually devoid of water or other life, moist areas with wide temperature extremes, in soil, and in fresh water or salt water. All are either saprophytic (obtaining food from dead organic material) or parasitic (feeding on viable tissue).

Fungi are known to be a significant cause of allergic disease. Proteases in fungal extracts have been shown to interact with epithelial cells, leading to production of proinflammatory cytokines. Several important fungal allergens have been identified. Those most extensively studied include allergens from *Alternaria alternata* (*Alt a* 1, *Alt a* 2), *Cladosporium herbarum* (*Cla h* 1, *Cla h* 2, *Cla h* 3), *Aspergillus fumigatus* (*Asp f* 1) and *Penicillium*. Enolases, which are enzymes required for glycolysis and gluconeogenesis, have been obtained from *Cladosporium*, *Alternaria*, *Saccharomyces cerevisiae*, and *Candida albicans* and have been shown to be highly conserved fungal allergens. With technological advancements in molecular biology, much has been learned regarding fungal allergenicity, especially in regard to *Alternaria*. Using molecular biology techniques, *Alternaria* allergens have been cloned which can aid in the standardization of extracts.

A. **Structure of fungi.** Despite the enormous number of fungal species, only two basic structural forms exist: **Yeast forms** grow as single cells and reproduce by simple division or "budding" to form daughter cells; **hyphal forms** grow as a network of interconnecting tubes. Some hyphae are specialized to produce reproductive spores, which are dispersed by water, wind, insects, or other animals. Most fungi have hyphae.

B. **Classification of fungi.** The mode of sexual reproduction has been chosen as the basis for classification of fungi. During the life cycle of most fungal species, reproduction is accomplished by **fragmentation** of the hyphae, or by **production of spores**, or by both processes. Spores may be produced asexually (simple division of a cell) or sexually (fusion of two compatible cells to form a zygote followed by reduction-division). Most fungi reproduce both asexually (the **imperfect stage**) and sexually (the **perfect stage**). On the basis of the morphology of their sexual spores, fungi are grouped into three major classes: **Ascomycetes**, **Basidiomycetes**, and **Zygomycetes**. Formerly, a fourth large class was referred to as **Deuteromycetes**, or Fungi Imperfecti, because only asexual spores were identifiable. This class included most of the known allergenic fungi. Current classification places many fungi in one of the three main classes. *Alternaria*, *Penicillium*, and *Aspergillus* (important allergenic fungi) have been identified as asexual spores in the class Ascomycetes and are now placed in a subclass called *Hyphomycetes*. Subclassifications within this group are based on morphologic differences of spores (form classification); such classification may be expected not to reflect true botanical groupings and probably **does not reflect antigenic similarities** (Table 3.1).

C. **Distribution of fungi.** The enormous diversity of these organisms and their remarkable adaptations result in unavoidable human exposure regardless of geographic region. However, because a small amount of moisture and oxygen is a basic requirement for fungal growth, arid regions or areas of high altitude are relatively free of fungi by conventional sampling and culture methods. Fungal dormancy is also observed in subfreezing climates. In the northern parts of the United States, fungal spores typically appear as the snow cover disappears, increase as it warms, and peak in the late summer months. In the south, spores can appear year round with peak concentration in the summer or early fall. Beyond these generalities, **it is difficult to predict fungi prevalence by geographic locale**.

Table 3.1. Common molds and their relative clinical importance

ASCOMYCETES

Greater than 15,000 species; prevalent in wood pulp mills and on bark and deadwood; locally heavy clouds of spores are sometimes seen.

Alternaria: Perhaps the most common fungus identified in air samples, often exceeding pollen counts; saprophytes of leaves, plants, and other decaying organic material; high counts on hot, dry, windy days; indoor concentration reflects outdoor concentration usually by a factor of 25%; major problem for allergic patients, especially in the late summer months.

Aspergillus: Most common indoor fungus; substrate is spoiled food and other organic debris; very thermotolerant, especially where humidity is high; may colonize the respiratory tract and cause major hypersensitivity problems (allergic bronchopulmonary aspergillosis).

Penicillium: Indoor concentrations often exceed *Aspergillus* concentrations; natural substrate includes spoiled food, cheeses, and other organic debris; allergic sensitivity to *Penicillium* not predictive of penicillin sensitivity.

Cladosporium (includes *Hormodendrum*): Saprophyte on compost and decaying vegetables; counts often exceed counts of *Alternaria;* hot, dry, windy days; indoor concentration usually 25 percent of outdoor concentration; major problem in late summer months.

Helminthosporium: Prevalence level generally lower than that for *Alternaria* and *Cladosporium*, but skin reactivity is frequent; especially common in southern states; parasite of many plants.

Aureobasidium: Found in soil and on leaves, but also colonizes lumber and paper; widespread in distribution, but levels usually lower than those of the other prominent outdoor molds.

BASIDIOMYCETES

Greater than 12,000 species; colonize wild and cultivated plants. These are among the most prevalent fungi identified by most states in the American Academy of Allergy, Asthma and Immunology aeroallergen network. Positive skin prick tests to these allergens may be seen in 19% to 30% of individuals tested. Identification of a specific cause and effect relationship between these molds and clinical allergic situations has not yet been made.

Smuts: High concentrations on contaminated fields of grain; significant respiratory allergen, especially in rural atopic people.

Rusts: Lower concentrations than smuts around contaminated fields, but significant exposure for rural workers, especially in dry, windy situations.

Mushrooms: Prevalent in damp, forested areas, especially in wet weather; allergenic importance undetermined.

ZYGOMYCETES

Relatively few species ($N = 250$) are important allergens.

Rhizopus: Prominent in damp interiors; contaminant of bread and sugary foods; moderate allergic importance.

Mucor: Found in damp interiors; contaminant of bread and sugary foods; moderate allergic importance.

OOMYCETES

Greater than 250 species identified in air samples; include "downy mildews," which infect grasses and grape or onion crops; spores become airborne in dry, breezy weather; not a proven aeroallergen.

From Ausdenmoore RW, Lierl MB, Fischer TJ. Inhalant aerobiology and antigens. In: Weiss EB, Stein M, eds. *Bronchial asthma mechanisms and therapeutics*. 3rd ed. Boston: Little, Brown, 1993:552, with permission.

Fungi are found in **houses** and can be a source of perennial allergic symptoms. Spoiled food, soiled upholstery, and garbage containers are favorite substrates for home mold growth. Other common sites include damp basements, shower curtains, plumbing fixtures, and contaminated cool-mist vaporizers and console humidifiers.

D. Exposure patterns to fungi. Fungal sensitivity in allergic persons is commonly characterized by sporadic exacerbations that reflect local, concentrated exposures (e.g., visiting a farm, harvesting and storing hay, picking corn, cutting weeds or grass, raking leaves, or hiking in the woods) or periods of maximal fungal growth (e.g., during moist, warm summers and falls, especially with leaves on the ground) (Table 3.1). Many occupations predispose workers to a high risk of fungal exposure (e.g., grain farmers, fruit pickers, and paper mill workers). Heavy fungal growth on cut Christmas trees brought indoors can produce a distinctly seasonal pattern in fungal-sensitive patients. Combined with the irritant pine scent and dusty stored decorations, this fungal exposure can initiate allergic symptoms. For general measures toward improving fungal control, see Chapter 4.

E. Assessment of fungal exposure. Empiric fungal-control methods are mandatory for allergic patients to prevent reactions and/or sensitization. In selected situations, identification and semiquantitative determinations of mold exposures are helpful. These situations include: (i) patients with hypersensitivity disease requiring fungal identification for more accurate diagnosis and treatment (e.g., hypersensitivity pneumonitis), (ii) monitoring the success of fungal eradication measures, and (iii) determining fungal types in locales where prevalence data are unavailable.

Measurement of airborne fungus is accomplished by microscopic identification of samples obtained by volumetric collectors or by cultured mold plates. General-purpose mold plates can be made with Sabouraud glucose, potato dextrose, corn meal, or V-8 agars. Certain conditions of temperature, humidity, and barometric pressure also can favor growth of molds that are not clinically relevant. Fungal identification requires time, equipment, and mycologic expertise. References are available (see Selected Readings); fungal-identification services are also available through manufacturers of allergen extracts (Appendix XII). Table 3.1 lists important allergenic fungi and their common sources. Individual fungus prevalence by region in the United States can be found in Appendix VI.

V. Animal allergens

Inhaled dander (epithelial scales) from animal species (other than human) can sensitize an allergic person. Any foreign animal dander could conceivably be responsible for sensitization, but the most common epidermal allergens come from dogs, cats, and hair or feathers (cattle, horse, sheep, goat, duck) used for stuffing materials. Because the soluble dander, rather than the hair, produces allergic reactions, finished material without dander is less allergenic (e.g., furs used as clothing). Many of the allergens found in the dander are also found in urine and saliva. Studies have characterized the more common allergens. Examples include cat (*Fel d* 1), dog (*Can f* 1, *Can f* 2), and horse (*Equ c* 1, *Equ c* 2).

Sensitivity is often exquisite, especially with cat dander, requiring only a brief or unexpected exposure to create a marked allergic response. The major allergens in cat dander are present on particles that are very small (some less than 2.5 µm); therefore, they have a low falling rate that causes them to remain airborne for long periods of time even without air disturbance. Clinically, this probably accounts for the sudden onset of symptoms that characterizes encounters with cats or homes with cats. Dander concentrations may be cumulative within a home or other enclosed space; dispersal throughout the home is easily accomplished by the heating system. Vacuuming and pet cleansing are only mildly effective, temporary methods of control. Because the allergen is in the soluble dander, **short-haired breeds or nonshedding dogs** also cause allergy.

Occupational exposure to laboratory animals can be an important cause of difficulty for allergic individuals and can preclude their ability to function in this occupation. It is also possible that large exposures to rodent dander and urine in tenements and other poorly kept dwellings can account for a significant amount of allergic difficulty. Recent studies have shown that mouse allergen is widely distributed in inner-city homes and may be an important indoor allergen, especially for children with asthma.

VI. House dust mite

Dust from mattress stuffings is an important source of indoor allergens. In 1967, European investigators identified the house dust mite (*Dermatophagoides pteronyssinus*) as a highly allergenic fraction of mattress dust. *Dermatophagoides farinae*, a different species, is the most widespread mite in mattress stuffing samples in North America. House dust mites subsist on human epithelial scales, reaching a seasonal peak concentration in September and October. Secondary reservoirs include overstuffed furniture, rugs, and pillows.

Mite allergenicity does not depend on viability of the mite. Specific mite allergens have been characterized and isolated (*Der p* 1 and *Der p* 2 from *D. pteronyssinus*; *Der f* 1 and *Der f* 2 from *D. farinae*). *Der p* 1 is considered the most immunodominant house dust mite allergen. It has been shown to have cysteine protease activity, which plays a major role in its allergenicity. The proteolytic activity facilitates transepithelial allergen delivery by disruption of tight junctions, and also cleaves clusters of differentiation (CD)23 and CD25, which induces immunoglobulin E (IgE) synthesis.

The highest concentrations of mite allergens are found in mite feces; however, some studies have shown that mite allergens can also be carried on a variety of other particles. Therefore, preventive measures include not only destruction of the mite, but also physical removal of the mite, or placing a barrier between mite antigen and the susceptible person, or both. Studies have shown that effective mite elimination can be of clinical significance.

Because of the larger size, the falling rate of mite allergen particles is more rapid than that of cat dander, so exposures to mite particles result in more subtle reactions over a greater period of time. Brief periods of intense mite exposure can occur during vacuuming or other activities that disturb rugs, bedding, or upholstery.

VII. Cockroaches and other insects

Allergic persons can show sensitivity by skin testing to a wide variety of insects, suggesting that inhalation of insect parts can play a role in symptom production. The cockroach, in particular, is known to be an important allergen, especially for allergic individuals living in crowded and poorly kept dwellings, or working in warehouses or other storage facilities. *Periplaneta americana* and *Blattella germanica* are two species of cockroaches important in atopic diseases. Allergens for both species have been isolated and characterized: *Per a* 1 and *Bla g* 1. Studies have shown cross-reactivity between these species.

Inhalation of insect parts, especially in endemic areas, is suspected as a cause of respiratory disease in atopic individuals. Epidemics of asthma from the caddis fly, moth, mayfly, butterfly, and midge are documented. Absolute proof of this association is lacking because of the inability to identify insect parts microscopically. Current interest in studying the role of insects in allergic disease is increasing with the ability to use immunologic assays on air samples.

Environmental Factors

I. Climatic factors

It is difficult to isolate and separately study the complex interaction of temperature, humidity, and barometric pressure in producing or exacerbating allergic symptoms. It appears that allergic disease, especially asthma, tends to be adversely affected by **high humidity**, by **sudden temperature changes** (particularly from warm to cold), and by **drops in the barometric pressure**. Intolerance to these factors is highly individual. Dry, cold air commonly precipitates exertional dyspnea.

II. Outdoor air pollution

A. **Industrial smog** results from the combustion of liquid or solid fossil fuels and is usually measured by the levels of carbon monoxide, particulate matter, and sulfur dioxide.

1. **Carbon monoxide** has been linked to certain health problems, including decreased exercise tolerance in ischemic heart disease and atherosclerotic arterial disease in smokers. However, even at peak levels measured in urban rush-hour traffic (120 ppm), it cannot be shown to affect respiratory function adversely in normal persons or asthmatic patients.

2. **Particulate matter** is made up of several components including silica, metal ions, organic residues, and endotoxins. The inhalable particulate matter is made up of particles less than 10 mm in diameter (PM 10) or of particles less than 2.5 mm in diameter (PM 2.5). Inhalable particulate matter can cause coughing and reflex bronchoconstriction and can lead to direct stimulation of small-airway receptors causing bronchiolar constriction. It is also known to potentiate the effect of other pollutants and may act as carriers for other well-described allergens. Particulate matter has also been associated with increased risk of death from all causes, especially in individuals with cardiovascular and respiratory illnesses.

3. **Sulfur dioxide** does not have a large inflammatory effect at levels found in the atmosphere. However, in very high experimental concentrations it causes increased airway resistance and suppression of mucosal ciliary activities in humans and other animals. At higher concentrations (from 0.25 to 0.50 ppm) it has been shown to have potent bronchoconstrictive effects especially noted in those patients with underlying asthma. These effects are typically easily reversed with beta-adrenergic agonists and do not cause delayed effects.

B. **Photochemical smog.** Photochemical smog is produced by ultraviolet radiation on hydrocarbons (emitted by automobile exhaust) with the formation of **ozone**, **nitric oxide**, and other **oxidants**. Average urban levels of oxidants may be in the range of 0.2 to 0.5 ppm, with a peak at 1 ppm. Low levels (0.25 ppm) can cause eye irritation and coughing. High concentrations have been associated with diminished vital capacity, forced expiratory volume, and diffusion capacity (even in normal persons). Most of the oxidants measured are ozone (greater than 90%), but nitrogen dioxide is often present in significant concentrations. Nitrogen dioxide, in addition to its direct toxic effect on the lung, may produce irreversible pulmonary changes in smokers. Ozone has been fairly extensively studied, especially in regard to its effect on asthma. Ozone has been found to cause a relatively rapid decrease in forced vital capacity and forced expiratory volume in 1 second. It has also been shown to cause a neutrophil inflammatory response. Some studies have also shown that ozone can potentiate bronchial responsiveness to allergens.

III. Indoor air pollution

Closed ventilation in modern office buildings and homes may increase exposure to common indoor inhalants that are no longer infinitely diluted by outside air. Passively inhaled tobacco smoke, in particular, is being linked to more respiratory difficulty than previously suspected in co-workers, family members (particularly infants and toddlers), and even house guests. Environmental tobacco smoke has been associated with several increased health risks, including otitis media, upper and lower respiratory tract infections, and wheezing. Environmental tobacco smoke may also help to potentiate atopy through a variety of mechanisms. One possibility includes its effect on increasing the airway mucosal permeability. Another possibility is a direct effect on immune function, including an alteration in monocyte function and a suppression of functions mediated through gamma-interferon, such as phagocytosis of opsonized antigens.

Aerosols and smoke fumes from kerosene heaters, coal stoves, gas stoves (and pilot lights), fireplaces, and space heaters, plus noxious odors from solvents (e.g., formaldehyde in glues for carpeting and paneling), may all reach higher levels in closed structures. In homes where natural gas is used, another important agent to consider is nitrogen dioxide. Increased levels of nitrogen dioxide have been associated with increased respiratory symptoms. To some extent, this may be due to its role in ozone production.

Many new homes have been constructed in an attempt to conserve energy. Such homes may develop increased relative humidity levels (dampness) because of poor ventilation, the so-called "tight-home." Increased rates of respiratory symptoms, including wheezing, have been reported in these dwellings. High concentrations of house dust mite allergens may partly explain this occurrence, but other mechanisms, including fungal sensitivity, require further study.

IV. Viruses and bacteria

No proof can be given to support the views of some that true allergic reactions exist toward infectious antigens. It is well known, however, that such infectious agents may frequently trigger and/or complicate allergic reactions (e.g., sinusitis preceding or complicating asthma).

Conclusion

Allergic diseases may affect multiple target organs, including nasal mucosa, skin, and the airways, which can lead to significant morbidity. A key feature in the pathogenesis of allergies is inflammation triggered by allergen exposure. With this in mind, the traditional mainstay of treatment has been allergen avoidance. For us to understand the pathogenesis and decrease the morbidity associated with allergic diseases, it is essential that we become familiar with the aeroallergens and environmental factors that can initiate the inflammatory process.

Selected Readings

Aden E, Weber B, Bossert J. Standardization of Alternaria alternata: extraction and quantification of Alt a 1 by using an mAb-based 2-site binding assay. *J Allergy Clin Immunol* 1999;103:128–135.

Bascom R, Bromberg P, Costa D, et al. Health effects of outdoor air pollution part I. *Am J Respir Crit Care Med* 1996;153:3–50.

Breitenbach M, Simon B, Probst G, et al. Enolases are highly conserved fungal allergens. *Int Arch Allergy Immunol* 1997;113:114–117.

Bush RK. The role of fungal allergens. In: Bush RK, Lenfant C, eds. *Environmental asthma: lung biology in health and disease*, New York: Marcel Dekker, 2001;153:69–90.

Bush RK, Sanchez H, Geisler D. Molecular cloning of a major Alternaria alternata allergen, rAlt a 2. *J Allergy Clin Immunol* 1999;104:665–671.

De Lucca S, Sporik R, O'Meara T, et al. Mite allergen (Der p 1) is not only carried on mite feces. *J Allergy Clin Immunol* 1999;103:174–175

Deviller P, Pauli G. Crossreactions involving plant allergens. *Clin Rev Allergy Immunol* 1997;15:405–413.

Frenz DA. Volumetric ragweed pollen data for eight cities in the continental United States. *Ann Allergy Asthma Immunol* 1999;82:41–46.

Frenz DA, Palmer MA, Hokanson JM, et al. Seasonal characteristics of ragweed pollen dispersal in the United States. *Ann Allergy Asthma Immunol* 1995;75:417–422.

Friedmann P, Tan B. Mite elimination—clinical effect on eczema. *Allergy* 1998;53:97–100.

Gough L, Schulz O, Sewell H, et al. The cysteine protease activity of the major dust mite allergen Der p 1 selectively enhances the immunoglobulin E antibody response. *J Exp Med* 1999;190:1897–1901.

Gregoire C, Rosinski-Chupin I, Rabillon J, et al. cDNA cloning and sequencing reveal the major horse allergen Equ c 1 to be a glycoprotein member of the lipocalin superfamily. *J Biol Chem* 1996;271:32957–32959.

Helm R, Cockrell G, Stanley S, et al. Isolation and characterization of a clone encoding a major allergen (Bla g Bd90K) involved in IgE-mediated cockroach hypersensitivity. *J Allergy Clin Immunol* 1996;98:172–180.

Ipsen H, Lowenstein H. Basic features of crossreactivity in tree and grass pollen allergy, *Clin Rev Allergy Immunol* 1997;15:389–396.

Jorres R, Nowak D, Magnussen H. The effect of ozone exposure on allergen responsiveness in subjects with asthma or rhinitis. *Am J Respir Crit Care Med* 1996; 153:56–64.

Kauffman H, Tomee J, Van de Riet M, et al. Protease-dependent activation of epithelial cells by fungal allergens leads to morphologic changes and cytokine production. *J Allergy Clin Immunol* 2000;105:1185–1193.

Kehrl H, Peden D, Ball B, et al. Increased specific airway reactivity of persons with mild allergic asthma after 7.6 hours of exposure to 0.16 ppm ozone. *J Allergy Clin Immunol* 1999;104:1198–1204.

Konieczny A, Morgenstern J, Bizinkauskas B, et al. The major dog allergens, Can f 1 and Can f 2, are salivary lipocalin proteins: cloning and immunological characterization of the recombinant forms. *Immunology* 1997;92:577–586.

Melen E, Pomes A, Vailes L, et al. Molecular cloning of Per a 1 and definition of the cross-reactive group 1 cockroach allergens. *J Allergy Clin Immunol* 1999;103:859–864.

Nightingale J, Rogers D, Barnes P. Effect of inhaled ozone on exhaled nitric oxide, pulmonary function, and induced sputum in normal and asthmatic subjects. *Thorax* 1999;54:1061–1069.

Ormstad H, Johansen B, Gaarder P. Airborne house dust particles and diesel exhaust particles as allergen carriers. *Clin Exp Allergy* 1998;28:702–708.

Phipatanakul W, Eggleston P, Wright E, et al. Mouse allergen. I. The prevalence of mouse allergen in inner-city homes. *J Allergy Clin Immunol* 2000;106:1070–1074.

Phipatanakul W, Eggleston P, Wright E, et al. Mouse allergen. II. The relationship of mouse allergen exposure to mouse sensitization and asthma morbidity in inner-city children with asthma. *J Allergy Clin Immunol* 2000;106:1075–1080.

Platts-Mills TAE, Solomon WR. Aerobiology and inhalant allergens. In: Middleton E Jr, et al., eds. *Allergy: principles and practice*, 5th ed. St. Louis: Mosby, 1998:367–403.

Samet JM, Marbury MC, Spengler JD. Health effects and sources of indoor air pollution, part I. *Am Rev Resp Dis* 1987;136:1486–1508.

Samet J, Dominici F, Curriero F, et al. Fine particulate air pollution and mortality in 20 US cities, 1987–1994. *N Engl J Med* 2000;343:1742–1749.

Schulz O, Sewell H, Shakib F. Proteolytic cleavage of CD25, the alpha subunit of the human T cell interleukin 2 receptor, by Der p 1, a major mite allergen with cysteine protease activity. *J Exp Med* 1998;187:271–275.

Shakib F, Schulz O, Sewell H. A mite subversive: cleavage of CD23 and CD25 by Der p 1 enhances allergenicity. *Immunol Today* 1998;19:313–316.

Smith EG. *Sampling and identifying allergenic pollens and molds. An illustrated manual for physicians and lab technicians*. San Antonio, TX: Blewstone Press, 1984.

Spitzauer S. Allergy to mammalian proteins: At the borderline between foreign and self? *Int Arch Allergy Immunol* 1999;120:259–269.

Tan B, Weald D, Strickland I, et al. Double-blind controlled trial of effect of house dust mite allergen avoidance on atopic dermatitis. *Lancet* 1996;347:15–18.

Van Ree R, Van Leeuwen WA, Aalberse RC. How far can we simplify in vitro diagnostics for grass pollen allergy?: a study with 17 whole pollen extracts and purified natural and recombinant major allergens. *J Allergy Clin Immunol* 1998;102:184–190.

Wan H, Winton H, Soeller C, et al. Der p 1 facilitates transepithelial allergen delivery by disruption of tight junctions. *J Clin Invest* 1999;104:123–133.

Wu C, Wang N, Lee M, et al. Cloning of the American cockroach Cr-PII allergens: evidence for the existence of cross-reactive allergens between species. *J Allergy Clin Immunol* 1998;101:832–840.

4. RHINITIS, NASAL POLYPS, SINUSITIS, AND OTITIS MEDIA

Mark S. Dykewicz and Jonathan Corren

Chronic rhinitis is extremely common, with upwards of 25% of the population report-ing persistent nasal symptoms at some time in their life. Chronic rhinitis, which may be allergic or nonallergic, is frequently associated with other upper airway dis-orders, including nasal polyposis, sinusitis, and otitis media. In total, these diseases have significant physical, social, and economic impact, necessitating effective treatment for prolonged periods of time.

Allergic Rhinitis
I. Pathophysiology
In genetically susceptible individuals, exposure to airborne allergens results in sensitization with the production of specific IgE. Upon subsequent exposures, al-lergen binds to immunoglobulin E (IgE), which is fixed to tissue mast cells, and mast cell degranulation results. Within minutes of binding, preformed mediators (e.g., histamine) are released, followed shortly thereafter by newly synthesized, lipid-derived mediators (e.g., leukotrienes C4, D4, and E4, and prostaglandin D2). These mediators cause acute mucosal edema, mucus secretion, vascular leak, and stimulation of sensory neurons. Chemotactic factors (e.g., eotaxin, interleukin-5 [IL-5]) are also released, resulting in the influx of inflammatory cells, particularly eosinophils, over several hours.

II. Diagnosis
Appropriate therapy for allergic rhinitis requires differentiation of this syn-drome from other forms of chronic rhinitis. A thorough history and physical ex-amination are frequently all that is required to make an initial diagnosis and begin therapy.

A. History
1. **Primary symptoms.** Allergic rhinitis typically presents with symp-toms of intermittent nasal congestion, clear rhinorrhea, sneezing, and itching of the nose, palate, and/or ears. A significant number of patients also report tearing, redness, and itching of the eyes, usually when nasal symptoms are most active. Nasal and ocular pruritus are among the most helpful symptoms in differentiating allergic from other forms of chronic rhinitis.

2. **Secondary symptoms.** In many patients, mucous membranes of the eustachian tubes, middle ears, and sinuses may become involved, causing ear fullness or popping, muffled hearing, facial pressure, and headache. Significant postnasal drainage may result in sore throat and chronic cough. A number of central nervous system (CNS) complaints may also occur, including malaise, fatigue, irritability, anxiety, and depression, which are most common at the height of the pollen season and improve after pollen exposure ends. Recent research also suggests that allergic rhinitis is associated with decreased school performance in children, which may either be improved (by nasal steroids or nonsedating antihistamines) or worsened (by sedating antihistamines) with concomitant therapy.

3. **Differentiating seasonal and perennial allergic rhinitis.** In sea-sonal allergic rhinitis (also referred to as pollinosis or hay fever), this constellation of symptoms occurs during predictable, defined seasons, depending on which allergens the patient has become sensitized to. This temporal pattern is a key feature in distinguishing seasonal allergic from other forms of rhinitis. In general, trees pollinate in the spring (February through April), grasses in the late spring and early summer (May and June), and weeds in the late summer and fall (August through October). In perennial allergic rhinitis, however, aeroallergens are present in the

environment throughout the year (e.g., house dust mites and animal proteins), causing symptoms to vary little between seasons, and making differentiation from other types of rhinitis more difficult. In addition, patients who have perennial allergic rhinitis (particularly due to dust mites) tend to be more affected by persistent nasal congestion and rhinorrhea, and less by ocular symptoms, making it difficult to discriminate allergic from nonallergic causes.

B. Physical examination

  1. Inspection of the face often reveals periorbital darkening, or "allergic shiners," due to the chronic venous pooling. However, this particular finding may also be seen in nonallergic rhinitis. Children frequently rub their noses upward in response to itching ("allergic salute"), which may produce a persistent horizontal crease across the nose. The conjunctivae commonly appear mildly injected, with either watery or gelatinous exudate present. Ocular findings are helpful in differentiating allergy from other causes of rhinitis. **Anterior rhinoscopy** with a hand-held otoscope or headlamp with nasal speculum allows visualization of the anterior one-third of the nasal airway. Patients with allergic rhinitis typically have pale, swollen inferior and middle turbinates, and clear discharge. When severe mucosal edema is present, it may be helpful to spray the nose with a topical decongestant, such as oxymetazoline (Afrin), in order to visualize structures located more posteriorly. Better visualization of the nasal cavity may allow the examiner to detect a variety of obstructive abnormalities, including posterior deviation of the septum, septal spurs, and nasal polyps.

C. Laboratory testing

  1. Assessments of allergen-specific immunoglobulin E

   a. Principal indications for allergy skin testing or *in vitro* measures of specific IgE (e.g., radioallergosorbent testing [RAST]) are the determination of allergic sensitivities prior to the institution of allergen avoidance measures or allergy immunotherapy. All patients with perennial allergic rhinitis should undergo a basic screen for perennial allergens, including dust mites, relevant animal danders, cockroaches, and select molds. However, assays for specific IgE are not necessary in patients who respond well to and tolerate simple empiric medical therapy for seasonal allergic rhinitis of limited duration. It is important that skin or *in vitro* testing be done in the context of the patient's geographic location and specific home environment, in order to include all relevant allergens.

     (1) Immediate skin testing is the preferred method of investigation, because of greater sensitivity, broader variety of available antigens, and lower cost compared with *in vitro* testing. In most situations, prick or puncture tests are sufficient to assess specific sensitivities in allergic rhinitis, and intradermal testing should be reserved for special circumstances (e.g., highly suggestive history with negative skin prick tests).

     (2) *In vitro* allergy testing should be employed in patients who suffer from widespread dermatitis or dermatographism, who have poorly reactive skin (as seen in some infants and elderly patients), or who cannot withhold antihistamines, tricyclic antidepressants, or phenothiazines that inhibit skin testing. In addition, *in vitro* allergy testing may be a practical first step when assessing a small number of allergens in the home environment prior to starting allergen avoidance measures. Results often vary greatly among laboratories performing these assays, making interpretation difficult.

   b. Other tests. Peripheral white blood counts with differentials and absolute blood eosinophil counts may demonstrate an increased number of circulating blood eosinophils. However, allergic rhinitis may occur in the absence of peripheral eosinophilia and nonallergic forms of rhinitis may be associated with significant blood eosinophilia (e.g., NARES, see D.1.b. below). Therefore, it is not recommended that blood eosinophils be used to screen for allergic rhinitis. Similarly, total serum IgE concentrations are frequently normal in patients with allergic rhinitis and therefore should not be used to screen for nasal allergy.

2. **Cytologic examination** of nasal scrapings can be helpful if the diagnosis has not been made from other information. Significant eosinophilia in nasal secretions (greater than 5 eosinophils per high-power field) is an excellent clue to the presence of allergy. Although the detection of nasal eosinophilia is suggestive of allergic rhinitis, it is not diagnostic, because eosinophils are also found in nonallergic rhinitis with eosinophilia (NARES). Large numbers of neutrophils, without eosinophils, would alert the clinician to the possibility of a viral upper respiratory infection or bacterial sinusitis (see Appendix III).

D. **Differential diagnosis**

The symptoms and signs of allergic rhinitis frequently overlap with those of other forms of rhinitis and various anatomic abnormalities of the upper airway (Table 4.1).

1. **Nonallergic rhinitis syndromes**

   a. **Nonallergic rhinitis without eosinophilia** is characterized by perennial nasal symptoms of rhinorrhea and/or congestion that are unrelated to allergen exposure. Nasal symptoms are often provoked by sudden changes in the environment, airborne irritants or dietary factors (see page 66).

   b. **Nonallergic rhinitis with eosinophilia syndrome.** NARES is characterized by perennial nasal symptoms (particularly nasal congestion) with nasal and occasionally blood eosinophilia in the absence of documentable allergen sensitivity (see page 66).

   c. **Hormonal rhinitis** is most often characterized by nasal congestion and is usually secondary to thyroid disease (hyperthyroid or hypothyroid), pregnancy, or oral contraceptive use.

   d. **Drug-induced rhinitis** usually presents with symptoms of chronic nasal congestion and occurs following the use of both oral and topical medications. Responsible oral medications include many antihypertensive drugs (most common of which are beta-blockers and methyldopa), and nonsteroidal antiinflammatories. Use of topical vasoconstrictors (e.g., oxymetazoline, phenylephrine) for longer than 3 days may result in a state of rebound nasal congestion termed rhinitis medicamentosa. Repeated use of intranasal cocaine and methamphetamines may also cause rebound congestion and occasionally septal erosion and perforation.

Table 4.1. Differential diagnosis of allergic rhinitis

	AR	NAR	CS	NP
Prominent congestion	+/−	+/−	+/−	+
Prominent itch	+	−	−	−
Prominent sneezing	+	−	−	−
Ocular symptoms	+/−	−	−	−
Color of nasal turbinates	Pale	Pale/red	Red	Pale
Color of secretions	Clear	Clear	Purulent	Clear
Nasal cytology	Eos	−/Eos*	−	Eos

AR, allergic rhinitis; NAR, nonallergic rhinitis; CS, chronic sinusitis; NP, nasal polyps; Eos, eosinophils.

* Eosinophils usually are present only in a subset of patients, i.e. non-allergic rhinitis with eosinophils syndrome.

  e. Food-related rhinitis may occur because of vagally mediated mechanisms (gustatory rhinitis) or IgE mediated reactions.
2. **Infectious rhinosinusitis**
  a. Acute viral upper respiratory infection presents with symptoms of rhinorrhea, congestion, sneezing, and constitutional symptoms (fever, myalgias, malaise). Usually, pruritis is notably absent and symptoms resolve within 7 to 10 days.
  b. **Bacterial sinusitis.** Acute bacterial sinusitis most often presents with symptoms of purulent anterior rhinorrhea or postnasal drip, facial pain or pressure, and persistence or worsening of nasal congestion. Chronic bacterial sinusitis usually presents with chronic (longer than 8 weeks) symptoms of nasal congestion, purulent postnasal drip, facial pressure, and cough (see sinusitis III.B.1. on page 67). However, no single symptom or sign is reliable for distinguishing rhinitis from sinusitis
3. **Anatomic abnormalities** usually present with obstructive symptoms without other symptoms of rhinitis, such as sneezing, rhinorrhea, or itching.
  a. **Septal deviation** can be visualized with an otoscope. It is most often asymptomatic; severe deviation may cause symptoms of unilateral congestion.
  b. **Adenoidal hypertrophy** is typically seen in young children, causes bilateral nasal obstruction, and is often associated with nocturnal mouth-breathing and snoring. Diagnosis requires a mirror examination of the nasopharynx, flexible anterior rhinopharyngoscopy, or computed tomography (CT) scanning of the nasal airway.
  c. **Nasal polyps** are benign, inflammatory growths that may result in unilateral or bilateral nasal obstruction and rhinorrhea (see Nasal Polyps on page 65).
  d. **Nasal carcinoma** should be suspected in elderly patients who complain of unilateral epistaxis and nasal pain.
  e. **Intranasal foreign bodies**, often consisting of a small plastic toy part, usually occur in young children. Foreign bodies usually cause unilateral nasal obstruction with or without rhinorrhea, and may eventuate in acute sinusitis.
4. **Systemic diseases involving the upper airway**
  a. **Wegener granulomatosis** is a systemic necrotizing vasculitis that often presents with nasal and sinus complaints (see Chapter 7). These symptoms frequently include purulent rhinorrhea and occasionally septal erosions and perforations.
  b. **Sjögren syndrome** is an autoimmune disease that destroys exocrine glands and impairs mucous gland function. Occasionally, the nose may be prominently involved, with symptoms of congestion, dryness, and crusting.
  c. **Sarcoidosis**, a disease characterized by systemic granuloma formation, may present with nasal granulomata and congestion (see Chapter 7).
III. **Treatment**
  A. **Allergen avoidance measures**
   Avoidance of aeroallergens is an effective, nonpharmacologic method for treating allergic rhinitis. These measures will ultimately limit long-term expense and potential adverse effects of medications. Because environmental control measures may be inconvenient and expensive to implement, allergy testing should be performed first to confirm suspected allergic sensitivities (Table 4.2).
   1. **Outdoor aeroallergens.** For patients who have strictly seasonal rhinitis caused by exposure to plant pollens or seasonal molds, avoidance of outdoor activity during peak pollen hours (late morning to early afternoon) may be helpful. For patients who are allergic to grass pollen, wear-

Table 4.2. Recommended allergen avoidance measures

Dust mites
    Allergen-impermeable encasings on bed and all pillows
    Wash bedding in hot water (>130° F)
    Remove carpet or consider spraying with tannic acid solution
    Frequent vacuum cleaning of carpet (HEPA-type)
Animals
    Remove animal from home, followed by removal of carpet and thorough house
        cleaning
    All other measures have unproven efficacy
Indoor mold
    Identify, remove, and replace mildewed wood and plaster
    Correct sources of water intrusion (plumbing, roof, windows)
    Reduce indoor humidity (dehumidifiers)
Pollen
    Avoid outdoor activity during peak pollen hours (11 a.m. to 3 p.m.)
    Keep windows shut and use air conditioner

---

ing a surgical-type mask while mowing the lawn or gardening may help
avert symptoms. Keeping the windows closed throughout the day is important, and the use of an air conditioner prevents airborne pollen from
entering the home. If windows are kept open during the day, high-
efficiency particulate air (HEPA) filters placed in the home also reduce
indoor pollen counts.

2. **Indoor aeroallergens**
    a. **Dust mites.** For patients who have perennial symptoms, the most
        common source of allergen sensitization is the house dust mite. Large
        reservoirs of these microscopic insects are usually found in bedding,
        mattresses, and carpeting. Down-filled comforters and wool blankets
        should be eliminated. Washing of all sheets, mattress pads, pillow-
        cases, and blankets every week in hot (greater than 130°F) water ef-
        fectively kills these organisms. Both down-filled pillows and polyester
        fiberfill pillows serve as reservoirs for house dust mites. The most im-
        portant intervention is to use specially constructed pillow, mattress,
        and box spring covers made of fabrics or plastic that act as a barrier
        between the interior of these furnishings and the patient. Carpeting
        can be treated with a commercially prepared tannic acid spray, which
        denatures allergenic mite proteins, but mites reaccumulate rapidly
        and frequent re-treatment is required. Available acaricides that kill
        house dust mites, such as benzoic acid, have been demonstrated to
        provide only minimal benefit to mite-allergic patients.
        If these measures do not result in satisfactory improvement, pa-
        tients can consider removing the carpeting from the bedroom, pro-
        viding there are hardwood or linoleum floors underneath. Vacuuming
        with conventional vacuum cleaners does not significantly reduce mite
        numbers in carpeting, and often increases the number of airborne
        mite allergen for short periods of time. Vacuum cleaners with at-
        tached HEPA filters are therefore preferable.
    b. **Pets.** Domestic pets are an important source of allergen exposure in
        many atopic patients. The first and most important step in allergen
        avoidance is removal of the animal from the home environment. Once
        the animal has been placed outside of the house, it is then best to re-
        move all carpeting and thoroughly clean the walls. Because patients
        are often reluctant to take this step, other, less drastic methods of
        environmental control have been tried but are of unproven efficacy.
        The animal should be kept out of the bedroom at all times, and cen-
        tral air vents to the bedroom should be kept closed. Following re-

moval of the pet from the bedroom, consideration should be given to removing upholstered furniture and carpeting and replacing it with plastic or leather. A HEPA filter reduces the quantity of airborne animal allergens. Washing the pet is of questionable value. The patient should be informed that it might take several weeks to even months for indoor levels of animal dander to return to low levels.

c. **Indoor fungi**, such as *Aspergillus* and *Penicillium* species, are usually found in homes that have experienced water damage. However, in some regions of the country, molds such as *Alternaria* have been found to be perennial indoor allergens even in homes without water damage. Leaky roofs and ceilings, flooded basements, damaged plumbing, and wet crawl spaces are common sites of mold growth within homes. The only effective way to reduce indoor levels of fungal spores is to repair water-damaged areas. For damp spaces where mold growth is a potential problem, a high-intensity heat lamp can be turned on for 1 to 2 hours. Although most indoor plants do not elevate household levels of mold spores, wicker basket planters should be avoided.

d. **Cockroaches can be a major allergen**, particularly in inner city and rural areas. Professional extermination may be required.

B. Medications

A large number of therapeutic options exist, and each has different effects on symptoms of rhinitis (Table 4.3).

1. H1-antihistamines

a. **General.** H1-antihistamines are frequently used as first-line therapy for patients who have allergic rhinitis (Table 4.4). These medications effectively reduce rhinorrhea, sneezing, and nasal and ocular pruritus, but have little effect on nasal congestion. Antihistamines are effective when taken on an as-needed basis, although they work best when administered before the onset of symptoms.

b. **Antihistamine classification.** Older, first-generation antihistamines (e.g., chlorpheniramine, diphenhydramine), are generally available over the counter and have been associated with significant adverse events (see c. below). Newer, second-generation antihistamines (e.g., azelastine, cetirizine, fexofenadine, loratadine) bind more specifically to the H1-histamine receptor and generally cause fewer side effects than first-generation agents. Because fexofenadine is a metabolite of terfenadine, it technically represents a third-generation antihistamine, but this distinction is not clinically important. Although cetirizine, fexofenadine, and loratadine are all administered as oral drugs, azelastine is the only available topical antihistamine in the United States.

c. **Adverse effects.** First-generation antihistamines have several possible **CNS side effects**, the most common of which are somnolence and fatigue. Other subjective CNS effects include irritability,

Table 4.3. Effects of medications on nasal and ocular symptoms

	AH	D	INS	INC	INIB	IAH	LTRA
Congestion	−	+	+	−	−	+	+
Sneezing	+	−	+	+	−	+	+
Discharge	+	+	+	+	+	+	+
Itching	+	−	+	+	−	+	+
Ocular symptoms	+	−	+	−	−	−	+

AH, oral antihistamine; D, decongestant; INS, intranasal steroid; INC, intranasal cromolyn; INIB, intranasal ipratropium bromide; IAH, intranasal antihistamine; LTRA, leukotriene receptor antagonist.

Table 4.4. Antihistamines commonly used for allergic rhinitis

	Dose/interval	Sedating	Anticholinergic
First generation			
Chlorpheniramine	4–8 mg q.d.	+	+
Diphenhydramine	12.5–50 mg q.i.d.	+	+
Clemastine	1.25 mg b.i.d.	+	+
Second generation			
Azelastine	2 sprays b.i.d. intranasally	+	±
Cetirizine	10 mg q.d.	+	−
Fexofenadine	30–60 mg b.i.d./180 mg q.d.	−	−
Loratadine	10 mg q.d.	−	−

anxiety, and depression. Although 30% to 50% of patients report that they experience sedation, most patients without subjective complaints still demonstrate objective evidence of mental impairment. These effects may manifest as reductions in divided attention ("multitasking") and slowing of reaction time. These effects are of practical importance, because they may result in increased accidents at home, at the workplace, or while the patient is driving. Clinical studies have also demonstrated that children learn less effectively at school while taking these drugs. In addition to CNS effects, first-generation antihistamines have significant **anticholinergic effects**, including dryness of the mouth and eyes, blurred vision, constipation, urinary retention, and precipitation of glaucoma.

Neither fexofenadine nor loratadine causes CNS or anticholinergic effects at prescribed doses. Although cetirizine and is devoid of anticholinergic effects and azelastine has only negligible effects, they may both result in sedation. Although they are not as sedating as first-generation agents, physicians should be aware of this potential side effect with both of these agents.

2. **Decongestants.** Alpha-adrenergic agonists are potent vasoconstrictors that are available in both topical and systemic forms. These medications significantly reduce nasal swelling and rhinorrhea, but do not affect other symptoms of allergic rhinitis.

a. **Topical decongestants** include oxymetazoline and phenylephrine nasal sprays. In patients who have severe nasal congestion, these medications enhance the penetration of other topical drugs, such as intranasal corticosteroids. Systemic side effects are not usually observed with these intranasal agents. Use should be limited to 3 to 5 days to avoid rebound nasal congestion and rhinitis medicamentosa.

b. **Oral decongestants,** such as pseudoephedrine and phenylephrine, are also effective in relieving nasal blockage, and do not cause rebound nasal swelling after prolonged periods of use. They are most often combined with antihistamines for treatment of allergic rhinitis and are superior in clinical efficacy to either drug used alone. Oral decongestants frequently cause CNS stimulation, including nervousness and insomnia. For this reason, they should be avoided during the evening hours in susceptible patients. They may also cause significant cardiac stimulation, and should be avoided in patients with unstable hypertension, and used only with caution in patients with cardiac arrhythmias or ischemic heart disease. Finally, this class of drugs may also cause urinary retention, and should be avoided in patients with any form of bladder outlet obstruction.

3. **Intranasal corticosteroids**

a. **General.** Corticosteroid nasal sprays are an extremely effective form of therapy for allergic rhinitis. When used on a regular basis before allergen exposure, these medications reduce mast cell mediator release (e.g., histamine, prostaglandin D2) and retard eosinophil influx into nasal tissue. They have been approved for use in seasonal and perennial rhinitis in children and adults. Unlike many other available treatments for nasal allergy, topical corticosteroids are effective in controlling nasal congestion. Although these drugs are most beneficial when used on a regular schedule, there is recent evidence suggesting that most of the compounds have a relatively rapid onset of action and may be beneficial when used on an as-needed basis.

   b. **Specific formulations.** There are several formulations currently available (Table 4.5). Although these products range widely in potency on the basis of *in vitro* assessments, in most clinical trials they have proven equally effective in treating both seasonal and perennial allergic rhinitis. Systemic bioavailability differs between the agents, with the two newest compounds (fluticasone propionate, mometasone furoate) having much lower bioavailability (less than 1%) than the older agents. Although the significance of these differences in bioavailability is not entirely clear, it appears to have clinical relevance with respect to systemic adverse effects (see Adverse effects on page 62).

   Some of the compounds are available as aqueous preparations, some as aerosols, and some as both. Some of the formulations are now available without alcohol or fragrances, both of which may be irritating in some patients. Determining whether or not to use an aqueous or aerosol formulation, or one that is alcohol- or fragrance-free, is largely a matter of patient preference.

   c. **Adverse effects** are usually local in nature and include transient stinging, occasional mild epistaxis, nasal dryness, and pharyngeal irritation. Stinging and dryness may be lessened by switching from an aerosol to one of the aqueous preparations, or by using a saline nasal spray before administering the corticosteroid. Epistaxis will usually resolve if the patient stops using the spray for 2 to 3 days; adverse effects are sometimes aided if a topical ointment is applied to the nasal septum. With long-term use, there do not appear to be any significant atrophic effects on the nasal mucosa. Septal perforations have been reported only rarely with use of intranasal corticosteroids, but the nasal septum should be periodically examined to ensure that there are no mucosal erosions that may precede development of nasal septal perforations.

   With respect to systemic adverse effects, cataracts, glaucoma, and clinically meaningful hypothalamic–pituitary–adrenal axis suppres-

Table 4.5. Nasal corticosteroids

Compound	Formulation	mcg/spray	Daily dose
Budesonide	Aqueous	32 mcg	1–2 sp. q.d.
	Aerosol	32 mcg	2 sp. b.i.d. or 4 sp. q.d.
Beclomethasone dipropionate	Aqueous	42 mcg	1–2 sp. b.i.d.–t.i.d.
		84 mcg	1–2 sp. q.d.
	Aerosol	42 mcg	1–2 puffs b.i.d.–t.i.d.
Flunisolide	Aqueous	25 mcg	1–2 sp. b.i.d.–t.i.d.
Fluticasone propionate	Aqueous	50 mcg	1–2 sp. q.d.
Mometasone furoate	Aqueous	50 mcg	1–2 sp. q.d.
Triamcinolone acetonide	Aqueous	55 mcg	1–2 sp. q.d.
	Aerosol	55 mcg	2 puffs b.i.d.

sion have not been reported. Linear growth suppression in young children has been reported with intranasal beclomethasone taken for 1 year, but did not occur with mometasone furoate used for that period of time.

4. **Intranasal cromolyn sodium**, given as a 4% topical nasal spray, is available as an over-the-counter medication and appears to work by stabilizing mast cells as well as by direct anti-inflammatory effects on granulocytes. It controls symptoms of seasonal and perennial allergic rhinitis, but is only partially effective in reducing nasal congestion. For chronic symptoms, nasal cromolyn needs to be used on a prophylactic basis, one to two sprays per nostril four-times daily. It can also be used as an acute prophylactic treatment, two sprays per nostril 30 to 60 minutes before a known allergen exposure. Except for mild, transient stinging, nasal cromolyn is well tolerated by most patients and has one of the best safety records of any medication. Therefore, it can be given without concerns of any toxicity to pregnant women and young children.

5. **Intranasal ipratropium bromide** reduces watery nasal secretions in allergic rhinitis, nonallergic rhinitis, gustatory rhinitis, and viral upper respiratory infections. Ipratropium bromide has no significant effect on nasal congestion, sneezing, and pruritus, and is best used as a supplemental medication in allergic rhinitis when rhinorrhea has not responded to other measures. An initial starting dose is one spray per nostril, three times daily, which may be increased to two sprays per nostril, three times per day, as tolerated. As might be expected, the principal side effect is mucosal dryness, which can be reduced by adjusting the dose and by premedicating with nasal saline. There appears to be no significant systemic absorption at the above doses, given intranasally.

6. **Leukotriene receptor antagonists**, including montelukast and zafirlukast, have both been approved for the treatment of bronchial asthma. Both drugs have also been shown to have beneficial effects in allergic rhinitis. In recent trials, montelukast was demonstrated to significantly reduce nasal allergy symptoms, particularly nasal congestion and rhinorrhea.

7. **Systemic corticosteroids** should be used infrequently in patients with allergic rhinitis. If symptoms are florid, particularly with severe nasal congestion that prevents the topical administration of intranasal corticosteroids, then a short (3 to 5 day) course of prednisone, 30 mg per day in adults, is usually sufficient in controlling the acute disease process. It is important that an intranasal corticosteroid be started at the same time, so that symptoms do not quickly recur after the oral steroid is stopped. Intramuscular corticosteroids should be avoided because of the risk of prolonged adrenal suppression.

8. **Antiimmunoglobulin E therapy** has been shown to be reduce symptoms of both seasonal and perennial rhinoconjunctivitis as well as allergic asthma. There is no evidence that the long-term course of allergic rhinitis is modified by anti-IgE, unlike specific allergen immunotherapy.

C. **Allergen immunotherapy/allergy vaccination**

1. **Mechanisms.** Although the mechanisms by which allergen immunotherapy works are still unclear, it has been documented to reduce mast cell mediator release, eosinophil infiltrations, and circulating levels of specific IgE.

2. **Efficacy.** Numerous placebo-controlled studies have documented efficacy with a variety of allergens, including dust mite, cat dander, and multiple grass, tree, and weed pollens. Approximately 80% of patients will experience symptomatic improvement after 1 to 2 years, and therapy should be continued for a total of 4 to 5 years. Although the beneficial effects of immunotherapy persist for several years in some patients, in others the effects may be lost once the injections are stopped.

The success of immunotherapy depends on accurate confirmation of allergic sensitivities with skin or *in vitro* testing, and a history suggestive of clinical worsening after allergen exposure. The cumulative dose of extract is also important; low-dose immunotherapy has been shown to be no more effective than placebo.

3. **Indications.** Allergen immunotherapy should be considered in patients who do not respond to allergen avoidance or medications, who have significant adverse side effects from medications, or who have difficulty adhering to a complex regimen of multiple drugs. Because immunotherapy has also been shown to be effective in allergic asthma, patients who have concomitant rhinitis and asthma should be strongly considered as candidates for immunotherapy.

4. **Adverse effects.** As the dose of the extract is increased, local reactions are common and systemic reactions can occasionally occur. For this reason, it is important that immunotherapy be administered by practitioners who are skilled in adjusting the dose of immunotherapy and treating untoward reactions.

D. **Considerations for treating allergic rhinitis in select populations**

1. **Children.** When prescribing intranasal steroids, practitioners should attempt to use formulations with lower bioavailabilities, and should always use the lowest dose required to maintain symptoms. When symptoms remit, the intranasal corticosteroid may be stopped and restarted when symptoms return. Finally, the patient's height should be monitored at least once yearly to ensure that significant linear growth suppression is not occurring.

2. **Elderly.** The elderly may have increased susceptibility to the adverse CNS and anticholinergic effects of first-generation antihistamines (as well as cetirizine and azelastine nasal spray). Similarly, oral decongestants should generally be avoided because of their CNS and cardiac effects, as well as effects on bladder function. Therefore, fexofenadine and loratadine are the antihistamines of choice in these patients, and are usually given without pseudoephedrine. Intranasal ipratropium bromide also has an excellent side effect profile in the elderly and is well suited to the treatment of watery rhinorrhea in these patients.

3. **Pregnancy.** Nasal cromolyn has the most reassuring safety profile in pregnancy. Chlorpheniramine and tripelennamine have developed a long safety record in pregnancy (U.S. Food and Drug Administration [FDA] pregnancy category B) and have been the antihistamines of choice in pregnancy. The newer antihistamines loratadine and cetirizine have also been rated as category B drugs, whereas fexofenadine is rated as category C. All intranasal corticosteroids have been rated as category C; however, beclomethasone dipropionate has a long safety record in pregnancy and has been the preferred drug in its class during pregnancy. Oral decongestants are best avoided in the first trimester because of the risk of gastroschisis in the newborn. Allergen immunotherapy without dose escalation may be continued in patients during pregnancy, but should not be started.

Nasal Polyps

Nasal polyps are chronic inflammatory growths that usually emanate from the ethmoid sinuses and most often develop in patients with long-standing rhinosinusitis. Nasal polyps may develop in patients with either allergic or nonallergic rhinitis. Allergy may predispose to polyp formation, and between 10% and 15% of patients with allergic rhinitis also have nasal polyps. Histopathologic studies suggest that nasal polyps are the result of chronic T helper 2 (Th2) lymphocyte activation with eosinophil infiltration.

Common findings associated with nasal polyps include nasal congestion, which may gradually worsen over time, and loss of taste and smell. Other symptoms, including sneezing, itching, and clear, mucoid, or purulent rhinorrhea are also frequent. When large, the polyps may be visualized with an otoscope; smaller polyps and those high in the nasal airway may only be seen via flexible rhinoscopy or CT scanning. Polyps are unusual in children with the exception of those afflicted with cystic fibrosis. Therefore, observation of polyps in a young child should prompt a sweat chloride test. In adolescents and adults, the presence of polyps suggests aspirin intolerance, which may occur with concomitant asthma. In patients with nasal polyps and asthma, nonsteroidal anti-inflammatory drugs should be empirically avoided. If these drugs are needed by a patient (e.g., coronary artery disease), specialized aspirin challenge testing and possible desensitization should be conducted by an allergist.

Treatment. If polyps are small to moderate in size, they should be treated with an intranasal corticosteroid for a minimum of 2 to 3 months. Although the steroid spray may be stopped in some cases, chronic use of nasal corticosteroids may be required to prevent recurrence of polyps. For large, obstructing polyps, a short (5 to 10 day) course of prednisone, 30 to 40 mg per day, will usually shrink them considerably; a nasal steroid spray can then be instituted to maintain control. When polyps are refractory to medical therapy, or CT scanning of the sinuses demonstrates significant evidence of hyperplastic sinusitis, the patient should be referred for evaluation by an otolaryngologist. After surgical polypectomy, nasal corticosteroids are generally required to prevent recurrence of nasal polyps.

Nonallergic Rhinitis With and Without Eosinophilia

Nonallergic rhinitis without eosinophilia, also called idiopathic rhinitis or vasomotor rhinitis, is a condition of unknown origin. Clinically, patients have year round nasal congestion, and/or anterior rhinorrhea, and/or postnasal drip, which may be triggered by a number of nonspecific stimuli, including changes in environment (temperature, humidity, barometric pressure, or weather); airborne irritants (odors, fumes); dietary factors (spicy food, alcohol); sexual arousal; and emotional factors. In general, sneezing and itching are not prominent and ocular symptoms are unusual. On examination, the nasal mucosa may vary in color from pink to erythematous, along with varying amounts of turbinate swelling. Mucus secretions may range from clear and watery to thick and cloudy. Allergy skin tests or *in vitro* tests should be performed to exclude the possibility of allergic rhinitis, and imaging studies of the paranasal sinuses should be conducted if indicated. In patients with predominant congestion, oral decongestants and/or intranasal corticosteroids may be tried and are usually partially successful. Patients should be cautioned not to use topical decongestants chronically for this condition. In patients with rhinorrhea, treatment with intranasal ipratropium is often very effective. If the rhinorrhea is episodic and triggered by known stimuli (e.g., food causing gustatory rhinitis), the spray may be given prophylactically 30 minutes prior to an anticipated exposure.

Nonallergic rhinitis with eosinophilia, (NARES) also referred to as eosinophilic nonallergic rhinitis, is characterized by perennial symptoms of congestion, sneezing, itching, and rhinorrhea, occasionally with eye symptoms. On examination, the nasal mucosa is pale and boggy, and nasal cytologic examination demonstrates eosinophilia. Despite the clinical resemblance to allergic rhinitis, allergy skin tests or *in vitro* tests are negative. Often, NARES is associated with bronchial asthma, and in some cases, nasal polyposis. For treatment, intranasal corticosteroids are very effective.

Sinusitis

I. Definitions and epidemiology

Sinusitis is a clinical condition characterized by mucosal inflammation of the paranasal sinuses. Acute sinusitis is a rapid-onset bacterial infection that has been present for less than 4 weeks and most commonly affects the maxillary sinuses. Chronic sinusitis is defined as symptoms lasting longer than 8 weeks. The role of infection is less clearly defined in chronic sinusitis.

Sinus disease is frequently encountered in general practice, and it has been estimated that 0.5% of viral upper respiratory infections result in acute sinusitis. Chronic sinusitis is also a very common condition and afflicts at least 31 million people in the United States.

II. Pathogenesis

Four host factors determine the susceptibility to **acute sinusitis**; patency of the ostia, ciliary function, quality of secretions, and local host immunity. Obstruction of the sinus ostium leads to reduced oxygen content and the development of mucosal edema and serum transudation within the sinus cavity. These alterations foster bacterial growth, reduce ciliary movement, and alter leukocyte function. If an acute episode of sinusitis occurs, the sinus will usually return to normal following

Table 4.6. Conditions associated with sinusitis

Acute and chronic inflammatory conditions
  Viral upper respiratory infection
  Allergic rhinitis
  Nonallergic rhinitis
  Nasal polyposis
Anatomic obstructive lesions
  Septal deviation
  Concha bullosa (aerated middle turbinate)
  Adenoidal hyperplasia
  Foreign body
Barotrauma
Dental infection
Systemic diseases (rare)
  Cystic fibrosis
  Wegener granulomatosis
  Antibody deficiency syndromes
  Ciliary dyskinesia syndrome

effective antibiotic treatment. However, if therapy is incomplete or underlying etiologic factors are not treated, persistent changes may occur in sinus anatomy and physiology.

Histopathologic studies of **chronic sinusitis** usually demonstrate mucosal hyperplasia, often with associated nasal polyps, and dense infiltration with eosinophils. Similar to allergic rhinitis and asthma, Th2 lymphocytes and their cytokines (e.g., IL-5) appear to play a key role in sustaining these pathologic changes.

Factors that have been associated with sinusitis are listed in Table 4.6.

III. **Clinical presentation**
  A. **Acute sinusitis**
    1. **History.** The most consistent feature distinguishing acute bacterial sinusitis from a viral respiratory infection is persistence of symptoms beyond 7 to 10 days. Cough and nasal discharge are the two most common complaints in children, whereas headache and facial pain are unusual in children younger than the age of 10 years. Adult patients with acute sinusitis most often complain of discolored nasal discharge or postnasal drip, unilateral facial pain or pressure, and nasal congestion. A history of purulent secretions and maxillary tooth pain has the highest positive predictive value of all symptoms.
    2. **Physical examination.** On examination, high temperature and signs of toxicity are unusual and should prompt a search for complications, such as meningitis or periorbital abscess. Anterior rhinoscopy using an otoscope frequently reveals erythematous, swollen turbinates and purulent secretions on the floor of the nose. However, the absence of pus does not rule out active infection, because sinus drainage may be intermittent. Facial tenderness elicited by palpation is an unreliable sign in differentiating sinusitis from acute rhinitis. Transillumination is not reliable in diagnosing sinusitis. Visualization of purulent secretions has the highest positive predictive value of all physical signs.
  B. **Chronic sinusitis**
    1. **History.** Patients suffering from chronic sinusitis usually present with indolent symptoms of nasal congestion, thick postnasal drip, and cough. Adult patients may also complain of facial fullness and headache. Secondary eustachian tube obstruction or middle ear fluid may result in popping of the ears and muffled hearing. In addition to these chronic complaints, patients may also experience recurrent exacerbations of symptoms resembling acute sinusitis.

      2. **Physical examination** often demonstrates swelling and erythema of the inferior and middle turbinates, and occasional mucopurulent secretions on the floor of the nose and middle meatus. Nasal polyps may be present and usually originate from the middle meatus. In children, middle ear effusions are present in half of all cases, and serve as excellent clues to the presence of sinusitis. Flexible fiberoptic rhinoscopy is occasionally an adjunct to the routine physical exam that can help identify anatomic lesions that may predispose to chronic sinusitis. These include posterior deviation of the nasal septum, nasal polyps, enlargement or inflammation of the adenoid, or tumor.

III. Diagnostic tests

In nearly all patients who present with acute sinusitis, diagnosis and subsequent therapy are based upon the history and physical findings. However, in patients with chronic disease, signs and symptoms may be equivocal, and additional testing is required to make a diagnosis.

  A. Laboratory tests. A number of ancillary laboratory tests have been used to assist in diagnosing sinusitis. Nasal cytology may be helpful in differentiating sinusitis from exacerbations of allergic rhinitis (see allergic rhinitis on page 56). Other commonly used tests, including the peripheral white blood count/differential, sedimentation rate, and nasal swab cultures have no utility in determining the presence of infection or in accurately identifying pathogenic bacteria in sinusitis.

  B. Imaging studies

    1. **Plain radiography** has largely fallen out of favor because of poor sensitivity in evaluating the ethmoid and sphenoid sinuses. The Waters projection plain film continues to be useful in young children for evaluating possible chronic maxillary sinusitis, because the test is moderately sensitive for maxillary disease and is simple and inexpensive to perform. Plain films are of limited utility in adults with suspected chronic sinusitis.

    2. **Computed tomography** of the sinuses provides a detailed view of all of the paranasal sinuses, including the ethmoid and sphenoid sinuses, as well as the ostiomeatal complex regions. To reduce both radiation dose and cost, most patients require only a single orientation (coronal or axial) "screening" study (4 to 10 cuts) rather than a complete study. Sinus CT should be considered in the following three circumstances: (i) to establish the diagnosis in equivocal cases of chronic sinusitis before starting antibiotic therapy; (ii) to assess the sinuses following failed medical therapy; and (iii) to evaluate possible cranial extension of sinus disease (although magnetic resonance imaging [MRI] may be preferable if accessible). Of note, CT scanning should be delayed if a viral upper respiratory infection has recently occurred, because 85% of the patients have transient abnormalities on CT scanning following a cold. CT imaging of the sinuses should always be used judiciously, because even the "screening" scan remains a relatively expensive test and requires sedation for most children younger than 8 years of age.

    3. **Magnetic resonance imaging** is extremely sensitive in detecting subtle soft-tissue abnormalities of the paranasal sinuses. For this reason, it is the technique of choice in imaging suspected sinus neoplasms, fungal infections, and complicated infections that extend intracranially. An MRI should not be used for routine diagnosis of sinusitis, because it is very costly and does not adequately visualize the bony landmarks required for surgical planning.

    4. **Sinus ultrasound** is rarely used as a diagnostic test, owing to its poor sensitivity and specificity in patients who have both acute and chronic sinusitis.

  C. Maxillary aspiration and culture

Referral should be made to an otolaryngologist for maxillary aspiration and culture when acute maxillary sinusitis is associated with signs of severe toxicity (particularly in hospitalized or immunosuppressed patients), or if acute sinusitis is unresponsive to an adequate trial of appropriate antibiotics.

Maxillary aspiration has not been found to be useful in assessing the bacteriology of chronic sinusitis.

IV. Microbiology

A. Acute sinusitis

The most commonly identified organisms in children with acute sinusitis are *Streptococcus pneumoniae* in 30% to 40%, *Haemophilus influenzae* in 20% to 25%, and *Moraxella catarrhalis* in 20%. In adults, *S. pneumoniae* and *H. influenzae* are the two leading causes of acute sinusitis, whereas *Moraxella* is unusual. Anaerobic organisms are primarily identified in cases of acute sinusitis originating from dental root infections, but are otherwise uncommon. Hospital-acquired sinusitis is most often seen as a complication of nasogastric tube placement, and is typically caused by gram-negative enteric organisms, such as *Pseudomonas* and *Klebsiella* species.

B. Chronic sinusitis

1. **Bacteria** cultured from children with persistent symptoms are usually the same as those seen in acute disease. In children with more severe and protracted symptoms, anaerobic species (such as *Bacteroides*) and staphylococci are cultured more frequently. In adults with refractory symptoms, *Staphylococcus epidermidis* is frequently cultured from intraoperative specimens. The exact role of this species in the pathogenesis of chronic sinusitis is unclear. Although anaerobic organisms were once implicated in adults with chronic sinus disease, more recent evidence casts doubt upon those data.

2. **Fungi**, such as *Aspergillus* species, are a common cause of sinus disease in immunocompromised hosts, including diabetics and patients who have defective cell-mediated immunity. Increasingly, fungi have been identified as causes of sinusitis in patients who are otherwise healthy and should, therefore, be considered in cases of refractory sinusitis. Allergic fungal sinusitis is a syndrome that occurs in adults with asthma and has been attributed to *Aspergillus*, *Bipolaris*, and *Curvularia* species. It is characterized by severe, hyperplastic sinusitis and nasal polyposis, and is associated with significant eosinophilia of sinus tissue and blood.

V. Medical therapy

A. Acute sinusitis

1. **Antibiotics** are the primary form of treatment for acute sinusitis (Table 4.7).

   For mild acute sinusitis, amoxicillin remains the initial drug of choice. However, in patients with moderate to severe discomfort and in regions where there are very high rates of beta-lactamase-producing strains of *H. influenzae*, a beta-lactamase-resistant antibiotic (e.g., amoxicillin–

Table 4.7. Antibiotic recommendations for acute bacterial sinusitis

---

First line
  Amoxicillin
  In cases of penicillin allergy, trimethoprim–sulfamethoxazole, clarithromycin, azithromycin
Second line
  Amoxicillin–clavulanate[a]
  Cefuroxime axetil[a]
  Cefpodoxime[a]
Third line
  Levofloxacin
  Amoxicillin or clindamycin plus cefixime

---

[a]May be used as first-line drug in more moderate cases, in patients who have received antibiotics in the prior 4 to 6 weeks, and in areas with very high prevalence of beta-lactamase-producing *Hemophilus influenzae*.

clavulanate, cefuroxime) should be used as a first-line antibiotic. Although the newer fluoroquinolones (e.g., levofloxacin) provide excellent coverage of the relevant pathogens, particularly penicillin-resistant *S. pneumoniae*, these antibiotics should be reserved for patients who have not responded to amoxicillin–clavulanate or second- or third-generation cephalosporins, or who are allergic to these antibiotics. Symptoms begin to improve with these antibiotics within 3 to 5 days in 70% of cases. Therapy should be continued for a minimum of 10 to 14 days, and many specialists recommend treating the infection for 7 days beyond the day of initial improvement. If patients demonstrate no improvement with the initial antibiotic after 5 days, they should be started on an alternative beta-lactamase-resistant agent for 10 to 14 additional days. In patients who do not respond to two trials of empiric therapy, consultation with an otolaryngologist is indicated for consideration of sinus aspiration and culture.

2. **Adjunctive agents**
   a. **Topical and oral decongestants** reduce nasal congestion associated with acute sinusitis and may reduce ostial edema, allowing for improved sinus drainage.
   b. **Mucolytic agents**, such as guaifenesin, are occasionally helpful in patients who complain of abundant, thick secretions.
   c. **Antihistamines** have not been shown to reduce symptoms of acute sinusitis. Older antihistamines with strong anticholinergic effects, such as diphenhydramine and hydroxyzine, may cause mucus inspissation and impede sinus drainage. However, the newer, second-generation antihistamines have virtually no anticholinergic effects and can be continued in patients who require those agents for concomitant allergic rhinitis.

B. **Chronic sinusitis**
   1. **Antibiotics.** Although there are few published data regarding antimicrobial therapy for chronic sinusitis, anecdotal evidence suggests that patients should be treated for 3-6 weeks. In patients who have not been previously treated with antibiotics, amoxicillin is a cost-effective choice for first-line therapy. In patients who are allergic to penicillin, clarithromycin provides good coverage against most relevant pathogens. If the patient has not responded to these drugs within 10 days, a beta-lactamase-resistant antibiotic should be given for an additional 3 weeks. In a small number of children and adults who do not respond to these antibiotics, an agent with increased anaerobic coverage, such as clindamycin, may occasionally be effective.
   2. **Adjunctive therapies**
      a. **Topical intranasal corticosteroids** should be prescribed for 3 to 6 weeks to reduce mucosal edema and inflammation.
      b. **Prednisone** (0.5 mg per kg q.d., given in two to three divided doses for 5 to 7 days) may be useful. Both topical and oral cortico-steroids appear to be safe in chronic sinusitis, and there is no evidence that they increase the risk of intracranial extension or fulminant infection when given to patients who have normal immune function. In allergic patients and patients who have nasal polyposis, chronic use of nasal corticosteroids may be helpful in preventing recurrences of sinusitis.
      c. **Nasal irrigations**, performed two to three times daily with a bulb syringe and saline, can be very helpful in removing dried secretions. Other methods to increase nasal humidification (hot showers, room humidifiers, and steam inhalers) are easy to use and may provide symptomatic relief for short periods of time.

VI. **Surgical therapy**
   A. **Refractory disease.** Patients who have chronic sinusitis that is refractory to medical therapy and confirmed by CT should be referred to an otolaryngologist for consideration of surgery. In children who have persistent maxillary sinus

disease, antral lavage (with or without adenoidectomy) effectively removes purulent material and often provides long-lasting symptom relief. In adults, however, functional endoscopic surgery has largely supplanted other surgical procedures, and is effective in 50% to 80% of patients. Patients who have aspirin-sensitive asthma, nasal polyposis, and pansinusitis are more likely to have recurrent disease and should be discouraged from undergoing multiple/repeat surgeries.

    B. Suspected intracranial complications. Patients who are suspected of having intracranial complications of acute sinusitis (e.g., periorbital abscess, brain abscess, or meningitis), should be referred for immediate surgical consultation. Cardinal signs and symptoms include a high fever, severe headaches, proptosis, and changes in mental status.

VII. Evaluation of possible predisposing factors

Fifty percent of children, and 30% to 40% of adults with recurrent or chronic sinusitis are sensitized to common aeroallergens, such as plant pollens, house dust mite, and animal danders. Allergy skin testing should be performed in those patients, because they often benefit from a comprehensive program of allergen avoidance, antiallergic drug therapy, and in selected cases, immunotherapy. Patients who have severe, recurrent episodes of sinusitis associated with other infections (e.g., otitis, bronchitis, and pneumonia), may suffer from one of the antibody deficiency syndromes, and should undergo a screening assessment of their immunoglobulin levels. If a deficiency is noted or is still suspected after the initial testing, these patients should be referred to an allergist/immunologist for further evaluation.

Otitis Media

I. Definitions and epidemiology

Acute otitis media (AOM) refers to an acute suppurative infection of the middle ear space, which usually lasts for 3 weeks or less. **Otitis media with effusion** (OME) (previously referred to as "secretory" or "serous" otitis media) represents persistent middle ear fluid that most often follows an episode of AOM and may last for many months. **Recurrent acute otitis media** is defined as three or more episodes of acute otitis.

AOM is typically diagnosed in young children and is unusual in adult patients. It occurs in roughly 60% of children by age 1 year, and in 80% of children by the age of 3 years. Half of all children have had three or more episodes of AOM by the age of 3 years. Otitis medial with effusion is similarly common, noted in approximately 50% of patients during the first year of life.

Epidemiologic risk factors associated with middle ear disease include: male gender, absence of breast feeding, race (Native Americans more often than Caucasians more often than African Americans), overcrowding, air pollution, and cigarette smoking by the mother.

II. Pathogenesis

The two factors that contribute most significantly to otitis media are eustachian tube dysfunction and bacterial proliferation in the nasopharynx. The functions of the eustachian tube include pressure equalization, protection of the middle ear from nasopharyngeal secretions, and mucociliary clearance of the middle ear. Eustachian tube obstruction results in the development of negative pressure, which is followed by serum transudation into the middle ear. This sterile effusion may become infected by bacteria refluxing from the nasopharynx into the middle ear. Incomplete eradication of an initial infection, or prolonged underventilation of the middle ear, may ultimately result in a chronic mucoid effusion. Some of the conditions associated with otitis media are listed in Table 4.8.

III. Clinical presentation

    A. Acute otitis media

        Children who have AOM typically complain of acute unilateral ear pain, which occurs several days after a viral upper respiratory infection. The symptoms frequently start early in the morning and are associated with irritability and fever, although nausea, vomiting, and diarrhea may also occur.

Table 4.8. Conditions associated with otitis media

Acute and chronic inflammatory diseases
Viral upper respiratory infection
Allergic rhinitis
Chronic sinusitis
Anatomic obstruction
Tonsillar and adenoidal enlargement
Variants of eustachian tube anatomy
Cleft palate disease
Systemic diseases (rare)
Immunodeficiency
Cystic fibrosis
Ciliary dyskinesia syndrome
Down syndrome

Otoscopy usually reveals a red, thickened, and bulging tympanic membrane. Insufflation (pneumatic otoscopy) generally demonstrates poor mobility of the drum. It is important that the drum may also appear red in a crying child (owing to increased vascularity of the tympanic membrane) and may lead to an incorrect diagnosis of AOM.

B. Otitis media with effusion

Children with this chronic condition are usually asymptomatic, but may have a subtle loss of hearing. There is usually no recent history of fever, irritability, or other systemic symptoms. The eardrum may appear yellow, orange, or blue, and is often retracted. Air–fluid levels or bubbles may be present, and the drum moves poorly with insufflation. Unfortunately, if middle ear fluid is very thin, mobility may appear normal, even to highly trained observers. Physical findings suggestive of allergic rhinitis, sinusitis, or tonsillar hypertrophy should be sought, because these conditions may play important pathogenic roles in OME.

IV. Diagnostic tests

  A. Electroacoustic impedance (tympanometry) is a convenient, simple procedure that is extremely sensitive in detecting middle ear fluid. Middle ear fluid can be confidently ruled out when tympanometry is normal.

  B. Audiometry is an important test in children older than 18 months of age in determining whether OME has resulted in hearing loss. This test should be employed when middle ear fluid has been present for at least 3 months and before deciding whether ventilation of the middle ear is necessary.

  C. Diagnostic tympanocentesis with culture of middle ear fluid is indicated in children who are extremely ill with AOM, children who have not responded to an adequate trial of appropriate medical therapy, and children in intensive care nurseries.

V. Microbiology

The three principal organisms identified in middle ear effusions from both AOM and OME are the same as those isolated from patients with acute sinusitis; *S. pneumoniae*, non-typable *H. influenzae*, and *M. catarrhalis* are isolated in 35%, 23%, and 14% of effusions, respectively. Other organisms that are occasionally cultured include *Staphylococcus aureus*, alpha streptococcus, and group A streptococcus. Special exceptions include very young infants and children in intensive care nurseries, in whom group B streptococci and gram-negative organisms are very common causes of AOM.

VI. Medical therapy

  A. Acute otitis media

    1. Antibiotics. Although placebo-controlled studies have demonstrated that many children will recover from AOM without treatment, antibiotics do reduce the duration and severity of signs and symptoms. More important, antibiotics have reduced the incidence of, and death rate from, suppurative complications of AOM. For initial episodes, amoxicillin is the drug of choice, and should be given for 10 to 14 days. Trimethoprim–sulfamethoxazole is a good alternative in penicillin-allergic patients. In most cases, symptoms should improve significantly within 2 to 3 days. If symptoms persist, a second-line antibiotic with beta-lactamase resistance (see Acute sinusitis on page 69) should be given for an additional 10 to 14 days.

2. **Adjunctive measures**, including antihistamine–decongestant combinations and topical nasal corticosteroids, have not been proven to be effective in children with AOM. However, these agents may have a beneficial effect upon concomitant allergic rhinitis.

B. **Recurrent acute otitis media**

1. **Prophylactic antibiotics.** Prophylactic antibiotics have been shown to be effective in reducing the number of episodes of AOM in children who are prone to recurrence. Amoxicillin (20 mg per kg q.d.) and sulfisoxazole (50 mg per kg q.d.) are used most commonly, and treatment should be continued through the high-risk upper respiratory infection seasons (late fall to early spring).

2. **Pneumococcal vaccine** should also be encouraged in all children over the age of 2 years who suffer from recurrent otitis media.

C. **Otitis media with effusion**

Although at least 80% of effusions resolve spontaneously within 2 months, effusions that persist longer than 3 months will not usually improve with therapy. The most effective medical therapy for OME is probably a 14-day trial of amoxicillin. More potent antimicrobial agents or longer courses of antibiotics have not been shown to be helpful. Adjunctive measures (antihistamine–decongestants, topical corticosteroids) have also not been shown to be effective. Antibiotic therapy for OME should be considered in children with associated sinusitis, or those who have a documented conductive hearing loss, vertigo, tinnitus, structural changes in the tympanic membrane or middle ear, or in infants who are unable to describe symptoms. Following antibiotic therapy, the effusion must be followed carefully to ensure resolution.

VII. **Surgical therapy**

If medical therapy for recurrent AOM or OME is ineffective or poorly tolerated, a patient should be referred for evaluation by an otolaryngologist. Myringotomy with tube placement is effective in reducing the frequency of acute infections and in decreasing the course of chronic effusions and their associated hearing loss. If tube placements are not effective, or a child has persistent adenoidal infection or enlargement, adenoidectomy with repeat tube placement has been shown to be beneficial in children older than age 4 years. Tonsillectomy has not been shown to provide any additional benefit over adenoidectomy alone.

VIII. **Evaluation of possible predisposing factors**

Thirty percent to 40% of children with recurrent AOM and OME have associated nasal allergy. These patients should undergo allergy testing and, if indicated, a complete program of allergen avoidance and antiallergic drug therapy, prior to surgical intervention. Children with very severe, recurrent episodes of AOM, associated with intracranial complications or bronchial infections, should undergo an evaluation of their humoral immunity.

Suggested Readings

Allergic Rhinitis

Bousquet J, Lockey R, Malling HJ. Allergen immunotherapy: therapeutic vaccines for allergic diseases. A WHO position paper. *J Allergy Clin Immunol* 1998;102:558–562.

Corren J. Allergic rhinitis: treating the adult. *J Allergy Clin Immunol* 2000;105: S610–S615.

Corren J. Intranasal corticosteroids for allergic rhinitis: how do different agents compare? *J Allergy Clin Immunol* 1999;104:S144–S149.

Day J. Pros and cons of the use of antihistamines in managing allergic rhinitis. *J Allergy Clin Immunol* 1999;103:S395–S399.

Dykewicz M, Fineman S, Skoner DP, et al. Diagnosis and management of rhinitis: complete guidelines of the Joint Task Force on Practice Parameters in Allergy, Asthma and Immunology. American Academy of Allergy, Asthma, and Immunology. *Ann Allergy Asthma Immunol* 1998;81:478–518.

Platts-Mills T, Vaughan JW, Carter MC, et al. The role of intervention in established allergy: avoidance of indoor allergens in the treatment of chronic allergic disease. *J Allergy Clin Immunol* 2000;106:787–804.

Nonallergic Rhinitis

Settipane RA, Lieberman P. Update on nonallergic rhinitis. *Ann Allergy Asthma Immunol* 2001;86:494–507.

Nasal Polyposis

Blomqvist EH, Lundblad L, Anggard A, et al. A randomized controlled study evaluating medical treatment versus surgical treatment in addition to medical treatment of nasal polyposis. *J Allergy Clin Immunol* 2001;107:224–228.

Sinusitis

Hadley JA. The microbiology and management of acute and chronic rhinosinusitis. *Curr Infect Dis Rep* 2001;3:209–216.

Rao VM, el-Noueam KI. Sinonasal imaging. Anatomy and pathology. *Radiol Clin North Am* 1998;36:921–939.

Otitis Media

Berman J. Otitis media in children. *N Engl J Med* 1995;332:1560–1565.

Jacobs RF. Judicious use of antibiotics for common pediatric respiratory infections. *Pediatr Infect Dis J* 2000;19:938–943.

5. ALLERGIC AND IMMUNOLOGIC DISORDERS OF THE EYE

Leonard Bielory

The eye is a frequent site of inflammatory responses induced by local and systemic immunological hypersensitivity reactions. Inflammatory ocular conditions resulting from immune responses are highly prominent because of the eyes' considerable vascularization and the sensitivity of the vessels in the conjunctiva that are embedded in a transparent medium. The eye and its surrounding tissues are also involved in a variety of other immunologically mediated disorders. When such reactions occur, they are not infrequently seen first by the clinical allergist/immunologist, who then is in the position to correlate ocular and systemic findings, and to coordinate therapy so as to treat underlying disease (if present), rather than only local eye symptoms.

I. Anatomy
  A. Cross section
  The eye is essentially constructed of four layers from the mast-cell-rich anterior to the vascular contents of the posterior section of the eye (see Fig. 5.1): (i) the anterior portion, consisting of the **conjunctiva** and the tear fluid layer are the eye's primary barrier against environmental aeroallergens, chemicals, and infectious agents; (ii) the collagenous **sclera** is commonly involved in "collagen" vascular disorders such as rheumatoid arthritis; (iii) the highly vascular **uvea**, the site of aqueous humor production, is the most common site for systemically active immune disorders mediated by circulating immune complexes (e.g., vasculitis) and lymphocyte-mediated disorders (e.g., sarcoid); and (iv) the posterior portion composed of the **retina and the optic nerve**, which are involved in central nervous system disorders (e.g., multiple sclerosis).

  B. Conjunctiva
  The **conjunctiva is the most immunologically active tissue of the external eye**. It is composed of two layers: the epithelial and substantia propria. Mast cells (6,000 per mm^3) and other inflammatory cells normally are found in the substantia propria, just below the junction with the epithelium. Normal ocular epithelia do not contain any mast cells, eosinophils, or basophils, although in ocular inflammatory disorders (e.g., vernal conjunctivitis and giant papillary conjunctivitis) such cells are seen.

  C. Uvea
  The **uvea is the most immunologically active tissue within the eye**. The uvea comprises a continuous layer of iris, ciliary body, and choroid, and a characteristic vascular architecture within the alymphatic globe of the eye. The ciliary body is the production site of a filtrate, the aqueous humor, and is similar to other structures that produce a filtrate, which include the renal glomerulus (urine) and the choroid plexus (cerebrospinal fluid). These filtration sites are clinically involved in clinical disorders associated with circulating immune complexes. Although there is a paucity of mast cells within the uveal tissue, there is a notable increase in mast cell numbers in uveitis. The predominant inflammatory cell type in uveitis is the lymphocyte.

Ocular Symptoms and Examination
  D. Ocular history
  A detailed history commonly reveals recent exposure to individuals with conjunctivitis or upper respiratory tract infections, sexual activity, and association with animals that may cause various forms of infectious conjunctivitis. Direct questioning will often reveal the frequent use of over-the-counter medications, such as vasoconstrictors or artificial tears, cosmetics, or contact lens wear, which can cause conjunctivitis medicamentosa. A knowledge of sys-

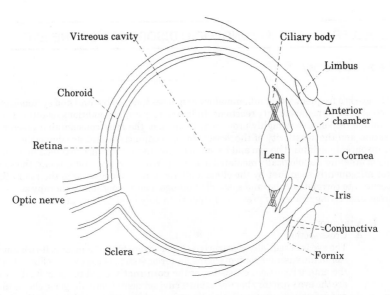

FIG. 5.1. Sagittal cross-section view of the human eye revealing the parts commonly involved in immunological hypersensitivity reactions: eyelids (blepharitis and dermatitis), conjunctiva (conjunctivitis), cornea (keratitis), sclera (lepiscleritis and scleritis), optic nerve (neuritis), iris (iritis), vitreous cavity (vitreitis), choroid (choroiditis), and retina (retinitis). Uveitis involves inflammation of uveal tract (iris, vitreous, and choroid).

temic diseases such as rheumatoid arthritis will heighten the awareness of associated ocular conditions such as keratoconjunctivitis sicca (KCS) or scleromalacia.

   E. **Ocular symptoms** are often nonspecific, such as tearing, irritation, stinging, burning, and photophobia.

      1. **Itching** is the hallmark of allergic conjunctivitis that can last hours to days and can be described as mild to severe. Burning may signify other forms of pathology such as dry eye.

      2. Review of the type of **ocular secretions** is recommended, in which discolored and "sticky" secretions (which may cause eyelids to become "glued") or morning crusting are associated with infectious etiologies, and a clear, white, stringy or ropy discharge are consistent features with allergic etiologies.

      3. Most environmental allergen exposures are associated with **bilateral** symptoms, whereas a unilateral conjunctival involvement commonly signifies an infectious etiology and is also commonly associated with preauricular node involvement.

      4. **Pain** is commonly associated with an intraocular inflammatory process, especially when it is associated with photophobia. It is commonly described as sharp and sometimes piercing in character. Sinusitis is associated with retroorbital dull pain. Pain is not a feature of acute seasonal or perennial allergic conjunctivitis.

   F. **Ocular examination**

      1. External

         a. **Examination of the eye** starts with a careful examination of the periorbital tissue for evidence of **eyelid involvement** in the form of blepharitis and/or dermatitis, as well as "**allergic shiners**" associated with allergic rhinoconjunctivitis. One then directly examines the bulbar conjunctiva for evidence of **chemosis, hyperemia,** and **papillae** formation. One then examines the palpebral conjunctiva by everting the upper and lower eyelids. The eversion of the upper eyelid requires experience to accomplish correctly. The conjunctival fornix is examined for the presence of increased or abnormal-appearing **secretions.** Finally, a fundoscopic examination should be done for the presence of **cataracts** (associated with atopic disorders and chronic corticosteroid use) and/or intraocular inflammation, and if detected, the patient should be referred to an ophthalmologist for a more detailed examination with a biomicroscope.

    b. When **conjunctival inflammation** is noted, a more careful examination is then performed to verify the presence of **follicles** or **papillae** involving the bulbar and tarsal conjunctiva. For the clinician to determine an acceptable (nonpathological) level of follicular and papillary reactivity, the upper and lower tarsal plates and bulbar conjunctiva should be examined on a routine basis.

    c. Examination of the palpebral conjunctiva is performed by grasping the upper lid at its base with a cotton swab on the upper portion of the lid, and then pulling out and up. The patient should be looking down during the examination. To return the lid to its normal position, have the patient look up.

    d. The **anterior chamber** is examined for clearness or cloudiness of the aqueous humor. Check for the presence of blood, either diffuse or settled out (hyphema) or the settling out of pus (hypopyon). **A shallow anterior chamber suggests narrow-angle glaucoma, which is a contraindication for the use of mydriatic agents.** Illuminating the anterior chamber from the side with a penlight can provide a crude estimate of the anterior chamber depth. If the iris creates a shadow on the far side from the light, a high index of suspicion exists for increased intraocular pressure (IOP, glaucoma).

    e. The presence of palpable preauricular and cervical lymph nodes supports an infectious etiology and helps one differentiate it from an allergic etiology (see Table 5.1)

2. Internal

    a. Ophthalmoscopy. The direct (hand-held) ophthalmoscope provides approximately 14× magnification. One may need to adjust the ophthalmoscope power setting to accommodate for the patient's or the clinician's own refractive errors: Minus (red numbered) lenses correct for nearsightedness, whereas the positive (green numbered) lenses correct for farsighted errors. Using the lens settings of +8 with the ophthalmoscope held close to the patient's eye will assist the physician in focusing on the anterior segment to reveal corneal opacities or changes in the iris or lens. Decreasing the power of the lens from +8 to −8 will increase the depth of focus so that the examiner can move from the anterior segment progressively through the structures including the vitreous and reach the retina. The red-free (green) light filter is employed to sharply delineate small aneurysms and hemorrhages as black in color in patients with autoimmune disorders (e.g., systemic lupus erythematous [SLE], vasculitis). Eyes that have had cataracts removed (aphakia) should be examined with a +8 for view of the fundus.

    b. Surface lesions can best be demonstrated by applying fluorescein dye to the eye, preferably following the instillation of a topical anesthetic drop. The end of the fluorescein strip is touched to the marginal tear meniscus. When the patient blinks the dye is dispersed throughout the ocular surface and stains wherever an epithelial defect exists— as in a corneal or conjunctival abrasion. A light utilizing a cobalt filter will best demonstrate the abnormal accumulations of the dye.

Table 5.1. Differential diagnosis of conjunctival inflammatory disorders[a]

	AC	VC	AKC	GPC	Contact	Bacterial	Viral	Chlamydial	KCS	BC
SIGNS										
Predominant cell type	Mast cell, Eos	Lymph, Eos	Lymph, Eos	Lymph, Eos	Lymph	PMN	PMN, Mono, Lymph	Mono, Lymph	Lymph, Mono	Mono, Lymph
Chemosis	+	+/−	+/−	+/−	−	+/−	+/−	+/−	−	+/−
Lymph node	−	−	−	−	−	+	++	+/−	−	−
Cobblestoning	−	++	++	++	−	−	+/−	+	+/−	−
Discharge	Clear, mucoid	Stringy, mucoid	Stringy, mucoid	Clear, white	+/−	Muco purulent	Clear, mucoid	Muco purulent	Mucoid	Muco purulent
Lid involvement	−	+	+	−	++	−	−	−	−	++
SYMPTOMS										
Pruritus	+	++	++	++	+	−	−	−	−	+
Gritty sensation	+/−	+/−	+/−	+	−	+	+	+	+++	++
Seasonal variation	+	+	+/−	+/−	−	+/−	+/−	+/−	−	−

a The differential diagnosis of the red eye includes various inflammatory conditions that involve the outside and the inside of the eye. The list focuses on the signs and symptoms of external causes of the red eye, which include the predominant cell type found in the conjunctival scraping, the presence or absence of chemosis, lymph node involvement, cobblestoning of the conjunctival surface, discharge, lid involvement, pruritus, gritty sensation, and seasonal variation.
AC, Allergic conjunctivitis; VC, vernal conjunctivitis; AKC, atopic keratoconjunctivitis; GPC, giant papillary conjunctivitis; KCS, keratoconjunctivitis sicca; BC, blepharoconjunctivitis; PMN, polymorphonuclear cell; Mono, monocyte; Lymph, lymphocyte; and Eos, eosinophil.

Most modern ophthalmoscopes are equipped with a cobalt blue filter, and many penlights have an attachable adapter. A Wood lamp, used to demonstrate tinea infections, will also cause the dye to fluoresce. Mucous adhering to the corneal or conjunctival surfaces is considered pathologic.

Common Clinical Signs of Ocular Disease

3. **Trichiasis** (in-turned eyelashes) usually results from the softening of the tarsal plate within the eyelid leading to an **entropion**. An entropion is an inward turning or inversion of the margin of the eyelid. Although this condition commonly results in minor conjunctivitis, it can be associated with corneal scarring.

4. **Epiphora** (excessive tearing) can result from increased tear production in response to allergic reactions (e.g., mast cell-mediated hypersensitivity reaction) or obstruction of the nasolacrimal drainage system commonly seen in chronic sinusitis and/or rhinitis. Obstruction of the nasolacrimal drainage system can be evaluated with the placement of a 2% fluorescein solution in the conjunctival sac that should disappear within 1 minute after placement.

5. **Subconjunctival hemorrhages** often occur spontaneously, but can follow vigorous rubbing of the eye, vomiting, coughing, or Valsalva maneuvers. If the hemorrhages are recurrent, check for a possible coagulation abnormality.

6. A **pinguecula** is a common, benign, yellowish elevation more commonly located on the nasal portion of the conjunctiva. Pinguecula, composed of subepithelial deposits of collagen and senile elastic tissue, are slightly yellow and caused by benign degeneration of elastic tissue. They are almost always asymptomatic and become more prominent with age. A pinguecula is often confused with a **pterygium**, which is a triangular growth of hyalinized conjunctiva encroaching on the nasal portion of the cornea.

7. A **phlyctenula** is the formation of a small, gray, circumscribed lesion at the corneal limbus and has been associated with staphylococcal colonization that may be due to the release of staphylococcal exotoxins or superantigenic stimulation. It has also been associated with tuberculosis infection and malnutrition.

8. **Blepharitis** is inflammation of the eyelids.

9. A **chalazion** is a chronic, granulomatous inflammation of the **meibomian gland**. A **hordeolum** is synonymous with a "sty" (a small abscess that forms on the conjunctival or cutaneous surface of the eyelid, resulting from infection of a sebaceous gland adjacent to an eyelash follicle).

10. **Episcleritis** and **scleritis** are inflammatory reactions involving the tunic that surrounds the ocular globe. The sclera is continuous with the cornea and the lamina cribosa of the optic nerve.

11. **Leukocoria** is a white pupil and is seen in patients with **cataracts**, **Chédiak-Higashi syndrome** (an immune deficiency syndrome with a neutrophil defect) (see Chapter 17), **retinoblastoma**, and **retrolental fibroplasia**.

12. **Follicles** are smaller than papillae and appear as grayish, clear, or yellow bumps varying in size from pinpoint to 2 mm in diameter, with conjunctival vessels on their surface. These can generally be distinguished from **papillae** that contain a centrally located tuft of vessels.

II. Ocular allergy

A. **Overview.** Ocular allergy includes four overlapping conditions that include seasonal and perennial allergic conjunctivitis, vernal conjunctivitis, giant papillary conjunctivitis, and atopic keratoconjunctivitis, all of which appear to be part of a clinical spectrum ranging from acute non-sight-threatening to chronic sight-threatening disorders. This clinical spectrum can best be viewed from the perspective of immunologic changes that occur in the conjunctival surface. In seasonal allergic conjunctivitis, the change is a visible increase in the type and number of cells provoking allergy symptoms at particular times of the year. These cells include mast cells, eosinophils and other cells that interact and release a variety of allergic mediators including histamine, leukotrienes, and prostaglandins when exposed to various airborne allergens (aeroallergens). In contrast, perennial allergic conjunctivitis is associated with a persistent increase in the number of these allergy-mediating cells throughout the year. In vernal conjunctivitis, there is a seasonally recurrent increase in mast cells, eosinophils, and lymphocytes. Giant papillary conjunctivitis has similar features but is directly related to the presence of objects irritating the eye, such as contact lenses. Finally, in atopic keratoconjunctivitis, there is chronic invasion of the immune cells into the conjunctiva that is seen in middle-aged and older patients with extensive allergic disorders, specifically eczema and asthma. Although contact conjunctivitis is purely a lymphocytic-mediated type of reaction like other delayed type hypersensitivity reactions, it is also presented in this section as a common clinical hypersensitivity reaction seen by the allergist/clinical immunologist (Table 5.2)

B. Allergic conjunctivitis (seasonal and perennial)

1. **Basic mechanisms.** Because of the direct exposure of the ocular mucosal surfaces to the environment, mast cell and immunoglobulin E (IgE)-mediated reactions are the most common hypersensitivity responses of the eye. (There are an estimated 50 million mast cells in the ocular and adnexal tissue of one human eye.) The conjunctiva is a commonly involved site for the development of angioedema in a variety of hypersensitivity reactions. A conjunctival late-phase reaction can occur.

2. **History, physical examination, laboratory findings, and differential diagnosis.** Seasonal and perennial allergic conjunctivitis are the most prevalent forms of ocular allergy, with seasonal allergic conjunctivitis being more common. Grass pollens appear to produce more ocular symptoms than other aeroallergens. The conjunctival symptoms of itching, tearing, and burning can also include corneal symptoms of photophobia and blurring of vision. Clinical signs of allergic conjunctivitis include milky or pale pink conjunctivae with vascular congestion, which may progress to conjunctival swelling (chemosis). A white exudate can form during the acute state, which becomes stringy in the chronic form. Tears can contain histamine and a small number of eosinophils.

C. Vernal conjunctivitis

1. **Basic mechanisms.** Histopathologically, vernal conjunctivitis is characterized by conjunctival infiltration with eosinophils, degranulated mast cells, basophils, plasma cells, lymphocytes, and macrophages, supporting the hypothesis that vernal conjunctivitis is a combined mast cell-, IgE-, and lymphocyte-mediated hypersensitivity reaction. As the disease progresses, fibrous tissue proliferates to generate the **giant papillae**. Mucosal mast cells are increased in the conjunctiva of these patients. Degranulated eosinophils and their toxic enzymes (e.g., major basic protein) are found in the conjunctiva and in the periphery of corneal ulcers, suggesting an etiologic role in many of the associated problems.

2. **History, physical examination, laboratory findings, and differential diagnosis.** Vernal conjunctivitis commonly begins in the spring, thus the name **vernal catarrh**. Symptoms include intense pruritus exacerbated by length of exposure, type of exposure (wind, hot weather, dust, or bright light), or physical exertion associated with sweating. Associated symptoms involving the cornea include **photophobia, foreign body sensation, and lacrimation**. Signs include conjunctival hyperemia with papillary hypertrophy (**"cobblestoning"**) reaching 7 to 8 mm in diameter of the upper tarsal plate; a thin copious milk-white fibrinous secretion composed of eosinophils, epithelial cells, and Charcot-Leyden granules; limbal or conjunctival yellowish-white points known as **Horner points** and **Trantas dots** lasting 2 to 7 days; an extra lower eyelid

Table 5.2. An overview of the spectrum of ocular allergic disorders, their signs and symptoms, and their salient features

Type	Signs/symptoms	Salient features
Seasonal allergic conjunctivitis	Moderate to severe pruritus Mild to moderate diffuse conjunctival injection Usually seasonal in nature Lid swelling and conjunctival chemosis	Family and personal history of atopy Most common type of ocular allergy More than 50% of allergic rhinitis patients also have ocular symptoms Pollen sensitivity is the most common cause
Perennial allergic conjunctivitis	Conjunctival injection and edema Year-round symptoms Majority of patients have seasonal exacerbations Eosinophils in scrapings	Family and personal history of atopy Predominantly seen in adults Often associated with a specific environment (pollen, animal dander, dust mites at home, industrial allergens at work)
Vernal conjunctivitis	Severe pruritus Ropy, stringy discharge Palpebral variety: cobblestone papillae covering upper tarsus Limbal variety: limbal infiltrates and nodules Trantas dots (Horner points) Untreated corneal complications (shield ulcer) may result in scarring and permanent visual impairment Appears from early spring until fall	80% of patients <14 years old Usually outgrown by late teens or early 20s 75% patients are male More common in dry, warm climates (e.g., Mediterranean basin, northern Africa)
Giant papillary conjunctivitis	Decreased tolerance to contact lenses Blurred vision Conjunctival hyperemia Late stage: giant papillae or follicles (up to 0.3 mm), pain, foreign body sensation, increased mucus production	Trauma induced by contact lenses, ocular prosthetics, exposed sutures
Atopic kerato-conjunctivitis	Severe itching, burning, photophobia Erythematous, eczematous eyelids Superficial punctate keratitis Superficial corneal infiltrates Perennial symptoms May be exacerbated in winter	Food, dust mite, pollen, animal dander sensitivity Associated with atopic dermatitis activity Begins in late teens or early 20s

crease, or a **Dennie line**; **corneal ulcers** infiltrated with Charcot-Leyden crystals; or pseudomembrane formation of the upper lid when everted and exposed to heat (**Maxwell-Lyon sign**). Although vernal conjunctivitis is a bilateral disease, it can affect one eye more than the other. The most common corneal degenerative change seen is **pseudogerontoxon** (**arcus senilis**), whereas the most severe is corneal ulceration. Tears contain histamine, major basic protein, Charcot-Leyden crystals, basophils, IgE and IgG specific for aeroallergens (e.g., ragweed pollen), and eosinophils (in 90% of cases). The tear-specific IgE level does not correlate with positive immediate skin tests.

3. **Natural history.** Vernal conjunctivitis is a disease of childhood appearing more commonly in males before puberty. Onset after puberty is equally distributed among the sexes, and dissipates by the third decade of life (about 4 to 10 years after onset).

4. **Treatment** requires a multidisciplinary approach in consultation with an ophthalmologist. Cool compresses to the eyes can benefit the patient. Immunotherapy and cromolyn sodium have been reported in studies to be an adjunctive treatment modality in patients clearly having a seasonal component.

D. **Giant papillary conjunctivitis**

1. **Basic mechanisms.** Infiltrations of basophils, eosinophils, plasma cells, and lymphocytes suggest a mixed mast cell- and lymphocyte-mediated process associated with the continued use of contact lenses.

2. **History, physical examination, laboratory findings, and differential diagnosis.** There is typically an increase of symptoms during the spring pollen season. The major symptom is itching. Signs include a white or clear exudate upon awakening that chronically becomes thick and stringy, and the patient may develop Trantas dots, limbal infiltration, and bulbar conjunctival hyperemia and edema. Upper tarsal papillary hypertrophy (cobblestoning) has been described in 5% to 10% of soft and 3% to 4% of hard contact lens wearers. Although this condition is most commonly seen in patients wearing contact lenses, it is also seen in patients with other foreign materials around the orbit such as ocular sutures, scleral buckles, or prosthetics. The contact lens polymer, preservative (thimerosal), and proteinaceous deposits on the surface of the lens have been implicated as the etiology of giant papillary conjunctivitis. The etiology remains controversial.

3. **Treatment** primarily involves the avoidance of the inciting process (i.e., removal of the contact lens), but when this is impractical, cromolyn sodium and topical corticosteroids assist in controlling the localized inflammatory process.

E. **Atopic keratoconjunctivitis**

1. **Basic mechanisms.** Atopic keratoconjunctivitis is mediated by a mixture of mast cell, IgE, and lymphocytic interactions along with infiltrations of basophils, eosinophils, plasma cells, and lymphocytes.

2. **History, physical examination, laboratory findings, and differential diagnosis.** A family history of atopy and its association with atopic dermatitis is common. Symptoms include itching, burning, and tearing. Signs include pale conjunctivae and limbal infiltration (Horner points or Trantas dots). Tears can contain IgE, eosinophils, and mononuclear cells with a paucity of basophils and mast cells. Other abnormalities include increased basophil histamine release, eosinophilia, and an elevated serum IgE.

3. **Complications.** Corneal ulceration and scarring, retinal detachment, keratoconus, and cataract formation (8%) can occur in patients with atopic keratoconjunctivitis. Cataracts are associated with this disease and predominantly involve the **anterior portion of the lens**, and can evolve rapidly into complete opacification within 6 months. Many patients may develop secondary staphylococcal blepharitis.

4. **Treatment** usually requires a multidisciplinary approach in consultation with an ophthalmologist. **Cool compresses** are often of some benefit to the patient. **Cromolyn sodium** or lodoxamide can be adjunctive treatment modalities in a small subset of patients. Topically applied and oral corticosteroids are the mainstay of treatment. Immunotherapy has no apparent effect on the progression of the disease. Topical cyclosporine has been used with some success in severe cases.

F. **Contact dermatitis**

1. **Basic mechanisms.** This is primarily a delayed-type hypersensitivity reaction invoking at times an intense lymphocyte-mediated conjunctival reaction.

2. **History, physical examination, laboratory findings, and differential diagnosis.** Delayed hypersensitivity reactions involving the eyelids frequently causes the patient to seek medical attention for a cutaneous reaction that elsewhere on the skin would be less of a concern. The eyelid skin being soft, pliable, and thin increases the eyelid's susceptibility to contact dermatitis. The eyelid skin is capable of developing significant swelling and redness with minor degrees of inflammation. There is a significant incidence of conjunctival and eyelid contact hypersensitivity to neomycin sulfate, in patients treated with this medication topically for conjunctivitis. This may lead to excessively prolonged conjunctivitis or presumed lack of therapeutic response and the addition of unnecessary topical antibiotics. Preservatives such as thimerosal that are found in contact lens cleaning solutions have been shown by patch tests to be one of the major culprits. This condition responds when the patient changes to the cleaning solutions that are preservative free. Interestingly, epinephrine hydrochloride itself, in the form of propine, used in the control of glaucoma has been implicated in the development of a local ocular delayed-type hypersensitivity reaction in some patients, as supported by patch testing to epinephrine.

   Contact dermatitis is the most common eruption of the eyelid, which is most often caused by cosmetics applied to the hair, face, or fingernails rather than by cosmetics directly applied to the eye area. It is important to bear in mind that the sites to which some of these cosmetics are applied may not be affected. This is particularly true for hair dye and nail polish. Allergic and irritant reactions to face creams, makeup (foundation lotions and bases), and blushes may likewise be limited to the eyelids. Stinging and burning of the eyes and lids on application of an eye-area cosmetic are the most common complaints. These subjective symptoms are usually transitory and unaccompanied by objective signs of irritation. Evaporation of volatile components (such as mineral spirits, isoparaffins, and alcohol) and the presence of potential irritants (such as propylene glycol and soap emulsifiers) in eye-area formulations are among the principal causes. In some instances, tolerance increases with subsequent applications, so that the offending product does not have to be discarded.

3. **Diagnosis.** The patch-test response to allergens and irritants may likewise be indistinguishable. Either allergens or irritants may elicit erythema and/or edema at the patch-test site. An eczematous vesicular reaction diagnostic of delayed allergic hypersensitivity in response to potential allergens in eye makeup is by no means the rule. Interpretation of patch-test results may consequently be difficult, and the likelihood of irritant false-positive reactions must be borne in mind.

III. **Ocular allergy treatment**

A. General considerations of treatment of ocular allergic disorders include the following (Table 5.3):

1. **Avoidance** remains the primary foundation for allergy treatment.

2. **Cold compresses** provide considerable symptomatic relief, especially from ocular pruritus. This relief is most likely due to a decrease in neural stimulation.

Table 5.3. A therapeutic overview for the treatment of the ocular allergic disorders

Therapeutic intervention	Clinical rationale	Pharmaceutical agents	Comments
PRIMARY			
Avoidance	Effective Simple in theory Typically difficult in practice		>30% symptom improvement
Cold compresses	Decrease nerve C fiber stimulation Reduce superficial vasodilation		Effective for mild to moderate symptoms
Preservative-free tears	Lavage Dilutional effect	Artificial tears	Extremely soothing Recommend refrigeration to improve symptomatic relief Inexpensive OTC Safe for all ages Comfortable Use as needed
SECONDARY			
Topical antihistamine and decongestants	Antihistamine relieves pruritus Vasoconstrictor relieves injection	Antazoline–naphazoline Pheniramine–naphazoline	Quick onset More effective than systemic antihistamines Limited duration of action Frequent dosing required
Topical antihistamine and mast cell stabilizer	Single agent with dual action Has immediate and prophylactic activity Eliminates need for two-drug therapy Comfort enhances patient compliance	Olopatadine (Patanol™) Ketotifen (Zaditor™) Azelastine (Optivar™)	B.i.d. dosing Dual-acting agents Antihistamine, mast cell stabilizer, inhibitor of inflammatory mediators More effective at relieving symptoms than other classes of agents Longer duration of action Safe and effective for patients 3 years and older

Category	Drugs	Notes
Topical mast cell stabilizers	Cromolyn (Crolom™) Lodoxamide (Alomide™) Nedocromil (Alocril™) Pemirolast (Alamast™)	Safe and effective for allergic diseases affecting corneal changes Cromolyn relives mild to moderate symptoms of vernal keratoconjunctivitis, vernal conjunctivitis, vernal keratitis Lodoxamide is highly potent Dosing 1–4 times daily Safe and effective for patients 3 years and older
Topical antihistamines	Levocabastine (Livostin™) Emedastine (Emadine™)	Relieves signs and symptoms of pruritus and erythema
Topical NSAIDs	Ketorolac (Acular™)	Relieves pruritus Stinging and/or burning on instillation experienced up to 40% of patients
TERTIARY		
Topical corticosteroids	Loteprednol (Lotemax™, Alrex™) Rimexolone (Vexol™) Fluorometholone (FML™)	Relieves all facets of the inflammatory response including erythema, edema, and pruritus Appropriate for short-term use only Contraindicated in patients with viral infections
Immunotherapy		Identify and modulate allergen sensitivity Adjunctive, although may be considered in secondary treatment in conjunction with allergic rhinitis
ANCILLARY		
Oral antihistamines	Loratadine Fexofenadine Cetirizine	Mildly effective for pruritus May cause dry eyes and worsening of ocular symptoms (especially first generation) May not effectively resolve the ocular signs and symptoms of allergy

OTC, over the counter; NSAIDs, nonsteroidal antiinflammatory drugs.

   3. **Lubrication** with artificial tears can be applied topically 2 to 4 times a
      day as necessary (the solution should be refrigerated before application
      to improve symptomatic relief) (Table 5.4).
   4. **Decongestants** (vasoconstrictors) may be applied topically 2 to 4 times
      a day as necessary. Oxymetazoline has a faster onset of action, longer
      duration of action, and better decongestant effect than naphazoline and
      tetrahydrozoline.
   5. **Topical antihistamines** such as levocabastine (Livostin 0.05%) and
      emedastine (Emadine 0.05%) are extremely selective H1-receptor antag-
      onists that have been shown to be excellent for ocular pruritus. Livostin
      dosage is for individuals 12 to 65 years old—one drop instilled in each eye,
      two times daily. The dose may be increased to one drop three to four times
      daily. Levocabastine has been reported to be more effective than oral ter-
      fenadine for treatment of seasonal allergic conjunctivitis. Emadastine
      (Emadine 0.05%) dosage is one drop in the affected eye up to four times

Table 5.4. Artificial tear preparations

Major component	Concentration	Trade name	Preservative/EDTA
Carboxymethylcellulose	0.5%	Cellufresh	None
	1%	Celluvisc	None
Hydroxyethylcellulose		Lyteers	Benzalkonium Cl + EDTA
		TearGard	sorbic acid + EDTA
Hydroxyethylcellulose + polyvinyl alcohol		Neo-Tears	Thimerosal + EDTA
Hydroxyethylcellulose + povidone		Adsorbotear	Thimerosal + EDTA
Hydroxypropyl cellulose		Lacrisert (Biodegradable insert)	None
Hydroxypropyl methyl-cellulose	0.5%	Isopto Plain	Benzalkonium Cl
		Isopto Tears	Benzalkonium Cl
		Tearisol	Benzalkonium Cl + EDTA
	1%	Isopto Alkaline	Benzalkonium Cl
		Ultra Tears	Benzalkonium Cl
Hydroxypropyl methyl-cellulose + dextran 70		Tears Naturale	Benzalkonium Cl + EDTA
		Tears Naturale II	Polyquad
		Tears Naturale Free	None
Hydroxypropyl methyl-cellulose + gelatin A		Lacril	Chlorobutanol + Polysorbate 80
Methylcellulose	1%	Murocel	Methyl- + propylparabens
Polyvinyl alcohol	1.4%	Akwa Tears	Benzalkonium Cl + EDTA
		Just Tears	Benzalkonium Cl + EDTA
		Liquifilm Tears	Chlorobutanol
		Liquifilm Forte	Thimerosal + EDTA
Polyvinyl alcohol + PEG-400 + dextrose	1%	Hypotears	Benzalkonium Cl + EDTA
		Hypotears PF	EDTA
Polyvinyl alcohol + povidone	1.4%	Murine	Benzalkonium Cl + EDTA
	0.6%	Refresh	None
		Tears Plus	Chlorobutanol

EDTA, ethylenediaminetetraacetic acid; PEG, polyethylene glycol.

daily. Over-the-counter antihistamine eye drops such as Naphcon-A, Vasocon-A, and Opcon-A contain either pheniramine or antazoline as a decongestant (e.g., naphazoline). These older antihistamines appear to have limited efficacy and the use of combination products for more than a few days can cause rebound congestion. Some topical antihistamines have other antiinflammatory effects (see Topical mast cell stabilizers below). Combined use of topical antihistamines and vasoconstricting agents is more effective than either agent alone for the relief of ocular itching.

6. **Oral antihistamines** also have a clinical effect on ocular symptoms of allergic rhinoconjunctivitis, but some patients may complain of worsening due to the excessive drying effect that is commonly seen with the use of the first-generation oral antihistamines, although increasing the doses of certain later-generation oral antihistamines (nonsedating) has also been observed to have a similar effect.

7. **Topical mast cell stabilizers** include cromolyn, lodoxamide, pemirolast, and nedocromil. Olopatadine, azelastine, and ketotifen have H1-receptor blocking activity as well as mast cell stabilizing activity.

   a. **Cromolyn sodium 4% ophthalmic solution** (Crolom) applied four to six times a day with the dosage being decreased incrementally to twice a day as symptoms permit (pregnancy category B). Cromolyn sodium acts by inhibiting the release of histamine and leukotrienes from sensitized mast cells. It is used for prophylaxis of allergic and vernal keratoconjunctivitis, is commonly initiated in patients with moderate symptoms, and may infrequently cause transient ocular burning and stinging.

   b. **Lodoxamide 0.1%** (Alomide) is a mast cell stabilizer 2,500 times more potent than cromolyn sodium in the prevention of histamine release in several animal models. Lodoxamide inhibits antigen-stimulated release of histamine and leukotrienes, and eosinophil chemotaxis. Clinical trials have shown lodoxamide delivers greater and earlier relief than cromolyn sodium in patients, and is used for prophylaxis of allergic and vernal keratoconjunctivitis. Lodoxamide is a 0.1% ophthalmic solution applied topically to adults and children older than 2 years of age. The usual regimen is 1 to 2 drops to each eye four times a day for up to 3 months (pregnancy category B). The most common side effects are transient local irritation, burning, and itching.

   c. **Pemirolast 0.1%** (Alamast), a pyridopyrimidine compound, is a mast cell stabilizer that is 100 times more potent than disodium cromoglycate. It has been approved in Japan for use in the treatment of bronchial asthma, allergic rhinitis, and allergic/vernal conjunctivitis. The usual regimen is one to two drops to each eye four times a day.

   d. **Nedocromil 2%** (Alocril) is a pyranoquinolone mast cell stabilizer that has been previously used in the treatment of asthma and is indicated for the treatment of ocular pruritus. It has been shown to relieve both the early- and late-phase symptoms of allergic conjunctivitis by inhibiting the release of histamine, decreasing chemotaxis, and inhibiting inflammatory cell actions. An environmental study reflects an onset of action within 15 minutes. Headache was increased, but does not appear to be clinically significant (pregnancy category B)

   e. **Olopatadine 0.05%** (Patanol) is another agent with multiple mechanisms of action that affects H1-receptor binding, with inhibition of mast cell mediator release shown to be greater than 90% in *in vitro* studies and with effects on a variety of other inflammatory cells, including eosinophilic infiltration. Olopatadine combined with oral loratadine produced greater relief of ocular itching than loratadine alone. The half-life of the drug is about 3 hours and the drug is administered in a usual dosage of one to two drops in each affected eye twice daily at an interval of 5 to 8 hours. Olopatadine can be administered to children as young as 3 years old and is well tolerated (pregnancy category C).

      f. Azelastine 0.05% (Optivar) appears to have a triple-action effect. It is an H1-receptor antagonist (antihistamine effect), stabilizes mast cells (mast cell stabilizing effect), and inhibits inflammation (anti-inflammatory effect). The dosage is twice a day because of the long duration of the drug's effectiveness (8 to 10 hours) in individuals 3 years and older. It has an onset of action within several minutes after application (pregnancy category B).

      g. Ketotifen 0.025% (Zaditor) also has several actions focusing on the H1-receptor and mast cell stabilization, as well as eosinophil chemotaxis and adhesion molecules. The recommended dosage for individuals 3 years and older is one drop in the affected eye every 8 to 12 hours (pregnancy category C).

8. **Nonsteroidal antiinflammatory drugs** (NSAIDs) administered orally (aspirin) as well as topically applied inhibitors of the cyclooxygenase system (1% suprofen) have been used in the treatment of vernal keratoconjunctivitis. Another topically applied NSAID (0.03% flurbiprofen) has been examined in the treatment of allergic conjunctivitis and decreased conjunctival, ciliary, and episcleral hyperemia and ocular pruritus. The primary benefit of these medications in the eye may be related to the control of pruritus. Flurbiprofen (Ocufen), ketorolac (Acular), and diclofenac (Voltaren) are three topical nonsteroidal medications approved for the treatment of ocular conditions. Further studies are underway for NSAIDs in the treatment of allergic conjunctivitis, including flurbiprofen and ketorolac tromethamine, which have been shown in clinical studies to significantly diminish the ocular itching and conjunctival hyperemia associated with allergic conjunctivitis. Topical ocular NSAIDs, unlike topical corticosteroids, do not mask ocular infections, affect wound healing, increase IOP, or contribute to cataract formation. NSAIDs derived from indole (indomethacin, sulindac, tolmetin), pyrazolon (phenylbutazone, oxyphenabutazone, apazone, ketorolac), propionic acid (ibuprofen, flurbiprofen, ketoprofen, naproxen), and fenamate have been developed for topical treatment of inflammatory conditions of the eye, but have been associated with a low to moderate incidence of burning and stinging.

9. **Topical ocular corticosteroids.** When topically administered medications such as antihistamines, vasoconstrictors, or cromolyn sodium are ineffective, milder topical steroids are a consideration. Topical corticosteroids are highly effective in the treatment of acute and chronic forms of allergic conjunctivitis and are regretfully required for control of some of the more severe variants of conjunctivitis, including atopic keratoconjunctivitis, vernal conjunctivitis, and giant papillary conjunctivitis. However, the local administration of these medications is not without possible localized ocular complications, including increased IOP (i.e., glaucoma), viral infections, and cataract formation. Topically or systemically administered steroids will produce a transient increase in IOP in susceptible individuals; this trait is thought to be genetically influenced. Two "modified" steroids rimexolone (Vexol) and loteprednol (Lotemax 0.5%; Alrex 0.2%) have shown excellent efficacy with minimal side effects in the treatment of allergic conjunctivitis. They have also been used for anterior uveitis.

10. **Allergen immunotherapy** is a well established treatment for allergic conjunctivitis. Studies have shown that children receiving immunotherapy to specific mold allergen, *Cladosporium*, ragweed, Japanese cedar, or animal dander (*Fel d* I allergen), were found to require less medications and required higher doses of topically applied allergen to induce allergic symptoms of redness, pruritus, and swelling in ocular challenges.

11. **Contact lens wear and topical medications** The general recommendation is not to apply any medication to the eyes while wearing contact lenses. However, in the practical day-to-day use where patients are using disposable lenses and when their eyes are not injected, they could

be advised to either use their topical medications but frequently dispose of their disposable contact lenses, or wait at least 10 minutes after instilling topical ocular medication before they insert their contact lenses. This will decrease the likelihood of developing an adverse reaction to the medication as it is absorbed into the predominantly water matrix of the contact lenses, while increasing the longevity of the extended-wear soft contact lens.

B. Ophthalmological consultation should be obtained for:
- The evaluation of any patient using ocular corticosteroids for more than 2 weeks for the presence of cataracts and increased intraocular pressure.
- Any persistent ocular complaint.
- The consideration of using strong topical or systemic corticosteroids.

IV. Other forms of the "red eye"

A. Keratoconjunctivitis sicca. KCS and other dry eye syndromes are the most common entities confused with ocular allergic disorders. KCS is commonly associated with underlying systemic immune disorders such as Sjögren syndrome, rheumatoid arthritis, human immunodeficiency virus (HIV) infection, and notably, in postmenopausal women. It is characterized by an insidious and progressive dysfunction of the lacrimal glands. Patients initially complain of a mildly injected eye with excessive mucus production. Symptoms include a gritty, sandy feeling in the eyes as compared to the itching and burning feeling many patients complain with ocular allergy. The symptoms worsen throughout the day as the limited portion of the aqueous tear film evaporates. Exacerbation of symptoms also occurs in the winter months when heating systems decrease the relative humidity in the household to less than 25%.

   1. The **Schirmer test** generally demonstrates decreased tearing with 0 to 1 mm (normal is greater than 4 mm) of wetting at 1 minute and 2 to 3 mm (normal is greater than 10 mm) at 5 minutes. Rose Bengal staining providing a distinct staining pattern over the central portion of the eye also assists in identifying the defect in tear film production. Biopsy of the lacrimal or minor salivary gland reveals an abnormal infiltration of lymphocytes. Treatment has primarily focused on the replacement of tear fluid constituents with a variety of lubricants and artificial tears.

B. Pemphigoid and pemphigus. Pemphigoid of the eye, known as **cicatricial pemphigoid**, has a similar histopathologic picture to bullous pemphigoid of the skin, in that the desmosomal attachments between epithelial cells are lysed. IgG and IgA bind to the basement membrane in 80% of patients. When the subepidermal blister ruptures, an overgrowth of fibrous tissue occurs, leading to severe corneal damage, dry eyes, neovascularization with fibrosis, and subsequent loss of vision. In the eye, the denuded conjunctival epithelium leads to adhesions termed symblepharons, which can obliterate the mechanical closing of the eyelids and the mucous-producing goblet cells. Similar to pemphigoid, **pemphigus vulgaris** is mediated by complement-fixing IgG to intercellular cement substance producing acantholysis and intraepithelial blisters all over the body, including the skin, mouth, and eyes. Lesions of the eye commonly involve the conjunctivae. The bursting of the bullae is painful but the area usually heals without sequelae.

C. Uveitis. Ocular inflammation is associated with increasing visual loss as one proceeds from the anterior portion to the posterior pole. Although ocular allergy is the most common form of ocular inflammation, anterior uveitis is the most common form of intraocular inflammation. Intraocular inflammation is normally described by location, with **anterior uveitis** involving all structures anterior to and including the lens–iris diaphragm and posterior segment intraocular inflammation (posterior uveitis) including structures behind the lens–iris diaphragm such as the ciliary body, retina, and choroid. Some disorders involve both portions and are called **panuveitis**. Anterior uveitis is commonly classified as (i) autoimmune (idiopathic) affecting the eye only, (ii) associated with a systemic disease, or (iii) associated with trauma. Anterior uveitis is frequently unilateral and may be self-limiting, but when it is associated with a systemic immune disorder it is often more chronic, recurrent, and may be bilateral. Uveitis is not to be confused with another form of intraocular inflammation called **endophthalmitis** that is usually limited to **infectious** forms of uveitis, i.e., where the infection is the major cause of inflammatory response leading to tissue damage. However, some forms of infections may cause intraocular inflammation predominantly through a cross-reaction to antigens versus a direct infection as is suspected with uveitis associated with tuberculosis or syphilis. However, a staphylo-coccal infection causes major destruction through direct tissue invasion. The choroid contains a sparse collection of B and T lymphocytes, mast cells, and fibroblasts. When inflamed, it becomes densely populated with plasma cells, phagocytes, and B and T lymphocytes, which may form pseudolymphoid follicles or granulomas with some cells entering the aqueous humor. A variety of specific uveal antigens have been isolated and shown to be capable on inducing uveitis, and include the soluble **S antigen** (molecular weight 55 kD) and **opsin retinal proteins**.

1. **Clinical features, symptoms, and signs**
   a. Common clinical features of anterior uveitis include inflammatory cells and protein exudate floating in the anterior chamber, with deposition of cells and protein on the endothelial surface of the cornea (corneal deposits—**keratic precipitates**) when there is an intense process. Some have further classified the inflammatory process based on cell type as nongranulomatous (predominantly neutrophil) versus granulomatous (predominantly lymphocyte and macrophage). Involvement of the ciliary body is commonly accompanied with miosis, dilatation, and engorgement of the ciliary vessels (ciliary injection).
   b. The symptoms of anterior uveitis are dependent upon the inflammatory processes that occur and their location. Blurring of vision occurs from infiltration of cells and protein into the anterior chamber. Photophobia and glare occurs from corneal epithelial edema, infiltration of cells and protein into the anterior chamber, and ciliary muscular spasm. Pain is an important sign indicating intraocular inflammation. Pain is not associated with conjunctival inflammation as seen in ocular allergies. Pain can vary from mild to severe. Severe pain is often associated with ciliary muscle spasm. As the pain persists the patient may develop a dull aching sensation in the eye or a generalized headache. Periorbital pain and pain or tenderness on rubbing or touching the eye should raise the concern for increased intraocular pressure, i.e., glaucoma. Pain on palpation or movement of the eye is also a sign of inflammation of the outer sheath of the eye, i.e., scleritis. Tearing is a common symptom and is related to the stimulation of the parasympathetic nerves.
   c. The signs of anterior uveitis include lid edema or even pseudoptosis, injection with a ciliary distribution, i.e., increasing intensity of the injection from the periphery to the corneal–scleral junction, and the injection appears to have a more purplish hue. Notably, the conjunctival surface remains clear, whereas conjunctival injection appears more intense and distributed throughout the periphery than at the corneal–scleral junction. Conjunctival injection also involves both the conjunctival and palpebral surfaces. When the inflammation is intense, a large number of inflammatory cells accumulate in the form of a hypopyon. Miosis is usually a sign of ciliary muscle spasm, but may also be due to adhesion of the inflamed iris to the anterior lens capsule (posterior synechia). Synechia can also form between the iris and the cornea readily within hours, especially in the presence of miosis. Severe inflammation of the iris leads to engorgement of the fragile iris blood vessels and possibly a localized hemorrhage that forms a hyphema. Direct iris infiltration with accumulation of inflammatory cells can lead to nodular lesions within the iris (Busacca nodules) or at the rim of the pupil (Koeppe nodules). Increased intraocular pres-

sure is not uncommon for a variety of reasons including inflammatory infiltration, edema, and ciliary body detachment. Cataract is the most common complication of anterior uveitis.

2. **Clinical immunological investigation**

   a. The immunological investigation of the patient with anterior uveitis includes asking about a history of recent infection with gram-negative organisms or viral infections, history of symptoms associated with systemic disease, such as joint symptoms, mucosal lesions (aphthous ulcerations), respiratory symptoms, and a history relevant to assess a state of immunosuppression, including exposure to HIV. The following tests are recommended in the evaluation and the preparation for further systemic immunomodulatory treatment: complete blood count with differential and platelets; 24 hour urine collection for protein, creatinine (creatinine clearance) for evidence of glomerulonephritis associated with various autoimmune disorders, and calcium (for hypercalciuria associated with sarcoid); erythrocyte sedimentation rate and C-reactive protein (general markers of inflammation associated with rheumatoid arthritis and vasculitis); serum chemistries including blood urea nitrogen, liver enzymes, electrolytes, angiotensin converting enzyme levels (associated with chronic granulomatous disorders such as sarcoid or granulomatous infections); a urinalysis for glucose; a chest radiograph and a tuberculin skin test with a full anergy panel for the possible infection with tuberculosis or histoplasmosis and to assess for anergy that can be seen in sarcoid, HIV infection, and the possible pathergic response seen in Behçet disease. One should also consider doing specific tests that focus on the presence of certain physical findings, such as:

      (1) Cutaneous eruptions and arthritis: include various antibody assays for autoimmune disorders such as systemic lupus erythematosus, Wegener granulomatosis, anticardiolipin syndrome, and infectious disorders such as Lyme disease or syphilis (antinuclear antibodies, antineutrophilic cytoplasmic antibodies, lupus anticoagulant, anticardiolipin antibodies, serology for Lyme and syphilis);

      (2) Genitourinary tract symptoms: include culture for nonspecific urethritis (chlamydial and gonococcal infections);

      (3) Gastrointestinal symptoms: include endoscopy and colonoscopy/biopsy to evaluate for possible inflammatory bowel disease (Crohn disease).

   b. Close cooperation with the ophthalmologist is necessary to maximize the clinical outcome.

V. **Adverse reactions to ocular medications**

   A. **Topical beta-adrenergic receptor antagonists** are commonly the agents of choice for the treatment of glaucoma. The presumed mechanism of action is the decreased production of aqueous humor in the anterior chamber of the eye, which subsequently decreases IOP. Some of the topical beta-blockers currently available include cardioselective agents (e.g., betaxolol) and nonselective agents (e.g., levobunolol, metipranolol, and timolol). Topical betaxolol has been shown to cause less bronchospasm in patients with asthma when compared with the nonselective agents. However, all of the topical beta-blockers have been reported to produce respiratory symptoms in certain patients. The development of respiratory symptoms with minute quantities of topical beta-adrenergic blocker medications may be due to higher serum concentrations of drug that bypass hepatic degradation and directly enter the pulmonary vascular bed.

   B. **Intravenous fluorescein** (i.e., fluorescein angiograms) is used for a more thorough examination of the retinal and choroidal vasculature. Anaphylactoid reactions have been reported with an overall incidence of 5% increasing to about 50% for patients who have had a previous history of reactions to fluorescein angiograms. The mortality rate has been reported to be 1 per 220,000 fluorescein procedures (0.5% on initial exposure), resulting in several deaths each year in the United States. Intravenous fluorescein reactions are associated with the development of nausea (2.9%), vomiting (1.2%), flushing and urticaria (0.2%), and systemic features consistent with anaphylactic shock similar to those caused by high osmolar contrast media. Elevated plasma levels of histamine have been found in patients receiving intravenous fluorescein. Immediate skin testing in patients with prior history of intravenous fluorescein reactions is not helpful. Premedication protocols with H1- and H2-receptor blockers and prednisone have been anecdotally successful (see Chapter 10 for information on treatment for anaphylaxis).

Selected Readings

1. Berdy GJ, Hedqvist B. Ocular allergic disorders and dry eye disease: associations, diagnostic dilemmas, and management. *Acta Ophthalmol Scand Suppl* 2000; 230:32–37.
2. Bielory L. Allergic and immunologic disorders of the eye. Part II: ocular allergy. *J Allergy Clin Immunol* 2000;106:1019–1032.
3. Friedlaender MH. The current and future therapy of allergic conjunctivitis. *Curr Opin Ophthalmol* 1998;9:54–58.
4. Trocme SD, Raizman MB, Bartley GB. Medical therapy for ocular allergy. *Mayo Clin Proc* 1992;67:557–565.

6. ASTHMA

Ali I. Musani, Rodolfo M. Pascual, and Stephen P. Peters

I. Introduction

In 1998, there were 5,438 deaths from asthma in the United States. It has been estimated that nearly 17 million Americans are affected and it was the principal diagnosis listed for more than 12.9 million visits to office-based physicians in 1998. In addition, asthma results in nearly 2 million emergency department visits, 3 million lost workdays, and more than $6 billion in healthcare costs each year. The incidence and prevalence of asthma in developed countries seems to be increasing, and importantly, a disproportionate burden of asthma morbidity and mortality is born by ethnic minorities, the very young, the very old, and the poor. It is an especially important public health problem because much of the potential morbidity and mortality attributable to asthma is avoidable.

II. Definition

The definition of asthma has evolved as our understanding of the pathogenesis has become more sophisticated. In 1997, a National Institutes of Health (NIH) consensus group defined asthma on the basis of the current understanding of its pathogenesis. Asthma is a chronic inflammatory disorder of the airways in which many cells and cellular elements play a role, in particular, mast cells, eosinophils, T lymphocytes, macrophages, neutrophils, and epithelial cells. In susceptible individuals, this inflammation causes recurrent episodes of wheezing, breathlessness, chest tightness, and coughing, particularly at night or in the early morning. These episodes are usually associated with widespread but variable airflow obstruction that is often reversible, either spontaneously or with treatment. The inflammation also causes an associated increase in the existing bronchial hyperresponsiveness to a variety of stimuli. Moreover, recent evidence indicates that subbasement fibrosis may occur in some patients with asthma, and that these changes contribute to persistent abnormalities in lung function.

A. Asthma is a chronic inflammatory disorder of the airways

As implied in the above general definition, there is no question that inflammation plays a crucial role in the pathogenesis of asthma, and recognition of this fact has led to a paradigm shift in asthma management. Numerous studies have demonstrated that varying degrees of chronic inflammation are present in the airways of all asthmatics, including those with clinically mild disease. Moreover, significant inflammation has even been demonstrated in the airways *in vivo* of asthmatics during symptom-free periods. Importantly, there is mounting evidence that asthmatics have greater annual declines in lung function than the general population, and that failing to treat this inflammation may lead to increased morbidity and mortality.

In susceptible individuals, this inflammation causes recurrent episodes of wheezing, breathlessness, chest tightness, and coughing, particularly at night or in the early morning. Asthma is a disease characterized by exacerbations, and although atypical symptoms may be present, the majority of patients will have one or more of these cardinal symptoms. In addition, there is no question that the presence of symptoms correlates with the presence of airway inflammation *in vivo*, and this has been demonstrated in numerous studies.

B. Bronchial hyperresponsiveness

The inflammation also causes an associated increase in the existing bronchial hyperresponsiveness to a variety of stimuli. Bronchial hyperreactivity (BHR) is an important concept to understand because its presence may be key in establishing a diagnosis of asthma in a given patient. Clinical studies have shown that the degree of BHR strongly correlates with the amount of inflammation and symptoms, as well as overall asthma severity in most patients.

C. Airway remodeling

Recent evidence indicates that subbasement fibrosis may occur in some patients with asthma and that these changes contribute to persistent abnormalities in lung function. The classic teaching about asthma was that the resultant airflow obstruction was completely reversible or nearly so. Many authorities now believe that the airways are remodeled as a result of an unbalanced inflammation–repair response. Recent studies suggest that both structural and functional changes in the airway may result in persistent declines in lung function.

III. Pathophysiology

Asthma is a chronic inflammatory disease involving the airways, and many cells and mediators play key roles. Postmortem studies in patients who died from their asthma demonstrate large and small airways containing mucus plugs/casts, cellular debris, and proteins. Histopathologic changes involve the whole thickness of the airway and include epithelial denudation, edema, mast cell activation, subbasement membrane collagen deposition, and mucosal and submucosal infiltration by eosinophils, neutrophils, and lymphocytes. In addition, the airway smooth muscle is often hypertrophied and vascular proliferation and mucous gland hypertrophy are present. Experimental models suggest that changes in the layers of the airway alter its geometry and subsequent function. The contributions of various cell types and mediators have been studied in a number of models both *in vitro* and *in vivo*. Bronchoscopy and airway challenge studies have added much to our understanding about the control and consequences of airway inflammation.

A. Asthma associated with atopy

Asthma often begins in childhood and is frequently associated with atopy. Atopy refers to the genetic susceptibility to develop specific immunoglobulin E (IgE) antibodies against common environmental allergens. Atopy is also strongly associated with allergic dermatitis (eczema) and rhinitis. Extrinsic asthma refers to asthma that is associated with atopy; this terminology is older, confusing, and is less commonly used. Epidemiological studies have shown that asthma is more prevalent in "Western," industrialized countries. A number of theories have been offered to explain this. One theory under intense investigation suggests that increased use of antibiotics in childhood, cleaner drinking water, improved sanitation, as well as widespread vaccination practices have led to a lower cumulative exposure to microbial pathogens. In other words, conditions that are found in industrialized nations could be associated with an increase in asthma prevalence. T-helper lymphocytes or cluster of differentiation 4 (CD4$^+$) lymphocytes are key regulators of both cell-mediated and humoral immunity. Naïve T-helper lymphocytes (Th0) cells differentiate into either Th1 or Th2 phenotypes based on their local milieu. Th1 cells are more prevalent in the presence of infections and they secrete interferon-gamma while Th2 cells seem to play a prominent role in allergic disease and secrete IL-3, IL-4, IL-5 and GM-CSF. Th2 cells are found in increased numbers in the airways of asthmatics. It is believed that in normal subjects there is a balance between Th1 and Th2 lymphocytes, whereas in asthma there is an imbalance favoring the so-called Th2 or allergic phenotype. Because there is a decreased exposure in childhood to infection, the Th1 phenotype may be underexpressed and the Th2 phenotype relatively overexpressed. This imbalance has been blamed on improved sanitation and cleaner living conditions and forms the basis of the hygiene hypothesis for asthma. For more about this Th1/Th2 paradigm, refer to Chapter 1 and/or recent reviews.

B. Intrinsic/extrinsic asthma

In population studies the incidence of atopy and hence total IgE levels declines with age. Asthma that occurs in the absence of atopy frequently used to be called "intrinsic asthma." Like "extrinsic asthma," this term is now infrequently used. Asthma that first occurs in adults is not as closely linked to atopy, and when it occurs in older adults, it tends to be more severe and less responsive to standard therapy. The pathogenesis of asthma first expressed in adulthood is poorly understood compared to childhood onset disease. However, it is increasingly recognized that many of these patients likely had asthma as children that was misdiagnosed or undiagnosed. Studies of the pathogenesis and clinical features of atopic versus nonatopic asthma suggest some important differences between these two asthma subtypes.

IV. Relationship of pulmonary function and airway inflammation

  A. Airway hyperresponsiveness or BHR is a cardinal manifestation of asthma. A patient with BHR will develop bronchoconstriction in response to a provocation or stimulus that would otherwise elicit little or no response in a normal person. Numerous studies have shown that asthmatics have a greater degree of bronchial responsiveness than do normal subjects. In addition, asthmatics that are currently experiencing symptoms or an exacerbation exhibit greater BHR than when they are asymptomatic.

  B. Airflow obstruction
  Airflow obstruction is also a cardinal manifestation of asthma. Some degree of airflow obstruction is present in nearly all patients with asthma when acute symptoms are present. Reversibility refers to the rapid relief of obstruction upon treatment with a bronchodilator. In fact, at least partial reversibility of obstruction, if present, is required to diagnose asthma. *In vivo* studies using bronchoscopy have demonstrated that the degree of airflow obstruction, much like the degree of BHR, directly correlates with the severity of airway inflammation. It was thought that airflow obstruction was completely reversible in asthma, but that is not true in every case. There is a significant subset of patients who never smoked cigarettes and who have at least some component of irreversibility to their airflow obstruction. Moreover, some patients with asthma seem to lose lung function at an accelerated rate, that is, their annual decline in forced expiratory volume in 1 second (FEV_1) is greater than age matched controls. These clinical observations have led to a great deal of research and many authorities believe that the asthmatic airway undergoes changes or remodeling that can lead to progressive reductions in airflow over time. How this process can be modulated or controlled has been an area of active research. Whether control of airway inflammation might attenuate the annual decline in FEV_1, and perhaps ameliorate the development of irreversible airflow obstruction, is an area of passionate debate. This airway-remodeling paradigm has led to the hypothesis that inflammation associated with asthma, if left unchecked, can lead to irreversible losses of lung function and thus has important therapeutic implications.

V. Clinical features and initial diagnosis
  Because there is no single gold-standard test that defines asthma, it remains a clinical diagnosis. Therefore, the combination of history, physical examination, and laboratory findings is used to make the diagnosis. When features consistent with asthma are present, the clinician may make the diagnosis with confidence.

VI. Risk factors
  The phenotypic expression of asthma is the result of the interplay of multiple genetic and environmental factors. Population studies suggest that gender, atopy, bronchial hyperresponsiveness, perinatal factors, and genetics all play a role. Further studies suggest that exposure to aeroallergens, outdoor pollution, respiratory infections, and tobacco smoke can be factors as well.

  A. Childhood asthma as a male disease
  Childhood asthma is predominantly a male disease and this may be due in part to the increased prevalence of atopy in male children. Morphometric studies also indicate that the airways of male children tend to be smaller and hence more vulnerable to airflow obstruction. However, by the second and third decade, the prevalence is similar in the sexes and the prevalence then reverses later in life so that more females have asthma in the fourth decade and beyond.

B. Bronchial hyperresponsiveness and asthma

Not all people who have BHR have symptoms of asthma, although patients with asthma and current symptoms nearly always have BHR when tested. However, BHR is not unique to asthma and is present in many patients with other diseases of the airways, including chronic obstructive pulmonary disease (COPD) and bronchiectasis. Therefore, BHR cannot be equated with asthma. However, one cohort study in children suggested that the presence of BHR was a risk factor for the subsequent diagnosis of asthma on follow-up visits. Viewed in another way, BHR might be a precursor to full-blown asthma.

C. Criteria of atopy

Atopy is closely linked to asthma. Atopy is diagnosed using three criteria: skin test reactivity, eosinophilia, and serum IgE levels. Large population studies demonstrate that the prevalence of self-reported asthma correlates strongly with serum IgE levels. There is also a positive correlation with skin test reactivity, though it is not as robust. Similarly, elevated IgE levels are a risk factor for the subsequent diagnosis of asthma in children. Whether IgE causes asthma or is a marker of a phenotype that expresses asthma is a matter of debate.

Population studies suggest that the atopy seems to be strongly linked to genetic factors. Asthma also appears to be linked to genetic factors, but perhaps to a lesser extent. Nonetheless, depending on the population under study, the presence of asthma in one or both parents seems to be an important risk factor, with the maternal factor probably being more important than the paternal.

D. Genetics

Asthma is a clinical diagnosis, and because the diagnosis has been applied inconsistently, efforts at isolating specific genetic factors have been hampered. Studies of family pedigrees suggest that there are genetic factors, but they do not follow a simple mendelian pattern; that is, asthma is probably not monogenetic. Linkage analysis has suggested a link with atopic asthma and the long arm of chromosome 5 (5q). Notably, the loci of several Th2 cytokines and the beta$_2$-adrenergic receptor (B2AR) are located on chromosome 5 as well. Much work has been done studying polymorphisms of the B2AR as well as the interleukin 4 (IL-4) receptor gene; however, the role of such polymorphisms in the genesis or expression of asthma is not clear. It is becoming more apparent that asthma is a heterogeneous disease in its phenotypic expression, so it is likely that the genotypic expression will be heterogeneous as well. Nonetheless, eliciting a family history of asthma or atopy lends further strength to the diagnosis.

E. Aeroallergen exposure

Aeroallergen exposure is a risk factor for the development of asthma. It is becoming clear that indoor allergens play a significant role in many cases. Indoor allergens include house dust mite, animal allergens (especially dog and cat), cockroach, and fungi. It is therefore appropriate to ask patients suspected of having asthma if they have any pets or moldy odors in their home or in the workplace. House dust mites are found in increased concentrations in bedrooms, especially those that are carpeted, so asking questions about furnishings and coverings may be helpful. Similarly, cockroach antigen is also ubiquitous, but especially so in urban settings. Surprisingly, there is no evidence that outdoor air pollution contributes to the pathogenesis of asthma. However, industrial pollution does increase the incidence of bronchitis and other respiratory illness and can contribute to exacerbations of preexisting asthma.

F. Cigarette smoking

Cigarette smoking and BHR have been linked in population-based studies, however, the role of smoking in the pathogenesis of asthma in the adult asthmatic is not clear. In fact, asthmatics are probably less likely to start smoking than their nonasthmatic counterparts. Cohort studies suggest that perinatal maternal smoking and childhood environmental tobacco smoke exposure may contribute to the pathogenesis of asthma in childhood. Notably, environmental cigarette smoke (second-hand smoke) is a nonspecific asthma trigger in many patients with BHR and asthma.

G. Occupational risk factors

Asthma is the most prevalent occupational lung disease in developed countries. There are two major categories of asthma in the workplace: occupational asthma (OA) and work-aggravated asthma. Stated simply, OA is caused by conditions in a particular work environment; i.e., asthma that develops because of exposure to a particular factor in the workplace. Host factors, exposure to certain types of substances, and the intensity of exposure probably determine the risk of OA. In most patients a latency period of several months to several years is present before the development of asthma. The reactive airways-dysfunction syndrome (RADS) is a unique and interesting form of occupational lung disease. Typically with RADS, asthma symptoms and BHR develop immediately after a brief intense exposure. In this situation the intensity of the exposure is the most important factor. Population prevalence studies suggest a broad range of prevalence rates for OA. This broad range of prevalence is due in part because even though many workers will report symptoms suggestive of OA, a minority will have occupational asthma confirmed by objective measures such as specific inhalation challenge. More common than asthma that develops because of the workplace is preexisting asthma that is exacerbated by workplace exposures.

VII. History

The types of symptoms, as well as their pattern, are important clues because the manifestations of asthma are manyfold and the diagnosis is made on clinical grounds. The most common symptoms include cough, wheezing, shortness of breath, chest tightness, and sputum production. Classically, the triad of cough, wheezing, and dyspnea occur together during an exacerbation of asthma. However, any symptom can occur singly or in combination with another. Furthermore, the symptoms of asthma are nonspecific, that is, they occur in many other respiratory diseases. This is even true of wheezing, which is often considered a cardinal symptom. For example, the postnasal drip syndrome can present with cough, wheeze, dyspnea, and sputum expectoration just like asthma. In fact, in one study of patients who presented to a pulmonary outpatient clinic with the complaint of wheezing, more patients were subsequently diagnosed with postnasal drip than asthma. However, asthma was diagnosed in more than one-third of patients in the series and should be considered strongly in the differential diagnosis of any patient who is wheezing.

The pattern of symptoms can also suggest the diagnosis. Many patients with asthma have atopy, so symptoms tend to show a seasonal variation. In other words, the atopic asthmatic will have increased airflow obstruction and BHR during increased exposure to aeroallergen to which he or she is allergic. The clinical correlate will be a seasonal variation in the amount of cough, dyspnea, and wheeze that the asthmatic experiences. Asthmatics have increased BHR at baseline when compared to normal subjects and this difference is even more pronounced during a period of exacerbation. As a result, many asthmatics will develop symptoms of airflow obstruction when they are exposed to "specific triggers" such as aeroallergens, cold air, strong odors, cigarette smoke, and other forms of air pollution. Again, one must recognize that sensitivity to triggers can occur with other disease states. Finally, most asthmatics display a diurnal variation in airflow obstruction manifest by a greater prevalence of symptoms in the early morning hours. As a result, many patients will complain of cough and wheeze that awakens them from sleep. Conversely, many asthmatics will state that they feel best in the late afternoon/early evening time period. This diurnal variation in symptoms has been correlated both with variations in lung function measured with spirometry, and with airway inflammation *in vivo* using bronchoalveolar lavage (BAL) and bronchoscopic biopsy sampling techniques.

VIII. Physical examination

When asthma is suspected on the basis of the history, the physical examination should include a careful assessment of the upper and lower respiratory tracts and the skin. Asthma is a disease characterized by BHR and airflow obstruction that is mediated by inflammation. Although it is an inflammatory disease, constitutional symptoms such as fever, weight loss, and arthralgias are not common and should suggest an alternative diagnosis. It should be recognized that asthma exists concurrently with other diseases where constitutional symptoms may be prominent, such as allergic bronchopulmonary aspergillosis or Churg-Strauss vasculitis. Moreover, upper and lower viral respiratory infections are common triggers of asthma exacerbations and these may cause prominent constitutional symptoms.

A. Wheeze

Wheeze during normal breathing is recognized as a classic manifestation of airflow obstruction and it is commonly heard on auscultation when asthma is present. It is important to note that because airflow obstruction is often intermittent, so too will be the finding of wheeze. In addition, wheezing heard on forced exhalation is a nonspecific finding when wheezes are not heard with normal breathing. High-pitched musical end-expiratory wheezes are most frequently heard in asthma. Often there is concurrent mucus production and the correlate would be rhonchi or wheezes with a "wet" or coarse quality. Wheezes are more commonly heard in children. Some adults, particularly those with so-called "cough-variant asthma," will not wheeze. Sometimes wheezes are not present even when airflow obstruction is present. A prolonged expiratory phase or a quiet chest with decreased airflow is also frequently observed. In fact, one should not take solace when wheezes are absent, because more severe airflow obstruction and hyperinflation may be present. Generally, other clues such as hyperresonance/hyperinflation, nasal flaring, intercostal retractions, and other accessory muscle use are present when this is the case. Conversely, the presence of wheeze is not always indicative of asthma. Wheeze is frequently heard with acute or chronic bronchitis, emphysema, postnasal drip syndrome, acute viral upper and lower respiratory tract infections, vocal cord dysfunction syndrome, and upper airway obstructing lesions, among other conditions (Table 6.1). Notably, persistent wheeze, especially when it does not respond to therapy, should raise the suspicion of upper airway neoplasm or obstruction.

B. Manifestations of atopy

Because asthma is often an atopic disease, other manifestations of atopy are often present. Examination of the skin may reveal atopic dermatitis/eczema or another rash. Similarly examination of the nose might reveal allergic rhinitis manifested by increased secretions, mucosal swelling, or nasal obstruction. Nasal polyps are associated with asthma, especially in patients with aspirin sensitivity.

C. Physical signs

The physical examination of severely ill asthmatics deserves mention. In children, certain physical signs are ominous and indicate a more severe attack. Signs of a severe asthma flare in children include an anxious appearance with signs of air hunger, and distressed children tend to sit upright. Other ominous signs include diaphoresis, pallor, cyanosis, and accessory muscle use. Accessory muscles include the intercostal, subcostal, and sternocleidomastoid muscles. Similarly, adult physical findings of severe asthma might include any alteration in consciousness, fatigue, upright posture, diaphoresis, and the use of accessory muscles of breathing. Tachypnea (respiratory rate greater than 30 per minute), tachycardia (pulse greater than 120 per minute), and a decrease of more than 15 mm Hg in systolic blood pressure during inspiration (pulsus paradoxus) are more common in severe attacks. It is important to appreciate, however, that the absence of these findings does not exclude even immediately life-threatening airflow obstruction, especially if the patient is exhausted or obtunded.

Table 6.1. Selected causes of wheeze or noisy breathing

Upper airway obstruction
  Extrathoracic causes
    Anaphylaxis/angioedema
    Postnasal drip syndrome
    Nasal polyps
    Rhinitis
    Vocal cord dysfunction
      Vagal/recurrent laryngeal nerve compression
      Vocal cord dysfunction syndrome
      Cricoarytenoid dysfunction
        Cricoarytenoid dislocation
        Cricoarytenoid arthritis
    Laryngeal edema
      Gastroesophageal reflux
    Upper airway tumors
    Goiter
    Hypertrophied tonsils
    Obesity
  Intrathoracic causes
    Tracheal stenosis
      Wegener granulomatosis
      Postintubation
      Relapsing polychondritis
    Tracheal and bronchial tumors
    Tracheobronchomegaly
    Goiter
    Foreign body aspiration
    Tracheobronchitis
Lower airways obstruction
  Eosinophilic lung diseases
    Asthma
    Eosinophilic bronchitis
    Allergic bronchopulmonary aspergillosis
    Churg-Straus vasculitis
    Hypereosinophillic syndrome
    Simple pulmonary eosinophila
    Acute eosinophilic pneumonia
    Chronic eosinophilic pneumonia
    Tropical pulmonary eosinophilia
  Chronic obstructive pulmonary disease
  Bronchiectasis
  Cystic fibrosis
  Anaphylaxis
  Aspiration
  Pulmonary edema
  Carcinoid syndrome
  Pulmonary embolism
  Bronchiolitis

IX. Laboratory findings

    A. Arterial blood gases

In the outpatient setting the measurement of arterial blood gasses (ABG) in the initial assessment of asthma is usually not useful. However, the ABG may be useful when a concurrent disorder or alternative diagnosis is suspected. The ABG can be helpful when a patient presents with severe acute asthma or status asthmaticus (SA). Generally, a derangement of gas exchange indicated by hypercapnia, hypoxia, or a widening of the alveolar–arterial oxygen gradient is not seen until severe airflow obstruction is present. This is typically seen when the FEV_1 is less than 1.0 L or the peak expiratory flow (PEF) is less than 120 L per minute. As illustrated in Fig. 6.1 the P_aO_2 is linearly related to the severity of airflow obstruction. Early in SA mild hypoxemia and a respiratory alkalosis with hypocapnia (decreased P_aCO_2) may be seen. As the degree of airflow obstruction worsens there is a worsening of the ventilation–perfusion relationships marked by normalization of the P_aCO_2 (eucapnia) followed by hypercapnia. Although hypercapnia indicates severe airflow obstruction, it alone is not an indication for intubation. Conversely, the absence of hypercapnia does not exclude the possibility of severe airflow obstruction and impending respiratory failure. Refer to Fig. 6.1, which illustrates that the CO_2 level may be low, with moderate to severe degrees of obstruction, and increases only when quite severe obstruction is present. With prolonged hypocapnia there will be compensatory renal bicarbonate wasting and resultant hypocarbia (low HCO_3^-). Lactic acidosis may be seen with more severe airflow obstruction because of tissue hypoxia, increased acid generation by fatigued muscles, and beta-agonist administration. Although ABG measurements can be useful in the assessment of the severity of SA, they are not a substitute for careful clinical evaluation and serial examinations.

    B. Other serum or blood laboratory measurements generally are not useful in the initial diagnosis or subsequent management of asthma. This is because these measurements generally are neither sensitive nor specific when asthma is present. Because atopy is frequently associated with asthma, serum or sputum eosinophilia is frequently seen. However, eosinophilia is present in nonallergic asthma as well. The serum IgE levels may be abnormal as well. Eosinophilia and elevated IgE levels are not specific to asthma and are seen in several of the other eosinophilic lung diseases.

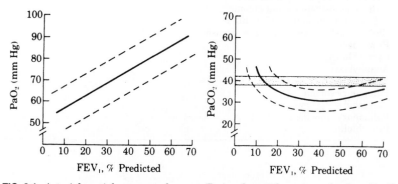

FIG. 6.1. Arterial partial pressure of oxygen (PO_2) and partial pressure of carbon dioxide (PCO_2) values in asthma in relation to airflow obstruction of varying severity (indicated by percentage of predicted forced expiratory volume in 1 second [FEV_1]). Area between broken lines represents normal range of partial arterial pressure of carbon dioxide (P_aCO_2) values.

However, when alternative diagnoses are being considered, these tests can be of considerable value.

C. Pulmonary function tests

1. Spirometry and peak expiratory flow

According to the 1997 National Asthma Education and Prevention Program (NAEPP) Expert Panel Report 2 guidelines, three key features must be demonstrated in order for a diagnosis of asthma to be established. These are as follows: (i) Episodic symptoms of airflow obstruction are present. (ii) Airflow obstruction is at least partially reversible. (iii) Alternative diagnoses are excluded. In the report it was recommended that history, physical examination, and spirometry be used to establish the diagnosis.

Spirometry is valuable for three reasons. First, history and physical examination findings are not completely reliable in establishing the presence of airflow obstruction. Second, history and physical examination are similarly imprecise in establishing or ruling out alternative diagnoses. Finally, although many clinicians can predict when restrictive or obstructive patterns will be seen based on findings of physical examination, they do poorly when trying to predict the degree of airflow limitation. It should be noted that spirometry may be normal in mild forms of asthma and that bronchial provocation testing may be needed in selected cases (see section IX.D on page 104). Peak expiratory flow (PEF) measurements are best used for monitoring response to therapy and assessing control. PEF should not routinely be used to establish the diagnosis because there is inherent variability and imprecision with this technique. However, when asthma is strongly suspected on clinical grounds, measurement of PEF, particularly PEF variability, may be useful when the FEV_1 is normal (i.e., when mild disease is present) (see section IX.C on page 104).

Spirometry typically measures the total volume of air that can be forcibly expelled from the point of maximum inhalation (forced vital capacity [FVC]) as well as the amount of air expelled in the first second of the FVC maneuver (FEV_1). Airflow obstruction is demonstrated when there is a reduction in the ratio of the FEV_1 to FVC volumes (FEV_1/FVC) and in the FEV_1 when compared to predicted values or reference values. Spirometry should be performed both before and after the inhalation of a short- to intermediate-acting beta$_2$-agonist bronchodilator to establish reversibility. Reversibility is established when there is an increase of at least 12% and 200 mL in the FEV_1 after the administration of a bronchodilator. Some patients who do not initially demonstrate reversibility of airflow obstruction will show reversibility after a 2-week course of oral steroids (approximately 0.5 mg per kg of prednisone or the equivalent).

2. Other pulmonary function tests

It is important to recognize that airflow limitation that is reversible can be seen in other conditions. In nearly all cases the history and physical exam are sufficient to exclude alternative diagnoses. When other diagnoses are suspected, other pulmonary function tests may be useful. In the smoker with airflow limitation, the carbon monoxide diffusion capacity is useful in distinguishing between asthma and emphysema. The diffusing capacity should be normal in asthma, whereas it may be decreased in emphysema. It obviously should be noted that both diseases commonly coexist. Flow volume loops (FVL) may be used to characterize patterns of airflow limitation. See Fig. 6.2 for representative loops demonstrating restrictive and obstructive patterns when compared to normal airflow. Lower-airways obstruction is characterized by a reduction in expiratory airflow at all lung volumes (Fig. 6.3A) and this is the pattern seen in asthma when bronchospasm is present. When central/upper airway obstruction (UAO) is suspected the flow-

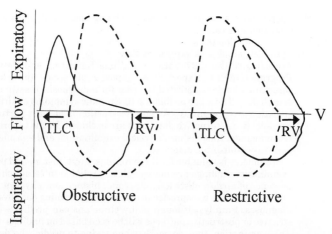

FIG. 6.2. Obstructive versus restrictive flow-volume loops (FVL). Representative FVL *(solid lines)* illustrate airflow obstruction and restriction. Flow (volume per second and *y*-axis) is plotted as a function of volume (*x*-axis). Obstructive disease is characterized by reduced expiratory flows at all lung volumes, as well as increased total lung capacity (TLC) and residual volumes (RV). Restrictive lung disease is characterized by a reduction of TLC and RV. Superimposed normal loops are shown with *dashed lines.*

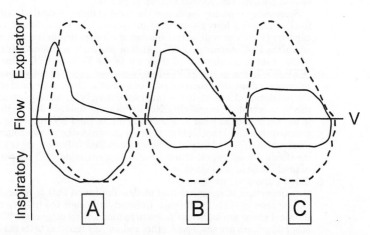

FIG. 6.3. Patterns of airflow obstruction. Representative flow-volume loops *(solid lines)* illustrate lower airway obstruction (A), variable intrathoracic upper airway obstruction (B), and fixed upper airway obstruction (C).

volume loop (FVL) can be diagnostic. Upper airway obstruction is often classed as variable (Fig. 6.3B) or fixed (Fig. 6.3C). Note also that air trapping, resulting in an increased residual volume (RV) and hyperinflation (increased total lung capacity [TLC]), are often present when there is airflow obstruction. There is a resultant leftward shift of the FVL because of increased lung volume. In contrast, with variable UAO there is a resultant decrease in inspiratory airflow at all lung volumes; the corresponding reductions in expiratory flows are due to the dependence of expiratory airflow on lung volume, and not due to lower airway obstruction, per se (Fig. 6.2B). Note that the shape of the expiratory loop is normal in variable UAO. When the UAO is fixed, there are reductions in flow on both limbs of the FVL (inspiratory as well as expiratory limbs), and it typically has a characteristic "squared off" appearance.

As airflow obstruction worsens there is concomitant air trapping with an increase in RV and increased TLC. As illustrated in Fig. 6.4, the TLC does not increase proportionately with the increased RV, so there is a subsequent loss of vital capacity with more severe airflow obstruction. With severe airflow limitation there may also be a reduction in FVC because of air trapping. Because the FVC maneuver is typically performed for only 6 to 10 seconds, very slowly emptying areas of the lung may not contribute to the measured FVC. This so-called "pseudorestriction" can most accurately be differentiated from true reductions in lung volumes by measuring lung volumes in a pulmonary function laboratory. Sometimes the experienced observer can distinguish pseudorestriction from restriction by examining the shape of the FVL or by determining if there is a plateau in the volume–time graph (spirogram). It is important to keep in mind that the predictive value of the FVC maneuver is highly dependent on the correct performance of the maneuver, and accurate spirometry is most dependent on a maximal effort by the patient. The American Thoracic Society has published guidelines on quality control of spirometry.

Another feature of asthma is an exaggeration of the normal diurnal variation in PEF. Normally, the PEF is lowest when the patient first

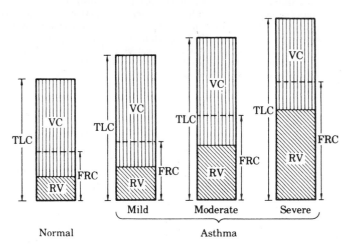

FIG. 6.4. Pattern of abnormalities in various subdivisions of lung volume in asthma of varying severity. VC, vital capacity; RV, residual volume; FRC, functional residual capacity; TLC, total lung capacity.

arises from sleep and is greatest several hours before the midpoint of the waking day (between noon and 2 p.m.). The peak flow should be measured as close to those times as possible. The a.m. PEF should be obtained prior to inhalation of a beta$_2$-agonist bronchodilator, whereas the afternoon value should be measured after inhalation of a bronchodilator. A greater than 20% difference between the two PEFs is suggestive of asthma. The NAEPP recommends that PEF variability be determined when the spirogram is normal if symptoms compatible with asthma are present. The diurnal variation should be observed over a 1- to 2-week period to maximize diagnostic accuracy.

D. Bronchial provocation testing

This technique is useful when spirometry is normal and asthma is suspected. A nonspecific agent such as methacholine or histamine is typically used. Increasing concentrations of the provocative agent are inhaled and the post-inhalation FEV$_1$ is compared to the pre-challenge value. The provocative concentration causing a 20% decline in FEV$_1$ is noted as the PC$_{20}$. Patients with asthma will typically have a PC$_{20}$ of 8 mg per mL or less. Furthermore, the degree of BHR in a symptomatic person correlates well with asthma severity. The lower the provocative concentration, the greater is the degree of BHR. Bronchial provocation testing may have diagnostic and prognostic value. It is perhaps most useful when ruling out the diagnosis of asthma. Failure to elicit a response in a patient with current symptoms essentially rules out asthma; in other words, it has a good negative predictive value. Both the American Thoracic Society and the European Respiratory Society have published procedures for methacholine challenge. Methacholine is a particularly safe agent and has been safely used even when there was a significant reduction in baseline FEV$_1$.

Exercise-induced bronchospasm (EIB) is common in asthmatics and exercise can be used as a bronchial provocation test. Typically, a patient is exercised on a treadmill or bicycle ergometer until they reach 85% of their maximal heart rate; the goal is to reach the target heart rate within 6 to 8 minutes. The electrocardiogram (ECG) should be monitored during the study as well. After exercising, the patient is rested for 5 to 10 minutes and then serial measurements of FEV$_1$ are obtained and compared to baseline. A patient will typically experience a decrease in the FEV$_1$ within 10 to 15 minutes after exercising. Inhalation of cold dry air during the test can increase the sensitivity, especially when the patient reports that exercising in cold air precipitates their symptoms. Some patients will only experience bronchospasm during exercise. Most important is that bronchodilators not be used for 8 to 12 hours prior to the test, because they are effective at preventing bronchospasm. An inadequate exercise stimulus can result in a false-negative test, so it is important to ensure adequate exercise intensity. It is generally agreed that exercise challenge is not as sensitive as methacholine challenge testing to establish the presence of bronchial hyperresponsiveness.

Other "specific" bronchial provocation tests include food additive challenges and antigen challenge tests. These tests should only be performed in specialized centers by physicians familiar with the technique because of the possibility of severe reactions. These tests can be useful especially when a patient is unwilling to avoid a suspected stimulus. Demonstration of a positive challenge is helpful in counseling patients about avoidance of a specific trigger. Antigen challenge testing has also been used to identify antigens in the workplace that may be responsible for occupational asthma.

E. Radiographic findings

Plain chest radiographs (CXR) and computed tomography (CT) of the chest are not particularly useful except to exclude alternative diagnoses (see Differential diagnosis of asthma on page 105). Hyperinflation of the chest may be seen with flattening of the diaphragmatic contours. This is especially true of infants and children. Hyperinflation also occurs in adults with an acute exacerbation of asthma. Excessive mucus production can lead to plugging of small and large airways and is usually not apparent on CXR. Segmental or lobar atelectasis can occur when larger airways are plugged with tenacious mucus. The CXR may also be useful to exclude infections that might exacerbate asthma, but because a viral infection is generally the culprit, the CXR is typically clear.

X. Differential diagnosis

Recurrent episodes of cough and wheezing are usually due to asthma. Underdiagnosis is a problem particularly in children, because they will often wheeze with respiratory infections. Infants with atopy who wheeze when they have respiratory infections are more likely to have asthma that continues during childhood. Nonatopic children are less likely to have recurrent symptoms and thus are less likely to develop asthma. Misclassification of wheezing illnesses in adults is quite common. Asthma should be suspected in the adult with recurrent respiratory illnesses that are often prolonged. The asthmatic may be told that they have bronchitis, "walking pneumonia," or allergic bronchitis when they actually have asthma. The differential diagnosis of asthma is broad and includes all respiratory disorders that can cause recurrent cough, wheezing, or breathlessness. A list of diseases that cause wheezing is listed in Table 6.1.

Vocal cord dysfunction (VCD) is being increasingly recognized. It has also been termed Munchausen's stridor, paradoxical vocal cord motion syndrome, or factitious asthma. These patients are felt to have abnormal adduction of the vocal cords during inspiration. This disorder is more common in adults with psychiatric disorders. Patients with VCD may present with sudden, severe dyspnea, wheeze, a quiet chest, and distress. Such patients will often present with "difficult-to-control" asthma. They sometimes undergo endotracheal intubation because their respiratory distress appears to be so profound. Clues to the diagnosis include a monophonic wheeze heard best over the glottis and during inspiration, and a complete resolution of wheezing with intubation. A completely normal blood gas without hypoxemia, particularly in a patient who otherwise might be felt to be in extremis, also suggests this diagnosis. Demonstration of adduction of the vocal cords throughout the respiratory cycle or during inspiration using flexible fiberoptic laryngoscopy can confirm the diagnosis. However, the examination typically needs to be done during an attack or when symptoms are present. Similarly, examination of the FVL may demonstrate extrathoracic upper airway obstruction during an attack. The diagnosis is important because unnecessary medication side effects can be avoided and good responses to speech therapy and voice training have been reported.

XI. Clinical classification

Assessment of Severity

The NAEPP Expert Panel recommends that asthma severity should be classified. The classification of asthma severity is based on both the pattern of symptoms and lung function (Table 6.2). In addition to eliciting a history of symptoms compatible with asthma, an assessment of the severity and frequency of symptoms should be obtained. At the initial visit, patients should be questioned about the frequency of symptoms, and whether the symptoms affect activity. The presence of nocturnal symptoms and frequent use of a short-acting bronchodilator indicates poor asthma control and more severe inflammation. However, there is a loose correlation between symptoms, activity limitation, and lung function, so measured lung function should also be used to classify asthma severity. More severe disease mandates more aggressive treatment and monitoring. In contrast, aggressive pharmacological therapy with its attendant side effects is not warranted in milder cases. When asthma is under control, a step-down in therapy is also appropriate. The asthma patient may migrate from one category to another, so that frequent reassessment of severity is appropriate.

XII. Modification of risk factors

    A. Recognition that certain modifiable factors contribute to both the pathogenesis of airway inflammation and BHR allows one to modify exposure to these factors, and hence improve clinical outcomes. First, many asthmatics

Table 6.2. Classification of asthma according to the NAEPP

Classification	Symptoms	Nighttime symptoms	Lung function
Step 4: severe persistent	Continual symptoms Limited physical activity Frequent exacerbations	Frequent	FEV_1 or PEF ≤60% predicted PEF variability >30%
Step 3: moderate persistent	Daily symptoms Daily use of inhaled short-acting beta$_2$-agonists Exacerbations affect activity Exacerbations ≥2 times a week; may last days	>1 time a week	FEV_1 or PEF >60% to <80% predicted PEF variability >30%
Step 2: mild persistent	Symptoms >2 times a week but <1 time a day Exacerbations may affect activity	≥2 times a month	FEV_1 or PEF ≥80% predicted PEF variability 20% to 30%
Step 1: mild intermittent	Symptoms ≤2 times a week Asymptomatic and normal PEF between exacerbations Exacerbations brief (from a few hours to a few days); intensity may vary	≤2 times a month	FEV_1 or PEF ≥80% predicted PEF variability <20%

NAEPP, National Asthma Education and Prevention Program.
Adapted from Fig. 1-3, National Asthma Education and Prevention Program. Expert panel report 2: Guidelines for the diagnosis and management of Asthma, NIH publication no. 97-4051. Available from: National Heart, Lung and Blood Institute, National Institutes of Health, Bethesda, MD, 1997, with permission.

are atopic and most who are atopic are allergic to one or more common indoor and outdoor aeroallergens. Second, BHR is a cardinal feature of asthma so that nonspecific triggers can lead to exacerbations. Third, viral upper respiratory infections commonly lead to exacerbations. Fourth, certain medications and substances are known to elicit IgE-mediated inflammation in some patients, whereas others can cause non-IgE-mediated responses. Finally, other modifiable comorbid conditions may cause exacerbations. It should be recognized that exhaustive evaluations of the above-mentioned factors are not needed in all patients. Rather, focused history taking can be used to screen for pertinent factors, particularly in those with moderate to severe disease, those who have an unsatisfactory response to therapy, or patients with difficult-to-manage disease.

B. Allergens

There is a wealth of data demonstrating that sensitization to common indoor allergens such as house dust mite, animal dander, cockroach, and the mold *Alternaria*, among genetically susceptible populations, is a risk factor for the development of asthma in children. Seasonal asthma is also a well-described phenomenon, although allergy to seasonal allergens such as grass and ragweed carries a lower risk for asthma than allergy to indoor allergens. For patients with persistent symptoms and the need for daily maintenance therapy, an assessment of allergen exposure is appropriate. Seasonal variation of symptoms or symptoms that worsen when the patient is outdoors suggest allergy to tree pollen (spring), grass (spring to early summer), or ragweed (late summer and early fall). Allergy to molds such as *Alternaria* has been associated with seasonal asthma exacerbations. Questions about exposures to pets or animals (work or home related) should be asked. When appropriate, skin testing or *in vitro* testing can be used to confirm sensitivity to one or more of a panel of allergens. Only those personnel who are well versed in the technique and who are trained to support the rare patient who develops a severe reaction should perform skin testing. *In vitro* testing (radioallergosorbent tests [RAST]) to detect antigen-specific IgE in serum avoids the risk of systemic reactions, but is less sensitive and more costly.

C. Indoor allergen control

When it has been determined that atopy is present, the treatment is avoidance when possible, and there is evidence that avoidance can improve asthma control. This is even true for the ubiquitous house dust mite. Encasement of the mattress and pillow in allergen-impermeable covers can improve asthma control. It is also recommended that linens be washed in hot water (greater than 130°F). Pets are another major source of allergen and the dander, saliva, and urine of any warm-blooded animal can be a source. Removal of the pet to which the patient is allergic from the home is the best treatment. When the pet cannot be removed, it should be recommended that pets not sleep in the patient's bedroom and that pets be kept outside if possible. The use of air purification devices has proven beneficial for certain indoor airborne allergens, such as pet dander. Cockroaches present a major problem, especially in urban areas. Traps, baits, and hygiene control are recommended to control infestation, because sprays may exacerbate asthma. Controlling indoor humidity can reduce symptoms when mold is a problem, and lowering humidity also helps to reduce dust mite allergen levels. It is recommended that the patient remain indoors and that air conditioning be used during the problem season when seasonal allergens are an issue.

XIII. Asthma monitoring

Asthma is a chronic disorder that, in most patients, is characterized by periods of exacerbation interspersed with periods that are relatively symptom free. It has been long recognized that when an exacerbation of airway inflammation occurs there often is a decline in lung function prior to a worsening of symptoms. Important too is the fact that aggressive treatment of inflammation in its early stages can abort more severe attacks that lead to physician visits or hospitalization. Therefore, the early detection of an exacerbation can result in a significant reduction in morbidity as well as a reduction in costs. Other equally important goals of asthma care include the maintenance of normal or near-normal lung function, minimization of medication side effects, prevention of symptoms, maximizing exercise and activity tolerance, improving quality of life (QOL), and ensuring patient satisfaction.

A. Periodic assessment

Current strategies mandate periodic assessment and evaluation of the following aspects of asthma: symptoms, signs, lung function, QOL, pharmacotherapy, and history of exacerbation. The patient should be instructed about recognizing symptoms and signs that would indicate a worsening of asthma control. These would include exertional dyspnea, wheezing, cough, chest tightness, and nocturnal awakenings for asthma. Patients should be instructed to use their short-acting inhalers and to make a note of how often they are using their inhalers. The patient should also note when their symptoms occur, especially if they occur at night. Any persistence of symptoms suggestive of worsening airflow obstruction should be reported to a physician. Several authorities also advocate the regular monitoring of the peak flow with a personal device. Monitoring the peak flow can lead to early detection of worsening airflow obstruction and can prompt early intervention prior to the development of overt symptoms. The peak flow should be obtained at the same time each day (usually on first awakening) and it should be compared to the individual patient's personal best. The personal best should be obtained from a series of daily or twice-daily measurements over a period of 2 weeks during which the patient feels well. Self-monitoring, either by noting symptoms or combining symptoms with peak flow measurements, is an important part of asthma self-management, especially in patients with moderate to severe disease severity.

B. Asthma self-management

Some data suggest that asthma action plans may improve outcomes. "Asthma self-management" is a term that has been coined to describe the use of self-monitoring coupled with the use of a written action plan and regular reviews of medication used. Asthma self-management reduces morbidity, healthcare system utilization, and lost days from work. All patients with persistent asthma, particularly those who have had a severe exacerbation, should be instructed on the recognition of serious or worsening symptoms (in conjunction with PEF monitoring, if appropriate) and the implementation of an asthma action plan if asthma control worsens. Essentially, the patient is given instructions to follow if his symptoms and/or peak flow are within certain parameters. Evidence of a severe exacerbation should lead the patient to begin therapy, usually with systemic corticosteroids, and to seek immediate medical attention. A less severe exacerbation may be treated with stepped-up therapy in the outpatient setting with close follow-up care. The NAEPP expert panel recommends a step-up in care whenever the patient's PEF decreases below 80% of their personal best. A more recent review suggests that setting PEF action points a certain number of standard deviations below the patient's mean during a period of stability (i.e., using quality control analysis), results in more effective use of the patient's personal PEF data. Finally, if an action plan is used, it should be written using explicit language that the patient can clearly understand. Figure 6.5 provides an example of a written asthma action plan.

C. Follow-up physician visits

Periodic assessment by a physician is also essential. The follow-up visit serves several functions. It allows for an assessment of asthma symptom control. The asthma patient should be asked about the frequency and pattern of symptoms as well as their effect on daily activities. The health care provider should also ask about medication usage patterns and determine if the quick relief medications provide relief. Metered-dose inhaler (MDI) technique should be reviewed frequently as well. Patients should be asked about their asthma in a global sense and questioned about recent exacerbations. Finally, lung function should be checked initially, after initiation of treatment, and at least every 1 or 2 years in all but the mildest cases. Lung function (spirometry) should be monitored frequently in severe asthma (every few months) and these patients require intensive education, close monitoring of medication usage, and frequent follow-up visits.

XIV. Pharmacological management of asthma

A. General principles

Successful management of the asthmatic patient demands an appreciation of certain guiding principles. First, is an understanding that within the overall asthmatic population, there is a considerable heterogeneity with respect to clinical presentation, severity, natural history, response to therapy, and pathogenetic factors. Asthma should be considered as a syndrome rather than a single nosologic entity, because it probably consists of multiple disorders having common clinical manifestations. Good asthma management is based on the following:

Making the correct diagnosis
Identifying and avoiding or minimizing asthma triggers
Educating the patient and family

Action Plan for _____
Your treatment goals:
•Be free of symptoms
•Sleep through the night
•Maximize Lung Function
•Be able to perform desired activities
•Not need to use emergency room
•Use medications with minimal side effects

Daily Monitoring:
•Measure peak flow each morning and
record
•Monitor for symptoms like shortness of
breath, chest tightness, cough or limitation
of exercise
•When symptoms are present measure
PEF and act according to the PEFR

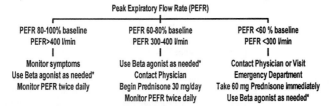

Peak Expiratory Flow Rate (PEFR)

PEFR 80-100% baseline	PEFR 60-80% baseline	PEFR <60 % baseline
PEFR>400 l/min	PEFR 300-400 l/min	PEFR <300 l/min
Monitor symptoms	Use Beta agonist as needed*	Contact Physician or Visit
Use Beta agonist as needed*	Contact Physician	Emergency Department
Monitor PEFR twice daily	Begin Prednisone 30 mg/day	Take 60 mg Prednisone immediately
	Monitor PEFR twice daily	Use Beta agonist as needed*

FIG. 6.5. Asthma action plan. An action plan should be written, concrete, and include goals of therapy and parameters that trigger specific responses depending on the severity of an exacerbation.

Selecting appropriate medications
Close monitoring and modification of management for effective long-term
    control
Aggressive treatment and prevention of asthma exacerbations

The differential diagnosis of asthma, identification and modification of risk factors, and patient monitoring have been discussed above. The treatment of asthma should address both short- and long-term goals. Therapeutic objectives for the short term include the immediate relief of symptoms and airflow obstruction. Long-term objectives include preventing chronic and troublesome symptoms; the maintenance of as "normal" pulmonary function as possible; maintaining normal activity levels; preventing exacerbations, emergency department visits, and hospitalizations; minimizing the side effects of medications; and meeting the patient's and family's expectations for asthma treatment.

Current guidelines emphasize the stratification of asthmatics by disease severity, classifying asthma as intermittent or persistent, and persistent asthma as mild, moderate, or severe (Table 6.2). Table 6.3 summarizes an overview of the pharmacology of asthma therapy as outlined by NAEPP, Expert Panel Report according to this classification. To avoid needless long-term medication side effects, the minimal amount of medication that is re-

Table 6.3. Stepwise treatment of asthma

	Long term (preventive)	Short term (quick relief)

Step 4: severe persistent	Daily medications
	  Inhaled corticosteroids, 800–2000 µg or more and
	  Long-acting bronchodilators
	Either long-acting inhaled β_2-agonist and/or sustained-release theophylline, and/or long-acting β_2-agonist tablets or syrup, and corticosteroids tablets or syrup long term
		Short-acting bronchodilator
		  Inhaled β_2-agonist as needed for symptoms

Step 3: moderate persistent	Daily medications
	  Inhaled corticosteroids, ≥500 µg and, if needed
	  Long-acting bronchodilator either long-acting inhaled β_2-agonist, sustained-release theophylline, or long acting β_2-agonist tablets or syrup
	  Consider adding antileuko-trienes, especially for sensitive patients and for preventing exercise induced bronchospasm
		Short-acting bronchodilator
		  Inhaled β_2-agonist as needed for symptoms, not to exceed 3–4 times in 1 day

Step 2: mild persistent	Daily medication
	  Either inhaled corticosteroids, 200–500 µg, or cromoglycate, nedocromil, or sustained-release theophylline. Antileukotriene may be considered, but their position in therapy has not been fully established.
		Short-acting bronchodilator
		  Inhaled β_2-agonist as needed for symptoms, not to exceed 3–4 times in 1 day

Step 1: inter-mittent	None needed	Short-acting bronchodilator
		  Inhaled β_2-agonist as needed for symptoms
		  Intensity of treatment will depend on severity of attack
		  Inhaled β_2-agonist or cromoglycate before exercise or exposure to allergen

Adapted from Fig. 3-4b, National Asthma Education and Prevention Program. Expert panel report 2: Guidelines for the diagnosis and management of asthma, NIH publication no. 97-4051. Available from: National Heart, Lung and Blood Institute, National Institutes of Health: Bethesda, MD, 1997, with permission.

quired to provide control of inflammation, symptoms, and airflow limitation should be used. The key principle is that severe asthma requires aggressive pharmacological therapy, whereas mild or improving asthma requires less medication. In other words, as symptoms and lung function worsen, there is a step-up of therapy; as symptoms improve, therapy is stepped down. However, in newly diagnosed symptomatic asthmatics, it is often recommended that asthma therapy begin at one step higher than the patient's current status. Therapy is then stepped down cautiously once the patient is clinically stable. Refer to Table 6.4 for the glossary of asthma medications.

B. Beta$_2$-adrenergic receptor agonists

    1. Short- and intermediate-acting beta$_2$-agonists

The most important class of quick-relief medications is the β_2-adrenergic receptor agonists (beta$_2$-agonists). Agonist-mediated stimulation of β_2-adrenergic receptors activates adenylyl cyclase, causing formation of intracellular cyclic-adenosine monophosphate (cAMP) with resultant bronchial smooth muscle relaxation. Significant effects of β-adrenergic stimulation in asthma include bronchodilation, facilitation of mucociliary clearance, and inhibition of mast cell mediator release, although whether β-agonists produce significant inhibition of mast cell mediator release *in vivo* is questionable. Several selective β_2-agonists are available, including metaproterenol, terbutaline, and albuterol, with albuterol being the preferred agent in most cases because of its longer duration of action. In general, these agents are safe, with few toxic effects even when used in high doses. However, some dose-dependent side effects are seen with β_2-selective agents, particularly when they are used orally.

The delivery and pharmacodynamics of these agents has been an area of active research. When compared to systemic administration, local/aerosol delivery provides a more rapid onset of action with fewer side effects. When used properly, the traditional MDIs, dry powder inhalers (DPIs), and nebulized forms provide comparable effects. However, the current Expert Panel Report 2 recommends the use of nebulized forms of bronchodilators for acute asthma in the emergency room. Because of environmental concerns, MDIs are undergoing a change of propellant from chlorofluorocarbons (CFCs) to hydrofluorocarbon (HFC)-like hydrofluoroalkanes (HFA). Nonpropellant or DPIs are gaining popularity also.

Beta-adrenergic agonists are derived from adrenaline, which exists as a mixture of two enantiomers, levo- (R) and dextro- (S), rotatory isomers. The R-isomer is mainly responsible for the desirable pharmacological activity, whereas the S-isomer may be associated with side effects. Recently, R-albuterol (levalbuterol) (without its S-isomer) was approved for use in nebulized form (Xopenex).

Several earlier epidemiological studies suggested that the chronic, regular use of inhaled β_2-agonists might result in deterioration of asthma control, while other studies went so far as to suggest a potential increase in mortality among severe asthmatics related to β_2-agonist use. These early studies, however, were retrospective and thus subject to bias. Recently published studies in mild (on no additional medication) and moderately severe asthmatics (most taking inhaled corticosteroids [ICSs]) concluded that there was no difference in asthma control when albuterol was used on a regular basis compared to when albuterol was used as needed. Most experts currently recommend the use of quick-relief medications on an as-needed basis (p.r.n.).

    2. Long-acting beta-agonists

These agents provide a longer duration of bronchodilation (greater than 12 hours) when compared to the short- and intermediate-acting bronchodilators. By virtue of their long lipophilic side chain, these agents are believed to bind with the beta-receptor for longer periods of time.

Table 6.4. Glossary of asthma medications

Class	Generic name	Mechanism of action	Side effects	Comments
Corticosteroids Adrenocorticoids Glucocorticoids	Inhaled Beclomethasone Budesonide Flunisolide Fluticasone Triamcinolone (Mometasone) (Ciclesonide)	Antiinflammatory agents	Inhaled: >1 mg a day may be associated with skin thinning, easy bruising, adrenal suppression, and cataracts. Minor growth delay or suppression (average 1 cm) may occur in children; especially in doses >400 μg/day	Inhaled: Potential but small risk of side effects is well balanced by efficacy. Spacer devices and mouth washing after inhalation decrease oral candidiasis. Preparations not equivalent on per-puff or microgram basis
	Systemic—tablets or syrups: Methylprednisolone Prednisolone Prednisone		Systemic—tablets or syrups: Used long term may lead to osteoporosis, hypertension, diabetes, cataracts, adrenal suppression, obesity, and skin thinning or muscle weakness. Consider coexisting conditions that could be worsened by *oral steroids*, e.g., herpes virus infections, *Varicella*, tuberculosis, hypertension	Systemic—tablets or syrups: Long-term use: alternate day a.m. dosing produces less toxicity. Short-term use; 3–10 day "bursts" effective for gaining prompt control; administer until PEF >80% predicted or symptoms resolve
Cromones	Sodium cromoglycate	Antiinflammatory agent	Minimal side effects. Cough may occur upon inhalation	May take 4–6 weeks to determine maximum effects
	Nedocromil	Antiinflammatory agent	Similar to Cromolyn. About 10% of subjects experience a bitter taste	

Long-acting β$_2$-agonists Long-acting beta-adrenergics Sympathomimetics	Inhaled Salmeterol Formoterol Sustained-release tablets Salbutamol Terbutaline Albuterol	Bronchodilator	Inhaled: β$_2$-agonists have fewer and less significant side effects than tablets. Tablets: β$_2$-agonists may cause cardiovascular stimulation, anxiety, pyrosis, skeletal muscle tremor, headache, and hypokalemia	Not to be used to treat attacks. Always use in combination with antiinflammatory therapy. Combining with low to medium dose of inhaled steroid usually gives more effective control than higher doses of inhaled steroid alone. Available in a fixed combination with inhaled steroid, Advair
Methylxanthines	Sustained-release theophylline Aminophylline	Bronchodilator (with uncertain anti-inflammatory effect)	Nausea and vomiting are most common. Serious effects occurring at higher serum concentrations include seizures, tachycardia, and arrhythmias	Theophylline monitoring is often required. Absorption and metabolism may be affected by many factors, including febrile illness
Antiallergics	(Ketotifen)	Antiallergic agent	May cause sedation and weight gain	Not available in the United States for asthma
Antileukotrienes Leukotriene modifiers	Montelukast Zafirlukast (Pranlukast)	Leukotriene receptor antagonist	Data are limited; no specific adverse effects to date at recommended doses. Churg-Strauss syndrome (1 in 10,000 reported, but does not appear to be due to drug)	The position of antileukotrienes in asthma therapy is not fully established; further study and clinical experience is required
	Zileuton	5-Lipoxygenase inhibitor	Elevation of liver enzymes possible. Limited case reports of reversible hepatitis and hyperbilirubinemia	

continued

Table 6.4. *Continued*

Class	Generic name	Mechanism of action	Side effects	Comments
QUICK-RELIEF MEDICATIONS				
Short-acting β_2-agonists Adrenergics β_2-stimulants Sympathomimetics	Albuterol Bitolterol (Fenoterol) Isoetharine Levalbuterol Metaproterenol Pirbuterol Salbutamol Terbutaline	Bronchodilator	Inhaled β_2-agonists have fewer and less significant side effects than tablets or syrups. Tablet or syrup β_2-agonists may cause cardiovascular stimulation, skeletal muscle tremor, headache, and irritability.	Drug of choice for acute bronchospasm. Inhaled route has faster onset and is more effective than tablet or syrup. Increasing use, lack of expected effect, or use of >1 canister a month indicates poor asthma control; adjust long-term therapy accordingly
Anticholinergics	Ipratropium bromide (Oxitropium bromide) (Tiotropium bromide)	Bronchodilator	Minimal mouth dryness or bad taste in the mouth.	May provide additive effects to β_2-agonist but has slower onset of action. Is an alternative for patients with intolerance for β_2-agonist. Dose delivered by MDI is low.
Short-acting theophylline Aminophylline		Bronchodilator	Nausea, vomiting; at higher serum concentrations: seizures, tachycardia, and arrhythmias.	Aminophylline may be considered if inhaled β_2-agonist not available. Theophylline blood level monitoring may be required.
Epinephrine/adrenaline		Bronchodilator	Similar, but more significant side effects than β_2-agonist. In addition: convulsions, chills, fever, and hallucinations.	In general, not recommended for treating asthma attacks if inhaled β_2-agonists are available.

Parentheses indicate drugs not yet U.S. Food and Drug Administration (FDA)-approved at printing time.
PEF, peak expiratory flow; MDI, metered-dose inhaler.
Adapted from Fig. 3-1, National Asthma Education and Prevention Program. Expert panel report 2: Guidelines for the diagnosis and management of asthma, NIH publication no. 97-4051. Available from: National Heart, Lung and Blood Institute, National Institute of Health: Bethesda, MD, 1997, with permission.

Salmeterol xinafoate is available as both a MDI and DPI in the United States and has a similar incidence of adverse effects as albuterol. Formoterol has also been extensively studied, is available in Europe, and may eventually be commercially available in the United States. Notably, salmeterol, unlike formoterol, has a slow onset of action (30 to 60 minutes), and is not appropriate for use as a quick-relief agent. Oral sustained-release albuterol is also available in the United States.

Because these agents do not have significant antiinflammatory activity, they should not be used as controller agents, nor should they be used to treat exacerbations. Many patients will experience a significant and rapid improvement in symptoms when these agents are introduced, so it is very important to educate patients about their proper use. More specifically, they should be counseled not to discontinue ICSs while taking these drugs. It is important that patients not exceed the recommended daily dose (for salmeterol, four puffs daily) during an exacerbation of symptoms. In other words, patients should be specifically instructed against increasing long-acting beta-agonists (LABAs) doses or frequency of administration when acute symptoms develop; rather, they should be told to use their short-acting bronchodilator as needed for acute symptom control. The point that LABAs should not be used in emergency situations should be emphasized.

Generally, LABAs should be used as adjuncts to ICSs to further control symptoms in patients with moderate and severe persistent asthma. They are also particularly useful for the control of nocturnal symptoms and the prevention of EIB. Several studies show that the LABAs provide a more prolonged attenuation of EIB when compared to the short- and intermediate-acting beta-agonists. Similar to cysLT1 antagonists, the LABAs provide bronchoprotection to allergen and exercise challenge. However, some studies suggest that the bronchoprotective effect provided by LABAs might wane with time. Despite this, there seems to be no significant loss of bronchodilator efficacy with chronic LABA use, so the clinical relevance of the reduction in bronchoprotective effect is not clear.

C. Corticosteroids

Corticosteroids have broad antiinflammatory effects and represent the single most important class of controller medications presently used to treat asthma. Potential mechanisms of action of corticosteroids include the modulation of leukocyte functions, the synthesis of nuclear regulatory proteins, catecholamine receptors, eicosanoid synthesis and function, and vascular endothelial integrity. Steroids inhibit the transcription of several cytokines including IL-1, tumor necrosis factor-α (TNF-α), granulocyte macrophage colony-stimulating factor (GM-CSF) and IL-3, 4, 5, 6, and 8. Corticosteroids also increased the synthesis of lipocortin-1, which has an inhibitory effect on the production of lipid mediators such as leukotrienes (LTs), prostaglandins, and platelet activating factors via its inhibition of phospholipase A_2. Additional effects include the inhibition of mucus secretion in airways and upregulation of β_2-receptors. Steroids decrease airway inflammation with chronic use, as shown histologically by decreases in T lymphocytes, eosinophils, and mast cells in the lamina propria. Inhaled steroids also reduce BHR, as measured by methacholine, histamine, or exercise challenge.

1. Inhaled corticosteroids

Multiple well-controlled trials have shown that the regular use of ICS leads to significant reductions in the symptoms of chronic asthma, the use of rescue β_2-agonists, number of asthma exacerbations, and urgent care visits. Regular ICS usage results in improvements in pulmonary function as shown by increases in FEV_1, a.m. and p.m. peak flow, and modest improvements in BHR. A large randomized study involving more than 1,000 children showed that the regular use of ICS provided better asthma control (reduced acute care visits and hospitalizations) and reduced the need for oral steroids when compared to placebo or nedocromil.

Whether ICSs affect mortality has been a matter of great debate. However, a recent large retrospective study showed that the regular use of low-dose corticosteroids is associated with decreased risk of death from asthma. According to the authors' analysis of pharmacy data, for each additional canister of ICS steroid (primarily beclomethasone) used per year by an asthmatic, the relative chance of dying decreased 21%. Conversely, discontinuing the used of ICS resulted in a 4.6-fold increased risk of death during the 3 months immediately after ICS withdrawal.

Inhaled steroids continue to be a first-line agent for all forms of persistent asthma, but the dosing schedules have been undergoing modification. All ICSs can be effective when given on a twice-a-day (b.i.d.) dosing schedule. Recent studies have also shown that once daily administration of ICS can usually be used effectively when mild to moderate asthmatics are under good control on a b.i.d. schedule, although this approach does not appear to work in all asthmatics.

   a. The relative potency of ICSs based on receptor binding and skin blanching tests is summarized in Table 6.5. Of particular note is the higher potency of fluticasone propionate in comparison with the other agents. Although this is a good general guide to steroid potency, other factors, particularly the steroid formulation and the delivery system used, have important effects of the amount of drug delivered to the patient and its potential for beneficial versus adverse effects. The use of both DPIs and the introduction of HFA MDIs are two developments that could alter risk/benefit ratios. HFA-containing MDIs should eventually replace conventional CFC-propelled MDIs, because CFCs have been shown to have a detrimental effect on the atmospheric ozone layer and have been targeted for elimination. In addition to having advantages of a warmer temperature and a less harsh plume, HFA–beclomethasone (Qvar) and HFA–flunisolide have improved lung deposition and potency compared with CFC–beclomethasone and CFC–flunisolide, respectively.

   Factors contributing to adverse effects of ICS include the total dose, the dosing schedule, whether or not a spacer device is used, and whether mouth rinsing is used. Topical/local side effects of ICS include cough, oral candidiasis, and dysphonia. These can usually be avoided, minimized, or treated by using a spacer and good oral hygiene. More troubling systemic effects include skin thinning and easy bruising, cataract formation, ocular hypertension, suppression of the hypothalamic–pituitary–adrenal (HPA) axis, slowing of growth in children and adolescents, and osteoporosis. Skin changes, while uncommon, do occur in some asthmatics treated with ICSs; there is no effective treatment for this problem except to minimize the dose of ICS used, and perhaps to consider switching to a less potent ICS formulation. Evidence for both cataract formation and ocular hypertension caused by ICS use comes from epidemiological studies. Both the relative and absolute risks of these problems appear to be small. However, asthmatics taking ICSs should be told of this possibility and undergo regular eye examinations. It has been suggested that more than 800 µg per day of ICS (beclomethasone equivalent) in adults may suppress the HPA axis. However, corticosteroids differ in their ability to suppress the HPA axis. Any asthmatic taking more than this dose of ICS per day, particularly of a high-potency ICS such as fluticasone propionate, should be warned not to abruptly discontinue ICS use, and should be monitored for signs of adrenal insufficiency. However, clinically important HPA axis suppression with the use of ICSs is rare. Systemic corticosteroid supplementation may be considered in times of stress (e.g., general surgery). With ICS most side effects appear to be distinctly uncommon, particularly when doses less than 1,000 µg per day are used, but osteoporosis may be an important exception to this

Table 6.5. Estimated comparative daily dosages for inhaled corticosteroids

Drug	Low dose	Medium dose	High dose
ADULTS			
Beclomethasone	168–504 µg	504–840 µg	>840 µg
42 µg/puff	4–12 puffs	12–20 puff	>20 puffs
84 µg/puff	2–6 puffs	6–10 puffs	>10 puffs
Budesonide DPI	200–400 µg	400–600 µg	>600 µg
200 µg/inhalation	1–2 puffs	2–3 puffs	>3 puffs
Flunisolide	500–1,000 µg	1,000–2000	>2,000 µg
250 µg/puff	2–4 puffs	4–8 puffs	>8 puffs
Fluticasone MDI	88–264 µg	264–660 µg	>660 µg
44 µg/puff	2–6 puffs	6–15 puffs	
110 µg/puff	2 puffs	2–6 puffs	>6 puffs
220 µg/puff			>3 puffs
Fluticasone DPI	100–300 µg	300–600 µg	>500–600 µg
50 µg/inhalation	2–6 inhalations	6–12 inhalations	
100 µg/inhalation	1–3 inhalations	3–6 inhalations	>5–6 inhalations
250 µg/inhalation		1–2 inhalations	>2 inhalations
Triamcinolone	400–1,000 µg	1,000–2,000 µg	>2,000 µg
100 µg/puff	4–10 puffs	10–20 puffs	>20 puffs
CHILDREN			
Beclomethasone	84–336 µg	336–672 µg	>672 µg
42 µg/puff	2–8 puffs	8–16 puffs	>16 puffs
84 µg/puff	1–4 puffs	4–8 puffs	>8 puffs
Budesonide DPI	100–200 µg	200–400 µg	>400 µg
200 µg/inh		1–2 inhalations	>2 inhalations
Flunisolide	500–750 µg	1,000–1,250 µg	>1,250 µg
250 µg/puff	2–3 puffs	4–5 puffs	>5 puffs
Fluticasone MDI	88–176 µg	176–440 µg	>440 µg
44 µg/puff	2–4 puffs	4–10 puffs	>10 puffs
110 µg/puff		2–4 puffs	>4 puffs
220 µg/puff			>2 puffs
Fluticasone DPI			
50 µg/inhalation	2–4 inhalations		
100 µg/inhalation		2–4 inhalations	>4 inhalation
250 µg/inhalation			>2 inhalations
Triamcinolone	400–800 µg	800–1,200 µg	>1,200 µg
100 µg/puff	4–8 puffs	8–12 puffs	>12 puffs

Adapted from Fig. 3-5b, National Asthma Education and Prevention Program. Expert panel report 2: Guidelines for the diagnosis and management of asthma, NIH publication no. 97-4051. Available from: National Heart, Lung and Blood Institute, National Institutes of Health: Bethesda, MD, 1997, with permission.

statement, because several studies have shown accelerated bone loss even when doses less than 1,000 µg per day are used. It is reasonable to ensure adequate elemental calcium (1,000 to 1,500 mg per day), and vitamin D (600 to 800 IU) in all asthmatic patients taking any corticosteroid preparation. If bone loss is of particular concern, then assessment of initial bone density and rate of bone loss as well as the use of further pharmacological measures may be indicated. Expert consultation with a bone mineral specialist may be needed in particularly challenging cases (i.e., the rare oral steroid-dependent patient). Efforts to minimize both the dose of ICS used (see Combination therapy, section D below) and steroid available for systemic absorption (via spacers and good oral hygiene) should also be undertaken.

   b. Safety

Safety issues regarding the effects of corticosteroids on skeletal growth and development in children have been an area of intense interest and the results have been mixed. For example, the Childhood Asthma Management Program Research Group studied the effects of budesonide versus nedocromil or placebo over a 4- to 6-year period. Budesonide provided superior asthma control but at the expense of a small but statistically significant reduction in growth velocity during the first treatment year. Despite this result, there was no difference in final projected adult height or growth velocity at the end of the treatment period. There was no difference in bone mineral density or sexual maturation between groups during the treatment period. In another important study the effects of budesonide were studied over an average of more than 9 years and it was found that patients taking budesonide attained normal adult height. Nonetheless, children taking ICS, especially those on concomitant nasal corticosteroids, should have routine measures of growth using a stadiometer.

D. Inhaled corticosteroid combination therapy

The dose-response for ICS tends to plateau at moderate doses for many patients; in other words, high doses of ICS (i.e., 1,000 µg) provides little more benefit than moderate doses. Some asthmatics continue to have bothersome symptoms even when high doses of ICS are used. For this reason, ICSs have been studied in combination with several other classes of long-acting antiasthma agents.

   1. Beta-agonist

Several studies have shown that the addition of a LABA (salmeterol, formoterol) to a moderate dose of ICS results in greater improvements in FEV_1 and asthma symptom scores than use of higher doses of ICS alone. However, the degree of bronchodilation provided by LABAs when used alone was inferior when compared to moderate doses of ICS. Notably, the use of LABA with ICS does not appear to adversely affect the beneficial reductions in BHR and exacerbation seen with ICS usage. Because of the superior treatment effect of the LABA–ICS combinations, several combination preparations are under study. Advair (DPI fluticasone–salmeterol) is one such preparation that is available in the United States.

   2. Leukotriene modifiers

The cysteinyl–LT antagonists have also been examined in combination with ICS. In one placebo-controlled study in which zafirlukast was added to high-dose ICS, it appeared to provide an incremental improvement in PEF. Notably, zafirlukast also appeared to further reduce exacerbation rates, and this perhaps can be attributed to its antiinflammatory properties. In another randomized-controlled study conducted in patients taking ICS, montelukast similarly improved FEV_1 and reduced exacerbation rates when used in combination with ICS. However, in the study arm where ICSs were withdrawn and montelukast was used as monotherapy, lung function deteriorated. This finding suggests that cysteinyl–LT antagonists should not be substituted for ICS in patients already requiring ICS; they may be useful adjunctive agents when higher dose ICS are inadequate or undesired.

3. Theophylline has also been assessed in combination with ICS. In one controlled trial, theophylline, when used with low-dose budesonide, appeared to provide slightly better benefit when compared to monotherapy with high-dose budesonide.

E. Antileukotriene agents

LTs are synthesized via the 5-lipoxygenation of arachidonic acid. This pathway has a branch point which leads to the synthesis of either LTB_4 or the cysteinyl LTC_4, LTD_4, and LTE_4. LTD_4 and LTE_4 are derived from LTC_4 by the stepwise removal of single amino acids present in the LTC_4 glutathione moiety. LTB_4 is a potent chemoattractant for eosinophils and other granulocytes. The cysteinyl LTs exert their biological action by binding and activating specific receptors, either the CysLT1 or CysLT2, receptor. Most of the actions of cysteinyl LTs important in asthma are mediated by the CysLT1 receptor. These actions include the contraction of human airway smooth muscle, stimulation of mucus secretion, and increase in vascular permeability. In human lung tissue, LTC_4 and LTD_4 have equivalent potency to stimulate smooth muscle contraction by acting on the CysLT1 receptor. Abrogating the effects of the cysteinyl LTs can be accomplished either by inhibiting the 5-LO with a 5-LO inhibitor (which will also inhibit the synthesis of LTB_4) or by blocking the CysLT1 receptor. More than a dozen chemically distinct, specific, and selective antagonist drugs that block the binding of LTs to CysLT1 receptors have been identified. This class of molecules has been given the generic suffix "lukast"; three of them (zafirlukast, montelukast, and pranlukast) have proven to be effective treatment for asthma.

1. Properties of antileukotrienes

Several distinguishing properties of the antileukotrienes have emerged from clinical studies in asthmatics. First, although they produce modest improvements in pulmonary function (FEV_1 and PEF), this improvement is additive to that produced by β-agonists, but less than that observed with ICS. Second, they decrease circulating eosinophil levels, and in this regard, appear additive or synergistic to the effect produced by ICS. Third, they are effective in inhibiting exercise-induced asthma, and this effect does not diminish when these drugs are used regularly, unlike that observed with the regular use of an LABA. Because exercise stimulates bronchoconstriction in 70% to 80% of patients with asthma, these agents might be especially useful in asthmatics in whom exercise is an important trigger. Fourth, the antileukotrienes (montelukast is the best studied in this regard) appear to have a beneficial effect on nasal symptoms present in allergic rhinitis, particularly congestion. Fifth, cysteinyl LTs appear to be particularly important in at least some asthmatics whose symptoms are triggered by nonsteroidal antiinflammatory agents such as aspirin.

2. Aspirin-induced asthma

At least 3% to 8% of patients with asthma have aspirin-induced asthma (AIA). In patients with AIA ingestion of aspirin or other non-steroidal antiinflammatory drugs (NSAIDs) causes profound, sometimes life-threatening bronchoconstriction as well as nasal–ocular, dermal, and gastrointestinal responses. These patients may have increased LTC_4 synthase activity. Furthermore, CysLT1 receptor antagonists may improve lung function in aspirin-sensitive patients with asthma in the absence of aspirin challenge. Therefore, LT modifiers should be considered first-line therapy in the subgroup of asthmatics with aspirin sensitivity.

Oral administration of any of these drugs to patients with chronic persistent asthma has improved lung function in a number of published studies. The drugs decreased the need for rescue treatment with β-adrenergic agonists, relieved asthma symptoms, decreased the frequency of exacerbations requiring oral glucocorticoid therapy or study withdrawal, and decreased the dose of inhaled glucocorticoid required to maintain control of asthma. These agents thus may have a glucocorticoid-sparing effect.

3. Bronchial relaxation

LT modifiers improve airway function rapidly; oral administration of either CysLT1 receptor antagonists or 5-LO inhibitors results in improvements in airway function within 1 to 3 hours. The bronchodilator effect is greater in patients with more airway obstruction, and the magnitude of this effect is about half that of the response to β_2-agonists, although as noted above, the bronchodilator effects of LT modifiers and beta-adrenergic agonists are partially additive. This suggests that the two types of drugs have different mechanisms of bronchial relaxation and therefore, that administration of both may be indicated for some patients.

4. Safety

Several studies have shown that LT modifiers are safe drugs. However, postmarketing surveillance indicates that zileuton can cause elevations in serum aminotransferases. Most laboratory abnormalities occur during the first 3 months of therapy, and they often resolve spontaneously or with the discontinuation of therapy, although rare cases of liver failure have been reported. Serum aminotransferase levels should be measured when zileuton therapy is initiated, monthly for 3 months, and periodically thereafter. A syndrome similar to the Churg-Strauss syndrome with marked circulating eosinophilia, cardiac failure, and associated eosinophilic vasculitis, has been reported in a few patients treated with zafirlukast or montelukast in several case studies. This syndrome is rare, and has been thought to represent the clinical unmasking of already present Churg-Strauss syndrome in patients misdiagnosed with steroid-dependent asthma. The incidence has been estimated at less than 1 case per 20,000 patients. Refer to Table 6.6 for a list of the currently available antileukotrienes and some of their properties.

F. Cromolyn sodium and nedocromil

Cromolyn sodium was developed as a mast cell stabilizer using a rodent mast cell model, whereas nedocromil is a second-generation agent developed using human cells as a model. Whether these two agents derive most of their clinical benefit from their "antimediator release" activities, rather than from other activities, is not clear. Cromolyn sodium blocks both early- and late-phase asthmatic responses to allergen exposure, cold air, and exercise when given as prophylaxis. A number of the studies suggest a modest improvement in airway reactivity with a chronic use (6 weeks) of cromolyn, similar to that observed with ICS. Addition of cromolyn to ICS (beclomethasone) therapy has not shown to have any added benefit when compared to ICS therapy alone. Cromolyn is available both as a solution for nebulization and as an MDI, although many pediatricians feel that it must be given by nebulization for optimal effect. Nedocromil sodium (Tilade) has similar pharmacologic properties as cromolyn, and may have an additional benefit of suppressing cough. It is available as an MDI. A meta-analysis published in 1993 reviewed several trials regarding the efficacy of nedocromil. It concluded that nedocromil was more effective than placebo and is most beneficial when used with bronchodilator monotherapy. As with cromolyn, nedocromil was less potent than ICS. Both agents are particularly noteworthy because of their excellent safety profile. In some studies nedocromil has been shown to have modest steroid-sparing effects.

G. Methylxanthines

The mechanism of action of methylxanthines remains unclear. Although it is known that these drugs inhibit the enzyme phosphodiesterase, they typ-

Table 6.6. Drugs that act on the 5-lipoxygenase pathway

Drug class and name	Trade name	Recommended dose	Other information
LEUKOTRIENE RECEPTOR ANTAGONISTS			
Montelukast	Singulair	Adult: 10 mg orally each night Pediatric: (2–5 yr) 4 mg orally each night; (6–14 yr) 5 mg orally each night	
Zafirlukast	Accolate	Adult (>12 yr): 20 mg orally twice daily Pediatric: (7–10 yr) 10 mg orally twice daily	Take 1 h before or 2 h after eating
5-LIPOXYGENASE INHIBITOR			
Zileuton	Zyflo	Adult: 600 mg four times daily Pediatric: not available	Measure serum alanine amino-transferase before treatment, every month for 3 months, and periodically thereafter

ically do so at higher concentrations than are seen *in vivo* at usual doses. Because phosphodiesterase catalyzes the breakdown of cAMP, its inhibition should lead to increased intracellular cAMP in airway smooth muscle and resultant bronchodilation. Another proposed mechanism of action of methylxanthines is that they antagonize airway smooth muscle adenosine receptors, but these data have also been inconclusive. Nevertheless, these agents do provide bronchodilation, and may improve diaphragmatic function as well. However, the degree of bronchodilation provided by the methylxanthines is inferior when compared to that of inhaled β-agonists. These agents should be considered second-line adjuncts for the control of asthma symptoms, and may be useful when nocturnal symptoms are prominent or when inhaler technique or compliance with medications is an issue.

The most frequently used methylxanthines are theophylline and aminophylline. Aminophylline has been available for many years for parenteral use and is typically used to treat status asthmaticus. Recent data suggest that parenteral aminophylline adds little to the management of status asthmaticus if high-dose inhaled beta-agonists are already in use. High-dose beta-agonists are safer than aminophylline and more efficacious, and as a result, the use of parenteral aminophylline has declined. Theophylline is a mild to moderate bronchodilator with myriad potential adverse effects and drug interactions. In addition, the methylxanthines have a narrow therapeutic index, thus close monitoring of serum levels is required. A serum concentration of between 5 and 12 µg per mL is typically recommended for chronic theophylline therapy. Close monitoring of serum concentrations is necessary in patients with liver disease, congestive heart failure, pregnancy, and when certain drugs such as macrolide and quinolone antibiotics and cimetadine are being used. If close monitoring is impossible, the daily dose should not exceed 10 mg/kg/day in adults. Low-dose theophylline has been reported to provide significant benefit when added to ICS in patients who were inadequately controlled while taking ICS alone. Signs and symptoms of theophylline toxicity include nausea, vomiting, palpitations, and tremor.

Malignant arrhythmias, seizures, and even death have been reported, particularly with high serum levels.

H. Anticholinergic agents

Parasympathetic nerves are the dominant bronchoconstrictor neural pathways in human airways and cholinergic tone is the major reversible component in COPD. Cholinergic pathways via the vagus nerve contribute to the diurnal variation in airway tone seen in most asthmatics. However, anticholinergic agents are less potent bronchodilators than beta$_2$-agonists for asthma, and their efficacy in the long-term management of asthma has not been demonstrated. However, several studies have shown that inhaled ipratropium might provide additive benefit when used with inhaled beta$_2$-agonists for acute asthma and status asthmaticus. Ipratropium is a quaternary ammonium derivative of atropine without the side effects of atropine. Ipratropium has been best studied as an adjunctive medication used with beta-agonists (either nebulized or MDI) in patients with moderate to severe acute asthma who present to the emergency department. One meta-analysis suggests that ipratropium provides a small additional improvement in bronchodilation when compared to inhaled beta-agonist used alone, and may produce a small reduction in subsequent hospital admission rates as well.

Tiotropium bromide is a quaternary ammonium compound that has been available for use in Europe and it appears to have a much longer duration of action in both animal and *in vitro* studies. It also appears to be more potent than ipratropium and has greater muscarinic receptor subtype selectivity. One small, randomized, controlled study demonstrated that tiotropium provided a small increase in FEV$_1$ that persisted for greater than 24 hours when compared to placebo. Tiotropium also reduced bronchial responsiveness, and provided a bronchoprotective effect when compared to placebo. Larger studies that specifically examine clinical endpoints relevant to asthma are needed before tiotropium can be considered for the management of asthma.

XV. Immunological therapies

A. Antiimmunoglobulin E

IgE plays an important role in the development of allergy and atopic asthma. IgE initiates the mast cell inflammatory cascade and thus plays an early role in the immunological response to allergens. The key role of IgE in asthma pathogenesis is supported by epidemiological studies showing that serum IgE levels correlate closely with cutaneous reactivity to common allergens, and the prevalence of asthma and BHR. Because IgE plays a role early in the sequence leading to early and late responses to allergens, BHR, and possibly airway remodeling, it is a very attractive and specific target for asthma therapy.

Recombinant humanized monoclonal antibody directed against IgE, (rhu MAb-E 25, or E25, omalizumab), is one of many monoclonal antibodies now being developed for therapeutic purposes. E25 is a chimeric antibody composed of both human (95%) and murine elements. It is designed to be nonimmunogeneic; in other words, it does not provoke the synthesis of neutralizing antibodies. When E25 binds to free IgE, it forms an immune complex that cannot interact with the FcεI or FcεRII receptor on effector cells. Because little IgE is available for binding to the FcεRI receptor, the priming and degranulation of mast cells and basophils is blocked, and IgE-mediated inflammatory responses are attenuated. Treatment of humans with anti-IgE also has the potentially important effect of markedly decreasing FcεRI receptor numbers on circulating basophils, and could conceivably have a similar effect on mast cells. E25 serum concentrations peak between 3 and 14 days after subcutaneous administration. One physiological endpoint that has been studied in early studies evaluating E25 was responsiveness to airway challenge. The early asthmatic response to inhaled allergen is mediated via IgE in a classic type I hypersensitivity reaction. Late-phase asthmatic responses to allergens occur 2 or more hours after allergen exposure and are manifested as bronchoconstriction, increased airway inflammation, increased bronchial and vascular permeability, and increased bronchial hyperresponsiveness. E25 therapy suppressed allergen-induced early- and late-phase asthmatic responses in a few early studies.

In a recent double-blind, placebo-controlled study of 317 patients with moderate to severe perennial allergic asthma who required daily use of ICSs or oral corticosteroids, E25 in a dose-dependent manner reduced asthma symptom scores. Furthermore, treatment with E25 allowed for a reduction in both the use of corticosteroids and rescue beta$_2$-agonists. However, in this trial, although E25 had a modest effect on PEF values, it had no effect on FEV$_1$. E25 has also been shown to reduce asthma exacerbations and improve QOL. Similar results have been found in pediatric populations. In both adults and children E25 had a good safety profile in clinical trials. Because of cost and drug delivery issues, E25 may be considered as an adjunct medication in the management of patients with moderate to severe perennial allergic asthma. Promising data also exist for E25 in seasonal and perennial allergic rhinitis, so that it might be particularly useful when asthma and rhinitis are coexistent. Further studies need to be performed to further clarify its role in other asthma patient subgroups. E25 will be administered subcutaneously every 2 to 4 weeks based on body weight and baseline serum IgE level.

B. Soluble interleukin 4 receptor

IL-4 plays an important role in allergic diseases and is considered a "Th2 cytokine." It induces isotype switching of immunoglobulins to the IgE phenotype. IL-4, by increasing vascular cell adhesion molecule-1 (VCAM-1) expression on endothelial cells, promotes the recruitment of eosinophils to sites of allergic inflammation. By promoting the differentiation of naive Th0 lymphocytes into the Th2 subtype, IL-4 increases the synthesis of Th2 cytokines. On the cell surface IL-4 interacts with high-affinity receptors. IL-4 may bind to a secreted form of the IL-4 receptor (IL-4R) and hence is inactivated; one such recombinant, soluble, extracellular product has been developed (Nuvance, Immunex Corp., Seattle, WA) and tested in a small, randomized, double-blind Phase II trial. IL-4R was given as a single dose of nebulized solution to patients with moderate atopic asthma. Subjects in the IL-4 arm experienced an improvement in FEV$_1$ and forced expiratory flow at 25% to 75% of FVC (FEF$_{25\%-75\%}$), a decrease in use of β$_2$-agonist, and no deterioration of symptoms after a withdrawal of corticosteroids when compared to the placebo arm. However, negative results have also been found in clinical trials. Obviously, larger clinical trials need to be conducted to further clarify the place of IL-4 antagonists in asthma.

C. Antiinterleukin 5

IL-5 is another Th2 cytokine. However, this cytokine has specific effects important to eosinophils. It appears necessary for eosinophilopoiesis, and can cause eosinophil priming and activation. Because of the importance of eosinophils in asthma, agents with eosinophil-specific activities have been thought to be ideal for asthma treatment, because of their selectivity. In both animal and human model systems, humanized preparations of anti-IL-5 have been shown to markedly decrease circulating eosinophil concentrations, and eosinophil numbers in the lung as determined by either BAL or induced sputum. Anti-IL-5 has been shown to be very effective in animal models of antigen-induced airway inflammation and asthma. However, at least some early trials of anti-IL-5 in human asthma have not been encouraging. Although anti-IL-5 decreased eosinophils, no significant effects were found on asthma symptoms. Whether this possible lack of beneficial clinical effect in humans is due to dosing issues, or because this approach to asthma therapy is doomed to failure, has not been determined.

D. Future therapies

Knowledge of the immune system and lung inflammation will likely provide even more therapeutic targets for asthma. The IL-4R and E25 data highlight a trend toward the specific targeting of inflammatory mediators and pathways in the future management of asthma.

XVI. Management of acute asthma

An asthma exacerbation may be managed in a variety of settings. However managing asthma attacks successfully requires knowledge of the factors that put patients at a greater risk of mortality or morbidity. Patients with such risk factors need special attention. Factors identified in epidemiological studies that might increase the risk of death include:

Current or recent use of systemic corticosteroids
Prior intubation for asthma
Recent hospitalization (within 1 year) for asthma
History of noncompliance with asthma medications
History of social problems or denial of asthma or its severity

Patients who are well educated about their asthma and who demonstrate sound judgment in the past may often be safely treated in the outpatient setting, provided that they are not having a severe exacerbation. A severe exacerbation requires prompt identification and treatment and is most safely accomplished in the inpatient setting.

A. Management of asthma exacerbation in the outpatient setting

Patients should be instructed to recognize the symptoms of an asthma exacerbation in its early stages. Such warning signs include, but are not limited to, exertional dyspnea, nocturnal awakenings and coughing, and increased rescue-MDI usage. They should learn to recognize factors that may lead to an exacerbation, such as an oncoming allergic season or viral upper respiratory infections. Some experts advocate the monitoring of PEF on a daily basis for all asthmatics, but especially those with frequent exacerbations. Some data suggest that the PEF will decrease prior to the development of overt symptoms. The obvious advantage is that the early detection of an exacerbation can lead to a step-up in antiinflammatory therapy, thus aborting an exacerbation before it requires acute care. Chronic asthmatics at a low risk of dying from acute asthma may be managed at home. First, the health care professional should ascertain the severity of an asthma exacerbation. Patients should be questioned about the presence of symptoms such as cough, breathlessness, wheeze, and chest tightness. Knowing if nocturnal symptoms are present, if there is a significant decrease in PEF compared to baseline, and the amount of recent rescue MDI use can help the health care professional establish the severity of an exacerbation. In addition, prior to deciding to treat asthma in the home setting, one needs to decide if the patient has adequate social support and the ability to receive prompt medical attention in case there is deterioration in the face of intensified therapy. One strategy that may be used to assess if home therapy is appropriate is illustrated below.

One may begin treatment with an inhaled short-acting β_2-agonist (SABA), dosing up to three times in the first hour. On the basis of response, further management should be as follows. If the response to SABA is satisfactory (i.e., relief of symptoms within 4 hours and/or PEF improves to greater than 80% of predicted or personal best), continue SABA every 3 to 4 hours for 1 to 2 days and follow up. If the response to SABA is unsatisfactory (i.e., persistent or deteriorating symptoms despite SABA and/or PEF less than 60% of predicted or personal best), start oral corticosteroids (i.e., 1 mg per kg of prednisone), repeat SABA, and recommend a prompt visit to the emergency department. If the response to SABA is partial (i.e., initially good response but recurrence of symptoms within 3 hours and/or PEF between 60% to 80% of predicted or personal best), start corticosteroids (i.e., 1 mg/kg of prednisone), continue SABA, and follow up within 12 to 24 hours.

B. Management of asthma in the emergency department

When the chronic asthmatic presents to the emergency department, it is often because short-acting controller medications have failed to provide relief and more severe degrees of airway inflammation and bronchospasm are present. In addition to the usual initial assessment of "airway, breathing, and circulation" every effort should be made to quickly determine the severity of acute asthma so that proper management can be instituted in a timely manner. Studies have shown that the initial response to an adequate dose of a short- or intermediate-acting bronchodilator is predictive of the need for admission to the hospital. However, some patients with a less than complete response to the initial beta-agonist treatment will eventually respond after a few hours of treatment. When a moderate or severe exacerbation is suspected, or if there is not a good response to initial bronchodilator treatment, systemic corticosteroids should be given. Patients with severe degrees of airflow obstruction that do not respond to aggressive treatment should be considered for admission to the intensive care unit. Parenteral methylxanthines, parenteral beta-agonists, and epinephrine may be used as second-line agents when high-dose inhaled bronchodilators (i.e., nebulized albuterol 12 mg per hour given by continuous nebulizer) and systemic steroids fail to achieve the desired response. However, the data suggest that these parenteral bronchodilators add little if anything to high-dose inhaled bronchodilators, and their side effects may be significant. The addition of anticholinergics by MDI or nebulizer can provide additive bronchodilation. The use of LT blockers is under study, and preliminary results are promising. Sedatives are absolutely contraindicated in the treatment of acute asthma in nonintubated patients. Mucolytic agents (because they may cause deterioration of cough), magnesium sulfate (no data to support benefit), massive hydration, and antibiotics (unless there is evidence of pneumonia or sinusitis) are not indicated in the management of acute asthma.

XVII. Intensive care unit management

Mechanical Ventilation In Acute Severe Asthma

Mechanical ventilation during a severe asthma attack presents several challenges. First, the incidence of barotrauma, and hence mortality, was formerly very high. This was due to the use of large tidal volumes and the resultant high distending pressures that developed because of bronchospasm and hyperinflation. Though hypoxia must be avoided, it has been recognized that the risks of hypercapnia are manageable. This has led to the use of permissive hypercapnia and lung protective strategies that have dramatically reduced morbidity. In addition, modern ventilators allow for the use of rapid flow rates, thus shortening the inspiratory time, and hence lengthening the expiratory time. Longer expiratory times allow for improved gas emptying, reduced air trapping, and reduced airway pressures. Attention to airway pressures, coupled with the judicious use of a broad array of sedative agents and neuromuscular relaxants, has led to improved management of severe asthma requiring mechanical ventilation. All patients should receive intensive beta-agonist therapy and systemic corticosteroids.

Notably, recent studies suggest that the need for mechanical ventilation for an episode of severe asthma identifies a group at high risk for subsequent morbidity and mortality. These patients had greater than 10% mortality rate in one study. Surprisingly, another study revealed that such patients were often not seen by a specialist nor had lung function checked after being discharged from the hospital after their severe asthma attack. These data reiterate that asthmatics developing severe attacks do so in part because they have poorly controlled disease. They therefore should be targeted for intense outpatient education, therapy, and follow-up with monitoring of objective measures of lung function.

XVIII. Management of conditions that exacerbate asthma

    A. Gastroesophageal reflux disease

        Gastroesophageal reflux disease (GERD) is a very common disorder, however, the true prevalence as reported in observational studies is unclear because it presents with a variable symptom complex, it occurs intermittently, and there is no easily performed gold standard test. Heartburn (pyrosis) is used as the symptom that identifies patients with GERD in many studies, and most adults will occasionally experience heartburn. Many patients with GERD also frequently complain of dysphagia and/or regurgitation. It is not clear whether GERD causes asthma. However, it occasionally causes wheezing and chest pain, frequently causes chronic cough, and may cause dyspnea. GERD seems to be quite common in asthmatics with a reported prevalence of between 30% and 90% in several studies. Notably, some patients with asthma have significant reflux but lack esophageal symptoms, including pyrosis and dysphagia. How GERD contributes to the pathogenesis of asthma or to bronchoconstriction is incompletely understood. One attractive theory is that acid-reflux contributes to bronchoconstriction via a vagally mediated mechanism. In this model, acidification of the esophageal lumen increases bronchial smooth muscle tone. Animal data exist that support the vagal hypothesis, but studies in humans have given conflicting results. There are also data suggesting that an increase in respiratory symptoms with acid reflux may not be entirely due to bronchoconstriction. Intratracheal acid administration leads to bronchoconstriction, supporting a role for microaspiration in the pathogenesis. These observations have lead some to speculate that GERD might cause asthma in some patients, while others believe that GERD aggravates but does not cause asthma.

Nevertheless, all asthma patients should be questioned about reflux symptoms. Because reflux is often clinically silent, establishing a pattern of asthma symptoms related to meals or recumbence is sometimes helpful. If symptoms compatible with GERD are present in a patient with asthma, a 3-month trial of acid suppression is warranted. The proton-pump inhibitors are most effective in alleviating GERD symptoms. General measures such as elevating the head of the bed, losing weight, and avoiding recumbence for at least several hours after meals, should also be tried. If uncertainty exists or if a patient fails to improve with an empiric trial, a 24-hour esophageal pH study with symptom recall may be used to establish the presence of reflux. Referral to a gastroenterologist should be considered, particularly if severe symptoms are present, the presence of esophagitis is suspected, or if the patient fails to respond to standard therapy.

B. Aspirin sensitivity

Patients with classic AIA develop wheezing, facial flushing, and profound nasal symptoms after aspirin ingestion. Notably, AIA patients often have asthma that is more severe and difficult to treat than non-AIA asthmatics. AIA also seems to be more prevalent in steroid-dependent asthmatics and in those who have sinusitis and nasal polyps.

AIA was once thought to be due to an allergy to aspirin, but is probably due to a nonallergic mechanism for several reasons. First, AIA tends to develop in the third and fourth decades, a period of life when the prevalence IgE-mediated allergies tends to decline. Second, patients with AIA tend to have a slow onset of symptoms after aspirin ingestion, in contrast to the typical rapid response to inhaled aeroallergens. Finally, AIA patients often will react to other NSAIDs, which may be structurally distinct from aspirin. NSAIDs and aspirin act by inhibition of the isoenzymes cyclooxygenase 1 and 2 (COX-1 and COX-2); however, they may also increase LT levels perhaps by a direct activation of 5-LO. In addition, several lines of evidence suggest that AIA is caused by an abnormality of LT metabolism. Definitive diagnosis involves challenge with aspirin and a placebo control and/or the subsequent measurement of urinary LT metabolites. Because there is the potential for a serious reaction, patients should be carefully selected and only tested in specialized centers.

The treatment of patients with AIA is similar to that of any other asthma patient. NSAID avoidance is strongly advised. The selective COX-2 inhibitors rofecoxib (Vioxx) and celecoxib (Celebrex) seem to have a reduction in side effects related to COX inhibition. Until further studies have proven their safety in AIA, alternative agents should be used in patients with a history of bronchospasm with rhinoconjunctivitis, or urticaria/

angioedema associated with aspirin or other nonsteroidal antiinflammatory agents. Desensitization to ASA and NSAIDs may be carried out in specialized centers when their use is strongly desired or necessary. Acetaminophen, magnesium salicylate, and salicylic acid have a low affinity for the COX enzyme and all three drugs may be used with caution in most patients with AIA. Patients with AIA should have their sinus and nasal disease evaluated and treated. Nasal steroids may be effective in controlling nasal symptoms and polyp growth. Most promising has been the use of both 5-LO inhibitors and LTD_4 receptor antagonists. Both classes of drugs have been shown to blunt the development of symptoms in some AIA patients who were subsequently challenged with aspirin. Similarly, both classes of medications improve pulmonary function and reduce beta-agonist use when used by patients with AIA. Because of the demonstrable benefit, the LT-modifying drugs should be considered as first-line therapy in the subclass of asthmatic patients with AIA.

C. Upper airway disease and asthma

The incidence of allergic rhinitis in asthmatic adults is estimated to be about 58% and is thus twice as common as it is in the general adult population. Similarly, sinusitis and nasal polyps occur with asthma more frequently than would be expected by chance. Therefore, there are convincing epidemiological data linking the upper and lower airways. The airway is a contiguous structure and is lined throughout its length by pseudostratified columnar epithelium. Nasal washings, BAL, and histopathologic studies suggest that similar cells and mediators play a role in both rhinitis and asthma. In addition, both early- and late-phase reactions have been observed after bronchial allergen challenge in nonasthmatic patients with allergic rhinitis. Finally, similar medications are used at both airway levels to treat inflammation and symptoms. Because of these relationships between the upper and lower airways, and because of the morbidity associated with rhinitis and sinusitis per se, it is easily understood how treatment of the upper airway, when it is affected in the asthmatic, can markedly improve outcomes and patient satisfaction.

1. Sinusitis

Sinusitis and asthma have been associated for many years. Some studies suggest that nonspecific treatment of coexistent sinusitis (i.e., with antibiotics and decongestants) can reduce asthma symptoms. However, it has been difficult to show concomitant improvements in objective measurements of lung function, despite some small studies that have suggested such a benefit. Although the treatment of rhinosinusitis often leads to improvements in the symptom of dyspnea, it often fails to relieve wheeze and cough. One explanation for this observation is that a reduction in upper airway impedance reduces dyspnea while having no effect on inflammation in the lower airways. Nasal polyposis may lead to recurrent sinus infections. Most patients with polyps have negative skin-prick tests and tend to have more severe asthma. Many of these patients require high doses of ICS or even oral steroids for asthma control. There seem to be two subsets of patients with nasal polyps and asthma. Nasal polyps in some seem to respond to topical steroids, whereas in others there is no response. Nonresponders tend to have lower PC_{20} and FEV_1 levels and they often require surgical intervention for their sinusitis. Because poorly-controlled sinusitis results in significant morbidity and may exacerbate asthma, it should be aggressively managed in the asthmatic. Care should be taken to identify symptoms of lower airway inflammation and to treat these with specific medications when they are present.

2. Allergic rhinitis

Allergic rhinitis is very prevalent and it may affect up to 40% of individuals. Of these, about 75% have seasonal rhinitis or hay fever, whereas about 25% have perennial rhinitis. Although a nasal allergen challenge typically does not induce airflow obstruction in lower airways, it may increase BHR. As with other atopic diseases, allergic rhinitis is often found early in life and its prevalence decreases with age. Asthma that has a seasonal pattern has been linked to hay fever, whereas house dust mite asthma has been linked to perennial rhinitis. Indoor allergens including house dust mite, cockroach, and cat dander have been strongly linked to both asthma and perennial rhinitis. In epidemiological studies the association for asthma and outdoor allergens is weaker; however, increased mold counts have been associated with asthma exacerbations. These disparities suggest that asthma and rhinitis are distinctly different in some ways. NSAIDs and aspirin also act as triggers for symptoms in both the nose and lung. One important management question that remains to be fully answered is whether local treatment of rhinitis can improve asthma control. The most effective treatment for rhinitis includes topical corticosteroids. In some, but not all studies, topical corticosteroids improved symptoms, pulmonary function, BHR, or EIB. Notably, the treatment effect was usually modest. Although histamine antagonists (H1-blockers) are first-line treatment for allergic rhinitis, they are not routinely recommended as asthma controller medications. Finally, newer drugs that modify the LT pathway have been shown to reduce asthma symptoms, improve lung function, and block EIB. Although the data examining the efficacy of LT antagonists in allergic rhinitis are limited, some data show efficacy in rhinitis, and these drugs also may potentate the effectiveness of H1 antagonists as well.

XIX. Immunotherapy

The efficacy of specific immunotherapy is well established for seasonal allergic rhinitis and to a lesser extent for perennial rhinitis. Specific immunotherapy consists of administering increasing concentrations of allergen over a long period. It has varied and broad effects on the immune system. Allergen immunotherapy promotes the production of blocking antibodies (IgG) that reduce allergic inflammation. Immunotherapy also shifts T-cell-mediated cytokine production from a Th2 pattern to a more Th1-like pattern. For the patient with rhinitis, immunotherapy often reduces and sometimes obviates the need for other pharmacotherapy such as H1-blockers, corticosteroids, and LT antagonists. Immunotherapy may be indicated for an asthmatic without severe disease (FEV_1 greater than 70% after pharmacological treatment). It is especially indicated when symptoms are not adequately controlled by avoidance of the suspected antigen, when both nasal and bronchial symptoms are present, and when pharmacotherapy is either incompletely effective or not desired. Immunotherapy is contraindicated when severe asthma or other cardiopulmonary disease is present because of the increased risk of adverse event outcomes. Because most patients with allergic asthma also have rhinitis, immunotherapy would seem to be an especially attractive option because it may alleviate symptoms and improve the QOL.

A number of clinical studies have examined the efficacy of immunotherapy for atopic asthma. Although some of these studies have been randomized and placebo controlled, most have been small. It appears that immunotherapy can reduce asthma and rhinitis symptoms for some allergens. Animal-induced asthma is an important entity, and between 15% and 30% of asthmatics test positive to dog or cat antigens. Cat dander (*Fel d* 1) is an important and potent antigen and some studies have shown that allergen immunotherapy can alleviate asthma symptoms while reducing both nonspecific (methylcholine, histamine) and allergen-induced BHR. Some of these studies were conducted in patients who have occasional exposures to animals. Thus, the results may not apply to the patient who is allergic to a pet that they keep in the home. Similarly, studies of patients who are allergic to dust-mite antigen have shown benefit with regard to symptom scores and antigen-specific BHR. However, it appears that older patients and patients with more severe asthma (FEV_1 less than 70%

predicted) are less likely to benefit. This is also true of patients with chronic sinusitis and aspirin sensitivity. Nonatopic asthma probably explains the lack of benefit in these subgroups.

Seasonal antigens such as tree pollen, grass, and ragweed differ from perennial antigens in that a patient with seasonal allergies may often have asthma symptoms only during the allergic season. The symptomatic period for those who are allergic to tree pollen sometimes is quite short, making immunotherapy for these allergens difficult to justify. Nevertheless, because grass and ragweed have longer seasons, immunotherapy may be of some value in carefully selected patients, although the long-term effects of immunotherapy on lung function and asthma-specific symptoms appear to be modest.

XX. Occupational asthma and reactive airways dysfunction syndrome

  A. Occupational asthma

  Asthma has become the most prevalent occupational lung disease in developed countries. More than 250 agents have been associated with asthma in the workplace. Some estimate that up to 15% of all asthma cases are caused by an agent in the workplace or worsened by the work environment. Therefore, all patients with suspected asthma or patients with known asthma and clinical deterioration should be questioned about workplace exposures. Patients should be questioned about materials they are exposed to and how they are used at work; the temporal relationship between work and symptoms should also be explored. Refer to Table 6.7 for a representative listing of agents known to cause asthma in the workplace. When a workplace factor is suspected, the degree of impairment must be continually assessed. The American Thoracic Society has published guidelines on the evaluation of impairment or disability in patients with asthma.

  There are two categories of asthma in the workplace. OA is characterized by variable airflow obstruction and BHR caused by conditions in the work environment. This is contrasted with work-aggravated asthma, which is preexisting asthma aggravated by a workplace exposure. Furthermore, there are two major categories of OA. Occupational asthma with latency is the most common type and may develop after a variable period of exposure to an agent. The latency period can vary from a few weeks to a few years. High molecular weight compounds typically induce asthma with specific IgE antibodies. Low molecular weight (LMW) compounds may also act as haptens and induce IgE-mediated asthma. However, specific IgE has not been found for many LMW substances known to cause OA. The prototypic LMW substances that cause asthma are the isocyanates. Isocyanates are frequently implicated in OA and widely used in many industrial applications.

  B. Reactive airways dysfunction syndrome

  Occupational asthma without latency is sometimes referred to as irritant-induced asthma or RADS. The term RADS was initially coined to describe the development of airflow obstruction and BHR in the minutes or hours following an intense exposure to an irritant gas, aerosol, or particles. It is also appreciated that multiple exposures to a low concentration of an irritant can lead to bronchial mucosal injury and subsequent BHR. There are numerous reports in the literature of clustered cases related to large spills. After the acute exposure, patients with RADS often describe the sudden onset of a burning sensation in the throat and nose as well as dyspnea, cough, and wheezing. The other key clinical feature of RADS is the development of persistent airflow obstruction and BHR. The bronchoconstriction in RADS is typically not responsive to bronchodilators. Epithelial denudation and airway inflammation play a prominent role. These observations, in combination with data from animal models, have caused some physicians to recommend that therapy for RADS include oral steroids (40 to 80 mg prednisone daily for 2 weeks) followed by high-dose ICS.

  C. Diagnosis

  The diagnosis of OA or RADS can be challenging. Ideally, the history should suggest a link between symptoms and work. For example, a history

Table 6.7. Common causes of occupational asthma

Material	Occupation at risk
Chemical	
Isocyanates	
Toluene diisocyanate (TDI)	Polyurethane workers, insulators, laminators
Diphenylmethane diisocyanate	Laminators, polyurethane foam workers
Hexamethylene diisocyanate	Painters, plastics workers
Napthalene diisocyanate	Chemists, rubber workers
Anhydrides	
Trimellitic anhydride	Chemical workers
Phthalic anhydride	Painters, plastics workers
Hexahydrophthalic anhydride	Epoxy resins workers
Tetrachlorophthalic anhydride	Epoxy resins workers
Polyvinyl chloride vapor	Meat wrappers
Formaldehyde	Laboratory workers, embalmers, insulators, textile workers
Dimethylethanolamine	Paint sprayers
Ethylenediamine	Rubber workers, photographic processors
Persulfate salts	Chemical workers, beauticians
Ethylene oxide	Medical sterilizers
Pyrethrin	Fumigators
Ammonium thioglycolate	Beauticians
Monoethanolamine	Beauticians
Hexamethylenamine	Beauticians
Wood dusts	
Western red cedar	Woodworkers
Cedar of Lebanon	Woodworkers
Mahogany	Woodworkers
California redwood	Woodworkers
Oak	Woodworkers
Iroko	Woodworkers
Boxwood	Woodworkers
Cocabolla	Woodworkers
Zebrawood	Woodworkers
Mansonia	Woodworkers
Mulberry	Woodworkers
Metals	
Chromic acid	Chrome platers, welders
Potassium chromate and dichromate	Chrome workers, cement workers
Platinum salts	Platinum refiners
Chloroplatinic acid	Platinum refiners, chemists
Nickel sulfate	Nickel platers, welders
Nickel carboxyl	Chemical workers, nickel platers, welders
Vanadium	Boiler cleaners, turbine cleaners
Dyes	
Anthraquinone	Fabric dyers
Carmine	Cosmetics and dye workers
Paraphenyl diamine	Fur dyers
Hexafix brilliant yellow	Dye manufacturers
Drimaren brilliant blue	Dye manufacturers
Cibachrome brilliant scarlet	Dye manufacturers
Henna extract	Beauticians

Table 6.7. *Continued*

Material	Occupation at risk
Fluxes	
Colophony (soft-core solder)	Solderers, electronics workers
Aminoethylethanolamine	Aluminum solderers
Drugs	
Benzyl penicillin	Pharmaceutical workers
Ampicillin	Pharmaceutical workers
Sulfathiazole	Pharmaceutical workers
Tetracycline	Pharmaceutical workers
Psyllium	Pharmaceutical workers
Methyldopa	Pharmaceutical workers
Albuterol	Pharmaceutical workers
Piperazine dihydrochloride	Pharmaceutical workers
Chloramine T	Pharmaceutical and laboratory workers
Organophosphates	Farm workers, pesticide formulators, fumigators
Enzymes	
Pancreatic extracts	Pharmaceutical workers
Bacillus subtilis	Detergent manufacturers
Papain	Food processors
Trypsin	Plastics and rubber workers
Flaviastase	Pharmaceutical workers
Bromelain	Food processors
Pectinase	Food processors
Animals	
Domestic animals (hair, dander)	Farmers, veterinarians, meat processors
Birds	Poultry breeders, bird fanciers
Mice, guinea pigs (dander, urine)	Laboratory workers
Fish (glue)	Bookbinders, postal workers
Silkworms	Silk sericulturers
Insects, mites	Grain mill and storage workers, bakers
Plants	
Wheat	Farmers, grain handlers
Buckwheat	Bakers
Grain dust	Farmers, grain handlers, bakers
Rye flour	Bakers
Hops	Brewers
Tamarind seeds	Millers, spice processors
Castor beans	Farmers, castor bean workers
Coffee beans	Farmers, coffee bean workers
Wool	Textile workers
Tobacco dust	Cigarette manufacturers
Tea	Food processors
Cotton, flax, hemp	Textile workers
Vegetable gums	
Acacia	Printers
Tragacanth	Printers, food processors
Karaya	Food processors
Arabic	Printers
Latex	Pharmaceutical, laboratory, and healthcare workers

that suggests an improvement in symptoms during weekends and holidays with a worsening of symptoms upon returning to work is suggestive of OA. However, this type of history is neither sensitive nor specific in making the diagnosis of OA. Because the diagnosis of OA has important social and economic implications for both the patient and employer, objective tests should be obtained to support the clinical suspicion. One strategy is to monitor bronchial responsiveness. Similar to other forms of asthma, the measurement of BHR to nonspecific challenge has excellent negative predictive value. For example, the failure to demonstrate BHR after a patient has worked for 2 weeks under typical work conditions virtually excludes the diagnosis of OA. The gold standard test is a specific challenge test in which a patient is subjected to escalating inhaled doses of a suspected agent. This test is often impractical and poses some risks. The serial measurement of peak flow while the patient is at work can be compared to similar measurements while the patient is away from work. This has been shown to correlate with specific challenge results.

D. Treatment

The pharmacological treatment and monitoring of OA is similar to that of other forms of asthma. As a rule, if the etiologic agent is in the workplace, the worker must be removed from exposure to the agent. Complete removal is often needed because significant disability may result from prolonged exposure to an offending agent. In only a few cases can a patient with OA be protected with a respirator or improved ventilation, because people with OA tend to react to an extremely low concentration of an agent. In fact, many workers with OA do not make a full recovery and have permanent impairment. It is therefore essential to refer confirmed cases of OA to the appropriate employee compensation boards and health departments.

XXI. Issues in the pregnant asthmatic

Asthma is the most common respiratory disease in women of reproductive age. Pregnancy represents a unique physiological state that has effects on asthma. Roughly one-third of patients will experience a worsening of their asthma with pregnancy, one-third will improve, and one-third will not experience a change. Fortunately, labor and delivery do not worsen asthma in most patients. Prepregnancy asthma severity and measurements of BHR are not useful predictors of clinical deterioration. Asthma is generally less severe during the last month of pregnancy; however, those who worsen typically will worsen during the third trimester. Why patients deteriorate is not clear but may be due to the cessation of controller medications by expectant mothers after they realize they are pregnant. In addition, there seems to be a small increase in pregnancy-related complications in asthma patients. Nonetheless, asthma should not be considered a contraindication to pregnancy because the risks can be significantly modified with proper monitoring and therapy.

The goals of therapy in the pregnant patient are similar to those of any asthmatic. The proper use of controller medications should maximize lung function and activity, while minimizing symptoms and preventing exacerbations. Objective monitoring of lung function is of particular importance in pregnancy because when the asthmatic woman experiences dyspnea the symptom could be due to asthma, other cardiopulmonary disease(s), or the "dyspnea of pregnancy." One should be able to differentiate between asthma and the dyspnea of pregnancy by performing spirometry. If dyspnea is due to asthma and airflow obstruction, the FEV_1/FVC ratio usually decreases. The dyspnea of pregnancy is not caused by airflow obstruction, but by a combination of factors. While the gravid uterus changes the resting position of the diaphragm and reduces the functional residual capacity (FRC), diaphragmatic excursion remains unchanged. Moreover, the FVC, FEV_1, and FEV_1/FRC ratio remain normal. The pathogenesis of the dyspnea of pregnancy is poorly understood, but progesterone-mediated hyperventilation is probably at least partially responsible.

Treatment of asthma during pregnancy is similar to that for patients in the nonpregnant state. Standard pharmacological agents should be used with knowledge of their current categorization for use in pregnancy, and attention given to the risk-to-benefit ratio. Refer to Table 6.8 for a listing of U.S. Food and Drug Administration (FDA) pregnancy categories for drugs commonly used to treat asthma.

XXII. Asthma in the athlete and exercise-induced asthma

Exercise-induced asthma is really a misnomer; the term has been used to describe the onset of airflow obstruction precipitated by exercise. EIB is a more accurate term because exercise does not cause asthma per se, but rather induces bronchospasm in the person who has BHR and asthma. An exercise challenge study is actually a sensitive test for confirming asthma because EIB occurs in 70% to 80% of those with current symptomatic asthma. On occasion, exercise will be the only precipitant of symptoms and thus is managed differently than asthma with regular daily symptoms. The pathogenesis of EIB is not fully understood, but is believed to be a response to increased flow of drier and cooled air in the airways during exercise. The quicker flow rates do not allow the usual equilibration of temperature and humidity that takes place in

Table 6.8. Pregnancy risk categories of pharmacologic agents used in asthma

Drug[a]	Risk category[b]
Adrenergic agents	
Epinephrine	C
Metaproterenol	C
Terbutaline	B
Albuterol	C
Bitolterol	C
Pirbuterol	C
Salmeterol	C
Theophylline	C
Aminophylline	NC[c]
Ipratropium bromide	B
Cromolyn sodium	B
Nedocromil sodium	B
Inhaled corticosteroids	
Beclomethasone	C
Triamcinolone	C
Flunisolide	C
Fluticasone	C
Systemic corticosteroids	
Prednisone	B
Prednisolone	B
Dexamethasone	C
Methylprednisolone	NC[c]
Leukotriene modifiers	
Montelukast	B
Zafirlukast	B
Zileuton	C

[a] Category is the same for all routes of administration for each drug.

[b] Risk categories determined by the U.S. Food and Drug Administration (FDA) include: A, no risk in well-controlled studies; B, no adequate human studies and either some risk or no risk in animal studies; C, no adequate human studies and some risk in animal studies or no adequate human and animal studies available.

[c] NC indicates a noncategorized drug; in such drugs, use is acceptable but the risk must be weighed against the need for use.

the upper airway during quiet breathing. The laboratory testing for EIB is described in the Bronchial challenge testing (Section IX.D, page 104). There are interesting differences between EIB and bronchospasm elicited by specific triggers. First, although exercise can induce immediate or early-phase (similar to IgE mediated) bronchoconstriction, it has not been shown to cause late-phase bronchoconstriction in well-designed studies. Second, the episode of EIB is typically followed by a refractory period during which the airways are resistant to further EIB upon rechallenge with exercise. Typically, the airways will actually dilate with exercise and remain dilated for 2 to 3 minutes after exercise is stopped, then bronchoconstriction ensues, peaks in about 10 minutes, and resolves after an hour. There are several strategies used to prevent and treat EIB. First, because EIB is caused by high-minute ventilation breathing during exercise, a reduction in minute ventilation during exercise is helpful. This is not accomplished by avoiding exercise, but rather by training, because training reduces minute ventilation requirements at a given level of work. Second, avoiding exercise in cold, dry air or using a mask covering the mouth and nose is advisable because the development of EIB is related to the humidity and temperature of inspired air. Third, control of the underlying airway inflammation, usually with ICS, may be beneficial. Finally, medications can be used to prevent EIB (bronchoprotective effect), or reverse EIB once it ensues. Prophylaxis with a short- to medium-acting beta-agonist MDI is highly effective in preventing EIB. For example, two puffs of albuterol 5 to 10 minutes prior to exercise is usually efficacious. Similarly, cromolyn sodium or nedocromil sodium provides effective prophylaxis if used 15 to 20 minutes prior to exercise. In some patients, both agents used in combination provide superior protection compared to either used alone. For patients such as children who exercise at high intensity and intermittently, a longer acting agent may be appropriate. The LABA salmeterol and the LT antagonists zafirlukast, pranlukast, and montelukast are effective at blocking EIB. Some studies suggest that salmeterol loses some of its prophylactic efficacy with regular use. This "loss of bronchoprotection" does not seem to be a problem for the LT antagonists. Finally, patients with EIB should be instructed to use a rescue beta-agonist inhaler to reverse EIB if it does occur.

XXIII. Scuba diving in the patient with asthma

Boyle's law ($PV = k$) essentially states that that the volume of a gas is inversely proportional to its pressure. When a diver descends the lungs are exposed to hyperbaric conditions; with a breath-hold dive, the thoracic gas volume (TGV) cannot exceed the TLC. However, with a scuba dive, the TGV can exceed TLC if the breath is held during ascent. Rapid uncontrolled ascent can result in the dissection of gas along the pulmonary, perivascular sheaths and into the pleural space (pneumothorax) or pericardium (pneumopericardium). Similarly, gas can enter the pulmonary veins and cause arterial gas embolism. Except for drowning, gas embolism is the most common cause of accidental death during recreational diving.

In theory, the asthmatic may have areas of the lung that empty slowly (slow time-constants). Such areas may be predisposed to air trapping and subsequent barotrauma during ascent. Some retrospective data suggest that small-airways obstruction might increase the incidence of barotrauma in divers with asthma. Obstruction in the small airways can be assessed using maximal mid-expiratory flow rates ($FEF_{25\%}$, $FEF_{25\%-75\%}$). Other factors could also put the diving asthmatic at risk. The work of breathing during diving is increased. Diving also involves significant exercise while inhaling cold, dry air. The inhalation of cold, dry air is an effective trigger of BHR in many patients with asthma. All of these factors should be taken into account when assessing the risk to a given patient. Unfortunately, there are no population studies of any significant size that examine the risk of either barotrauma or mortality in divers with asthma.

Because of the lack of good data to give accurate risk estimates, and the fact that many thousands of patients with asthma dive without untoward effects, a pragmatic approach should be used. First, asthma must be well controlled in any patient considering diving. In addition, patients with anything other than mild asthma should be discouraged from diving. Second, the diver should be mature and knowledgeable enough to both recognize the warning signs of worsening asthma and to avoid diving when asthma is not well controlled. Third, because diving is an inherently dangerous sport, the diver should participate in the decision to dive, just as any patient would consider any procedure with inherent risk. In other words, rather than "clearing" a patient with asthma for diving, having the patient give informed consent encourages the patient to understand the risks associated with the activity and to take shared responsibility for the decision.

Acknowledgments

This work was supported in parts by grants AI24509, HL67663, and HL51810 from the National Institutes of Health (Stephen P. Peters, M.D., Ph.D.).

Selected Readings

Agertoft L, Pedersen S. Effect of long-term treatment with inhaled budesonide on adult height in children with asthma. *N Engl J Med* 2000;343:1064–1069.

ATS guidelines: Evaluation of impairment/disability in patients with asthma. *Am Rev Respir Dis* 1993;147:1056.

Aubier M, Pieter WR, Schlosser NJ, et al. Salmeterol/fluticasone propionate (50/500 microg) in combination in a Diskus inhaler (Seretide) is effective and safe in the treatment of steroid-dependent asthma. *Respir Med* 1999;93:876–884.

Borish LC, Nelson HS, Lanz MJ, et al. Interleukin-4 receptor in moderate atopic asthma. A phase I/II randomized, placebo-controlled trial. *Am J Respir Crit Care Med* 1999; 160:1816–1823.

Boulet LP, Chapman KR, Cote J, et al. Inhibitory effects of anti Ig-E antibody, E25 on allergen induced early asthmatic response. *Am J Respir Crit Care Med* 1997;155; 1835–1840.

Burrows B, Martinez FD, Halonen M, et al. Association of asthma with serum IgE levels and skin-test reactivity to allergens. *N Engl J Med* 1989;320:271–277.

Carey VJ, Weiss ST, Tager IB, et al. Airways responsiveness, wheeze onset, and recurrent asthma episodes in young adolescents. The East Boston Childhood Respiratory Disease Cohort. *Am J Respir Crit Care Med* 1996;153:356–361.

Chan-Yeung M, Malo JL. Occupational asthma. *N Engl J Med* 1995;333:107–112.

Colavita AM, Reinach AJ, Peters SP. Contributing factors to the pathobiology of asthma. The Th1/Th2 paradigm. *Clin Chest Med* 2000;21:263–277, viii.

Corbridge T, Hall JB. Status asthmaticus. In: Hall JB, Schmidt GA, Wood LDH, eds. *Principles of critical care,* 2nd ed. New York: McGraw-Hill, 1998.

Cowburn AS, Sladek K, Soja J, et al. Overexpression of leukotriene C4 synthase in bronchial biopsies from patients with aspirin-intolerant asthma. *J Clin Invest* 1998;101:834–846.

Creticos PS. The consideration of immunotherapy in the treatment of allergic asthma. *J Allergy Clin Immunol* 2000;105:S559–S574.

Creticos PS, Reed CE, Norman PS, et al. Ragweed immunotherapy in adult asthma. *N Engl J Med* 1996;334:501–506.

Cumming RG, Mitchell P, Leeder SR. Use of inhaled corticosteroids and the risk of cataracts. *N Engl J Med* 1997;337:8–14.

Dennis SM, Sharp SJ, Vickers MR, et al. Regular inhaled salbutamol and asthma control: the TRUST randomised trial. Therapy Working Group of the National Asthma Task Force and the MRC General Practice Research Framework. *Lancet* 2000;355: 1675–1679.

Drazen JM, Israel E, Boushey HA, et al. Comparison of regularly scheduled with as-needed use of albuterol in mild asthma. Asthma Clinical Research Network. *N Engl J Med* 1996;335:841–847.

Drazen JM, Israel E, O'Byrne PM, et al. Treatment of asthma with drugs modifying the Leukotriene Pathway. *N Engl J Med* 1999;340:197–204.

Edwards AM, Lyons J, Weinberg E, et al. Early use of inhaled nedocromil sodium in children following an acute episode of asthma. *Thorax* 1999;54:308–315.

Egan RW, Athwar D, Bodnar MV, et al. Effect of Sch 55700, a humanized monoclonal antibody to human interleukin-5, on eosinophilic responses and bronchial hyper-reactivity. *Arzneimittelforschung* 1999;49:779–790.

Evans Dl, Taylor DA, Zetterstrom O, et al. A comparison of low-dose inhaled budesonide plus theophylline and high-dose inhaled budesonide for moderate asthma. *New Engl J Med* 1997;337:1412–1418.

Fahy JV, Fleming HE, Wong HH, et al. The effect anti Ig-E monoclonal antibodies on the early and late phase response to allergen inhalation in asthmatic subjects. *Am J Respir Crit Care Med* 1997;155:1828–1834.

Fish JE, Peters SP. Airway remodeling and persistent airway obstruction in asthma. *J Allergy Clin Immunol* 1999;104:509–516.

Gibson PG. Monitoring the patient with asthma: an evidence-based approach. *J Allergy Clin Immunol* 2000;106:17–26.

Greening AP, Ind PW, Northfield M, et al. Added salmeterol versus higher dose cortico-steroids in asthma patients with symptoms on existing inhaled corticosteroids. *Lancet* 1994;344:219–224.

National Asthma Education and Prevention Program. Expert Panel Report 2: Guidelines for the diagnosis and management of asthma, NIH publication no. 97-4057. Available from: National Heart, Lung and Blood Institute, National Institutes of Health: Bethesda, MD, 1997.

Harding SM, Richter JE, Guzzo MR, et al. Asthma and gastroesophageal reflux: Acid suppression therapy improves asthma outcome. *Am J Med* 1996;100:395.

Hopkin JM. Genetics of atopy. In: Busse WW, Holgate ST, eds. *Asthma and rhinitis*. Boston: Blackwell, 1995:988–992.

Israel E, Fischer AR, Rosenberg MA, et al. The pivitol role of 5 lipoxygenase products in the reaction of aspirin-sensitive asthmatics to aspirin. *Am Rev Respir Dis* 1993; 148:1447.

Kavaru M, Melamed J, Gross G, et al. Salmeterol and fluticasone propionate combined in a new powder inhalation device for the treatment of asthma: a randomized, double-blind, placebo-controlled trial. *J Allergy Clin Immunol* 2000;105:1108–1116.

Kay AB. Allergy and allergic diseases. Second of two parts. Allergic diseases and their treatment. *N Engl J Med* 2001;344:109–113.

Kips JC, O'Connor BJ, Inman MD, et al. A long-term study of the anti-inflammatory effects of low-dose budesonide plus formoterol versus high-dose budesonide in asthma. *Am J Respir Crit Care Med* 2000;161:996–1001.

Krieger BP. Diving: what to tell the patient with asthma and why. *Curr Opinion Pulm Med* 2001;7:32–38.

Laitinen LA, Laitinen A, Haahtela T. A comparative study of the effects of an inhaled corticosteroid, budesonide, and a beta 2-agonist, terbutaline, on airway inflammation in newly diagnosed asthma: a randomized, double-blind, parallel-group controlled trial. *J Allergy Clin Immunol* 1992;90:32–42.

Laviolette M, Malmstrom K, Lu S, et al. Montelukast added to inhaled beclomethasone in treatment of asthma. Montelukast/Beclomethasone Additivity Group. *Am J Respir Crit Care Med* 1999;160:1862–1868.

Leckie MJ, TenBrinke A, Khan J, et al. Effects of an interleukin-5 blocking monoclonal antibody on eosinophils, airway hyper-responsiveness, and the late asthmatic response. *Lancet* 2000;356:2144–2148.

Malo JL, Chan-Yeung M, Lemière C, et al. Reactive airways dysfunction syndrome and irritant-induced asthma. In: Rose, BD, ed. *UpToDate*, Wellesley, MA, 2000.

Marquette CH, Saulnier F, Leroy O, et al. Long-term prognosis of near-fatal asthma. A 6-year follow-up study of 145 asthmatic patients who underwent mechanical ventilation for a near-fatal attack of asthma. *Am Rev Respir Dis* 1992;146:76.

Martin RJ, Wanger JS, Irvin CG, et al. Methacholine challenge testing: safety of low starting FEV1. Asthma Clinical Research Network (ACRN). *Chest* 1997;112:53–56.

McFadden ER, Casale TB, Edwards TB, et al. Administration of budesonide once daily by means of turbuhaler to subjects with stable asthma. *J Allergy Clin Immunol* 1999;104:46–52.

Milgrom H, Fick RB, Su JQ, et al. Treatment of allergic asthma with monoclonal anti Ig-E antibody. *N Engl J Med* 1999;341:1966–1973.

Mofino NA, Nannini LJ, Rebuck AS, et al. The fatality-prone asthmatic patient. Follow-up study after near-fatal attacks. *Chest* 1992;101:621.

Nelson JA, Strauss L, Skowronski M, et al. Effect of long-term salmeterol treatment on exercise-induced asthma. *N Engl J Med* 1998;339:141–146.

O'Connor BJ, Tawes LJ, Barnes PJ. Prolonged effect of tiotropium bromide on metha-choline-induced bronchoconstriction in asthma. *Am J Respir Crit Care Med*. 1996; 154:876–880.

Pauwels RA, Lofdahl CG, Postma DS, et al. Effect of inhaled formoterol and budesonide on exacerbations of asthma. *N Engl J Med* 1997;337:1405–1411.

Peters SP. Risk-benefit issues in using glucocorticoids in adult and geriatric patients. *Clin Asthma Rev* 1997;1:115–121.

Platts-Mills TAE, Sporik RB, Chapman MD, et al. The role of indoor allergens in asthma. *Allergy* 1995;50:5.

Platts-Mills TAE, Tovey ER, Mitchell EB, et al. Reduction of bronchial hyperreactivity during prolonged allergen avoidance. *Lancet* 1982;2:675–678.

Pratter MR, Hingston DM, Irwin RS. Diagnosis of bronchial asthma by clinical evalua-tion: an unreliable method. *Chest* 1983;84:42–47.

Robinson DS, Hamid Q, Ying S, et al. Predominant TH2-like bronchoalveolar T-lymphocyte population in atopic asthma. *N Engl J Med* 1992;326:298–304.

Scadding G. The effect of medical treatment of sinusitis upon concomitant asthma. *Allergy* 1999;54:136–140.

Sears MR, Burrows B, Flannery EM, et al. Relation between airway responsiveness and serum IgE in children with asthma and in apparently normal children. *N Engl J Med* 1991;325:1067–1071.

Spector SL. Allergic inflammation in upper and lower airways. *Ann Allergy Asthma Immunol* 1999;83:435–444.

Standardization of spirometry, 1994 update. American Thoracic Society. *Am J Respir Crit Care Med* 1995;152:1107–1136.

Stoodley RG, Aaron SD, Dales RE. The role of ipratropium in the emergency man-agement of acute asthma: a metaanalysis of randomized clinical trials. *Ann Emerg Med* 1999;34:8–18.

Suissa S, Ernst P, Benayoun S, et al. Low-dose inhaled corticosteroids and the pre-vention of death from asthma. *N Engl J Med* 2000;343:332–336.

Sweet JM, Stevenson DD, Simon RA, et al. Long-term effects of aspirin desensitization— treatment for aspirin-sensitive rhinosinusitis-asthma. *J Allergy Clin Immunol* 1990; 85:59–65.

Szefler SJ, Weiss ST, Tonascia J. Long-term effects of budesonide or nedocromil in chil-dren with asthma. The Childhood Asthma Management Program Research Group. *N Engl J Med* 2000;343:1054–63.

Vignola AM, Chanez P, Godard P, et al. Relationships between rhinitis and asthma. *Allergy* 1998;53:833–839.

Virchow JC, Prasse A, Naya I, et al. Zafirlukast improves asthma control in patients receiving high dose inhaled corticosteroids. *Am J Respir Crit Care Med* 2000;162: 578–585.

Walker C, Bode E, Boer L, et al. Allergic and non-allergic asthmatics have distinct pat-terns of T-cell activation and cytokine production in peripheral blood and broncho-alveolar lavage. *Am Rev Respir Dis* 1992;146:109–115.

Weiss ST, Gold DR. Gender differences in asthma. *Pediatr Pulmonol* 1995;19:153–155.

Wolfe J, Rooklin A, Grady J, et al. Comparison of once- and twice-daily dosing of fluti-casone propionate 200 micrograms per day administered by diskus device in patients with asthma treated with or without inhaled corticosteroids. *J Allergy Clin Immunol* 2000;105:1153–1161.

Woolcock A, Lundbash B, Ringdal OL, et al. Comparison of addition of salmeterol to inhaled steroids with doubling of the dose of inhaled steroids. *Am J Respir Crit Care Med* 1996;153:1481–1488.

7. IMMUNOLOGIC DISEASES OF THE LUNG

Michelle Zeidler, Eric C. Kleerup, and Michael D. Roth

The lung is an important and vulnerable target in immunologic diseases. Not only does the lung participate in systemic immunopathologic processes, it is also capable of initiating local immune responses that may be beneficial or adverse to the host. With the exception of asthma, primary and secondary immunologic lung diseases are discussed in this chapter according to their presentation, immunologic features, pathologic features, diagnostic criteria, differential diagnosis, treatment, and prognosis. These various entities are either known or proposed to have immunologic mechanisms and include hypersensitivity pneumonitis, allergic bronchopulmonary aspergillosis (ABPA), eosinophilic lung diseases, Goodpasture syndrome, Wegener granulomatosis, sarcoidosis, and idiopathic pulmonary fibrosis of the lung.

Hypersensitivity Pneumonitis

Hypersensitivity pneumonitis (extrinsic allergic alveolitis) is a common and well-studied immunologically-mediated lung disease. It occurs after the inhalation of organic dusts and is an immunoglobulin G (IgG)-mediated response. The result is a diffuse pulmonary process consisting of reticulonodular or alveolar processes (or both) with poorly formed granulomas. In contrast to other granulomatous diseases (e.g., sarcoidosis, coccidioidomycosis), the immunopathologic process is localized in the lung, and there is no systemic involvement. Moreover, it can fully remit if the antigenic stimulus is removed. Hypersensitivity pneumonitis develops in only 5% to 15% of the exposed population, and the majority of patients are nonatopic and nonsmokers. The antigenic materials may be of animal, vegetable, fungal, bacterial, or chemical origin and must be less than 5 μm in diameter to penetrate to the alveoli. Reactions can be classified as acute or chronic. In general, there is no age, sex, or significant geographic predilections.

I. **Causative antigens**
   The antigens listed in Table 7.1 are recognized as capable of sensitizing susceptible persons and subsequently causing hypersensitivity pneumonitis. This is only a partial list, and new sources from occupational exposure, homes, and hobbies are reported annually. Despite this long expanding list, these conditions have striking similarities in their clinical, radiographic, and pathologic features.

II. **Clinical features**
   A. **Acute hypersensitivity pneumonitis** occurs when exposure is heavy but intermittent.
      1. **Symptoms and signs.** Acute symptoms mimic those of pneumonia and include fever, chills, dyspnea, chest tightness, and dry cough, appear 4 to 6 hours after each exposure, and remit when the agent is avoided. This is considered a late, or Arthus (type III), immune reaction (see Chapter 1). Physical exam reveals fever, tachypnea, tachycardia, and a few lung rhonchi or crackles.
      2. **Laboratory findings.** Peripheral neutrophilia (without eosinophilia) and increased IgG levels, including antigen-specific IgG, are common in the acute form. Serum IgE levels are usually within normal limits. Nonspecific markers of inflammation such as an elevated erythrocyte sedimentation rate (ESR), C-reactive protein, and rheumatoid factor may also be present.
      3. **Radiographic findings.** Radiographic abnormalities will typically develop with repeated antigen exposure, but may not parallel the severity of disease. Up to 4% of patients may have normal x-rays, whereas up to 45% may have very subtle changes. Initially, diffuse airspace opacification is present on x-rays. This resolves into a fine nodular or reticulonodular pattern. These changes may be completely reversible over 4 to 6 weeks if the initiating exposure is avoided. High-resolution com-

Table 7.1. Principal causes of hypersensitivity pneumonitis

Antigen source	Exposure history	Disease
Thermophilic bacteria		
Micropolyspora faeni, *M. polyspora*	Hay, straw	Farmer's lung
Thermoactinomyces candidus, T. vulgaris	Hay, straw	Farmer's lung
M. faeni	Grain	Grain handler's lung
T. sacchari	Pressed sugar cane	Bagassosis
T. vulgaris, *T. candidus, M. faeni*	Heated water reservoirs	Humidifier lung
Other bacteria		
Actinobifida dichotomica	Mushrooms	Mushroom worker's lung
Bacillus subtilis	Detergent manufacture	Detergent worker's lung
B. subtilis	Water reservoirs	Humidifier lung
True fungi		
Alternaria spp.	Various wood pulps	Wood worker's lung
Botrytis cinera	Wine grapes	Spaetlese lung
Cryptostroma corticale	Maple bark	Maple bark stripper's lung
Mucor stolonifer	Paprika pods	Paprika splitter's lung
Penicillium casei	Aged cheese	Cheese washer's lung
Trichosporon cutaneum	House dust	Summer type hypersensitivity (primarily recognized in Japan)
Animal proteins		
Parakeets, pigeons, canaries, ducks	Bird serum, excreta	Bird breeder's lung
Galliformes (poultry)	Feathers	Poultry worker's lung
Fox	Fur	Furrier's lung
Sitophilus granarius (wheat weevil)	Grain	Miller's lung
Vegetable matter		
Cork	Cork dust	Suberosis
Cotton	Bract of cotton flower	Byssinosis
Thuja plicata	Red cedar dust	Cedar worker's lung
Chemicals		
Copper sulfate	Vineyard antifungal	Vineyard sprayer's lung
Methylene diisocyanate or tolulene diisocyanate	Polyurethane foam or rubber manufacture	Chemical worker's lung
Trimellitic anhydride	Plastics	Chemical worker's lung

puted tomography (HRCT) has a higher sensitivity and specificity for detecting lung involvement and may be useful in cases where routine chest x-rays show only subtle findings or are normal. Findings on HRCT include scattered, small, rounded opacities in a centrilobular distribution as well as patchy airspace opacification.

4. **Physiologic tests.** Pulmonary function tests may show hypoxemia and a restrictive ventilatory defect, with reduced vital capacity, total lung capacity, diffusing capacity, and static compliance. Airway obstruction is not typical unless the patient is atopic or has a concurrent obstructive pulmonary disease. Nonspecific airway hyperreactivity can be seen.

B. **Acute hypersensitivity pneumonitis in asthmatic patients.** Approximately 10% of patients with hypersensitivity pneumonitis have atopy and asthma or asthmatic bronchitis. A two-stage reaction develops in these patients if they are exposed to organic dust. The immediate asthmatic (or type I) immune reaction will be manifested by dyspnea, wheezing, and an obstructive ventilatory defect. This reaction subsides and is followed in 4 to 6 hours by a type III immune reaction.

C. **Subacute hypersensitivity pneumonitis** occurs when an exposure is less intense but is consistent over a period of time.
  1. **Symptoms and signs.** Symptoms develop insidiously and include a productive, chronic cough, dyspnea on exertion, fatigue, anorexia, and weight loss. It is more difficult to correlate symptoms with an exposure to the inciting agent in subacute hypersensitivity pneumonitis. The physical exam may be the same as in acute hypersensitivity pneumonitis, although it lacks the explosive onset seen in the acute reaction. Physical findings may include tachypnea, tachycardia, and a few lung rhonchi or crackles.
  2. **Laboratory findings** are similar to those seen in acute hypersensitivity pneumonitis and include peripheral neutrophilia (without eosinophilia) and increased IgG levels. Serum IgE levels are usually within normal limits. Nonspecific markers of inflammation such as an elevated ESR, C-reactive protein, and rheumatoid factor may also be present.
  3. **Radiographic findings.** A fine nodular pattern is classically described on radiographs in subacute disease, but is not always present. The nodules are a manifestation of granulomas (poorly formed when reviewed pathologically), alveolitis, and a cellular ronchiolitis. HRCT shows intermittent ground glass opacities as well as small and poorly defined centrilobular nodules.
  4. **Physiologic tests** resemble those seen during acute disease. Pulmonary function tests may show hypoxemia and a restrictive ventilatory defect, with reduced vital capacity, total lung capacity, diffusing capacity, and static compliance. Airway obstruction is not typical unless the patient is atopic or has a concurrent obstructive pulmonary disease. Nonspecific airway hyperreactivity may also be seen in setting of concomitant asthma.

D. **Chronic hypersensitivity pneumonitis** occurs when the exposure is mild but more continuous (e.g., from a single parakeet).
  1. **Symptoms and signs.** Progressive dyspnea, decreased exercise tolerance, productive cough, and weight loss develop insidiously. Acute episodes of chills and fevers are less likely. Wheezing, bibasilar crackles, cyanosis, clubbing, and cor pulmonale develop as pulmonary inflammation and fibrosis progress.
  2. **Radiographic findings.** The diffuse nodular and reticulonodular pattern characteristic of the acute and subacute stages is superimposed on fibrosis and honeycombing, loss of lung volume, and compensatory overinflation (emphysema) of the less-involved lung zones. These changes are typical of diffuse interstitial fibrosis of any origin, and indicate irreversible damage to the lungs. HRCT may be useful for distinguishing hypersensitivity pneumonitis from idiopathic pulmonary fibrosis, which usually exhibits more extensive honeycombing and a predominance of changes in the peripheral and lower lung zones.
  3. **Physiologic testing.** Pulmonary function tests show severe restrictive disease, with variable airway obstruction and air trapping.

III. **Immunologic features**
  A. **Serum precipitins.** The characteristic immunologic feature of hypersensitivity pneumonitis is the presence of precipitating (usually IgG) antibody to the offending antigen. Serum antibodies or precipitins are readily and reproducibly demonstrated by the Ouchterlony double immuno-

diffusion technique. However, the presence of serum precipitins reactive to antigen present in the patient's environment is not prima facie evidence that it is the causal antigen in hypersensitivity pneumonitis. Although the **positive precipitin test** is clinically helpful, it actually indicates prior exposure and sensitization, not necessarily with clinical sequelae. Precipitins are observed in 90% of patients with active farmer's lung, but the percentage with detectable antibodies decreases as time passes. Serum precipitins without clinical pneumonitis can develop in up to 50% of asymptomatic patients. Conversely, there are rare patients with clinical disease and no demonstrable antibodies. Antibodies can be demonstrated by more sensitive techniques such as enzyme-linked immunosorbent assay (ELISA), immunoelectrophoresis, and immunofluorescence, although their specificity is lower. The correct antigen must be used to detect the antibodies, but many causative antigens have not been identified. Thus, a negative precipitin test in the face of convincing clinical evidence does not exclude the diagnosis, whereas a positive test without appropriate clinical findings does not establish a diagnosis.

B. Skin testing. Antigens for thermophilic actinomycetes and many molds result in a nonspecific irritant response that interferes with skin testing. Cutaneous anergy may also develop from increased suppressor T-cell activity. Many antigens provide a high percentage of positive responses even in exposed but unaffected individuals. Skin testing is therefore neither specific nor sensitive in determining the cause or presence of hypersensitivity pneumonitis. Skin testing for immediate, late-onset, or delayed reactions does not currently have a role in diagnosis or management of hypersensitivity pneumonitis.

C. Types III and IV immune reactions (and type I in atopic persons) are present in hypersensitivity pneumonitis. Acute exposure to an antigen (e.g., pigeon proteins) can induce intraairway immune complexes to form in sensitized individuals. This reaction, and complement activation, stimulates an acute influx of polymorphonuclear leukocytes (PMNs). By 48 hours, the infiltrate shifts to a lymphocytic predominance, which persists in the chronic stage. Both peripheral T cells and those obtained by bronchoalveolar lavage (BAL) from patients with hypersensitivity pneumonitis undergo blast transformation and cytokine release when exposed to the eliciting antigen *in vitro*, indicative of active cell-mediated immunity. BAL in patients with hypersensitivity pneumonitis shows up to a 5-fold increase in total cell recovery. Up to 70% of these cells are lymphocytes, with the majority being CD8+ lymphocytes. This results in a reversal of the usual CD4+:CD8+ ratio (less than or equal to 1:2) (normal 1.2:1 to 1.6:1), which is opposite of the alteration observed in sarcoidosis (CD4+:CD8+ ratio greater than or equal to 2:1). These CD8+ cells are composed of both activated suppressor (CD8+) and cytotoxic (CD8+ and CD56+) lymphocytes. BAL is not helpful in determining disease activity because asymptomatic exposed individuals can manifest similar changes in BAL cell recovery and CD4+:CD8+ ratios.

IV. Pathologic features

All forms of hypersensitivity pneumonitis have similar and nonspecific pathologic features regardless of the inciting agent. The histologic reflection of precipitating antigen–antibody complexes and activation of the complement cascade in lung tissue is best demonstrated in early hypersensitivity pneumonitis, because the causal antigen seen in the chronic phase is nonspecific. The histology of hypersensitivity pneumonitis includes: (i) a mononuclear interstitial infiltration with a bronchocentric distribution (100%), (ii) poorly formed noncaseating granulomas surrounding bronchioles (70%), and (iii) airway inflammation with foamy macrophages (65%), often associated with bronchiolitis obliterans (50%). Over the course of several months, the histology becomes nonspecific as the granulomas disappear and interstitial fibrosis and obliterative bronchiolitis predominate, resulting eventually in emphysema and a honeycomb lung.

V. Diagnostic approach

Hypersensitivity pneumonitis can be an elusive diagnosis and challenge even the experienced clinician. Because hypersensitivity pneumonitis can mimic multiple diseases, the diagnosis is founded on a high index of suspicion coupled with suggestive radiographic, physiologic, and immunologic findings.

A. **A high index of suspicion** is based on a detailed environmental history. Although patients often associate recurrent exposures with symptoms in the acute form of hypersensitivity pneumonitis, the chronic form is much more difficult to identify.

B. **Chest x-rays, high-resolution computed tomography, and pulmonary function tests** consistent with hypersensitivity pneumonitis.

C. **Serum precipitins and bronchoalveolar lavage** consistent with hypersensitivity pneumonitis. The finding of significant lymphocytosis should raise the index of suspicion of hypersensitivity pneumonitis. However, negative studies do not rule out disease, while positive studies do not necessarily confirm a diagnosis. BAL may be done as an adjunct to rule out infection, but is not a routine test required for the diagnosis of hypersensitivity pneumonitis.

D. **Histologic findings** consistent with hypersensitivity pneumonitis. This can usually be done with good transbronchial biopsies directed by radiographic findings, although occasionally (usually in the chronic form) an open lung biopsy is preferred. Special stains and cultures to rule out infectious etiologies should be sent.

E. **Trial of avoidance and controlled reexposure** to the suspected antigen or environment. Deliberate repetition of natural exposure to the suspected antigenic environmental source (e.g., barn, factory) and observing the clinical response (by physical examinations, chest x-rays, and/or spirometry before and after exposure) constitutes a simple, relatively safe diagnostic procedure, but is generally only useful in patients with acute hypersensitivity pneumonitis.

F. **Allergen inhalation challenge test.** When the specific diagnosis remains in doubt because the relevance of a particular exposure is questionable, allergen inhalation or bronchial challenge tests can be used to establish a definitive diagnosis. Various dusts or liquids in the home or workplace can be collected and cultured and extracts prepared from these for inhalation challenge studies in order to identify the responsible antigen. Positive reactions to aerosolized extracts of the appropriate antigen will produce symptoms and signs of hypersensitivity pneumonitis as immediate, late, or dual reactions. However, the patient can become severely ill during the procedure and require hospitalization and parenteral corticosteroids. Thus, this procedure should **not** be performed routinely and only in laboratories experienced in its administration.

G. **Differential diagnosis.** Both the acute and chronic forms of hypersensitivity pneumonitis can be confused with acute or recurrent pneumonias (viral, fungal, atypical), mycobacterial disease, drug-induced lung disease, organic dust toxic syndrome, ABPA, pulmonary mycotoxicosis, silo-filler's disease, pulmonary alveolar proteinosis, sarcoidosis, and collagen vascular disease. The latter two are most often accompanied by systemic, mediastinal, or pleural involvement not found in hypersensitivity pneumonitis. The many causes of interstitial fibrosis, summarized in Table 7.2, can also be confused with chronic hypersensitivity pneumonitis. Although the history and physical as well as radiologic findings can usually differentiate and limit the possibilities, open lung biopsy is justified in puzzling cases or patients without a correlating environmental history.

VI. Treatment

A. **General treatment measures**

1. **Avoidance.** Avoidance of the offending antigen is the most important treatment of hypersensitivity pneumonitis. Alterations in the work and home environment through adjustments in ventilation, heating, air con-

Table 7.2. Principal causes of diffuse interstitial pneumonitis and fibrosis

Chronic aspiration	Immune-mediated lung diseases
Collagen vascular diseases	Eosinophilic granulomatosis
Polymyositis–dermatomyositis	Eosinophilic pneumonia
Rheumatoid arthritis	Goodpasture's syndrome
Scleroderma	Sarcoidosis
Systemic lupus erythematosus	Wegener granulomatosis
Drugs and medical treatment	Gastrointestinal diseases
Antibiotics: nitrofurantoin	Chronic active hepatitis
Antiarrhythmics: amiodarone,	Cryptogenic cirrhosis
tocainide	Inflammatory bowel disease
Antiinflammatories: gold, penicillamine	Primary biliary cirrhosis
Anticonvulsants: phenytoin	Malignancy: lymphangitic carcinomatosis
Bone marrow transplant	Occupational and environmental
Chemotherapeutics: azathioprine,	exposures
bleomycin, busulfan, carmustine	Metals: aluminum oxide, antimony,
(BCNU), chlorambucil, cyclo-	barium, beryllium, cobalt, iron
phosphamide, cytosine arabinoside,	oxide, tin
lomustine (CCNU), melphalan,	Minerals: asbestos, diatomaceous
methotrexate, mitomycin C	earth, kaolin, shale, silica, talc
Dietary supplements: L-tryptophan	Organics: coal, silicone, paraquat,
Dopaminergic drugs: bromocriptine	polyvinyl chloride
Oxygen	Other
Radiation	Adult respiratory distress syndrome
Hereditary diseases	Alveolar microlithiasis
Familial idiopathic pulmonary fibrosis	Alveolar proteinosis
Lipid storage disorders	Amyloidosis
Neurofibromatosis	Lymphangioleiomyomatosis
Tuberous sclerosis	Lymphocytic interstitial pneumonitis
Hypersensitivity pneumonitis	Histiocytosis X
Infections: bacterial, fungal, myco-	Idiopathic pulmonary fibrosis
bacterial, viral	Mitral stenosis
	Pulmonary alveolar proteinosis

ditioning, and water-based systems may be useful. If avoidance is not possible, a trial of masks or dust filters can be attempted. Occasionally, patients must completely avoid the environment in which exposure to the offending agent occurs.

2. **Bronchodilators.** Beta-agonists, and nedocromil and chromolyn sodium usually alleviate or prevent acute bronchospasm in patients with asthmatic responses.

3. **Immunotherapy.** Immunotherapy is **not** useful or advisable because of the potential danger that parenteral injection of an antigen might increase levels of precipitins and set the stage for a severe reaction on reexposure to the airborne allergen.

B. **Corticosteroid therapy.** Corticosteroids are often used when the offending antigen cannot be avoided or when symptoms are severe or prolonged. In the acute episode the response to **prednisone**, 60 mg per day for a week, with tapering over a month, is often dramatic, with the chest x-ray and spirometric findings (except diffusing capacity) rapidly returning to normal. The initial pediatric dose of prednisone is 2 mg/kg/day in this disease and in other severe respiratory diseases (requiring pharmacologic antiinflammatory therapy) described subsequently in this chapter. The chronic form of the disease is more difficult to treat. A short trial of corticosteroids (prednisone at 0.5 to 1 mg/kg/day) is usually empirically given with the assumption that part of the interstitial disease is potentially reversible. If improvement is documented, the lowest effective dose should be continued for an extended course. If no improvement is documented, prednisone should be discontinued. The use of inhaled corticosteroids is of questionable value in hypersensitivity pneumonitis, although no studies of high-dose inhaled corticosteroids have been performed. Some patients, especially bird-keepers, will have a progressive course despite avoidance and oral corticosteroids. Although cytotoxic agents may be considered in these patients, the efficacy of this approach is unproven.

VII. Prognosis

Provided the antigen is avoided and/or corticosteroid therapy is initiated before irreparable tissue damage (fibrosis) occurs, the prognosis is excellent. In patients with acute disease, avoiding the offending antigen results in a return to normal pulmonary function. However, in chronic disease, pulmonary fibrosis and advanced respiratory failure often exist when the patients first present for treatment.

Allergic Bronchopulmonary Aspergillosis

ABPA represents the most commonly recognized cause of the allergic bronchopulmonary fungoses. It represents an exaggerated immunologic response to fungal colonization of the lower airways and results in subsequent bronchiectatic changes. It is classified as both an immediate hypersensitivity and immune complex disease. *Aspergillus fumigatus* is the most common causative agent of ABPA, although other *Aspergillus* species, as well as other fungal organisms, have been implicated. ABPA characteristically occurs in atopic patients and is **always associated with a history of asthma**. Up to 7% to 14% of steroid-dependent asthmatics and 10% of patients with cystic fibrosis may develop ABPA. In the majority of patients, the diagnosis is made after the age of 20 years and there is no gender predilection. The incidence is relatively high in the United Kingdom and low in the United States.

I. Clinical presentation

- **A. Symptoms and signs.** Patients typically present with episodes of fever, wheezing, productive cough, minimal hemoptysis, and shortness of breath, particularly in the winter months. Patients may expectorate brownish plugs or flakes (56%) and, occasionally, bronchial casts. Asthmatic and cystic fibrosis patients may occasionally have recurrent exacerbations of their disease that do not respond to conventional treatment. Physical exam may reveal wheezing or evidence of lobar or segmental collapse from mucous plugging.
- **B. Laboratory findings.** Peripheral blood eosinophilia (greater than 1,000 per mm^3) occurs in 90% to 100% of patients, whereas markedly elevated total serum IgE levels (greater than 1,000 IU per mL) occurs in 80% to 100% of patients. Serum precipitins (IgG and IgE) specific for *Aspergillus* are also elevated. Expectorated sputum casts contain the causative fungus, which is seen on microscopic examination and by culture, 67% of the time. A single sputum culture growing *Aspergillus* is not diagnostic because the organism is ubiquitous and can be a contaminant. Repeatedly positive sputum cultures, however, are suspicious.
- **C. Radiographic findings.** Mucoid impaction of involved airways frequently results in segmental or lobar atelectasis that is visualized as transient or fixed pulmonary infiltrates. Impaction of dilated bronchi with mucus plugs are classically described as "finger in glove" projections. Tram tracking, which represents thickened bronchial walls, is also described. HRCT has a higher specificity and sensitivity in detecting proximal bronchiectasis than plain x-rays. Upper lobe fibrosis occurs in patients with chronic disease.
- **D. Physiologic tests.** The presence of mucus plugging (mucus impaction syndrome) and airway damage is commonly, but not always, associated with evidence of reversible airways obstruction and lowered diffusing capacity on pulmonary function testing. This may wax and wane depending on the

changing mucous obstruction. A restrictive ventilatory pattern may occur with pulmonary fibrosis and may not reverse with corticosteroid therapy.

II. **Immunologic features**

Skin tests positive for *Aspergillus* show both an immediate wheal-and-flare reaction (type I) and a late reaction of erythema and edema, which may be a delayed type I and/or a type III (Arthus) reaction. After focal deposition of *Aspergillus* organisms in the lung, a type I (IgE-mediated) response occurs, resulting in local bronchial edema. This reaction is followed by immune complex deposition (IgG). Complement activation ensues, enhancing the inflammatory response. Fungal antigen-specific IgE, IgA, and IgG can be detected in bronchial lavage specimens. There is also recent evidence to suggest an active role of T cells of the Th2 phenotype in the inflammatory response to *Aspergillus*.

III. **Pathologic features**

The pathogenesis of ABPA likely includes damage from both the immune response to *Aspergillus* and direct proteolytic enzyme release from the fungus. Although thick, tenacious mucous plugs with fungal elements fill the affected bronchi, the organism does not invade the bronchial wall or lung parenchyma. In some patients, the bronchial wall damage is associated with intense parenchymal infiltration by eosinophils and mononuclear cells and the presence of granulomas (bronchocentric granulomatosis). Subsequently, proximal cystic bronchiectasis and upper lobe fibrosis develop.

IV. **Diagnostic approach**

   A. **Specific etiologic approach.** The diagnosis is certain if the following conditions (usually present in more than 90% of the patients) are present:

   1. **Episodic bronchial obstruction (asthma)**
   2. **Peripheral blood eosinophilia (more than 1,000 per mm³)**
   3. **Transient or fixed pulmonary infiltrates**
   4. **Proximal bronchiectasis.** Proximal bronchiectasis with normal tapering distal airways is specific for ABPA, but not absolutely essential because the bronchi may be normal or minimally altered early in the course of disease. HRCT is the preferred method for detecting proximal bronchiectasis.
   5. **Immediate skin reactivity** to *Aspergillus* antigen on prick or intradermal testing. Patients with a history of recurrent asthma and pulmonary infiltrates should be evaluated initially with a skin test for *Aspergillus*. If both prick and intradermal tests are negative, and assuming the *Aspergillus* antigen is reliable, it is very unlikely that ABPA is the cause of the symptoms.
   6. **Precipitating antibodies** against *Aspergillus* antigen. These precipitins are not diagnostic because they are also found in patients without active disease.
   7. **Elevated serum immunoglobulin E** by radioimmunoassay. Patients with positive skin tests should have confirmatory serum precipitins and IgE (total and antigen-specific) levels evaluated because they reflect disease activity.

   B. **Differential diagnosis.** Patients with ABPA frequently have had a prior diagnosis of intractable asthma, cystic fibrosis, chronic bronchitis, recurrent pneumonia, tuberculosis, or bronchiectasis from other causes. However, it is possible for some of these entities to coexist with the fungal hypersensitivity. ABPA may be confused with other conditions exhibiting pulmonary infiltrates with eosinophilia (Table 7.3).

V. **Treatment**

The goal of treatment is to prevent the progression of disease by controlling the inflammatory component of the asthma and suppressing the immune response to the fungus.

   A. **General treatment.** Bronchodilators and antibiotics (if bacterial infection is suspected) will improve the asthmatic component of the disease, especially during acute exacerbations. Immunotherapy with *Aspergillus* extracts is **not** recommended because it may accentuate local and asthmatic responses.

Table 7.3. Eosinophilic syndromes with pulmonary involvement

Syndrome	Etiology	Symptoms	Physical findings	Eosinophilia	Chest x-ray	Other features	Treatment	Prognosis
Simple pulmonary eosinophilia (Löffler syndrome)	Drugs, parasites, and others	None or mild cough, fever, myalgia	None or minimal	10%–30%	Transient, migratory, pleural-based infiltrates		None, usually self-limited	Excellent
Chronic (prolonged) pulmonary eosinophilia	Majority unknown; drugs and parasites	Fever, sweats, cough, dyspnea, wheezing, weight loss	Wheezes	20%–40% in two-thirds of patients	Dense peripheral infiltrates, recur in same location	Restriction on pulmonary function tests, may present with asthma	Corticosteroids	Good with prolonged therapy
Tropical eosinophilia	Filarial parasites	Dry cough, dyspnea, nocturnal wheezing, malaise, weight loss	Crackles, wheezes, lymph-adenopathy in children	20%–50%	Increased markings, 1–3 mm nodules or mottled opacities	IgE <1,000 IU/mL, antifilarial antibodies	Diethyl-carbamazine	Good
Churg-Strauss syndrome and poly-arteritis nodosa	Unknown	Wheezing, fever, weight loss, fatigue, neuropathy, sinus disease	Wheezes	>10% in Churg-Strauss, >20% in 20%–30% of poly-arteritis nodosa	Transient patchy infiltrates, consolidation nodules, effusions	Vasculitis of small and medium arteries	Corticosteroids, cyclophos-phamide	Poor
Eosinophilia–myalgia syndrome	Contami-nants in L-tryptophan	Cough, dyspnea, myalgias, fatigue	Wheezes, peripheral edema	>1,000/mm³	Interstitial and reticulo-nodular infiltrates		Corticosteroids, cessation of tryptophan	Fair

B. Corticosteroids

1. **Dose.** There is no standard recommended dose of corticosteroids in ABPA. Oral **prednisone** at 20 to 40 mg per day, or 0.5 mg/kg/day is an appropriate choice, which can usually be tapered over 2 to 4 weeks depending on clinical response. The efficacy of alternate-day corticosteroids or inhaled corticosteroids is limited because asymptomatic pulmonary infiltrates can continue to develop during either kind of therapy.

2. **Response.** Symptoms, expectorated plugs, positive cultures, and infiltrates seen radiographically resolve or rapidly decrease in frequency (in days to weeks) with daily prednisone therapy. Although the responses of precipitins and total serum IgG to corticosteroid therapy are variable, total serum IgE levels decrease significantly with remission and are of benefit in monitoring and predicting disease activity.

3. **Duration.** A 6-month course of prednisone therapy with subsequent tapering and monitoring (by history, chest x-ray, and serum IgE levels) will suffice in most patients. However, in some patients, the disease may be exacerbated after corticosteroids are discontinued, and after repeated courses they may require prednisone therapy indefinitely (e.g., at least 10 mg per day).

C. Antifungal therapy. Although the data are still limited, the use of antifungals in an attempt to eradicate fungal colonization may alter the course of ABPA. Itraconazole, in conjunction with corticosteroids, may hasten the time to recovery, as measured by IgE levels and pulmonary function, and reduce the required dose of steroids. An acceptable dose is itraconazole, 200 mg b.i.d. for 16 weeks.

VI. Prognosis

Pulmonary infiltrates and further lung destruction continue to develop in untreated patients. Irreversible bronchiectasis, pulmonary fibrosis, recurrent pneumonias, and eventually, respiratory failure result. However, effective treatment with corticosteroids is associated with significantly fewer recurrences of pulmonary infiltrates and less bronchial damage. Fungal invasion or extension in patients on long-term corticosteroid therapy has not been documented.

Eosinophilic Lung Disease

Eosinophilic lung disease is a generic term applied to a broad group of eosinophilic syndromes with pulmonary involvement. In this section, simple pulmonary eosinophilia (Löffler syndrome), chronic eosinophilic pneumonia, tropical eosinophilia, and pulmonary eosinophilias with vasculitis (Churg-Strauss syndrome [CSS] and polyarteritis nodosa) will be discussed (see Table 7.3). ABPA, another member of this spectrum of diseases, is discussed separately.

I. Simple pulmonary eosinophilia (Löffler syndrome)

Löffler syndrome is a constellation of mild pulmonary and systemic symptoms with peripheral eosinophilia. It is usually a response to an infectious or drug exposure and remits spontaneously.

A. Clinical presentation. Patients are usually asymptomatic or have mild cough, wheeze, and/or constitutional symptoms such as low-grade fever and myalgias. The syndrome likely represents a hypersensitivity response to one of numerous causative agents (para-aminosalicylic acid, sulfonamides, chlorpropamide, nitrofurantoin, phenytoin, bleomycin, tetracycline, nickel carbonyl, *Ascaris* and *Strongyloides* parasites, and several others) and a careful history of exposure can be important in establishing the diagnosis. Idiopathic cases also occur.

B. Laboratory findings. Peripheral blood eosinophilia is present in the range of 10% to 30%. Chest x-ray documents nonsegmental, bilateral or unilateral, transient, and migratory infiltrates which may be interstitial or alveolar. Stool examination can reveal parasites in cases due to *Ascaris* and *Strongyloides*. Although rarely required, biopsies show interstitial eosinophilic pneumonia without evidence of necrosis or vasculitis.

C. **Diagnostic approach.** No single feature establishes the diagnosis. A mildly symptomatic patient with eosinophilia, transient pulmonary infiltrates, and spontaneous resolution within a month meets the diagnostic criteria. An exposure history is helpful.

D. **Treatment and prognosis.** Simple pulmonary eosinophilia most often resolves spontaneously within a month of the onset of symptoms. Eliminating exposure to the offending agent, or treatment of the parasitic infection, is usually curative. A brief tapering course of prednisone may be required for more severe cases. The prognosis for a complete recovery is excellent.

II. **Chronic eosinophilic pneumonia**

Chronic eosinophilic pneumonia is a pulmonary and systemic disease generally affecting females in their fifth decade. The symptoms are insidious in onset, and time to diagnosis from onset of symptoms is, on average, 7.7 months. Peripheral eosinophilia may or may not be present. Although some cases are due to the same agents associated with simple pulmonary eosinophilia, the etiology remains unknown in the majority of cases.

A. **Clinical presentation.** Patients present with moderate to severe symptoms including cough (90%), fever (87%), dyspnea (57%), weight loss (57%), sputum production, sweats, malaise, and wheezing that have lasted for more than 1 month. A history of preexisting atopy is elicited in one-third of the cases and new onset asthma can be the presenting symptom. Asthma can persist even after treatment.

B. **Laboratory findings.** Peripheral blood eosinophilia ranging between 20% and 88% is present in two-thirds of patients. Chest x-ray shows progressive dense infiltrates that do not conform to lobar or segmental anatomy and are characteristically subpleural. This peripheral "butterfly" distribution, also described as the photographic negative of pulmonary edema, may be difficult to appreciate on some chest x-rays, but is universally documented by computed tomography (CT) scan of the chest. Opacities may disappear and recur in exactly the same location over time. Pulmonary function tests exhibit a restrictive ventilatory defect with a reduction in the diffusing capacity. Hypoxemia is noted on blood gases. Lung biopsy confirms the presence of eosinophils and mononuclear cells within the alveoli and interstitium. Occasionally, granuloma formation with eosinophilic abscesses and microangitis occur. Twenty-five percent of patients will have bronchiolitis or bronchiolitis obliterans.

C. **Diagnostic approach.** The finding of appropriate clinical symptoms and a characteristic chest x-ray is diagnostic in 75% of cases. The diagnosis is often made by radiographic findings alone. High levels of eosinophilia are confirmatory, but are not present in one-third of cases. BAL usually shows greater than a 25% eosinophilia. Lung biopsy may be required in the rare cases that lack characteristic chest x-rays or chest CT scans.

D. **Treatment and prognosis.** Early treatment is essential because less than 10% of chronic eosinophilic pneumonias resolve spontaneously and deaths have been reported. Therapy should begin with 30 to 60 mg per day of **prednisone** (1 to 2 mg/kg/day in children), with gradual tapering and maintenance on an individual basis. The clinical, x-ray, and histologic response is often dramatic and occurs within days, but relapses can occur if corticosteroids are decreased prematurely. No studies have yet been performed with high-dose inhaled steroids. The optimal duration of therapy is unknown and indefinite maintenance therapy may be necessary in difficult cases. Inhaled bronchodilators should be used to treat any bronchospastic component. The prognosis is good, but may necessitate protracted therapy.

III. **Tropical eosinophilia**

Tropical eosinophilia occurs in patients infected with the filarial parasites *Wuchereria bancrofti* and *Brugia malayi*. The filaria are transmitted through mosquitoes and the adult worm will eventually live in the lymphatic system and release microfilaria. The microfilaria travel to the lung and cause a marked inflammatory reaction. Patients are typically males (4:1 sex ratio) in their third or fourth decade and originate from endemic areas such as India, Africa, South America, and South East Asia.

A. **Clinical presentation.** Patients usually have an insidious onset of dry cough, dyspnea, nocturnal wheezing, malaise, anorexia, and weight loss. Course crackles, rhonchi, and wheezes are heard during symptomatic episodes. Moderate lymphadenopathy and hepatomegaly are common in children but not in adults.

B. **Laboratory findings.** The eosinophil count is extremely high (greater than 20% to 50% and greater than 3,000 per mm^3) and persists for weeks. IgE levels are elevated (greater than 1,000 IU per mL) and high levels of antifilarial antibodies are present in both serum and bronchial lavage specimens. No microfilaria are seen because the parasite is sequestered in the lung parenchyma. BAL reveals up to a 50% eosinophilia. Chest x-rays demonstrate increased bronchovascular markings and diffuse 1- to 3-mm nodules or mottled opacities. Pulmonary function tests show a restrictive ventilatory pattern and diffusing capacity impairment. Obstructive ventilatory defects are also seen in 25% to 30% of patients. Biopsy findings include eosinophilic bronchopneumonia with eosinophilic abscesses and interstitial granulomas surrounding degenerated microfilaria, or areas of necrosis.

C. **Diagnostic approach.** The diagnosis is usually made on clinical grounds in a patient that has had protracted exposure to an endemic area. The combination of diffuse nodular changes on chest x-ray, extreme eosinophilia, and high levels of serum IgE are important findings; a rapid response to treatment confirms the diagnosis. High titers of antifilarial antibodies are present, but are not specific for the disease.

D. **Treatment and prognosis.** Tropical eosinophilia requires specific treatment with diethylcarbamazine (6 to 12 mg/kg/day divided into three doses) for 21 days. Responses to therapy are generally rapid and associated with notable improvement in pulmonary function; however, 10% to 20% of patients either relapse or have unsatisfactory long-term responses. Another course of treatment is indicated in these cases, but some patients may still progress to chronic interstitial fibrosis.

IV. **Churg-Strauss syndrome**

CSS is a rare systemic vasculitis that involves small and medium blood vessels. CCS occurs in patients with a long-standing history of allergic disease (asthma, sinusitis, or rhinitis) and almost all patients with CSS have pulmonary involvement and peripheral eosinophilia. CSS affects men and women of all ages.

A. **Clinical presentation.** In CSS, patients with a known history of asthma usually present with paranasal sinus disease, mono- or polyneuropathy, and constitutional symptoms of fever, weight loss, and fatigue. Involvement of additional organs with vasculitis is common (e.g., skin [70%], gastrointestinal [59%], renal [49%], cardiac [47%], and central nervous system [27%]), although overt renal failure is rare. In the past few years there has been an association between use of the leukotriene receptor antagonists for the treatment of asthma (zafirlukast and monteleukast) and the development of CSS. Although the details of this association remain to be confirmed, this possible association should be recognized by clinicians.

B. **Laboratory findings.** In CSS, peripheral blood eosinophilia (greater than 10%) is present in 95% of patients and BAL eosinophil counts are elevated in one-third of patients. Because of the systemic vasculitis, these patients also commonly have anemia, leukocytosis, elevated ESR, elevated serum IgE levels, hypocomplementemia, and decreased renal function. Perinuclear staining of antineutrophil cytoplasmic antibody (P-ANCA) is positive in 35% to 50% of CSS. Radiographic abnormalities are almost always present in CSS and include transient patchy infiltrates, consolidations, pleural effusions, and nodules that rarely cavitate. High-resolution chest CT can demonstrate irregular pulmonary artery aneurismal changes as well as centrilobular and perivascular nodules. Lung biopsy in CSS is associated with eosinophilic vasculitis of small- and medium-sized arteries and veins with perivascular necrotizing granulomas and eosinophilic infiltrates.

C. **Diagnostic approach.** Diagnostic criteria established by the American College of Rheumatology for diagnosing CSS include patients who exhibit at least four of six well-defined criteria: (i) asthma, (ii) eosinophilia greater than 10%, (iii) mono- or polyneuropathy, (iv) nonfixed pulmonary infiltrates, (v) paranasal sinus abnormalities, and (vi) extravascular extension of eosinophils on lung biopsy. When obtaining lung tissue for diagnostic purposes, open lung biopsies are usually required because transbronchial biopsies rarely yield adequate tissue.

D. **Treatment and prognosis.** High doses of corticosteroids (**prednisone** 1 mg/kg/day for the first 2 months) are initially required in treating CSS and are tapered according to clinical improvement. In patients with primary lung involvement, **cyclophosphamide** (1 to 2 mg/kg/day adjusted for neutropenia) added to prednisone at the beginning of treatment more rapidly induces remission and reduces the incidence of relapse. However, because of a greater morbidity from infectious complications, cyclophosphamide should be reserved for those patients whose lung disease responds too slowly or relapses on prednisone alone. In addition, cyclophosphamide should be utilized in patients with concomitant involvement of the kidneys, nervous system, or gastrointestinal tract. The prognosis is generally poor, and 5-year survival rates range from 60% to 75%. Patients with multiorgan involvement tend to have a more fulminant course, and the majority of deaths occur in the first 3 months after diagnosis.

V. **Differential diagnosis of pulmonary disease and eosinophilia**

The combination of pulmonary infiltrates and eosinophilia (of the blood or tissue) raises a broad differential which includes the eosinophilic diseases discussed in this section; ABPA; drug reactions; a multitude of infectious processes including varied parasitic infections (*Strongyloides*, *Ascaris*, *Ancylostoma*, *Toxocara*, and others), mycobacterial and fungal infections, and brucellosis; malignancy; or collagen–vascular diseases that are occasionally associated with the hypereosinophilia syndrome, and less likely with Wegener granulomatosis. A detailed history and physical including special attention to a history of asthma or atopic disease, travel and exposures, and drug use is invaluable. This coupled with radiographic data and properly selected serology studies can lead to a diagnosis. Occasionally BAL or even open lung biopsy may be necessary. Biopsies in organs other than the lung may be necessary in various collagen vascular diseases.

VI. **Immunology of eosinophilic lung diseases.** The exact immunologic mechanisms responsible for eosinophilic lung disease are not known. Recent animal and human studies clearly suggest that these syndromes are T-lymphocyte mediated and that selective secretion of interleukin 4 (IL-4) and IL-5 by helper lymphocytes are responsible for the specific increases in serum IgE and eosinophils, respectively. The eosinophil undoubtedly plays a role in protection against parasites, but also likely plays a significant role in the inflammation and tissue injury observed in patients with eosinophilic lung disease. Stimulated eosinophils release granule-derived factors, including major basic protein (toxic for parasites, tumor cells, and respiratory cells, and which functions as a mast cell activator), eosinophilic cationic protein (toxic for parasites and nerve cells, and also is a mast cell activator) and eosinophil-derived neurotoxin. Stimulated eosinophils also release membrane-derived mediators including leukotriene C_4 (LTC$_4$), LTD$_4$, and platelet-activating factor (PAF) (see Chapter 2).

Goodpasture Syndrome

Goodpasture syndrome is one of the first diagnostic considerations raised when the clinician is confronted with the combination of pulmonary hemorrhage and nephritis. Its immunopathologic nature is underscored by its more accurate alternative name, **antiglomerular basement membrane disease**. Although Goodpasture originally described the syndrome as a sequelae of influenza, it is now well accepted as an antigen–antibody reaction (type II) against the alpha-3 chain of type IV collagen. This is a rare disease that typically affects males (male-to-female ratio 7:1) in their second to third decade of life, with occasional familial occurrence. There is also an atypical form that affects elderly females and has a renal predominance. Affected patients are usually smokers.

I. Clinical presentation

   A. Symptoms and signs. Hemoptysis, ranging from mild to life-threatening, is present in more than 90% of patients on presentation. Clinical manifestations of renal disease are often concurrent with, but may precede hemoptysis. Occasionally, there are only renal manifestations, whereas less often (less than 10%) lung involvement will occur without renal disease. Other symptoms include dyspnea (57%), fatigue (51%), cough (41%), chest pain (40%), fever (22%), and weight loss (14%). Symptoms attributed to a viral syndrome are found in 20% of patients. Physical findings commonly include pallor (50%), crackles and wheezes (37%), edema (25%), and occasionally mild hypertension and retinal hemorrhages and exudates.

   B. Laboratory findings. ELISA and radioimmunoassays for serum antiglomerular basement membrane (anti-GBM) antibodies are sensitive and relatively specific tests for Goodpasture syndrome. Up to one-third of patients may be P-ANCA positive. ESR is normal or minimally elevated. Iron-deficiency anemia is present in 98% of patients. Other laboratory findings include leukocytosis (50%), proteinuria (88%), red and white blood cell and granular casts (greater than 70%), and progressive azotemia. The urinalysis may be initially normal in up to 10% of patients.

   C. Radiographic findings. Following pulmonary hemorrhage, the chest x-ray will initially show widespread bilateral patchy airspace consolidation that simulates pulmonary edema or opportunistic infection in 90% of cases. Serial chest x-rays show either progressive acinar consolidation during continued pulmonary hemorrhage or a reticular pattern, the distribution of which matches that of the resolving airspace process, or both. The chest x-ray findings may return to normal in days after the acute episode. Progressive interstitial fibrosis results from repeated hemorrhage and increasing hemosiderin deposition within the lung interstitium.

   D. Pulmonary function tests. Pulmonary function tests often reveal a restrictive ventilatory defect. In the absence of recent hemorrhage, the diffusing capacity is reduced. With acute hemorrhage, blood is sequestered in the alveolar space where it can bind the test gas (carbon monoxide) and artificially increase the diffusing capacity by 30% or more above baseline.

II. Immunologic features

Anti-GBM antibodies are directed against the carboxy-terminal region of the alpha-3 chain of type IV collagen. It is postulated that alteration of the three-dimensional structure of collagen following an infectious or toxic exposure unveils this epitope and plays an important role in the initiation of the antibody response. This may explain the higher incidence of disease seen after viral infections and drug exposures. Once formed, anti-GBM antibody binds to the renal glomeruli, where subsequent fixation of complement and the attraction of neutrophils results in the characteristic renal pathology. Unlike the kidney, the lung is not directly damaged by circulating antibody, because the fenestrations in the basement membrane of the lung are not large enough to admit an IgG protein. It is not until a second insult occurs that there is an increased alveolar–capillary leak. This may explain the higher incidence of Goodpasture syndrome in smokers. There is a higher incidence of disease in patients with human leukocyte antigen DR2 (HLA-DR2), especially with the DRw15 haplotype (88% of patients versus 32% of controls), and with HLA-B7 (59% of patients versus 22% of controls). This may be due to alterations in antigenic processing by B cells, macrophages, and dendritic cells with these phenotypes.

III. Pathologic features

A. Lungs. The lungs reveal diffuse alveolar hemorrhage during an acute episode. Light microscopy reveals hemosiderin-laden macrophages, intact alveolar and endothelial cells, and a component of interstitial fibrosis in patients with chronic disease. Vasculitic changes are absent or minimal, but electron microscopy shows vascular damage with wide endothelial gaps and occasionally fragmentation of basement membranes. Immunofluorescence demonstrates linear deposits of IgG and, often, complement bound to the basement membranes of alveoli.

B. Kidneys. Renal biopsy shows focal and segmental glomerulonephritis with crescent formation and diffuse glomerular necrosis that progresses to interstitial inflammation and glomerular fibrosis without vasculitis. Electron microscopy reveals endothelial cell proliferation and swelling, increased basement membrane material, and fibrin deposition beneath the capillary endothelium. Linear deposits of IgG antibody along the capillary basement membranes demonstrated by immunofluorescence are seen more often in the kidney than in the lung. Deposition on IgA and IgM have also been reported.

IV. Diagnostic approach

A. Presentation. Goodpasture syndrome is diagnosed by the presence of **pulmonary hemorrhage, glomerulonephritis, and circulating anti-GBM**. Renal and pulmonary involvement may not manifest themselves concurrently, making the diagnosis more difficult in these cases.

B. Confirmation

1. **Renal biopsy** with immunofluorescence microscopy should be performed with the first manifestations of kidney involvement to determine the extent and severity of damage as well as to establish an early diagnosis.

2. **Serum antiglomerular basement membrane.** ELISA and radioimmunoassays for anti-GBM antibody are reliable and sensitive tests for Goodpasture syndrome and are useful in following the response to treatment. These tests may take several days to return from reference laboratories and should not delay treatment. There have been reports of false-positive anti-GBM antibody in human immunodeficiency virus (HIV)-negative patients with *Pneumocystis carnii* pneumonia (PCP), although the anti-GBM was not directed to the alpha carboxy portion of the protein.

3. **Lung biopsy.** Transbronchial lung biopsy will be helpful only if sufficient alveoli are obtained, and cannot be performed as easily and serially for accurate follow-up as can percutaneous renal biopsies.

C. Differential diagnosis includes exposure to trimellitic anhydride, hydrocarbons, mitomycin-c, penicillamine, or smoked crack cocaine, in addition to collagen vascular diseases such as microscopic polyangitis, Wegener granulomatosis, systemic lupus erythematosus, Henoch-Schönlein purpura, CSS, pulmonary capillaritis, idiopathic pulmonary hemosiderosis, uremic pneumonitis, acute (poststreptococcal) glomerulonephritis, and pneumococca viral pneumonia with nephritis. Several cases of pulmonary–renal disease similar to Goodpasture syndrome but without anti-GBM antibodies have been reported, and presumably involve other immunopathologic mechanisms.

V. Treatment

A. General measures. Emergency stabilization with blood transfusions, correction of fluid and electrolyte imbalances, supplemental oxygen, intubation and mechanical ventilation, and peritoneal or hemodialysis are often necessary.

B. Immunosuppressive therapy. Goodpasture disease is rapidly fatal if not treated aggressively and early. The current treatment of choice consists of early **plasmapheresis** (4 L every other day) to remove circulating anti-GBM antibody and a combination of **methylprednisone** (2 mg per kg intravenously q8) and **cyclophosphamide** (2 mg/kg/day intravenously, titrated to a leukocyte level of 5,000) to suppress further anti-GBM antibody production. Following acute treatment, prednisone treatment is continued at 1 mg per kg in a single morning dose for the first month, then tapered to 1 mg per kg on alternate days, and over the next 2 to 3 months is tapered off. Cyclophosphamide is continued at a dose of 1 to 2 mg per kg with the dose adjusted to maintain the total white blood cell count (WBC) between 3,000 and 4,000 per mL; it is maintained for 12 months after remission is achieved. Therapy with corticosteroids and cyclophosphamide is indicated in cases of pulmonary hemorrhage or rapidly progressive renal failure, but not in patients with end-stage renal failure. Pulmonary hemorrhage usually stops promptly, but recurrences require repeat plasmapheresis. Plasmapheresis should be continued for 2 weeks and then reevaluated. Chest x-rays and pulmonary function tests may return to normal in days to weeks, whereas renal function either improves or progresses to end-stage disease depending on the presenting severity of renal damage. Corticosteroid therapy alone may temporarily ameliorate the pulmonary hemorrhage, but not the glomerulonephritis. In patients who do not respond to the combination of corticosteroids, cyclophosphamide, and plasmapheresis, cyclosporine, 5 mg/kg/day in divided doses, has been advocated as an additional drug.

VI. Prognosis

Prognosis appears to be related to the severity of renal disease at presentation, as reflected by serum creatinine levels and percentage of crescent involvement on renal biopsy. No therapy, or brief immunosuppressive therapy alone, results in end-stage renal disease in up to 75% of patients, and death from pulmonary hemorrhage in 20% to 50% of patients. However, recent data suggest that the clinical course and the likelihood of survival are better than previously considered if early plasmapheresis and long-term maintenance with prednisone and cyclophosphamide are prescribed.

A 50% survival is estimated at 2 years for patients treated with all modalities, although a 50% survival at 6 months has been estimated for patients presenting with severe renal failure, even with aggressive treatment.

Wegener Granulomatosis

Wegener granulomatosis is necrotizing granulomatous vasculitis, the manifestations of which classically involve the upper and lower respiratory tracts and often the kidneys. It is one of the most common vasculitides involving the lung, with a prevalence of 3 in 100,000. **Generalized** Wegener granulomatosis is the term given when the manifestations are truly systemic, and is the most common form of the disease. In a minority of cases (less than 20%) the disease appears to be limited to either the upper airways and lungs, or lungs alone, indicating a limited form of Wegener granulomatosis. Wegener granulomatosis can occur at any age (reported cases from 9 to 78 years), but most commonly affects patients in the fourth and fifth decades of life. There is no sex predilection although affected persons tend to be Caucasian.

I. Clinical presentation

   A. Symptoms and signs. Wegener granulomatosis can involve virtually any organ system with vasculitis and/or granulomatous changes.

   1. Respiratory. More than 90% of patients seek medical attention because of upper and/or lower respiratory symptoms including sinusitis (50%), nasal complaints (36%), otitis media (25%), hearing loss (15%), cough (19%), hemoptysis (12%), and pleuritis (10%). About 92% of patients eventually develop ear, nose, or throat involvement, and 85% develop lung disease.

   2. Renal. Although glomerulonephritis eventually develops in 75% to 80% of cases, it is rarely the cause of presenting symptoms.

   3. Other. Musculoskeletal symptoms are prominent in two-thirds of patients, eye involvement in 50%, fever at some point in 50%, and skin lesions such as palpable purpura, ulcers, or nodules in 40% to 50%.

Thirty-five percent develop weight loss. About 5% to 15% of patients will develop symptoms from pericarditis, central nervous system mass effects, retroorbital pseudotumors, or mononeuritis multiplex.

B. Laboratory findings

1. **Antineutrophil cytoplasmic antibody.** Serum from 88% to 95% of patients with active systemic disease tests positive for diffuse granular cytoplasmic immunofluorescent staining of neutrophils for antineutrophil cytoplasmic antibody **(C-ANCA)**, which is highly specific for the diagnosis. This is reduced to 55% to 66% in the limited form of the disease. A minority of patients test positive for perinuclear staining **(P-ANCA)**, which occurs in other vasculitides and is not diagnostic for Wegener granulomatosis. ANCAs can also be detected by ELISA assay with specificity directed against either the proteinase 3 antigen (Pr3-ANCA), which correlates primarily with C-ANCA (90% of the time), or with specificity against myeloperoxidase (MPO-ANCA), which correlates primarily with P-ANCA immunofluorescence. The 1999 International Consensus Statement on Testing and Reporting of ANCA recommends that both neutrophil immunofluorescence and ELISA assays be performed in patients with suspected Wegener granulomatosis, because 5% to 10% of patients are positive for only one assay and not the other. C-ANCA and Pr3-ANCA titers parallel disease activity in only about 50% of patients and should not be used as the sole indicator to monitor disease or predict relapses.

2. **Blood and urine.** Anemia with normal indices, leukocytosis, hypergammaglobulinemia (particularly IgA and IgE), and an elevated Westergren erythrocyte sedimentation rate (average 71 mm per hour) are characteristically found before treatment. Peripheral eosinophilia, antinuclear antibodies, and cryoglobulinemia rarely occur and complement levels are normal or elevated. Elevated blood urea nitrogen (BUN) and creatinine are common, as are proteinuria, hematuria, and an increased urinary sediment.

C. Radiographic findings. Chest x-ray changes occur in 85% of cases but are often fleeting and asymptomatic. Unilateral or bilateral lung infiltrates are the most common finding (63%), followed by unilateral or bilateral nodules (31%). Cavitation of the nodules can occur. Computed tomography (CT) of the chest will better delineate the x-ray findings. Nodules may be seen perivascularly. Sinus x-rays or CT will also be abnormal at some point in up to 85% of cases.

D. Physiology studies. Pulmonary functions tests (PFTs) are variable in Wegener granulomatosis and can show either a restrictive defect with a decreased diffusion capacity or an obstructive defect due to endobronchial involvement.

II. Immunologic features

The target antigen of C-ANCA is serine protease 3 (Pr3), a component of the azurophilic neutrophil granule. *In vitro*, exposure of neutrophils to ANCA induces the release of primary granules and the production of oxygen radicals. ANCA also primes neutrophil and monocyte chemotaxis, signal transduction, and their potential to induce endothelial cell damage. These effects are enhanced by concurrent exposure to tumor necrosis factor. The high sensitivity and specificity of this antibody, its correlation with disease activity, and its capacity to activate neutrophils, suggest a pathologic role in the disease process.

III. Pathologic features

A. Lungs. Pulmonary involvement is characterized by parenchymal granulomas and necrosis (84%); granulomatous inflammation associated with a mixture of neutrophils, lymphocytes, plasma cells, histiocytes, and eosinophils (59%); and capillaritis (33%).

B. Kidneys. Renal biopsies show focal and segmental glomerulonephritis in the majority of cases. Proliferative changes and fibrinoid necrosis may also be seen. Crescentic and sclerotic lesions may be seen in end-stage renal disease. Vasculitis and granulomas are very rare, as is electron microscopy evidence of immune complex deposition.

IV. Diagnostic approach

A. Diagnostic criteria. Diagnosis of Wegener granulomatosis relies on the pathologic triad of necrosis, granulomas, and vasculitis. The granulomas are well formed and noncaseating, whereas the vasculitis involves medium-sized vessels. This diagnosis requires a large piece of tissue in order to identify the complete triad. The availability of C-ANCA and Pr3-ANCA serology, with its high level of sensitivity (90%) and specificity (95+%), provides an invaluable screening tool.

B. Tissue biopsies

1. **Lung biopsy.** Lung lesions are the sine qua non of both generalized and limited Wegener granulomatosis. Open lung biopsies will be diagnostic in 90% of patients. Transbronchial biopsies, on the other hand, are only diagnostic 5–7% of the time.

2. **Renal biopsy.** Renal biopsy provides a less invasive procedure to diagnose generalized Wegener granulomatosis. Although the focal glomerulonephritis itself is not pathognomonic, its presence in association with a positive C-ANCA serology and respiratory tract lesions is virtually diagnostic.

3. **Nasopharyngeal biopsy.** Although upper respiratory complaints are the most common presenting symptom, the diagnostic combination of vasculitis and necrosis and/or granulomatosis is found in less than 25% of nasopharyngeal biopsies. This is most likely due to the limited amount of tissue available from these biopsy sites.

C. Differential diagnosis. Wegener granulomatosis must be differentiated from other diseases exhibiting vasculitis, granulomas, glomerulonephritis, or a combination of these features. Hypersensitivity angiitis, polymorphic reticulosis, lymphomatoid granulomatosis, collagen vascular diseases, Goodpasture syndrome, infectious granulomatous diseases, sarcoidosis, and neoplastic diseases are the most important considerations. The availability of screening C-ANCA serology has dramatically improved the ability to differentiate Wegener granulomatosis from these conditions.

V. Treatment

A. Combined immunosuppression. In generalized Wegener granulomatosis, and probably also in most patients with limited Wegener granulomatosis, a combination of oral daily cyclophosphamide (2 mg/kg/day) and oral corticosteroids (prednisone 1 to 2 mg/kg/day starting dose) is considered the standard treatment of choice.

1. **Cyclophosphamide.** Higher initial doses of cyclophosphamide (3 to 5 mg/kg/day) should be considered in cases of fulminant or unresponsive disease. Daily maintenance therapy at 2 mg/kg/day (adjusted to keep absolute neutrophil count above 1,500 per mm^3) should be continued for at least 1 year after the patient achieves remission and then tapered by 25 mg every 2 to 3 months. Epidemiologic comparisons suggest that cyclophosphamide therapy results in a 2.4-fold overall increased risk for cancer; especially bladder cancer (33-fold increased risk) and lymphoma (11-fold increased risk). Lifelong screening is recommended.

2. **Corticosteroids.** A few days of intravenous corticosteroids (e.g., methylprednisolone up to 15 mg/kg/day) may be indicated in select patients with fulminant disease. Otherwise, daily prednisone at 1 mg per kg should be continued for 1 month and then changed over the next 2 to 3 months to 60 mg on alternate days. Therapy can then be tapered and discontinued as the symptoms of active disease resolve (average total course approximately 12 months). The incidence of infectious complications is greatest during daily corticosteroid therapy, decreases by more than 50% when corticosteroids are changed to alternate-day therapy, and decreases further when corticosteroids are discontinued altogether.

B. **Alternative therapies.** Patients with limited Wegener granulomatosis have been treated with corticosteroids alone, with variable success. Methotrexate in conjunction with corticosteroids has been shown to be effective. Trimethoprim–sulfamethoxazole has been reported to work in rare case reports, although only 1 in 9 patients treated at the National Institutes of Health responded to this approach. At this time, combined immunosuppression with cyclophosphamide and corticosteroids is recommended as the treatment of choice.

VI. **Prognosis**

A. **Untreated.** The prognosis in untreated generalized Wegener granulomatosis is extremely poor, with an average life expectancy of 5 months and a mortality rate of 93% at 2 years. The prognosis in limited Wegener granulomatosis is somewhat better, and spontaneous remissions have been reported, but death can occur rapidly due to progressive lung disease.

B. **Combined immunosuppression.** Combined therapy results in marked improvement or partial remission in more than 90% of cases and complete remission in 75% of patients. The median time to remission is about 12 months and approximately half of these cases experience a relapse; 13% of patients die from progressive disease despite maximal therapy, and 40% to 50% of patients experience a serious infectious complication during the course of treatment.

Sarcoidosis

Sarcoidosis is a systemic granulomatous disease of unknown origin, involving multiple organs with variable frequency and intensity, but invariably involving the lung. This manifests most commonly as isolated hilar lymphadenopathy, parenchymal infiltrates, or both. Sarcoidosis has an overall incidence of 11 in 100,000 in the United States, but has a much higher incidence in certain populations (e.g., African Americans [40 in 100,000], Puerto Ricans [36 in 100,000], and Scandinavians [64 in 100,000]). Patients usually present in the third to fourth decade of life. Although there is no documented patient-to-patient transmission, sarcoidosis has occurred in families, suggesting a constitutional susceptibility or a common exogenous mechanism.

I. **Clinical presentation**

A. **Symptoms and signs**

1. **General.** Approximately 80% of patients have symptoms at the time of diagnosis, the remainder being diagnosed from an incidental finding on chest x-ray. Constitutional symptoms (fever, weight loss, fatigue, malaise) develop insidiously in approximately one-third to one-half of patients. Patients presenting acutely with spiking fevers and erythema nodosum usually resolve most rapidly.

2. **Pulmonary.** Although more than 90% of patients have pulmonary involvement, respiratory symptoms occur in only 40% to 60% of patients and include shortness of breath, dry cough, substernal chest discomfort, and occasionally blood-streaked sputum. The physical findings are variable (depending on the stage) and nonspecific, consisting of tachypnea, crackles (diffuse or basilar), and sometimes wheezing (indicating endobronchial involvement).

3. **Extrapulmonary.** Adenopathy (32%), skin lesions (23%), hepatomegaly (less than 20%), uveitis (17%), peripheral nerve involvement (15%), splenomegaly (13%), arthritis (10%), arrhythmias (5%), salivary gland enlargement resulting in pain and/or dry mouth (5%), nasal mucosal edema (5%), and facial nerve palsy (2%) are seen clinically, but most are more commonly found on biopsy or at autopsy. Clubbing is very rare. All patients suspected of having sarcoidosis should have a careful slit-lamp examination to rule out uveitis.

B. **Laboratory findings.** Serum angiotensin converting enzyme (ACE) levels are elevated in 60% to 75% of all cases. However, mild elevations (up to two to three times normal) of ACE can be seen in multiple disease states. For this reason, ACE levels are not recommended for the workup of sarcoidosis. The erythrocyte sedimentation rate is usually elevated in active disease. Leukopenia is common, whereas anemia is unusual. Polyclonal hypergammaglobulinemia is present in 50% of cases. **Hypercalcinuria** with or without hypercalcemia may be present and appears to be due to secretion of 1,25-dihydroxyvitamin D_3 by the granuloma. Cutaneous anergy may be present. The **Kveim** test is an intradermal injection of sarcoid spleen suspension that results in a typical noncaseating granuloma in 4 to 6 weeks in affected patients. The Kveim test is not commonly used because of a lack of a standardized, specific antigen and concern about transmission of infection.

C. **Radiographic and nuclear medicine findings.** There are five described x-ray stages of sarcoid. A normal chest x-ray (stage 0) occurs in 5% to 10% of patients on presentation. Bilateral hilar lymphadenopathy without infiltrates (stage I) is found in 35% to 45% of presenting patients. Linear and reticulonodular infiltrates with bilateral hilar lymphadenopathy (stage II) and parenchymal infiltrates alone (stage III) are each observed in 25% of patients on presentation. End-stage patients develop fibrosis, hilar retraction, bronchiectasis, and bullae formation, which are irreversible (stage IV). Rarely, pneumothorax, unilateral pleural effusion, single or multiple cavities or nodules, or calcification of lymph nodes can be present. In 25% to 30% of cases x-rays are not specific or atypical, and HRCT can be used to aid in diagnosis. Classic findings of sarcoidosis on HRCT include symmetrical lymph node enlargement, and small nodules tracking in the peribronchial vascular regions, and adjacent to pleural surfaces, interlobular septae, and centrilobular areas. HRCT may also be useful in detecting early fibrosis not visible on x-rays. Gallium scintigraphy detects pulmonary inflammation of any etiology and correlates poorly with disease activity, limiting its usefulness.

D. **Physiologic tests.** PFTs commonly show a restrictive ventilatory defect with a decrease in vital capacity, total lung capacity, and diffusing capacity. If endobronchial sarcoidosis is present, an obstructive ventilatory defect may also occur.

II. **Immunologic features**

Sarcoidosis appears to be a cell-mediated (type IV) reaction, although the eliciting stimulus and etiology remain unknown. Pulmonary involvement is characterized by a lymphocytic infiltrate (alveolitis) of predominantly CD4+ (helper/inducer) T cells. BAL often reveals CD4+ : CD8+ T-cell ratios ranging from 2 : 1 up to 10 : 1 (normal 1.2 to 1.6 : 1). Cutaneous anergy is common and may be due to sequestration of peripheral helper T cells (CD4+) in the lung and at other granulomatous sites. These intrapulmonary T cells are activated as evidenced by their enhanced production of IL-2, gamma interferon, granulocyte macrophage colony-stimulating factor (GM-CSF), monocyte chemotactic factors, and soluble IL-2 receptors. Pulmonary macrophages are also activated with enhanced IL-1 and tumor necrosis factor (TNF) secretion and enhanced antigen-presenting capacity. Unfortunately, none of these immunologic markers or T-cell subsets sufficiently correlate with activity or prognosis to be clinically useful.

III. **Pathologic features**

The most characteristic pathologic feature of established sarcoidosis is the presence of well-formed, noncaseating granulomas composed of epithelioid and multinucleated giant cells surrounded by lymphocytes and monocytes. These are found in a lymphatic or perilymphatic distribution. Asteroid or Schaumann bodies are frequently seen in giant cells. A peripheral inflammatory response is absent. Granulomas may convert to nonspecific hyaline scars or resolve completely over time. These findings occur in multiple organs and are observed throughout the lung interstitium and bronchial walls even when the chest x-ray appears normal.

IV. Diagnostic approach
  A. Criteria. The diagnosis requires three primary criteria:
    1. A compatible clinical and radiographic presentation
    2. Histologic evidence of a noncaseating granuloma from tissue biopsy
    3. Careful exclusion of other disease processes, especially infectious diseases
  B. Biopsy. Choice of biopsy site depends both on clinical presentation and ease or risk of obtaining tissue from a particular site. All biopsies should be stained and cultured to exclude tuberculosis and fungal infections.
    1. **Lung.** Four to six transbronchial biopsies as obtained through a fiberoptic bronchoscope yield a positive diagnosis in 85% to 90% of cases, and is the procedure of choice for obtaining pulmonary diagnosis. Transbronchial biopsies are often positive even without clinical or radiologic evidence of pulmonary disease. Open lung biopsy is rarely necessary.
    2. **Reticuloendothelial sites.** Palpable lymph nodes (80% yield), liver (70%, especially if alkaline phosphatase is elevated), and spleen (50%) are more invasive sites for biopsy and rarely performed. Mediastinoscopy is usually diagnostic in cases with mediastinal adenopathy and can be employed when transbronchial biopsies are nondiagnostic.
    3. **Other sites.** Skin lesions, lacrimal and minor salivary glands, skeletal muscle, conjunctiva, and nasal mucosa all may yield positive biopsies with or without clinical involvement.
  C. Differential diagnosis. Noncaseating granulomas are **nonspecific** and are seen in tuberculosis, fungal infections, lymphoma, foreign-body reactions, berylliosis, hypersensitivity pneumonitis, primary biliary cirrhosis, leprosy, brucellosis, tertiary syphilis, granulomatous arteritis, and lymph nodes draining malignant tumors. Radiographic mimics of sarcoid include lymphangitic carcinomatosis, berylliosis, coal workers pneumoconiosis, and silicosis. Serum ACE levels are not specific and can be elevated in hyperthyroidism (81%), leprosy (53%), cirrhosis of the liver (28.5%), diabetes mellitus (24% to 32%), silicosis (21%), Lennert lymphoma, and berylliosis. Ordinarily, neither mycobacterial nor fungal infections are associated with elevated levels of ACE, but exceptions have been reported. Sarcoidosis is a diagnosis of exclusion.
V. Treatment
  A. Indications. Sarcoidosis is associated with both a variable clinical course and a high spontaneous remission rate, making assessment of therapeutic regimens difficult. It is appropriate to follow asymptomatic patients with bilateral hilar adenopathy and no extrapulmonary lesions with chest x-rays at 6-month intervals. Patients with symptomatic pulmonary disease, progressive or persistent parenchymal disease after 2 years, posterior ocular disease, persistent systemic findings, or clinically significant extrapulmonary disease are candidates for systemic corticosteroid therapy.
  B. Corticosteroids
    1. **Local.** Acute iridocyclitis or uveitis responds well to topical corticosteroids (triamcinolone acetonide 1%). Skin lesions may respond to intralesional corticosteroid injections.
    2. **Oral prednisone.** Although there are no controlled studies to support dosing regimens, prednisone at 20 to 40 mg per day in divided doses (1 to 2 mg per kg in children) is given for 3 to 6 months and then gradually tapered to 5 to 10 mg per day, if possible. Higher doses are used for cardiac and central nervous system disease. Therapy should continue for another 6 to 12 months with periodic attempts to further reduce the dosage or discontinue the drug. Alternate-day therapy (40 mg every other day) may also be an effective maintenance therapy and may be tapered by 10 mg every 3 months as tolerated. Lower doses and/or more rapid tapering may be possible in selected cases. Frequently, interruption or premature discontinuation of therapy results in relapse, which generally responds to increased doses of prednisone. Oral corticosteroids may or may not be effective in preventing fibrosis.

    C. **Alternative treatments.** Several cytotoxic agents have been used to treat sarcoidosis and were found to provide improvement, including methotrexate, azathioprine, and cyclophosphamide.

        1. **Methotrexate.** Several uncontrolled studies have reported response rates on the order of 60% when methotrexate (10 mg p.o. q. week adjusted for toxicity) was used alone, and 80% response rates when combined with low-dose corticosteroids (prednisone 10 mg per day). However, relapses were frequently reported upon discontinuation, suggesting that methotrexate suppresses but does not cure this disease. Administration of methotrexate may play a role in patients requiring a steroid-sparing agent.

        2. **Azathioprine.** The efficacy of azathioprine appears similar to that of methotrexate and it can be considered a second-line steroid-sparing agent for the treatment of sarcoidosis. Dosing in the range of 50 to 200 mg per day should be titrated according to the patient's absolute neutrophil count.

        3. **Other cytotoxics.** Cyclophosphamide (1 to 2 mg/kg/day) has been used in a limited number of patients with severe disease, but is associated with a significantly higher incidence of both short-term and long-term side effects. It should only be considered as a last alternative.

    D. **Monitoring of response.** No one test is optimal for following the response to therapy. The clinical picture in conjunction with some combination of objective tests (pulmonary function tests, diffusing capacity, chest x-rays) relevant to the patient's clinical situation is optimal. Lack of response may be present in inactive, fixed pulmonary fibrosis. Lung transplantation should be considered in patients with end-stage fibrosis.

VI. Prognosis

As many as 60% of patients have spontaneous clinical and physiologic resolution within 2 years. An additional 20% resolve with therapy, although 16% to 74% of these patients will relapse when the steroids are tapered. About 10% to 20% fail to resolve even with corticosteroid therapy, and a few present with irreversible disease. African American patients tend to have more progressive disease. Cases with rapid onset of disease, especially those with erythema nodosum, generally resolve most quickly and completely. Chronic extrathoracic and central nervous system sarcoidosis tend to respond poorly.

Idiopathic Pulmonary Fibrosis

The term pulmonary fibrosis is commonly applied to a heterogeneous group of pulmonary disorders characterized by interstitial inflammation and thickening, as well as varying degrees of parenchymal destruction and scarring. It is the common end pathway of many progressive interstitial lung diseases (ILDs). More than 160 different disease states have been associated with ILD and pulmonary fibrosis (Table 7.3). Despite this long list, an underlying etiology is not identified in greater than 50% of patients. These cases are referred to as idiopathic interstitial pneumonias. Idiopathic pulmonary fibrosis (IPF), also known as usual interstitial pneumonitis or cryptogenic fibrosing alveolitis, comprises one of the idiopathic interstitial pneumonias. Desquamative interstitial pneumonitis, respiratory bronchiolitis-associated ILD, nonspecific interstitial pneumonia, acute interstitial pneumonia, bronchiolitis obliterans with organizing pneumonia, and lymphocytic interstitial pneumonia comprise the remainder of the idiopathic interstitial pneumonias and represent distinct clinical entities. The exact prevalence of IPF is unknown, but is estimated to be approximately 10 to 20 in 100,000 in males and 7 to 13 in 100,000 in females. The prevalence increases with age (average age of diagnosis is 66 years) and may reach as high as 175 in 100,000 for individuals over the age of 75 years. Familial cases do exist and follow an autosomal-dominant pattern of transmission.

    I. **Clinical presentation**

        A. **Symptoms and signs.** The insidious and progressive development of shortness of breath, initially during exercise, and a nonproductive cough are the most common complaints (80% to 100%) and often exist for more than 6 months before presentation. A small percentage of patients may present with abnormal chest x-rays without respiratory symptoms, but invariably develop symptoms as the disease progresses. Up to 50% of patients develop systemic or constitutional symptoms (e.g., fatigue, weight loss, fever, myalgias, and arthralgias). Examination of the chest reveals late respiratory fine dry crackles ("Velcro rales") at the bases. Late in the course of disease, clubbing of the fingers (25% to 50%) and evidence of cor pulmonale and pulmonary hypertension (augmented P2, S3 gallop, right ventricular heave) are often found.

B. Laboratory findings. Hypergammaglobulinemia (80%), an elevated ESR (50%), positive rheumatoid factor (30%), positive antinuclear antibodies (15% to 20%), and circulating immune complexes are all relatively common with IPF but are nonspecific. Polycythemia rarely occurs even with hypoxemia.

C. Radiographic and nuclear medicine findings. The majority of patients with IPF will have an abnormal x-ray at presentation although a normal film does not rule out disease. Typical findings on x-ray include bilateral, peripheral, reticular opacities, greatest in the lower lobes and associated with low lung volumes. Alveolar infiltrates are rare and should raise suspicion for another disease process. HRCT has a higher sensitivity in detecting subtle disease and is used as an important diagnostic tool in IPF. A confident diagnosis of IPF by a trained HRCT reader can accurately predict the disease in about 90% of cases. However, because a confident diagnosis can only be made in about two-thirds of IPF cases, HRCT should not be the sole determinant in making the diagnosis. The pattern of IPF on HRCT includes subpleural, bibasilar, reticular infiltrates. There may be a minimal amount of ground glass noted as well as honeycomb lung and traction bronchiectasis in more advanced disease. There have been rare occurrences of normal HRCT with pathologically proven IPF. Gallium-67 lung scintigraphy does suggest active alveolitis when positive, but is nonspecific, and has no role in the diagnosis of IPF.

D. Physiologic tests. Pulmonary function studies invariably reveal a restrictive ventilatory defect, with reduction in vital capacity, total lung capacity, and diffusing capacity. Patients with obstructive disease and hyperinflation from cigarette smoking may present with normal lung volumes. Occasionally, reductions in diffusing capacity may precede reductions in lung volume. Arterial blood gas analysis may be normal initially and later reveal hypoxemia initially with exercise and later at rest, as well as a respiratory alkalosis (hyperventilation) induced by stimulation of intrapulmonary stretch-receptors. The hypoxemia at rest is secondary to ventilation/perfusion mismatch, whereas the hypoxemia with exercise is due to the alveolar–arterial oxygen gradient increase from diffusion impairment and ventilation/perfusion mismatch.

II. Immunologic features

IPF is an immunologically mediated inflammatory lung disease associated with activated pulmonary lymphocytes, macrophages, neutrophils, eosinophils, epithelial cells, and fibroblasts. The high prevalence of autoimmune antibodies, hypergammaglobulinemia, and circulating immune complexes also suggests a role for humoral immunity in the disease process. By definition, the initial triggering insult or antigen is unknown. Lymphocytosis is temporally associated with the earliest stages of the disease and is believed to initiate the immunologic cascade of events. Subsequent activation of pulmonary macrophages and endothelial cells appears to result in the expression of numerous cytokines involved in neutrophil recruitment and in fibrinogenesis. IL-8 is released by activated alveolar macrophages and is a major chemotactic factor for neutrophils and a potent angiogenic factor. In addition, bronchial epithelial and alveolar macrophages produce high levels of transforming growth factor beta (TGF-β), which directly stimulates fibroblast proliferation and collagen synthesis. The highest levels of TGF-β are found in the areas of greatest fibrosis. The progression of events from initial insult to end-stage fibrosis is only beginning to be understood. A better understanding of the pathogenesis of IPF will be essential in developing more effective forms of treatment.

III. **Pathologic features**

According to the International Consensus Statement published by the American Thoracic Society (ATS) in 2000, usual interstitial pneumonitis (UIP) is the defining pathologic pattern of IPF. The hallmark of UIP is the temporal concurrence of normal lung alternating with interstitial inflammation, fibrosis, and honeycomb changes. These changes are most prominent in the subpleural regions. The interstitial inflammation is composed of alveolar septal infiltrates of lymphocytes and plasma cells as well as type II pneumocyte hyperplasia. The areas of fibrosis have both dense collagen and areas of proliferating fibroblasts called "fibroblastic foci." The honeycombed zones consist of cystic fibrotic airspaces, which often are lined by bronchial epithelium and are filled with mucin. Recently, a subclassification of IPF termed nonspecific interstitial pneumonia has been described. This entity has both the inflammatory and fibrotic characteristics seen in IPF, although these components are of like age. There is some evidence to suggest that this is the earlier stage of IPF, although further studies are needed.

IV. **Diagnostic approach**

In 1999, the ATS adopted an international expert consensus statement in order to standardize diagnosis and treatment of IPF. The consensus statement delineated diagnostic criteria based on either surgical or clinical findings.

A. **Surgical diagnosis**

   1. Pathologic diagnosis of UIP on a surgically obtained specimen
   2. Exclusion of other causes of ILD
   3. Pulmonary function studies with evidence of restriction, and abnormal gas exchange or diffusion capacity
   4. Abnormalities consistent with IPF on chest x-ray or HRCT

B. **Clinical diagnosis.** Fulfillment of all the major criteria and three of the minor criteria is correlated with a high likelihood of IPF.

   1. **Major criteria**
      a. Exclusion of other causes of ILD
      b. Pulmonary function studies with evidence of restriction, and abnormal gas exchange or diffusion capacity
      c. Bibasilar reticular abnormalities with minimal ground glass opacities on HRCT
      d. Transbronchial lung biopsy or BAL excluding an alternative diagnosis

   2. **Minor criteria**
      a. Age greater than 50 years
      b. Insidious onset of unexplained dyspnea on exertion
      c. Duration of illness greater than 3 months
      d. Bibasilar dry crackles

C. **Bronchoscopy and lung biopsy.** Transbronchial biopsy and BAL using the fiberoptic bronchoscope may be useful in excluding alternative diagnoses, especially sarcoidosis and infection. However, the small sample size of the biopsy is often insufficient to make an accurate diagnosis of IPF, and the cellularity observed on the BAL is a poor indicator of the interstitial inflammatory response. Bronchoscopy, therefore, rarely gives a definitive diagnosis of IPF or an accurate assessment of its level of activity. A definitive determination of the cause and activity state of diffuse interstitial fibrosis can only be made by examining tissue obtained by surgical lung biopsy. Both thoracoscopic and open lung biopsy provide adequate tissue samples and thoracoscopic biopsy is the preferred approach because of its lower morbidity and its association with a shorter hospital stay.

V. **Differential diagnosis**

IPF is a diagnosis of exclusion but can be diagnosed with a high degree of accuracy on clinical and radiographic grounds. Many diseases affecting the lung result in similar clinical and histologic changes, making determination of the etiology and pathogenesis difficult unless there is historic or physical evidence of infection, occupational or environmental exposure, or multisystem involvement (e.g., collagen vascular disease). The many diseases that should be considered are listed in Table 7.2. Every effort should be made to identify treatable diseases such as tuberculosis and other infections, collagen vascular diseases, sarcoidosis, hypersensitivity pneumonitis, and the other idiopathic interstitial pneumonias including desquamative interstitial pneumonitis, nonspecific interstitial pneumonitis, and idiopathic bronchiolitis obliterans organizing pneumonia.

VI. Treatment

Traditional therapies have attempted to reduce inflammation and reverse fibrosis. These have consisted of corticosteroids, immunosuppressants (cyclophosphamide and azathioprine), and antifibrotic agents (colchicine and D-penicillamine). To date, none of these modalities have been shown to clearly halt or reverse the sequelae of IPF or to improve quality of life. The treatment recommendations issued by the ATS on IPF suggest that because there is no clear utility for treatment, it should only be offered if the potential benefits outweigh the risks. Patients at increased risk for complications of treatment include elderly and obese patients, as well as those with comorbid disease states such as cardiac disease, diabetes mellitus, osteoporosis, or marked pulmonary impairment. If treatment is undertaken it should be initiated early, include corticosteroids in conjunction with cyclophosphamide or azathioprine, and be continued for 6 months prior to reevaluation, barring complications.

A. Combination therapy

1. **Corticosteroids.** The current recommendation for prednisone dosing is initiated at 0.5 mg/kg/day for the first 4 weeks, 0.25 mg per kg for the following 8 weeks, and then 0.125 mg/kg/day every day or 0.25 mg/kg/day every other day. Prophylaxis for PCP should be given concurrently.

2. **Immunosuppressives.** Azathioprine is administered at 2 to 3 mg/kg/day to a maximum of 150 mg. Dosing should start at 25 to 50 mg per day and increase by 25 mg every 1 to 2 weeks until the target dose is achieved. The dose should be adjusted to keep the absolute neutrophil count greater than 1,500 and periodic hepatic transaminase panels should be monitored. **Alternatively,** cyclophosphamide is initiated at 2 mg/kg/day to a maximum of 150 mg per day. Dosing should start at 25 to 50 mg per day and increase by 25 mg every 1 to 2 weeks until the target dose is achieved. The dose is also adjusted for an absolute neutrophil count greater than 1,500 and periodic urinalysis should be monitored.

B. Adjunct and alternative therapy

1. **Colchicine.** Colchicine modulates the formation of collagen and the extracellular matrix and suppresses the release of fibronectin and macrophage-derived growth factors. Although clinical data documenting the efficacy of colchicine for the treatment of IPF are lacking, its side effects are limited and a trial of oral colchicine at 0.6 mg once or twice a day may be considered as a stand alone treatment or can be taken in conjunction with combination therapy.

2. **Interferon-γ.** Early clinical studies and *in vitro* models suggest that interferon-γ may provide a useful approach for the treatment of IPF by decreasing the expression of TGF-β, down-regulating fibrogenic activity, and by inhibiting the production of angiogenic chemokines. In 2000, a multicenter clinical trial was initiated to test this hypothesis, and recommendations regarding the use and dosing of this medication should wait for the conclusion of this study.

C. Predictors of response.

Currently, there is no staging system for IPF and no clear prognostic indicators. However, age less than 50 years, female sex, a short symptom time prior to prognosis, smoking at the time of diagnosis, ground glass on HRCT, a predominance of lymphocytes on BAL, and a response to steroids all bode for a longer survival. A failure to respond to ther-

Table 7.4. Response of idiopathic pulmonary fibrosis to treatment

Positive response to treatment
  Increase in level of exertion or decline in the frequency and severity of cough
  Improvement in the parenchymal abnormalities seen on chest x-ray or HRCT
  Improvement of two or more of the following PFT measurements:
      ≥10% increase in the TLC or VC
      ≥15% improvement in the DLCO
      ≥4% improvement in the P_aO_2 or S_aO_2
Stable response to treatment
  <10% change in the TLC or VC
  <15% change in DL_{CO}
  <4% change in P_aO_2 or S_aO_2
No response to treatment
  Increase in dyspnea or cough
  Increase in radiographic opacities on chest x-ray or HRCT or development of signs
    of pulmonary hypertension
  Decrease in two or more of the following PFT measurements
      ≥10% decline in the TLC or VC
      ≥15% decline in the DLCO
      ≥4% decline in the P_aO_2 or ≥4 mm Hg increase in the A_aO_2 at rest or during
        cardiopulmonary exercise testing

HRCT, high-resolution computed tomography; PFT, pulmonary function test; TLC, total lung capacity; VC, vital capacity; DLCO, carbon monoxide diffusion in the lung; P_aO_2, partial pressure of oxygen; S_aO_2, oxygen saturation of arterial blood; A_aO_2, alveolar-arterial O_2 gradient.

apy, increased fibrosis on HRCT, or a high percentage of neutrophils or eosinophils on BAL have been associated with a shorter survival time.

  D. Monitoring of response. A response to treatment may not be evident for at least 3 months. For this reason, reassessment at 6 months is recommended using standardized criteria (see Table 7.4). If the patient remains stable or improves on treatment, it should be continued and reassessed every 6 months. If deterioration is documented, the treatment should be altered or stopped. Patients who deteriorate on optimal therapy and are eligible candidates should be referred for transplantation as early as possible.
  E. Prognosis. The course of IPF is rapidly progressive, with only 20% to 30% of patients responding to conventional treatment. Current studies show a 5-year survival of 30% to 50%. The most common causes of death are respiratory failure, cor pulmonale, infection, and lung carcinoma.

Selected Readings
Hypersensitivity Pneumonitis
Ando M, Suga, M, Kohrogi, H. A new look at hypersensitivity pneumonitis. *Curr Opin Pulm Med* 1999;5:299.
Kaltreider HB. Hypersensitivity pneumonitis. *West J Med* 1993;159:570.
Lynch DA, et al. Can CT distinguish hypersensitivity pneumonitis from idiopathic pulmonary fibrosis? *Am J Roentgenol* 1995;165:807.
Sharma OP, Fujimura N. Hypersensitivity pneumonitis: a noninfectious granulomatosis. *Semin Respir Infect* 1995;10:96.
Zacharisen MC. Hypersensitivity pneumonitis: Knowing what to look for. *J Respir Dis* 1999;20:8.

Bronchopulmonary Aspergillosis
Angus RM, et al. Computed tomographic scanning of the lung in patients with allergic bronchopulmonary aspergillosis and in asthmatic patients with a positive skin test to *Aspergillus fumigatus. Thorax* 1994;49:586.

Cockrill BA, Hales CA. Allergic bronchopulmonary aspergillosis. *Annu Rev Med* 1999;50:303.

Kauffman JF. Review of fungus-induced asthmatic reactions. *Am J Respir Crit Care Med* 1995;151:2109.

Stevens DA, et al. A randomized trial of itraconazole in allergic bronchopulmonary aspergillosis. *N Engl J Med* 2000;342:756.

Stevens DA, et al. Practice guidelines for disease caused by Aspergillus. *Clin Infect Dis* 2000;30:696.

Pulmonary Infiltrates With Eosinophilia

Allen JN, Davis WB. State of the art: eosinophilic lung diseases. *Am J Respir Crit Care Med* 1994;150:1423.

Kim Y, et al. The spectrum of eosinophilic lung disease: radiologic findings. *J Comput Assist Tomogr* 1997;21:920.

Knoell DL. Churg-Strauss syndrome associated with zafirlukast. *Chest* 1998;114:332.

Lhote F, Guillevin L. Polyarteritis nodosa, microscopic polyangiitis, and Churg-Strauss syndrome. *Rheum Dis Clin North Am* 1995;21:911.

Masi AT, et al. The American College of Rheumatology 1990 criteria for the classification of Churg-Strauss syndrome (allergic granulomatosis and angiitis). *Arthritis Rheum* 1990;33:1094.

Ong RKC, Doyle RL. Tropical pulmonary eosinophilia. *Chest* 1998;113:1673.

Goodpasture Syndrome

Ball JA, Young KR. Pulmonary manifestations of Goodpasture's syndrome. *Clin Chest Med* 1998;19:777.

Kalluri R, et al. The Goodpasture's autoantigen: structural delineation of two immunologically privileged epitopes on a alpha 3(IV) chain of type IV collagen. *J Biol Chem* 1996;271:9062.

Kalluri R, et al. Reactive oxygen species expose cryptic epitopes associated with autoimmune Goodpasture syndrome. *J Biol Chem* 2000; 275:20027.

Wegener Granulomatosis

Duna GF, Galperin C, Hoffman GS. Wegener's granulomatosis. *Rheum Dis Clin North Am* 1995;21:949.

Harper L, Savage COS. Pathogenesis of ANCA-associated systemic vasculitis. *J Pathol* 2000;190:349.

Hoffman GS, et al. Wegener's granulomatosis: An analysis of 158 patients. *Ann Intern Med* 1992;116:488.

Rao JK, et al. The role of antineutrophil cytoplasmic antibody (c-ANCA) testing in the diagnosis of Wegener's granulomatosis. *Ann Intern Med* 1995;123:925.

Savige J, et al. International consensus statement on testing and reporting of anti-neutrophil cytoplasmic antibodies (ANCA). *Am J Clin Pathol* 1999;111:507.

Sarcoidosis

American Thoracic Society Statement on Sarcoidosis. *Am J Respir Crit Care Med* 1999;160:736.

Sarcoidosis. *Clin Chest Med* 1997;18:663.

Wells, A. High resolution computed tomography in sarcoidosis: a clinical perspective. *Sarcoidosis Vasc Diffuse Lung Dis* 1998;15:140.

Idiopathic Pulmonary Fibrosis

ATS International Consensus Statement: idiopathic fibrosis: diagnosis and treatment *Am J Respir Crit Care Med* 2000;161:646.

Coultas DB, et al. The epidemiology of interstitial lung disease. *Am J Respir Crit Care Med* 1994;150:967.

Orens JB. The sensitivity of high-resolution CT in detecting idiopathic pulmonary fibrosis proved by open lung biopsy: a prospective study. *Chest* 1995;108:109.

Ziesche R, et al. A preliminary study of long term treatment with interferon gamma-1b and low dose prednisone in patients with idiopathic pulmonary fibrosis. *N Engl J Med* 1999;341:1264.

8. ATOPIC DERMATITIS AND CONTACT DERMATITIS

Mark Boguniewicz and Vincent S. Beltrani

Atopic Dermatitis

Atopic dermatitis (AD) is a chronic, relapsing, highly pruritic, inflammatory skin disease that frequently precedes the development of asthma and/or allergic rhinitis. It is the most common chronic skin disease of young children, but can affect patients of any age. The associated sleep disruption, school absenteeism, occupational disability, and emotional stress can have a significant impact on the quality of life of patients and their families. AD may also be associated with significant morbidity, especially when complicated by erythroderma or concomitant infection. The prevalence of AD has continued to increase, affecting more than 10% of children at some point during childhood in most countries. Because wide variations in prevalence both within and between countries inhabited by similar ethnic groups have been documented, environmental factors may be critical in determining disease expression.

I. **Clinical aspects**
  A. **Natural history.** AD typically presents in early childhood with onset before 5 years of age in approximately 90% of patients. In adults with new onset dermatitis, especially without a history of childhood eczema, asthma, or allergic rhinitis, other diseases need to be considered (see Differential diagnosis, Table 8.2 on page 167). Although most children will have milder disease over time, they will often continue to have persistent or frequently relapsing dermatitis as adults.
  B. **Clinical features.** AD has no pathognomonic skin lesion(s) or unique laboratory parameters. Diagnosis is based on the presence of major and associated clinical features (Table 8.1). The principal features include **pruritus**, a chronically relapsing course, typical morphology and distribution of the skin lesions, and a history of atopic disease. The presence of pruritus is critical to the diagnosis of AD, and patients with AD have been shown to have a reduced threshold for pruritus.
    1. **Acute atopic dermatitis** is characterized by intensely pruritic, erythematous papules associated with excoriations, vesiculations, and serous exudate.
    2. **Subacute atopic dermatitis** is characterized by erythematous, excoriated, scaling papules.
    3. **Chronic atopic dermatitis** is characterized by thickened skin with accentuated markings (lichenification) and fibrotic papules. Patients typically have dry skin. Significant differences can be observed between the pH, capacitance, and transepidermal water loss of AD lesions compared with uninvolved skin in the same patients and with the skin of normal controls.
    4. During **infancy**, AD involves primarily the face, scalp, and extensor surfaces of the extremities, and the diaper area is typically spared. When involved, it may be secondarily infected with *Candida*, in which case, the dermatitis does not spare the inguinal folds. In contrast, infragluteal involvement is a common distribution in children.
    5. In **older patients** with long-standing disease, the flexural folds of the extremities are the predominant location of lesions. Localization of AD to the eyelids may be an isolated manifestation, but should be differentiated from an allergic contact dermatitis (ACD) (as discussed in Allergic Contact Dermatitis on page 179). Chronic rubbing of the skin can result in prurigo nodules.
  C. **Complicating features**
    1. **Infections.** Patients with AD have an increased susceptibility to infection or colonization with a variety of organisms.

Table 8.1. Clinical features of atopic dermatitis

Major features
  Pruritus
  Chronic or relapsing course
  Typical distribution of dermatitis
    Facial and extensor involvement in children <2 years old
    Flexural involvement in children >2 years old or adults
  Personal or family history of atopy
Associated features
  Early age of onset
  Course influenced by environmental or emotional factors
  Itch with sweating
  Intolerance to wools or other irritants
  Xerosis
  White dermatographism
  Infraorbital darkening
  Facial pallor or erythema
  Hand or foot dermatitis
  Hyperlinear palms
  Frequent cutaneous infections, especially by *Staphyloccocus aureus*

Adapted from Hanifin JM, Rajka G. Diagnostic features of atopic dermatitis. *Acta Dermatol Venereol (Stockh)* 1980;92:44–47, with permission.

a. **Viral infections** include *Herpes simplex* and molluscum contagiosum. This suggests that the T-cell-associated cytokine abnormalities seen in AD may enhance viral infections. Rarely, patients can have generalized dissemination of *H. simplex*, termed eczema herpeticum or Kaposi varicelliform eruption. Systemic antiviral therapy with acyclovir and hospitalization may be required. It is worth remembering that molluscum is a contagious disease, and although it often resolves spontaneously, it can spread and school-aged children need to be treated or their lesions need to be covered. Treatment options include cryotherapy, blistering agents, or curettage.

b. **Fungal infections** can also cause AD to flare. *Malassezia furfur* (*Pityrosporum ovale*) is a lipophilic yeast and IgE antibodies against *M. furfur* have been found predominantly in patients with head and neck dermatitis. The potential importance of *M. furfur* as well as other dermatophyte infections is further supported by the reduction in clinical severity of AD in patients treated with antifungal agents in some studies. Occasionally, resistant cheilitis or fissures may respond to antifungal therapy.

c. **Bacterial infections**, particularly *Staphylococcus aureus*, are frequent in patients with AD. *S. aureus* is found in more than 90% of AD skin lesions. In contrast, only 5% of healthy subjects harbor this organism. The importance of *S. aureus* is supported by the observation that even AD patients without superinfection show a reduction in severity of skin disease when an anti-staphylococcal antibiotic is added to their treatment regimen. Although recurrent staphylococcal pustulosis can be a significant problem in AD, invasive *S. aureus* infections occur rarely and should raise the possibility of an immunodeficiency such as hyperimmunoglobulin E (hyper-IgE) syndrome.

2. **Hand dermatitis.** Patients with AD often have a nonspecific hand dermatitis. This is frequently irritant in nature and aggravated by repeated wetting, especially in the occupational setting.

3. **Ocular problems.** Ocular complications associated with AD can lead to significant morbidity. Atopic keratoconjunctivitis is always bilateral and symptoms include itching, burning, tearing, and copious mucoid discharge. It is frequently associated with eyelid dermatitis and chronic blepharitis, and may result in visual impairment from corneal scarring. Vernal conjunctivitis is a severe bilateral recurrent chronic inflammatory process of the upper eyelid conjunctiva, usually occurring primarily in younger patients. It has a marked seasonal incidence often in the spring. The associated intense pruritus is exacerbated by exposure to irritants, light, or sweating. Examination of the eye reveals a papillary hypertrophy or "cobblestoning" of the upper inner eyelid surface. Keratoconus is a conical deformity of the cornea believed to result from persistent rubbing of the eyes in patients with AD and allergic rhinitis. Anterior subcapsular cataracts may develop during adolescence or early adult life.

4. **Psychological issues.** Patients with AD have been characterized as having high levels of anxiety and problems in dealing with anger and hostility, which can exacerbate the illness. Stress or frustration, in turn, can precipitate an itch–scratch cycle. In some cases, scratching is associated with significant secondary gain or with a strong component of habit. In addition, severe disease can have a significant impact on patients' self-esteem and social interactions.

D. **Differential diagnosis.** A number of diseases may be confused with AD (Table 8.2). Scabies can present as a pruritic skin disease, although distribution in the genital and axillary areas, presence of linear lesions, as well as skin scrapings may help to distinguish it from AD. It is especially important to recognize that an adult who presents with an eczematous dermatitis with no history of childhood eczema and without other atopic features

Table 8.2. Differential diagnosis of atopic dermatitis

Congenital disorders
  Netherton syndrome
Metabolic disorders
  Zinc deficiency
  Pyridoxine (vitamin B6) and niacin deficiency
  Multiple carboxylase deficiency
  Phenylketonuria
Immunodeficiencies
  Wiskott-Aldrich syndrome
  Severe combined immunodeficiency
  Hyper-IgE syndrome
Chronic dermatoses
  Seborrheic dermatitis
  Contact dermatitis
  Nummular eczema
  Lichen simplex chronicus
Infections and infestations
  Scabies
  HIV-associated dermatitis
Malignancies
  Cutaneous T-cell lymphoma (mycosis fungoides/Sézary syndrome)
Proliferative disorders
  Letterer-Siwe disease

IgE, immunoglobulin E; HIV, human immunodeficiency virus.

may have contact dermatitis. In particular, a contactant should be considered in those patients whose AD does not respond to appropriate therapy. Typical distribution for a suspected contactant may be suggestive. However, ACD complicating AD may appear as an acute flare of the underlying disease, rather than the more typical vesiculobullous eruption.

In older adults with a diffuse, pruritic, eczematous eruption, cutaneous T-cell lymphoma also needs to be ruled out. In such cases, biopsies should be obtained from three separate sites, because histology may show spongiosis and cellular infiltrate similar to AD. In addition, eczematous rash suggestive of AD has been reported with human immunodeficiency syndrome (HIV).

II. Immunopathologic aspects.

A. **General.** AD appears to result from a bone marrow-derived cell dysfunction rather than from a constitutive skin defect. Systemic immunoregulatory abnormalities include an increased frequency of both circulating and cutaneous allergen-specific interleukin 4 (IL-4) and IL-5 secreting T helper cells (Th2-type cells).

B. **Immunohistology**

1. **Acute lesions** are characterized by intercellular edema of the epidermis (spongiosis) and intracellular edema. A sparse lymphocytic infiltrate may be observed in the epidermis, whereas a marked perivenular infiltrate consisting of lymphocytes and some monocytes, with rare eosinophils, basophils, and neutrophils is seen in the dermis. Mast cells are found in normal numbers in different stages of degranulation.

2. **Chronic lesions** often demonstrate prominent hyperkeratosis of the epidermis with increased numbers of epidermal Langerhans cells and predominantly monocytes/macrophages in the dermal infiltrate. Mast cells are increased in number, but are not degranulated. Lymphocytes, in both acute and chronic lesions, are predominantly CD3, CD4, and CD45RO memory T cells that also express CD25 and human leukocyte antigen DR (HLA-DR) indicative of intralesional activation. In addition, almost all of the infiltrating T cells express high levels of the skin homing receptor, cutaneous lymphocyte antigen (CLA), which is a ligand for the vascular adhesion molecule, E-selectin. Langerhans cells found in the epidermis and dermis of chronic lesions are potent activators of autologous resting CD4 T cells and have been shown to express high affinity receptors for IgE. The latter appears to play an important role in cutaneous allergen presentation to Th2-type cells. Activated eosinophils are present in significantly greater numbers in chronic as compared to acute lesions. In addition, deposition of eosinophil major basic protein (MBP) can be detected throughout the upper dermis and to a lesser extent deeper in the dermis, especially in involved areas. MBP may contribute to the pathogenesis of AD through its cytotoxic properties and its capacity to induce basophil and mast cell degranulation.

C. **Immunoregulatory abnormalities** during acute AD include an increase in IL-4 expression, whereas chronic disease is primarily associated with IL-5 expression. IL-13 expression is also higher in acute lesions, whereas chronic lesions are characterized by increased IL-12 (a potent inducer of interferon γ [IFN-γ] synthesis) and IFN-γ (a Th1-type cytokine) expression. IL-16, a chemoattractant for CD4$^+$ T cells, is more highly expressed in acute than in chronic skin lesions. In addition, the C-C chemokines, RANTES, monocyte chemotactic protein 4 (MCP-4), and eotaxin are also increased in atopic lesions, and likely contribute to the chemotaxis of eosinophils and Th2-type lymphocytes into the skin. Cutaneous T cell-attracting chemokine (CTACK) may play an important role in the preferential attraction of cutaneous lymphocyte antigen (CLA$^+$T) cells into the skin.

III. Immunologic triggers

A. **Foods.** Double-blinded, placebo-controlled food challenges (DBPCFC) have demonstrated that food allergens can cause exacerbations in a subset of patients, primarily young children, with AD. Approximately one-third of children with chronic moderate to severe AD may have associated IgE-mediated food hypersensitivity. Seven foods (milk, egg, peanut, soy, wheat, fish, and tree nuts) account for nearly 90% of the positive DBPCFC. These data reaffirm the need to consider the role of food allergens in children with AD who do not respond readily to conventional therapy. Notably, elimination of proven food allergens results in amelioration of skin disease and a decrease in spontaneous basophil histamine release.

B. Aeroallergens. The evidence supporting a role for aeroallergens in AD includes the finding of both allergen-specific IgE antibodies and allergen-specific T cells. Exacerbation of AD can occur with exposure to allergens such as house dust mites. Direct contact with inhalant allergens can also result in eczematous skin eruptions. Environmental control measures have resulted in clinical improvement of AD.

C. Microbes. AD patients are frequently colonized by toxin-producing *S. aureus* that act as superantigens, which trigger expansion of antigen-specific lymphocytes. In addition, patients make specific IgE antibodies directed against the staphylococcal toxins found on their skin. *S. aureus*-specific IgE has been shown to correlate with clinical severity of AD and may contribute to persistent inflammation or exacerbations of AD.

IV. Treatment

A. Conventional therapy

1. **Education.** Education of patients and their families is an essential component of successful management of a chronic illness such as AD (Table 8.3). Adequate time and teaching materials are necessary to provide effective education, because most patients or parents will forget or confuse the skin care recommendations given them without written instructions. For many patients, a written step-care treatment plan will lead to improved outcomes and this should be reviewed and adjusted at follow-up visits. Educational brochures and videos can be obtained from the Eczema Association for Science and Education (800-818-7546 or www.eczema-assn.org) and information from the Lung Line (800-222-LUNG or www.njc.org).

2. **Identification and elimination of exacerbating factors**
   a. **Irritants.** Patients with AD have a lowered threshold of irritant responsiveness and need to avoid irritants including detergents, soaps, and chemicals. Cleansers with minimal defatting activity and a neutral pH should be used rather than soaps, especially after exposure to chlorine. Air temperatures at home and work should be temperate to minimize sweating. In addition, nonsensitizing sunscreens should be used to prevent sunburn.
   b. **Allergens.** Avoidance of foods confirmed by controlled challenges results in clinical improvement. More recently, the *in vitro* CAP

Table 8.3. First-line therapy for atopic dermatitis

Education
Avoidance of irritants and proven allergens
Hydration
Moisturizers and occlusives
Topical corticosteroids
Tacrolimus ointment[a]
Antibiotics (limited courses)
Antihistamines (primarily for sedative effects)
Stress reduction

[a] Tacrolimus ointment is currently indicated for moderate to severe atopic dermatitis not responsive to or at risk from conventional therapy.

assay has been shown to measure specific IgE to egg, milk, peanut, and fish allergens with clinically relevant predictive values. CAP IgE concentrations (measured in kUA per L) that have been shown to have a greater than or equal to 95% positive predictive value for an allergic reaction include: egg 7, milk 15, peanut 14, and fish 20. Recent data suggest that when the allergen-specific IgE level falls below 20% of these values, there is a greater than 60% chance that the patient will tolerate the food. In dust mite allergic individuals, environmental control measures aimed at reducing dust mite allergen loads (e.g., use of dust mite-proof covers for pillows and mattresses and washing sheets in hot water) have been shown to improve AD in patients allergic to dust mite allergen.

3. **Hydration.** Atopic skin shows an enhanced transepidermal water loss from both involved and uninvolved skin consistent with an impaired function of the water permeability barrier. Bathing helps restore skin water content and may also remove allergens from the skin surface and reduce colonization by *S. aureus*. Bathing or soaking the affected area should be done for approximately 15 to 20 minutes in warm water. Hydrating the face or neck can be done by applying a wet washcloth or towel to the involved area. The latter may be better tolerated when eye and mouth holes are cut out, allowing the patient to watch TV or engage in other activities while soaking. Isolated hand or foot dermatitis can be treated with soaks in basins. Baths may need to be taken on a long-term daily basis and may even need to be increased to several times daily during flares of AD. Showers may be appropriate for patients with milder disease. Addition of substances such as oatmeal to the bath water may be soothing to certain patients but does not promote skin hydration. Bath oils do not effectively add moisture to the skin and can make the tub dangerously slippery. After hydrating the skin, patients should be instructed to gently pat away excess water with a soft towel and immediately apply an occlusive preparation (see Moisturizers below). Because wet skin is more permeable to water, it is essential that the skin be covered within the first few minutes to prevent evaporation. Appropriate use of hydration and occlusives will help to reestablish the skin's barrier function.

4. **Moisturizers.** Use of emollients, especially when combined with hydration therapy, will help restore and preserve the stratum corneum barrier. Emollients may also decrease the need for topical corticosteroids. Moisturizers are available in lotions, oils, creams, and ointments. In general, ointments have the fewest additives and are the most occlusive, although in a hot, humid environment, their use may lead to trapping of sweat with associated irritation of the skin. Lotions and creams may be irritating because of added preservatives or fragrances. Lotions contain more water than creams and may have a drying effect due to evaporation. Oils are also less effective moisturizers. Moisturizers should be obtained in the largest size available because they typically need to be applied several times each day on a chronic basis. Crisco shortening can be used as an inexpensive moisturizer. Petroleum jelly (Vaseline) is not a moisturizer, but can be used as a sealer after hydrating the skin.

5. **Corticosteroids**

   a. **General.** Topical corticosteroids have been the mainstay of treatment for AD. They reduce inflammation and pruritus and are effective for both the acute and chronic phases of the disease. They impact multiple resident and infiltrating cells primarily through suppression of inflammatory genes. Topical corticosteroids are available in potencies ranging from extremely low (group 7) to high (group 1) (Table 8.4).

Table 8.4. Representative topical corticosteroid preparations

Group 1[a]
  Clobetasol proprionate (Temovate) 0.05% ointment/cream
  Betamethasone diproprionate (Diprolene) 0.05% ointment/cream
  Halobetasol propionate (Ultravate) 0.05% ointment/cream
Group 2
  Mometasone furoate (Elocon) 0.1% ointment
  Halcinonide (Halog) 0.1% cream
  Fluocinonide (Lidex) 0.05% ointment/cream
  Desoximetasone (Topicort) 0.25% ointment/cream
Group 3
  Fluticasone propionate (Cutivate) 0.005% ointment
  Halcinonide (Halog) 0.1% ointment
  Betamethasone valerate (Valisone) 0.1% ointment
Group 4
  Mometasone furoate (Elocon) 0.1% cream
  Triamcinolone acetonide (Kenalog) 0.1% ointment/cream
  Fluocinolone acetonide (Synalar) 0.025% ointment
Group 5
  Fluocinolone acetonide (Synalar) 0.025% cream
  Hydrocortisone valerate (Westcort) 0.2% ointment
Group 6
  Desonide (DesOwen) 0.05% ointment/cream/lotion
  Alclometasone diproprionate (Aclovate) 0.05% ointment/cream
Group 7
  Hydrocortisone (Hytone) 2.5% & 1% ointment/cream

[a] Steroids listed by group from 1 (super potent) through 7 (least potent).
From Stoughton RB. Vasoconstrictor assay-specific applications. In: Maibach HI, Surber C, eds. *Topical corticosteroids*. Basel: Karger, 1992:42–53, with permission.

b. Choosing the appropriate compound. Use of a particular drug
should depend on the severity and distribution of the skin lesions.
Patients should be informed of the strength of topical corticosteroid
they are given and the potential side effects. Patients often make
the mistake of assuming that the potency of their prescribed corticosteroid is based solely on the percent noted after the compound
name (e.g., believing that hydrocortisone 2.5% is more potent than
betamethasone dipropionate 0.05%) and may apply the preparations incorrectly. In general, the lowest potency corticosteroid that
is effective should be used, although using a topical corticosteroid
that is too low in potency may result in persistence or worsening of
AD. In such cases, a step-care approach with a mid- or high-potency
preparation (although usually not to eczema of the face, axillae, or
groin) followed by a low-potency preparation may be more successful. Often, patients are only prescribed a high-potency corticosteroid and told to discontinue use after a period of time, which can
result in rebound flaring of the AD, similar to what is often seen
with oral corticosteroid therapy. Occasionally, therapy-resistant lesions may respond to a potent topical corticosteroid under occlusion,
although this approach should be used with caution and reserved
primarily for eczema of the hands or feet. Of note, Lotrisone contains both clotrimazole, an antifungal, and beclomethasone dipropionate, a high-potency corticosteroid, and should rarely be used in
AD and never in the diaper area, face, or axillae.

c. **Choosing the appropriate vehicle.** The vehicle that the product is formulated in can alter the potency of the steroid and move it up or down in this classification. Generic formulations of topical steroids are required to have the same active ingredient and the same concentration as the original product. However, many generic products do not have the same vehicle formulation and their bioequivalence can vary significantly. In general the same steroid will be most potent in an ointment base, followed by emollient, gel, cream, and lotion. Topical steroids are available in a variety of bases including ointments, creams, lotions, solutions, gels, sprays, foam, oil, and even tape (Table 8.4). There is, therefore, no need for a pharmacist or patient to compound these medications. Ointments are most occlusive, have the fewest additives, provide better delivery of the medication, and decrease evaporative losses. During periods of excessive heat or humidity, creams may be better tolerated than ointments because the increased occlusion may cause itching or folliculitis. In general, however, creams and lotions, while easier to apply, may be less effective and can contribute to xerosis. Solutions can be used on the scalp or other hirsute areas, although the alcohol in them can be quite irritating when used on inflamed or excoriated lesions. Ingredients used to formulate the different bases may be irritating to individual patients and may cause sensitization.

d. **Other practical considerations.** Inadequate prescription size often contributes to poor compliance and a suboptimal outcome, especially in patients with generalized disease. In addition, dispensing the prescribed medication in larger (1 lb quantities when available) can result in significant cost savings for the patient. It is worth remembering that approximately 30 grams of medication is needed to cover the entire body of an average adult. The fingertip unit (FTU), defined as the amount of topical medication that extends from the tip to the first joint on the palmar aspect of the index finger, has been proposed as a measure for applying topical corticosteroids. It takes approximately 1 FTU to cover the hand or groin, 2 FTUs for the face or foot, 3 FTUs for an arm, 6 FTUs for the leg, and 14 FTUs for the trunk.

e. Always avoid placing an emollient either under or over an area of topical steroid application, as this will reduce the effectiveness of the steroid. **Side effects** of topical corticosteroids are infrequent with low- to medium-potency topical corticosteroids when used appropriately, even when applied for extended periods of time. More potent topical steroids cause thinning of the skin most commonly. Several weeks of topical corticosteroid application can lead to a decrease in collagen and elastin synthesis and subsequent skin fragility, dermal atrophy, striae, telangiectasia, purpura, and poor wound healing. In addition, hypopigmentation, secondary infections, and acneiform eruptions may occur. Local side effects are most likely to occur on the face and on the intertriginous areas, and therefore only low-potency corticosteroids should be used in these areas on a routine basis. Perioral dermatitis may also occur with the chronic use of topical corticosteroids on the face and is characterized by erythema, scaling, and follicular papules and pustules that occur around the mouth, alar creases, and sometimes on the upper lateral eyelids.

Systemic side effects are extremely rare with topical corticosteroids. However, prolonged use of high- and super-high-potency compounds, especially if used under occlusion, may cause systemic side effects and should therefore be used judiciously.

f. **Oral corticosteroids.** The use of oral corticosteroids should be avoided in a chronic disease such as AD. Although patients may experience rapid and dramatic relief with oral corticosteroids, this is all too often followed by rebound flaring of the dermatitis. Short courses of prednisone or prednisolone are occasionally used with the introduction of other treatment measures. Gradual tapering of the oral corticosteroid and intensification of topical skin care may decrease the occurrence of rebound exacerbations that can occur with systemic corticosteroid use.

6. **Tar preparations.** Although the antiinflammatory properties of tars are not as pronounced as those of topical corticosteroids, they may be useful in reducing the need for topical corticosteroids in chronic maintenance therapy of AD. Tars are used primarily in shampoos for scalp inflammation (T/Gel) or as bath additives (Balnetar). Newer coal tar products have been developed that are better tolerated with respect to odor and staining of clothes. A moisturizer applied over the tar product will decrease the drying effect on the skin. Some patients prefer a tar compounded in an ointment or cream base such as 5% liquor carbonis detergents (LCD) in Aquaphor ointment to avoid the need for multiple layers. Tar preparations may be used primarily at bedtime to allow the patient to remove the preparation in the morning and limiting staining to a few pairs of pajamas and bed sheets. Tar preparations should not be used on acutely inflamed skin, because this may result in irritation. Side effects associated with tars include inflammation of hair follicles and photosensitivity.

7. **Antiinfective therapy.**
   a. **Antibacterial therapy.** Systemic antibiotics may be necessary to treat AD secondarily infected with *S. aureus*. First- (e.g., cephalexin) or second-generation (e.g., cefuroxime axetil) cephalosporins given for 7 to 10 days are usually effective (e.g., cephalexin 500 mg twice daily or 25 to 50 mg per kg divided twice daily for pediatric patients). A semisynthetic penicillin (e.g., dicloxacillin) can also be used. Erythromycin-resistant organisms are common, which limits the usefulness of erythromycin and other macrolides. Long-term maintenance antibiotic therapy should be avoided because it may result in colonization by methicillin-resistant organisms. The topical antistaphylococcal antibiotic mupirocin (Bactroban) applied three times daily to affected areas for 7 to 10 days can be used to treat localized areas of involvement. In patients found to have positive nasal cultures for *S. aureus*, treatment with a nasal preparation of mupirocin twice daily for 5 days may reduce nasal carriage of *S. aureus*. On the other hand, use of topical neomycin can result in ACD, because neomycin is among the more common allergens causing contact dermatitis (see Contact Dermatitis on page 183). Although antibacterial cleansers have been shown to be effective in reducing bacterial skin flora, they can be irritating to the skin of atopic patients.
   b. **Antiviral therapy.** Patients with disseminated eczema herpeticum, also referred to as Kaposi varicelliform eruption, usually require treatment with systemic acyclovir. Recurrent cutaneous herpetic infections can be suppressed with a prophylactic oral antiviral (e.g., acyclovir 400 mg twice daily).
   c. **Antifungal therapy.** Superficial dermatophytosis and *P. ovale* can be treated with topical or rarely systemic antifungal drugs. A subset of patients with AD may respond to a course of empiric treatment with antifungal agents. However, the clinical significance of fungi as an etiologic factor in AD remains unresolved.

8. **Antihistamines.** Pruritus is the cardinal symptom of AD and even partial reduction can result in significant improvement in quality of life for patients with severe disease. In general, antihistamines do not have a large effect on pruritis associated with AD. First-generation

antihistamines appear to be most useful because of their tranquilizing effects, and can be dosed primarily in the evening to avoid daytime drowsiness. In patients with very severe pruritus and sleep disruption, the tricyclic antidepressant doxepin (which has both histamine H1- and H2-receptor binding affinity and a long half-life) may be given as a single 10- to 50-mg dose in the evening. Treatment of AD with topical antihistamines and local anesthetics should be avoided because of potential sensitization.

9. **Anxiolytics.** If sleep disruption caused by nocturnal pruritus remains severe, a sedative such as chloral hydrate or a benzodiazepine given at bedtime may be appropriate for short-term use.

10. **Psychosocial factors.** Counseling, relaxation, behavioral modification or biofeedback may be of benefit, especially in patients with habitual scratching. Patients and families should be counseled regarding the natural history and prognosis of the disease with appropriate vocational counseling.

B. **Novel topical therapy**

1. **Topical calcineurin inhibitors.** Calcineurin inhibitors (e.g., tacrolimus, ascomycin) are immunomodulators that act in part by binding to specific cytoplasmic proteins and interfering with gene transcription of proinflammatory cytokines. Tacrolimus 0.03% and 0.1% ointments (Protopic) have proven to be safe and effective and have been approved for short- and long-term intermittent use in both children and adults with moderate to severe AD. Protopic ointment 0.03% is indicated for adults and children aged 2 to 15 years and Protopic ointment 0.1% is indicated for adults. Patients should apply a thin layer of ointment twice daily and continue to use it for approximately 1 week after lesions clear. The most common adverse effect is cutaneous burning, which may be reduced by applying ice to the affected area before applying the ointment. In addition, patients should minimize or avoid sunlight (use a sunscreen), artificial tanning, or UV treatment during treatment with tacrolimus.

A new topical formulation of an ascomycin derivative has been shown to be safe and effective in adults and children with AD, and one of the compounds (pimecrolimus cream 1%) is currently undergoing U.S. Food and Drug Administration (FDA) review.

C. **Recalcitrant disease**

1. **Wet wraps.** Wet dressings can be used together with hydration and topical therapy in severe AD or to potentiate therapy with less potent topical corticosteroids. The prolonged hydration and occlusion provided by these wraps increases the absorption of topical medications and promotes healing. They can also serve as an effective barrier against the persistent scratching that often undermines therapy. Total body dressings can be achieved by using wet pajamas or long underwear with dry pajamas or sweatsuit on top. Hands and feet can be covered by wet tube socks under dry tube socks. Alternatively, the face, trunk, or extremities can be covered by wet gauze with dry gauze over it, and secured in place with an elastic bandage or by pieces of tube socks. Dressings may be removed when they dry out or they may be re-wetted. Wet wraps are often best tolerated and most convenient at bedtime. Overuse of wet dressings can result in chilling, maceration of the skin, or secondary infection.

2. **Hospitalization.** AD patients who are erythrodermic or who appear toxic may require hospitalization. This may also be appropriate for patients with severe generalized disease resistant to therapy. Removing the patient from environmental allergens or stressors, together with intense education and assurance of compliance with therapy results in marked clinical improvement in many cases. The patient can also un-

dergo appropriately controlled provocative challenges to help identify potential triggers while in the hospital.

3. **Phototherapy.** Ultraviolet (UV) light therapy can be a useful treatment modality for chronic recalcitrant AD. Patients who do not experience photoexacerbations of their AD and who are not fair complexioned may benefit from moderate amounts of natural sunlight. However, they should avoid both overexposure and overheating, which can induce pruritus. Sunlamp treatment at home is usually not recommended. UVB has been shown to be an effective treatment modality and addition of UVA to UVB can increase the therapeutic response. Alternatively, high-dose UVA1 has been found to be a fast-acting and effective phototherapeutic approach for patients with acute exacerbations.

   Photochemotherapy with oral methoxypsoralen therapy followed by UVA (PUVA) may be indicated for patients with severe disease, especially with failure of topical therapy or in patients with significant corticosteroid side effects. Short-term adverse effects may include erythema, pruritus, and pigmentation, whereas long-term adverse effects include premature skin aging and cutaneous malignancies. Topical PUVA has no risk of systemic side effects and may be especially useful for chronic hand eczema resistant to other treatment.

4. **Cyclosporin A.** Several short-term studies have demonstrated that patients with severe AD refractory to topical corticosteroids may respond to oral cyclosporin A (CsA) (5 mg/kg/day) with reduced skin disease and improved quality of life. However, side effects (including nausea, abdominal discomfort, paresthesias, hypertension, hyperbilirubinemia, and renal impairment with increased serum urea and creatinine) require close monitoring when this drug is used. Few patients have been evaluated on maintenance therapy. Studies in patients with severe AD treated with oral CsA (5 mg/kg/day) for 6 weeks, followed until relapse, then treated with a second 6-week course show that after both treatment periods, approximately half of the patients relapse, although a subset appears to have extended clinical benefit. Nevertheless, the potential for progressive or irreversible nephrotoxicity with extended treatment needs to weighed against the clinical benefit of this treatment.

D. **Experimental and unproven therapies**

Allergen desensitization, intravenous immunoglobulin, essential fatty acids (fish oil and evening primrose oil), traditional Chinese herbal therapy, and leukotriene modifiers have not been shown to be efficacious in patients with AD in double-blind, placebo-controlled studies. Humanized, monoclonal anti-IgE therapy has been shown to be effective in extrinsic asthma and allergic rhinitis. A multicenter, blinded, placebo-controlled, proof-of-concept study with subcutaneously administered anti-IgE is currently ongoing in pediatric patients with AD.

Contact Dermatitis

Contact dermatitis represents a spectrum of inflammatory skin reactions induced by exposure to external substances. Contact dermatitis is a common skin problem, resulting in nearly 8 million physician visits per year. It is estimated that there are more than 85,000 chemicals that may be encountered in the world environment. When applied to the skin, the majority of these agents will induce an irritant contact dermatitis and approximately 2,800 of these substances may act as contact allergens. Identifying the putative agent is essential for the appropriate management of patients with contact dermatitis. When avoidance is not achieved, the condition may become chronic, disabling, and lead to a major impairment in quality of life.

I. Types of contact dermatitis

A broad spectrum of adverse cutaneous reactions have been noted when an external agent comes into contact with skin. **Irritant contact dermatitis** is the most common type of reaction to a contactant and represents a nonimmunologic, irritant-induced reaction to an external substance. **Allergic contact dermatitis** (ACD) represents an immunologic, antigen-induced reaction, which may be acute, subacute, or chronic in duration. **Photocontact dermatitis** is a form of contact dermatitis which is caused by either irritants or allergens in combination with the effects of light. **Urticaria, acneiform eruptions, and pigmentary changes** may also occur in response to contactants and represent unusual presentations of contact allergy. Substances which commonly trigger irritant, allergic contact, and photocontact dermatitis are listed in Tables 8.5, 8.6, and 8.7.

II. **Pathogenesis**

A. **Irritant contact dermatitis** is a polymorphous syndrome that results from contact with agents that may chemically abrade, physically irritate, or damage the skin. Irritation is usually a cytotoxic event produced by a wide variety of external agents (e.g., chemicals, detergents, solvents, alcohol, creams, lotions, ointments, and powders) and by environmental factors such as washing, overhydration, improper drying, perspiration, and temperature extremes (Table 8.5). Epidermal keratinocytes play a key role in initiating tissue damage, followed later by mast cells and activated, nonsensitized T cells. The inflammatory response to irritants appears to be both dose- and time-dependent. Any impairment to the epidermal barrier layer (e.g., fissuring, overhydration, etc.) renders the skin more susceptible to an irritant effect. The clinical presentation of irritant contact dermatitis is usually restricted to the skin site directly in contact with the offending agents, with little or no extension beyond the site of contact. The evolution and resolution of irritant contact dermatitis is less predictable than that of ACD.

B. **Allergic contact dermatitis** is recognized as the prototypic cutaneous type IV delayed-type hypersensitivity reaction. The external agent, acting as an antigen, initiates sensitization at its site of contact with the skin. The antigen must be in the haptenic state and in solution (i.e., sweat) in order to reach the antigen-presenting cells in the epidermis. The thickness and integrity of the skin strongly influence the process of sensitization. Thus, thinner sites (i.e., eyelids, earlobes, and genital skin) are most vulnerable, whereas thicker skin (i.e., palms of hands and soles of feet) is more resistant.

Table 8.5. Important cutaneous irritants

Soaps, detergents
Janitorial cleaning agents
Disinfectants
Solvents, degreasers
Oils, greases
Plastic resins
Paints, inks, varnishes
Glues, adhesives
Gasoline, diesel and jet fuels
Metalworking fluids
Dust, dirt, sewage
Cement, mortar, plaster
Fiberglass
Acids, alkalis
Insects, fruits, vegetables
Grasses, weeds, shrubs
Shampoos
Permanent wave solutions
Pesticides, herbicides, fungicides
Fertilizers

Table 8.6. Important contact allergens

Plants	Carbamates
Rhus	*p*-Phenylenediamine antioxidants
Poison ivy	Plastic resins
Poison oak	Epoxies
Poison sumac	Acrylics
Compositae	Phenolics
Chrysanthemums	Formaldehyde resins
Ragweed	Hardeners, curing agents
Liverwort	Organic dyes
Feverfew	*p*-Phenylenediamine
Primula	Color developers
Primula obconica	Textile dyes
Tulips	Blocide preservatives
Tulip bulbs	Formaldehyde
Lichens	Quaternium 15
Frullania	Imidazolidinyl urea
Woods	Chloroisothiazolinone
Rosewood	*p*-Chloro-m-xylenol
Pine	Parabens
Cocobolo	Topical medications
Metals	Neomycin
Nickel	Bacitracin
Chromate	Thimerosal
Cobalt	Benzocaine
Gold	Miscellaneous
Mercury	Fragrances
Rubber chemicals	Colophony (rosin)
Thiurams	Ethylenediamine di-HCl
Mercapto compounds	

After the antigen penetrates the skin, keratinocytes are activated and initiate the immunologic response by releasing cytokines. The antigen is subsequently engulfed by antigen-presenting cells (Langerhans cells), which migrate to a draining lymph node during the next 12 to 48 hours. Langerhans cells then present the antigen to naïve T helper (Th0) cells, resulting in the development of antigen-specific Th1 cells. Following this period of sensitization, subsequent cutaneous exposure to the same antigen results in movement of these antigen-specific Th1 cells from regional lymph nodes to the systemic circulation and then to the affected area of skin. Within 12 to 36 hours, release of mediators from these Th1 cells causes a delayed-type inflammatory skin reaction (eczema). Further exposures to the same antigen result in progressive shortening of the period required for development of the skin reaction.

C. **Photocontact dermatitis** may be either phototoxic and photoallergic dermatitis in nature. Mechanisms resemble those in irritant or ACD except they require activation of an ultraviolet light-absorbing chemical substance on the skin surface before a toxic reaction in tissues can occur or a hapten–protein conjugate can be formed. Histopathologically, these reactions are identical to irritant or ACD reactions.

III. **Diagnosis of contact dermatitis**

A. **History**

A thorough history and physical examination will enable the physician to consider possible external causes of the patient's dermatitis. Several features will help make the distinction between contact and other causes of dermatitis.

Table 8.7. Important photocontact irritants and allergens

Coal tar	Mustard
Crude coal tar	Agrimony
Pitch	Goose foot
Creosote	Scurfy pea
Dyes	St. John's wart
Acridine	Oils and fragrances
Eosin	Angelica root oil
Fluorescein	Bergamot oil
Rhodamine	Lemon oil
Rose bengal	Lime oil
Plants	Bitter orange oil
Umbelliferae	Rue oil
Celery	Cedarwood oil
Carrots	Sandalwood oil
Bergamot	Lavender oil
Dill	Musk ambrette
Cow parsley	6-Methylcoumarin
Parsnip	Drugs
Fennel	Chlorothiazides
Giant hogweed	Phenothiazines
Angelica	Nonsteroidal antiinflammatory
Rutaceae	drugs
Limes	Tetracyclines
Lemons	Sulfonamides
Gas plant	Griseofulvin
Rue	Sunscreens
Bitter orange	*p*-Aminobenzoic acid, esters
Moraceae	Benzophenones
Figs	Antimicrobials
Compositae	Halogenated salicylanilides
Yarrow	Bithionol
Mayweed	Hexachlorophene
Miscellaneous	Dichlorophen
Buttercup	

1. **Time course and evolution of lesions.** A careful history should help establish whether the site of the dermatitis was in contact with the offending agent within 36 hours prior to the initial appearance of the rash. Although the history can strongly suggest the cause of contact dermatitis, history alone has been shown to confirm sensitization in only 10% to 20% of patients. The evolution of the skin reaction is influenced by many factors including the patient's skin, age, and color, and a number of ambient environmental conditions. Because the majority of contact reactions present as eczematous eruptions, it is essential to note the clinical evolution from acute vesiculation to chronic lichenification. The history should also consider responses to all prior treatment.

2. **Work history.** Because contact dermatitis is the second most common cause of worker's compensation cases, the work history must be closely examined. The exact nature of the work, duration of each activity, and effects on co-workers may be relevant. Recent changes in procedures and exposure to chemicals, vapors, and fumes must be sought. Frequency of hand washing and the cleansers used also should be noted. Material safety data (MSD) sheets are available for every

product used in the workplace, and should be reviewed in every case involving work-related dermatitis.

3. **Leisure activities** such as gardening, painting, carpentry, and photography may also be important in the etiology of contact dermatitis and should be reviewed in detail.

4. **Concomitant medical problems** may be a contributing factor, i.e., other allergic problems or defects in immune status. The impaired epidermal barrier layer of all atopic patients, with or without active dermatitis, subjects them to a greater risk for irritation and/or allergic sensitization.

B. **Physical examination**

The objective findings include the appropriate identification of all of the primary and secondary skin lesions (i.e., macules, papules, etc.), each of which may be secondarily affected by crusting and/or excoriations. Because eczema is a clinical symptom and not a specific disease, the clinician must be aware of the full differential diagnosis for all eczematous eruptions. It is not surprising that the body's exposed areas, especially the hands and face, are the sites most frequently and at times exclusively involved with contact dermatitis. Special clues regarding the etiology of contact dermatitis may be provided according to which part of the body is affected.

1. **Hands.** Hand dermatitis deserves special consideration not only because it is extremely common (10% of women and 4.5% of men), but also because the differential diagnosis can be challenging. Because the palmar skin is much thicker than the dorsum of the hands, ACD is rarely noted on the palms and occurs most often on the thinner skin between the fingers and the dorsum of the hands.

2. **Eyelids.** Eyelids are a common target for contact dermatitis because of frequent exposures, increased susceptibility to irritants and allergens, and easy accessibility to rubbing. In evaluating patients with eyelid dermatitis, one must note whether other areas of the body are involved. Chronic eyelid dermatitis is more often due to cosmetics applied to other areas of the body (i.e., nails, scalp) than to cosmetics directly applied to the eye area. The history should also take note of the use of eyelash curlers (especially in nickel-sensitive patients) and paper tissues (which may contain fragrances, formaldehyde, or benzylkonium chloride). Shampoos, conditioners, hair sprays, gels, and mousses may cause eyelid dermatitis without causing scalp or forehead lesions.

3. **Face.** Similar to eyelid dermatitis, facial dermatitis may occur secondary to allergens transferred to the face from other regions of the body. Although most commercially available cosmetics today are virtually free of sensitizing components, ACD to moisturizers, sunscreens, foundations, and powders do occur and usually produce a symmetrical dermatitis. Rubber-sensitive individuals may react to rubber sponges, masks, balloons, children's toys, etc., that come into contact with the face. A spouse's fragrance and cosmetics may produce a unique, unilateral facial eruption (via contact during sleep).

4. **Scalp.** The skin of the scalp is relatively resistant to penetration of antigens that are found in shampoos and hair dyes, and therefore the dermatitis may manifest strictly on the face or eyelids. The manufacturers of hair dyes recommend that all dye-users be patch tested with the product prior to each application.

5. **Neck.** The thin intertriginous skin of the neck is quite vulnerable to irritant reactions from chemicals used in curling preparations, hair dyes, shampoos, conditioners, and perfumes. In addition, sensitivity to nail polish often presents as localized areas of eczema on the neck rather than hand dermatitis. Nickel-sensitive individuals may react from wearing a necklace or from zippers.

6. **Axilla.** ACD can be caused by deodorants but is not seen with antiperspirant use. Deodorants cause a dermatitis involving the entire

axillary vault, whereas ACD due to clothing always spares the apex of the vault. Irritant contact dermatitis can be caused by both shaving and depilating agents.

7. **Legs.** Patients with chronic stasis dermatitis who apply topical medications to their inflamed skin are at high risk of developing ACD to these medications. Shaving creams, moisturizers, and elastic socks are frequent causes of ACD of the legs.

8. **Anogenital area** Topical medications, solutions for douching, fragrances (in liners, toilet paper, soap, and bubble baths), contraceptive devices (condoms and diaphragms), and spermicides may cause contact dermatitis in the anogenital region. Ammonia and/or the acidic nature of urine may cause an irritant dermatitis, especially in incontinent patients. The ingestion of spices, antibiotics, or laxatives may cause anal itching and result in a secondary irritant dermatitis. Finally, chemicals transferred from the hands are also an important source of potential irritants and allergens.

9. **Sun-exposed areas.** An eczematous rash on any sun-exposed area, such as the face, the anterior aspect (supraclavicular area) of the neck, the back of the hands, and the dorsal forearms suggest the possibility of photocontact dermatitis. These eruptions are often sharply demarcated, especially below on the arms below the sleeves.

C. **Patch testing**

The value of any test depends on whether it is used for an appropriate indication, administered correctly, interpreted accurately, and the results utilized to affect the patient's condition. The patch test remains the gold standard for differentiating ACD from other forms of dermatitis and for diagnosing the cause of ACD. Although the application of antigens for patch testing is rather simple, antigen selection and test interpretation requires experience and expertise on the part of the clinician.

1. **Who to patch test.** The greater the level of suspicion for ACD, the more frequently the correct diagnosis will be made. Therefore, a thorough history eliciting potential environmental sensitizers plays a key role in diagnosis. The majority of patients are allergic to a single allergen or a single group of allergens. Patch testing is warranted for any patient with a chronic, pruritic, or recurrently eczematous or lichenified dermatitis. Virtually any eczematous lesion can be caused or aggravated by a contactant.

2. **How and when to patch test.** Standardized criteria for the application, removal, and interpretation of patch tests have been established by the American Academy of Dermatology. The only available standardized patch test panel is the T.R.U.E. Test, which contains 23 standardized antigens and a negative control (Table 8.8). The testing materials are suspended in a vehicle and attached to an adhesive backing, which is applied to the patient's back. Other purified materials not included in this panel may be compounded in standardized concentrations and vehicles at specialized laboratories (Trolab, Pharmascience, Inc., Montreal, Canada, and Chemotechnique, Dormer Labs, Toronto, Canada). Specially compounded antigens are supplied in a syringe, which are placed onto aluminum Finn chambers and applied to the back. In addition, other materials used by patients may be patch tested using Finn chambers (Table 8.9).

Products obtained from the workplace should be tested with great caution. The employer should have an MSD sheet for each agent they use in the workplace, and it should be reviewed for toxicity, including effects upon the skin. When tested, toxic agents must be diluted similarly to the agents listed above, and also applied to at least two "control" subjects.

Patch testing should be done when the dermatitis is clear or at least quiescent.

Table 8.8. T.R.U.E. Test panel of standard antigens

Substance	Source
Nickel sulfate	Metal objects
Wool alcohols (lanolin)	Ointments, creams, lotions, soaps
Neomycin sulfate	Antibiotic creams, lotions, ointments
Potassium dichromate	Cement, industrial chemicals
Caine mix (benzocaine, tetracaine hydrochloride, dibucaine hydrochloride)	Topical anesthetic medications
Fragrance mix	Toiletries, perfumes, flavorings
Colophony	Adhesives, sealants, pine oil cleaners
Paraben mix	Cosmetics, skin creams, paste bandages
Negative control	
Balsam of Peru	Resin used in cosmetics, perfumes, flavoring agent in cough syrups, lozenges, chewing gum, and candles
Ethylenediamine dihydrochloride	Stabilizer, emulsifier, and preservative in topical fungicides, topical antibiotics, eye drops, and nose drops
Cobalt dichloride	Metal-plated objects and costume jewelry
p-tert-Butylphenol formaldehyde resin	Waterproof glues, leather goods
Epoxy resin	Adhesives, surface coatings, paints
Carba mix	Stabilizer in rubber products, pesticides, glues
Black rubber mix	Antioxidant and antiozonate in almost all black rubber products (e.g., tires, hoses)
Cl + Me–isothiazolinone	Antibacterial preservative in shampoos, creams, lotions, and other skin care products
Quaternium-15	Preservative in shampoos, lotions, soaps, and other skin care products
Mercaptobenzothiazole	Vulcanization accelerator used in most rubber products and some adhesives
p-Phenylenediamine	Permanent and semipermanent hair dyes
Formaldehyde	Building materials and plastics industry
Mercapto mix	Accelerators found in rubber products
Thimerosal	Mercury-containing preservative in cosmetics, nose drops, and eardrops
Thiuram	Antimicrobials and antioxidants found in rubber products

T.R.U.E. Test, thin-layer rapid use epicutaneous test

Table 8.9. Patch testing to nonstandard antigens

Agent	Test concentration
"Leave-on" products	As is
"Wash-off" products	1:10–1:100 dilution
Household products	1:100–1:1,000 dilution
Clothing, gloves, plants	As is
Industrial products	With great caution

3. **Reading the patch tests.** Patch test reagents and tape should be removed 48 hours after placement, with an initial reading at this time, and again 96 hours after placement. The reading at 96 hours is considered most clinically relevant. Patch test results should be evaluated 30 minutes after removal of the tape and patch test materials. Allowance for the irritative effect from the adhesive material must be considered. The standardized grading system should be used at both the 48- and 96-hour reading (Table 8.10).

4. **Factors that affect patch test results.** Oral corticosteroids (prednisone, 20 mg per day or more) and high-potency topical corticosteroids will significantly reduce patch test reactions. Therefore, if possible, oral corticosteroid doses should be reduced to less than 20 mg per day and potent topical corticosteroids should not be applied to patch test sites for 5 to 7 days prior to testing. Systemic and topical H1-antihistamines do not affect patch test results.

5. **Photopatch testing** involves performing patch tests with the addition of light and represents the gold standard for the diagnosis of photocontact dermatitis. It is a complex procedure and should be performed in specialized centers. Photopatch testing requires appropriate light sources, antigens, and light opaque shielding (necessary after patch tests are removed and before reading is performed). Generally, two sets of antigens are applied, one of which is irradiated after being in place for 48 hours; both sets are then read 48 hours later.

6. **Additional tests**
   a. **Repeat open application test** (ROAT) or exaggerated use test is performed by applying the antigen to the antecubital fossa twice daily for 1 week and observing for a reaction. This approach is most applicable to "leave-on" products but not useful for "wash-off" products.

Table 8.10. Grading and interpreting patch test results

Patch test grading
0	=	no reaction
+/–	=	mild erythema only
1+	=	50% of patch test site erythematous with edema
2+	=	50% of patch test site with papular erythema
3+	=	50% of patch test site with vesicles or bulla

Clinical interpretation of grading
0	=	no evidence of contact allergy
+/–	=	doubtful existence of contact allergy
1+	=	possible (or false-positive) contact allergy
2+	=	probable contact allergy
3+	=	definite contact allergy

  b. Immediate skin tests (prick or intradermal) are most useful in the evaluation of allergic contact urticaria. Contact urticaria can also be evaluated with an open patch test (interpreted at 15 minutes) as an alternative to the prick or intradermal skin test.

  c. Skin biopsy may be useful in diagnosing noneczematous conditions.

  d. Potassium hydroxide (KOH) preparations are helpful in assessing the presence of fungal elements in the skin lesion.

IV. Special considerations

A. Occupational contact dermatitis

More than 40% of worker's compensation cases involve skin disorders, and it is estimated that contact dermatitis constitutes 90% to 95% of all occupational skin diseases. Irritant contact dermatitis is the most common type of contact dermatitis in the workplace and most frequently involves the hands and face.

B. Dermatitis caused by natural rubber latex

Contact reactions to products containing natural rubber, particularly gloves, may include irritant contact dermatitis, ACD, and contact urticaria. Although irritant contact dermatitis associated with rubber gloves is caused by irritation from sweat retention and friction, ACD is due to type IV hypersensitivity to accelerators used in the rubber manufacturing process. Contact urticaria represents an IgE-mediated reaction to latex rubber proteins. Because these dermatoses may be difficult to distinguish on clinical grounds, particularly irritant and ACD, an accurate diagnosis requires a detailed history of the evolution of the lesions, physical examination, and appropriate skin testing. All patients with eczematous dermatitis related to rubber glove use should be tested with antigens that are commercially available as part of the TRUE test, along with pieces of latex glove, moistened on a Finn chamber. Contact urticaria due to immediate-type hypersensitivity reactions is best confirmed by *in vitro* tests measuring IgE to latex protein.

C. Dermatitis caused by topical medications

The topical of application of fragrances, lanolin, para-amino benzoic acid (PABA), topical anesthetics, antibiotics, and antiinflammatory drugs on the skin should be the cause of any persistent rash. Neomycin, nitrofurazone (Furacin), and iodochlorhydroxyquin (Vioform) are all potent sensitizers and frequent causes of ACD. Topical corticosteroids have also been shown to result in contact sensitization, which is more apt to occur during use for chronic dermatitis. It should be suspected in any patient whose skin condition worsens with the application of the corticosteroid. For diagnostic purposes, four representative topical corticosteroids are used for patch testing (see Table 8.11). Patch testing to corticosteroids is complicated by the therapeutic antiinflammatory nature of the corticosteroid itself, which may cause false-negative results. Once the diagnosis has been made, sensitized patients must also be instructed to avoid the systemic use of any implicated drug.

D. Contact dermatitis of the mucus membranes

Although oral and/or mucus membrane contact reactions are rare, contact sensitivity has been described as a factor in recurrent oral ulcerations.

Table 8.11. Topical corticosteroids used for patch testing

Tixocortol: for the lower potency topical corticosteroids

Triamcinolone: for mid-potency corticosteroids

Dexamethasone: for mid- to-high potency corticosteroids (betamethasone, desoximetasone)

Budesonide: for high-potency corticosteroids

Objectively, changes may be barely visible, or may vary from a mild ery-thema to a fiery red color, with or without edema. Dental and mouth care products contain abrasives and a number of sensitizing chemicals. Cinnamon flavorings and peppermint are probably the most common causes of allergic stomatitis from dentifrices and chewing gum. The metals used in dentistry that have been responsible for contact dermatitis include mercury, chromate, nickel, gold, cobalt, beryllium, and palladium. Among these metals, mercury (used in amalgam) has most often been implicated as a producer of oral allergic reactions. Gold has also been implicated in mucosal allergic disease.

E. **Contact dermatitis to surgical implants**

Allergic reactions to metals used in surgical implants, including cobalt, nickel, and chromium, are unusual and manifest as eczematous eruptions along with implant loosening. Fortunately, implants now being used most commonly contain titanium or plastic, both of which are relatively free of sensitization. If a patient is to undergo placement of an implant containing a potentially sensitizing metal, a prior history of metal allergy should be sought. Once an implant reaction has been determined, the implant must be removed and replaced with an implant free of the causative metal.

F. **Systemic allergic contact dermatitis**

Systemic contact dermatitis presents as a generalized eczematous eruption following the oral or parenteral administration of a drug or chemical that has previously caused ACD. A number of common examples are shown in Table 8.12.

G. **Contact dermatitis to cosmetics and personal hygiene products**

Cosmetics and/or personal hygiene products are common sources of contact allergens. It is not unusual for contact allergy to these personal products to manifest at sites distant from the site of contact, a phenomenon that is termed "ectopic contact dermatitis." Although there are hundreds of chemicals contained within these products, a relatively small number of substances consistently cause ACD. These include fragrances, preservatives, base chemicals, adhesives, and sun blocks. For purposes of patch testing, these antigens can be obtained in specifically labeled packages from Trolab Laboratories.

1. **Fragrances** are one of the most common causes of ACD in the United States. Although "fragrance-free" products do not usually contain fragrance ingredients, those that are labeled "unscented" often have masking fragrances added. The "fragrance mix" that is frequently used for patch testing contains eight different fragrances and will detect approximately 85% of fragrance allergic individuals. The proper identification of the sensitizing fragrance that is responsible is essential to a meaningful program of avoidance. Unfortunately, because many manufacturers do not label the specific fragrance present in their products,

Table 8.12. Common causes of systemic contact dermatitis

Topical sensitizer	Source of systemic reaction
Ethylenediamine	Intravenous aminophylline Oral piperazine/ethanolamine antihistamines
Diphenhydramine	Oral, parenteral diphenhydramine
Sulfonamides, benzocaine	Oral para-amino sulfonamide-containing hypo-glycemic agents (tolbutamide, chlorpropamide)
Corticosteroids	Oral, parenteral, intraarticular corticosteroids
Nickel	Nickel in tap water, foods cooked in nickel utensils, canned foods

consumers usually eliminate the use of many more products than would otherwise be necessary.

2. **Preservatives** are present in most aqueous-based cosmetics and personal hygiene products and can be grouped into those that release formaldehyde and those that do not (Table 8.13). Individuals who are patch test positive to formaldehyde should avoid contact with all of the formaldehyde releasers.

3. **Base chemicals/excipients** are inert substances that make up the base of a product and serve to solubilize, sequester, thicken, foam, or lubricate the active component in a product. Commonly used excipients include propylene glycol, ethylenediamine, butylene glycol, polyethylene glycol, triethanolamine, and lanolin. These substances can cause ACD or when used in higher concentrations, can act as irritants.

4. **Hair care products** are very common causes contact allergy. In addition to routine hair care products, such as shampoos and conditioners, hair dyes and permanent solutions are commonly used products and may be sensitizing. The active ingredient in hair dye is paraphenylene diamine (PPD) and is the most common cause of ACD in hairdressers; glycerol thioglycolate is the active ingredient in permanent wave solution and may also be highly sensitizing.

5. **Nail cosmetics** (including nail polish, artificial nails, and attachment glue) have become increasingly popular and contain a number of sensitizing chemicals, including methacrylate ester monomers, dimethacrylates, and trimethacrylates, as well as cyanoacrylate-based glues. Clinical allergy to acrylics in nails can present locally at the distal digit or ectopically on the eyelids and face. Patch testing to a variety of acrylates and nail polish resin may be necessary to delineate the causative agent.

6. **Sunscreens** may be used by themselves and are also frequently present in cosmetics such as moisturizers, "night" creams, lip and hair preparations, and foundation makeup. As a group they are the most common cause of photoallergic contact dermatitis. "Chemical-free" sunblocks employ physical blocking agents instead of photoactive chemicals, and they include titanium dioxide and zinc oxide, which rarely result in sensitization.

V. **Treatment of contact dermatitis**

   A. **Avoidance.** The mainstay of treating contact dermatitis is discontinuation of contact with the offending agent. Thus, the identification and avoidance of the putative agent remains the key to resolving the problem. All other measures, including mechanical barriers and medications, are palliative and temporary. Once the offending agent has been identified, careful education needs to be provided regarding sources of the offending material and avoidance practices.

Table 8.13. Preservatives

Releasers of formaldehyde	Nonreleasers of formaldehyde
Diazolidinyl urea	Parabens
Imidazolindinyl urea	Methylchloroisothiazolinone
Quaternium-15	Methylisothiazolione
DMDM hydration	Methyldibromoglutaronitrile
Bromonitropropane	PCMX/PCMC
	Benzalkonium chloride
	Thimerosal

B. Topical antipruritics. After removal of the offending agent, topical therapy should be instituted promptly. Cool compresses are usually soothing and mildly antipruritic. The addition of aluminum subacetate, milk, or other agents (e.g., calamine, colloidal oatmeal) is of questionable value; topical diphenhydramine should be strictly avoided because of the risk of cutaneous sensitization. In chronic eruptions, emollients may be used but they should be nonsensitizing and fragrance-free. Soaps and nonalkaline cleansers should be avoided.

C. Topical corticosteroids are effective when the dermatitis is localized to less than 10% of the body surface area. Patients with contact sensitivity to preservatives can use preservative-free corticosteroids such as Synalar ointment, Aristocort ointment, or Diprosone ointment. Low-potency corticosteroids are recommended for areas of thinner skin (particularly the face and eyelids) and high-potency corticosteroids are indicated for chronically thickened and lichenified lesions in other locations. Ointments are generally more potent, more occlusive, and contain less sensitizing preservatives than creams and lotions.

D. Systemic corticosteroids should be reserved for severe, acute cases, such as extensive *rhus* dermatitis (poison ivy). Because ACD may persist for 2 to 4 weeks, oral steroids should be generally given for at least 10 days (prednisone 0.5 to 1.0 mg/kg/day). Intramuscular corticosteroids do not offer significant advantages over oral preparations and may cause more prolonged periods of hypothalamic–pituitary–adrenal (HPA) axis suppression as well as other unusual but potentially serious side effects (e.g., aseptic necrosis of the femoral head).

E. Oral antihistamines, while very effective for urticarial reactions, offer minimal relief from pruritis for ACD.

Selected Readings

Bardana EJ, Montanaro A. Occupational asthma and allergies. *Ann Allergy Asthma Immunol* 1999;83:6.

Belsito DV. The immunologic basis of patch testing. *J Am Acad Dermatol* 1989;21:823.

Beltrani, VS. Contact dermatitis: irritant and allergic. *Immunol Allergy Clin N Am* 1997;17:3.

Beltrani VS, Beltrani VP. Contact dermatitis. *Ann Allergy Asthma Immunol* 1997; 78:160.

Boguniewicz M, Leung DYM. Atopic dermatitis. In: Leung DYM, Greaves MW, eds. *Allergic skin disease: a multidisciplinary approach*, 1st ed. New York: Marcel Dekker, 2000:125.

Fisher's contact dermatitis, 3rd ed. Reischel RL, ed. Philadelphia: Lea & Febiger, 2000.

Hamann CP, Sullivan KM. Natural rubber latex hypersensitivity. In: Charlesworth EN, ed. *Cutaneous allergy*. Cambridge MA: Blackwell Science, 1997:155.

Hanifin JM. Tacrolimus ointment: Advancing the treatment of atopic dermatitis. *J Am Acad Dermatol* 2001;44:1.

Harper J, Green A, Scott G, et al. First experience of topical SDZ ASM 981 in children with atopic dermatitis. *Br J Dermatol* 2001;144:781.

Kalish RS. Recent developments in the pathogenesis of allergic contact dermatitis. *Arch Dermatol* 1991;127:1558.

Leung DYM. Atopic dermatitis: New insights and opportunities for therapeutic intervention. *J Allergy Clin Immunol* 2000;105:860.

Long CC, Mills CM, Finlay AY. A practical guide to topical therapy in children. *Br J Dermatol* 1998;138:293.

Marks JG, DeLeo VA. *Contact and occupational dermatology*, 2nd ed. St. Louis: Mosby Year Book, 2000.

Sampson HA. Utility of food-specific IgE concentrations in predicting symptomatic food allergy. *J Allergy Clin Immunol* 2001;107:891.

9. CHRONIC URTICARIA AND ANGIOEDEMA: BACKGROUND, EVALUATION, AND TREATMENT

Ernest N. Charlesworth

Urticaria and angioedema will affect at least 15% of the general population at some time during their life span, and this remains one of the most vexing cutaneous conditions to evaluate and treat. Patients frequently go from one physician to another in hopes of finding an extraordinary healthcare provider who will be able to identify the cause, eliminate the culprit, and exorcise them from this ailment. Physicians treating hives are equally frustrated as they ponder the utility of obtaining a panel of screening laboratory tests that have previously been shown to have a low yield, or obtaining selected allergy tests in a group of patients who are no more prone to allergic disease than the general public. This review will attempt to put urticaria into a perspective in which the physician can understand the pathophysiology of the disease and then apply understanding of the disease to the formulation of an intelligent evaluation and treatment plan. The past decade has witnessed a bonanza of new information and an enhanced understanding of urticaria. In this review, the new information is put into a clinical context which will better define what workup might be appropriate in this new millennium.

I. Anatomy and physiology of the skin: A background to understanding urticaria. Urticaria and angioedema are skin reactive patterns in which pruritic raised erythematous plaques develop over the body. The lesions may be fleeting, coming and going within minutes or hours, or they may linger in the same location for beyond 12 to 24 hours, as observed in some patients with urticarial vasculitis. Usually the lesions occur in a random pattern, but they may favor the dependent areas in urticarial vasculitis or sites of constrictive pressure on the skin if there is a dermatographic component. The head and neck areas have an increased number of skin mast cells per unit area compared to other areas of the skin, and sometimes the urticaria and the itching is more intense in these areas. Angioedema occurs in approximately 50% of patients with chronic urticaria and may be both disfiguring and may compromise vital structures including the airway. Both urticaria and angioedema are characterized by the presence of tissue edema, with superficial edema resulting in clinical urticaria and deeper edema resulting in angioedema of the pharynx, face, or gastrointestinal tract. The clinical lesions are not difficult to recognize by the trained health care provider and the real challenge lies in the treatment, the evaluation, and the search for a potential cause. In fact, chronic urticaria is so frustrating for patients that they frequently go from one physician to another in hope of finding that extraordinary physician who will be able to identify the cause, eliminate the culprit, and cure their disease. Physicians treating urticaria are equally frustrated as they weigh the utility of obtaining a panel of screening laboratory tests that have previously been shown to have a low yield or consider an elimination diet with equally disappointing results. Therapy for chronic urticaria is frequently less than optimal and often leaves both the patient and the physician wondering whether the underlying cause was somehow overlooked.

It becomes critically important to understand that urticaria is a clinical reactive pattern and not simply a "disease," much like a fever is a symptom rather than being a disease. In this setting, it is important for the clinician to better understand the pathophysiology of the disease from the "inside out."

Mast cells play an important role in the immediate hypersensitivity reaction and they play a sentinel role with the pathogenesis of urticaria and angioedema. In allergic disease, mast cells are activated by the cross-linking of high-affinity immunoglobulin E (IgE) receptors on mast cells found in various tissues and on basophils found circulating in the peripheral blood. This activation of mast cells through the high-affinity IgE receptor results in the immediate release of histamine from the cell, which results in the development of a localized urticarial wheal and angioedema of the deeper tissues. The activation of the mast cell through the high-affinity IgE receptor ultimately results in the influx of myriad inflammatory cells including eosinophils, neutrophils, lymphocytes, and basophils several hours after mast cell activation. This "late" inflammatory event is observed in allergic rhinitis and asthma, and has been referred to as the late-phase response (LPR). This may be important in a recently characterized type of urticaria in which the high-affinity IgE receptors are activated by IgG autoantibodies directed against the high-affinity IgE receptors on mast cells and basophils. In these patients, the mature clinical urticarial lesions may persist for several hours, showing a polymorphic infiltrate on biopsy, which is quite similar to the histopathology observed in the skin during the LPR to antigen. Recent studies have suggested that this type of urticaria may account for as much as 40% of chronic urticaria, which has previously been classified as simply idiopathic. It is these patients who may also present the most challenge therapeutically because they may not respond to simple antihistamines.

Mast cells can also be activated without involving the IgE receptor. Direct mast cell releasers are capable of releasing preformed histamine, resulting in urticaria without the precipitation of an inflammatory response. For example, it is well known that codeine will activate the skin mast cell to release histamine without a resultant inflammatory cell infiltrate. Indeed, several studies have shown that mast cells in patients with chronic urticaria have an increased releasability to such substances as codeine, morphine, substance P, and compound 48/80. Although all individuals will develop a wheal and flare when skin tested with the above compounds, patients with chronic urticaria will develop significantly larger wheals and flares than individuals without urticaria. In this subpopulation of urticaria patients, the release of histamine from the cutaneous mast cell is the predominant trigger for urticaria.

Although the peripheral blood basophil also contains histamine, it appears that the mast cell is the usual source of the histamine in most patients with urticaria. A possible exception to this may be the patient who produces IgG autoantibodies directed against the high-affinity IgE receptors on both mast cells and basophils. In fact, there are data to suggest many patients with chronic urticaria may actually have a decreased releasability of histamine from their basophils. The fact that the mast cell, not the basophil, is the source of spontaneously released histamine in many patients with urticaria is further corroborated by the increase in tryptase levels in suction blister fluid from urticaria patients, because tryptase is a marker of the mast cell and not the basophil. The role of the mast cell becomes somewhat more complicated as we recognize that there is also a degree of mast cell heterogeneity, depending on the tissue from which the mast cells are obtained. For example, it has been noted that many noncytotoxic agents such as compound 48/80 cause the release of histamine only in the skin mast cell and not in mast cells located in the gut or the respiratory tree. The role of neuropeptides in causing the skin mast cell to release histamine is not totally clear. It may be that the microenvironment of the skin mast cell in patients uniquely enhances the liberation of cytokines, chemokines, and histamine releasing factors that then lower the "release threshold" for the cutaneous mast cell, resulting in an urticarial lesion. In addition to the role played by histamine in the pathogenesis of urticaria, it is conceivable that other mediators, such as leukotrienes, may also play a role.

II. Acute urticaria
  A. Definition and epidemiology
    By definition, acute urticaria has been present for less than 6 weeks. One is much more likely to identify a cause for acute urticaria than in the individual who has had urticaria persisting for months or years. Usually, acute urticaria is more likely to occur in a younger population and the causes may range from a medication to an infection (see Table 9.1). Acute urticaria occurs in as many as 15% to 24% of the U.S. population through-

Table 9.1. Causes of acute urticaria

Drug allergy
Food allergy
Insect sting allergy
Latex allergy
Contactants (e.g., animals)
Infection
   Viral
   Mycoplasma
   Bacterial
   Fungal
   Parasitic
Physical urticarias

out the course of their lifetime. The lesions are intensely pruritic and may be accompanied by angioedema in as many as 50% of the patients. When angioedema involves the upper respiratory tract, life-threatening obstruction of the laryngeal airway may occur, requiring emergency treatment.

B. Causes

The key to determining a potential cause for acute urticaria lies in a detailed medical history and physical examination. The medical history should focus on an exploration of recent medications, including herbal supplements and over-the-counter preparations. One should remember that many of the herbs and supplements are not considered to be "medications" by the patient and the medical questioning should be directed to these agents.

1. Foods

Although foods are an uncommon cause for chronic urticaria, foods should be explored as a possible cause, especially in acute urticaria. The most common foods associated with urticaria are nuts, milk, eggs, and fish. In this regard, one should try to establish a temporal relationship between the suspected food and the onset of the urticaria. Usually, if a food is the culprit cause of urticaria then the urticarial eruption will occur within 90 minutes of ingestion of the food, and certainly not the following day. This temporal association should be reproducible upon reexposure to the suspect food. Far more can be learned from a detailed medical history than from a series of skin or blood radioallergosorbent tests (RASTs) for IgE antibodies directed against various foods. The random screening for food allergies has the potential to add both expense and confusion to the evaluation.

2. Infections are a potential cause of urticaria and may occur as part of a viral prodrome. The urticaria may occur after the clinical infection has resolved, as part of a lingering immune-complex disorder. Localized bacterial infections in the sinuses, the lungs, the prostate, and even dental abscesses have been associated with acute urticaria. If the travel history suggests a possible exposure to parasites, then this should also be explored as a possible cause.

3. Autoimmune, lymphoproliferative, and endocrine disorders may also be associated with acute urticaria, although they are more likely associated with chronic urticaria.

4. Many patients with acute urticaria will also have a component of physical urticaria and relate an intensification of lesions at sites of constriction from garments. Some may relate an increase with heat exposure, cold exposure, or even an accentuation of the urticaria during the premenstrual time in some women.

5. Papular urticaria are localized pruritic papules secondary to insect bites. Some individuals have sensitivity to insect bites that leaves them with a localized urticarial wheal that is intensely pruritic and may remain for several days.

6. One must be cognizant that an allergic contact dermatitis may present with an urticarial-type lesion and may cause rather intense swelling of the eyes, which may be misdiagnosed as angioedema when it is secondary to an allergy to rhus found in poison ivy, poison oak, and poison sumac.

C. The physical examination should be a complete multisystem examination. Examination of the thyroid may help delineate an autoimmune thyroid disorder or a hormonal dysregulation. The lymphatic examination should include palpation of the liver and the spleen to rule out a lymphoma. Other areas of focus should include the joints, central nervous system, and the skin. The character of the cutaneous lesions should be noted, keeping in mind that urticarial vasculitis may present with lesions lasting longer than 12 to 24 hours and may burn and sting in addition to itching. Urticarial vasculitis may also have petechiae within and surrounding the urticarial lesions. The skin should be stroked as part of the physical examination to document a dermatographic component to the urticaria. In summary, the medical history may give certain clues to the etiology of the urticaria, and the physical examination may offer the opportunity to further define and characterize the urticaria.

III. Chronic urticaria

By definition, chronic urticaria is hives that have been present for longer than 6 weeks. There appears to be an inverse relationship between the length of time that the patients have had the urticaria and the probability of finding a specific trigger or cause for the urticaria. Much like acute urticaria, the lesions of chronic urticaria can occur almost anywhere on the skin including the scalp, palms, and soles. At least 50% of the patients may also have angioedema representing deeper involvement with edema of the soft tissues. The angioedema may result in alarming distortions of the lips and eyes and may result in compromise of the oropharynx. In should be noted that angioedema without urticaria is usually a distinct entity and will be discussed separately.

Chronic urticaria is more common in adults than it is in children. The course of chronic urticaria is variable, but 20% of patients will continue to have hives for 10 years or longer. As alluded to in the introduction, the skin mast cell is the primary cell that releases histamine into the surrounding dermal tissue, and this results in clinical urticaria. The causes and triggers for chronic urticaria are outlined in Table 9.2. As much as 80% of chronic urticaria is idiopathic, without a definable cause. Over 15 years ago, Grattan and his associates reported the presence of a serum factor that caused whealing on intradermal injection of autologous serum. This reaction to autologous serum was observed in approximately 40% of the patients with idiopathic urticaria. Subsequently, Greaves and his group in Great Britain identified this factor as an IgG antibody directed against the alpha chain of the high-affinity IgE receptor found on mast cells and basophils. Notably, this serum factor appears to have a greater affinity for the skin mast cells and does not usually provoke histamine release from mast cells found in the lung or gastrointestinal tract. This autoimmune paradigm of chronic urticaria is not surprising because it has been known for several years that there is an increased incidence of antithyroid antibodies in patients with chronic urticaria.

IV. Differential diagnosis of urticaria

It is sometimes helpful to approach urticaria as a symptom rather than a disease entity. Urticaria may vary clinically from a few fleeting urticaria wheals to large polycyclic annular plaques. Fixed urticarial plaques are characteristic of urticarial vasculitis and may be more pronounced on the dependent portions of the body. It should not be surprising that there are several dermatological disorders that may have urticarial lesions as part of their clinical presentation. Any

Table 9.2. Causes of chronic urticaria

Autoimmune
  IgG autoantibody directed against the high-affinity IgE receptor
    Mast cells
    Basophils
  Anti-IgE antibody
  Anti-thyroid antibody
Physical urticaria
  Cold urticaria
    Acquired
    Familial
  Aquagenic urticaria
  Cholinergic urticaria
  Solar urticaria
  Vibratory urticaria
  Delayed pressure urticaria
Chronic infection
  Dental abscess
  Chronic sinusitis
  Chronic parasitic infestation
Idiopathic

IgE, immunoglobulin E, IgG, immunoglobulin G.

disease that causes release of histamine into the skin may have an urticarial component with dermal edema (Table 9.3).

A. The spectrum of erythema multiforme frequently includes urticaria-like lesions, and conversely, urticaria may have polycyclic lesions with a "targatoid" appearance suggestive of erythema multiforme. Individual lesions of erythema multiforme usually last longer than the typical fleeting lesions of ordinary urticaria, and the lesions of erythema multiforme are more acrally distributed than usual urticaria. As the name implies, erythema multiforme is a cutaneous disease spectrum ranging from urticarial lesions to overt bullous lesions, and a skin biopsy may of help in establishing a diagnosis.

Table 9.3. Differential diagnosis of urticaria

Urticarial vasculitis
  Lesions persist beyond 24 h
  Purpuric component with residual hyperpigmentation
  Extracutaneous symptoms
    Arthralgia/arthritis
    Gastrointestinal symptoms
    Respiratory symptoms
Urticaria-like lesions
  Erythema multiforme
  Bullous pemphigoid
  Dermatitis herpetiformis
  Pruritic urticarial plaques and papules of pregnancy
  Schnitzler syndrome
    Urticaria
    Monoclonal gammopathy
  Papular urticaria

B. Bullous pemphigoid is an autoimmune blistering eruption in which immune complexes are directed toward an antigen located at the dermoepidermal junction, resulting in a generalized bullous eruption. In bullous pemphigoid, early lesions are frequently pruritic and may have a clear urticarial component. In patients with bullous pemphigoid in whom the disease is limited, it is possible that the urticarial plaque might not blister. In such a situation, a skin biopsy of perilesional skin for immunofluorescent staining should be diagnostic by demonstrating a deposition of IgG and complement along the dermoepidermal junction.

C. Dermatitis herpetiformis is another autoimmune vesiculobullous disorder in which the early lesions have a clear urticarial component. This disorder is markedly pruritic and the lesions usually appear on the elbows, knees, buttocks, shoulders, and sacral areas. These lesions frequently have an early urticarial appearance; however, they could also be easily confused with papular urticaria, cholinergic urticaria, or even scabies.

D. Hypersensitivity vasculitis may present with urticarial lesions that have the potential to be misdiagnosed as routine urticaria unless the clinician has a high index of suspicion and is willing to do a skin biopsy. The lesions of urticarial vasculitis tend to remain beyond the usual transient time period observed with ordinary urticaria. The clinical clues that should prompt the clinician to consider urticarial vasculitis are as follows.

  1. Lesions lasting longer than 24 hours.

  2. Lesions that are more prominent on the lower extremity than on the trunk or arms.

  3. Lesions that have a purpuric component.

  4. Lesions that leave a stippling of hemosiderin pigment in the wake of their healing.

  5. Lesions that are associated with constitutional symptoms such as arthralgia/arthritis, gastrointestinal complaints, low-grade fever, or respiratory complaints.

  Urticarial vasculitis may be confined to the skin or it may affect the synovia, kidneys, gastrointestinal tract, eyes, respiratory tract, or the central nervous system. The clinical spectrum of urticarial vasculitis may range from a relatively banal syndrome associated with mild constitutional symptoms to patients who have clear-cut systemic lupus erythematous with vasculitis.

E. Urticaria pigmentosa is a cutaneous disorder characterized by the proliferation of mast cells in the skin and other organs. Unlike the above-mentioned disorders, the lesions of urticaria pigmentosa are easily distinguishable from urticaria by their papular hyperpigmented character. The Darier sign is a characteristic diagnostic sign in which the individual lesions of urticaria pigmentosa form a linear wheal when the overlying skin is stroked. A skin biopsy, stained with a metachromatic stain such as alcian blue or Giemsa, will demonstrate abnormal collections of mast cells in the dermis, confirming the diagnosis.

  The above disorders are not frequently confused with urticaria but, nevertheless, one must consider urticaria as a clinical spectrum in which many other cutaneous disorders may have an urticarial component.

V. Physical urticarias

Physical urticarias are distinct urticarial eruptions triggered by a physical culprit which may range from temperature to physical pressure on the skin, or even to exposure to certain wavelengths of sunlight. Physical agents are responsible for 10% to 20% of all chronic urticaria reactions. Physical factors may aggravate idiopathic urticaria and urticaria from other causes, or the physical factors may be the primary disease pathology.

A. Dermatographism is the development of an urticarial wheal at the site of physical pressure on the skin from constricting clothes or from scratching the skin. This is probably the most common type of urticaria and affects between 4% and 5% of the general population. This type of urticaria is clearly secondary to the release of histamine from skin mast cells. Patients with symptomatic dermatographism respond well to regular dosing with a nonsedating, second-generation H1-antihistamine.

B. Delayed pressure urticaria (DPU) is a unique physical urticaria in which soft tissue swelling occurs several hours after prolonged pressure on the skin, such as on the feet or after carrying a handbag. The mean age is 33 years, although there is a broad range, and this disorder has the potential to interfere with daily activity and even impair one's ability to earn a living. Coexistent idiopathic urticaria occurs in 25% to 35% of patients.

DPU is unique and the dermal histology shows an inflammatory infiltrate of neutrophils and eosinophils, which suggests that this might represent more than simply skin mast cell histamine release. There may be an associated low-grade fever and malaise, and some investigators have shown an elevation in interleukin 6 (IL-6). The diagnosis can be established by suspending a 15-lb weight over the patient's shoulder for 15 minutes. A positive response is defined as erythema, edema, and tenderness at the site at least 2 hours after the challenge. The real challenge, however, is the treatment of DPU. Avoidance is not always feasible and antihistamines have not been shown to be uniformly helpful. Nonsteroidal antiinflammatory agents (such as aspirin, indomethacin, and ibuprofen) may be effective treatment for some patients with DPU, whereas they have been associated with triggering urticaria in other patients. In unusual cases, systemic corticosteroids may be required, although the potential for long-term side effects always looms as a possibility.

C. Vibratory angioedema is soft tissue swelling induced by vibration. This may be a problem in certain occupations such as manual laborers, carpenters, and metal grinders. Avoidance remains the primary modality of treatment and antihistamines may offer some degree of protection.

D. Cholinergic urticaria is the development of small urticarial wheals surrounded by a rather large macular erythema. Cholinergic urticaria results from physical activity, increased temperature (i.e., passive heating), and emotional stimuli. It is associated with intense pruritus and clearly is related to the release of histamine into the surrounding dermal tissues. Like many of the physical urticarias, daily nonsedating antihistamines can be quite effective in the control of cholinergic urticaria symptoms.

E. Solar urticaria is the presence of urticaria in sun-exposed areas that usually occurs within minutes following exposure to sunlight. This is probably a heterogeneous group of related disorders and may vary according to the specific spectrum of sun exposure that acts as the trigger (ultraviolet A [UVA], UVB, UVC, or the visible spectrum). One type may be secondary to IgE antibodies to a photoallergen (type I) and others may be secondary to a connective tissue disease or even erythropoietic protoporphyria (type VI). The history and physical examination is important to rule out a phototoxic drug reaction, a photoallergic drug reaction, or a connective tissue disease.

F. Aquagenic urticaria is the development of pinpoint hives precipitated by contact with water. The lesions may occur with bathing or showering and it usually occurs during the third decade of life. Usually, regular treatment with a nonsedating antihistamine will afford good relief of symptoms.

G. Cold urticaria (CU) syndromes are characterized by the development of urticaria or angioedema following exposure to cold. Although these conditions are generally considered to be benign, there are several instances reported of shock-like reactions during aquatic activities. Primary CU is usually acquired, although there is a rare familial form. It is important to remember that systemic disorders should be considered as potential causes for secondary CU, including cryoglobulinemia, mycoplasma infection, infectious mononucleosis, or vasculitis. It is interesting that the lesions of CU occur only following rewarming of the skin and one can easily test by using an ice-cube test on the forearm. The laboratory evaluation may include the following: complete blood cell count (CBC), erythrocyte sedimentation rate

(ESR), antinuclear antibody (ANA), heterophile agglutination, serologic test for syphilis (STS), RA latex, total complement, cold agglutinin, cold hemolysin, cryofibrinogen, and cryoglobulin.

VI. Evaluation of the urticaria patient

   A. In both acute urticaria and chronic urticaria, the most important part of the evaluation is the history and physical examination. It is sometimes helpful to evaluate patients based on broad categories of mechanisms (Table 9.4). IgE-dependent mechanisms would include drug allergies, food allergies, insect venom, and latex allergy. Complement-mediated mechanisms would include hereditary angioedema (HAE), serum sickness, and urticarial vasculitis. Physical causes would include dermatographism, cold-induced urticaria, heat-induced urticaria, cholinergic urticaria, delayed pressure urticaria, solar urticaria, and vibratory urticaria. Miscellaneous mechanisms would include autoimmune urticaria, hormonal dysfunction, malignancy, psychological stressors, and occupational exposures.

   B. The laboratory evaluation should be directed by the history and physical examination. Screening studies to be considered might include a CBC, ESR, urinalysis, and liver function tests. In the case of autoimmune urticaria secondary to the formation of IgG autoantibodies to the high-affinity IgE receptors, one might consider doing an intradermal skin test to autologous serum. This is done by injecting 0.05 mL of the patient's serum into their forearm with appropriate intradermal saline controls. More specific laboratory tests should be selective and based on diagnostic suspicions, such as a latex RAST for IgE in a clinical laboratory worker who develops urticaria and rhinitis that appears to be work related. If the ESR is elevated and if there is a history suggestive of an inflammatory arthritis, one may wish to obtain an ANA. In an older patient with weight loss and lymphadenopathy, one may wish to rule out a lymphoma or a monoclonal gammopathy. If there is a history of foreign travel to a third-world country, one may wish to obtain a stool specimen for ova and parasites. Beyond the history, physical examination, and a very basic laboratory screen, the evaluation of urticaria con-

Table 9.4. Evaluation of the urticaria patient

Medical history
Physical examination
Laboratory
   CBC
   ESR
   Urinalysis
   Liver function test
   Other
      Directed by history and physical examination
Skin Testing or Blood RAST
   Foods
      Based on history and physical examination
      Rare in adults
   Inhalant allergens and animals
      Based on history and physical examination
      Unusual cause for chronic urticaria
Skin testing to autologous serum
   40% of chronic urticaria patients
   Intradermal testing
   Read at 30 min

CBC, Complete blood cell count; ESR, erythrocyte sedimentation rate; RAST, radioallergosorbent test.

sists of a thoughtful follow-through on the clues obtained during the initial assessment of the patient.

C. A skin biopsy may be helpful as part of the evaluation of chronic urticaria. This is particularly helpful in patients in whom the lesions may linger at the same skin site for longer than 24 hours. In such a case, a skin biopsy may help to establish the diagnosis of urticarial vasculitis.

VII. Treatment of urticaria

A. Avoidance

The first priority in the treatment of urticaria is the elimination of the causative agent, stimulus or antigen. This is much easier said than done. Indeed, the routine management of autoimmune and nonautoimmune chronic urticaria is similar. Foods are often considered a cause for urticaria, but are rarely proven to contribute to chronic idiopathic urticaria. A careful history may give a clue to a food being a culprit in urticaria in children, and in such an instance an elimination diet can be helpful. When precipitating factors (such as hot baths or the ingestion of alcohol) are identified, they should be avoided.

B. Antihistamines

For the majority of chronic urticaria patients, symptomatic treatment with H1 antihistamines will remain the mainstay of management for their disease. The success of the classic antihistamines is somewhat limited by undesirable side effects such as daytime sedation and anticholinergic-induced dry mouth. Because it is well documented that the skin mast cell is triggered by various stimuli to release preformed mediators, such as histamine and tryptase, it is only logical that antihistamines function best when taken as a prophylactic medication rather than just at the time of flare of the urticaria.

The newer nonsedating or low-sedating antihistamines offer considerable benefit over the older sedating antihistamines (Table 9.5). Classical sedating antihistamines have the potential not only to promote sedation, but also to interfere with central nervous system reflex reaction times and globally suppress the central nervous system, comparable to the suppressive effects of alcohol. Other side effects that may be seen with traditional H1-antihistamines

Table 9.5. Management of urticaria and angioedema

Elimination of causative agents

Avoidance of precipitating stimuli

Antihistamines
  Classical/sedating
    Impair performance
    Anticholinergic side effects
  Second generation
    Loratadine 10 mg q.d.
    Cetirizine 10 mg q.d.
      Dose-related drowsiness
      May decrease eosinophils in skin
    Fexofenadine 60–180 mg q.d.
  Tricyclic antidepressants
  H2-antagonists (only in combination with H1-antagonists)

Antileukotrienes (experimental)

Corticosteroids
  Use with caution
  Significant side effects with long-term use

Experimental therapies

---

include dizziness, altered coordination, blurred vision, diplopia, and paradoxical symptoms of the central nervous system stimulation. All of these side effects are more common in young children and elderly patients. Seizure activity may be induced in patients with a propensity for seizures because these drugs readily cross the blood–brain barrier and bind with high affinity to H1-receptors in the brain and lower the seizure threshold. Anticholinergic effects such as dryness of mucous membranes, urinary retention, palpitations, agitation, and increased intraocular pressure are caused by the atropine-like antagonistic action of antihistamines on the muscarinic acetylcholine receptors. Lastly, the safety of the classical antihistamine in pregnancy has not been established because they cross the placental membrane with great proclivity. In the Collaborative Perinatal Project, an epidemiological investigation of possible teratogenic effects on pregnancy, brompheniramine was found to have an increased relative risk of birth defects. Therefore, most of the classical H1-antihistamines are classified as U.S. Food and Drug Administration (FDA) pregnancy category C, and should be used during pregnancy only if the expected benefits to the mother exceed the unknown risks to the fetus.

In 1985, terfenadine was approved for use in the United States as the first nonsedating H1-antihistamine. This drug enjoyed a reduced side effect profile *vis a vis* the classical antihistamines, and terfenadine quickly became the most commonly prescribed H1-antihistamine in this country. Because this drug was subsequently shown to be associated with a polymorphic ventricular tachycardia with prolongation of the QT interval (torsade de pointes), it was withdrawn from the market. For similar reasons, astemizole was removed from the market several years later. The remaining nonsedating antihistamines do not pose the same risks because they do not bind to K^+ channels in the heart. These newer antihistamines remain the first-line treatment for urticaria.

Because the newer antihistamines do not have the plethora of side effects observed with the classical antihistamines, they can be used in much higher doses (excluding those metabolized by the p450 34A hepatic enzymes). I favor the use of fexofenadine 180 mg or loratadine 10 mg in the morning and cetirizine 10 mg in the evening to control chronic urticaria in which an identifiable cause cannot be eliminated. Both the patient and the physician should have clear-cut therapeutic goals defined and the absolute elimination of all urticarial lesions may not be an achievable goal. For this reason, I try to define my goal as a degree of controlling itching, which allows the patient to work and live in relative comfort, despite the annoyance of an occasional urticarial lesion.

Fexofenadine is a nonsedating, long-acting drug that is highly selective for blocking peripheral histamine H1-receptors and may have some antiinflammatory effects *in vitro*. In one large multicenter study of 439 moderately severe urticaria patients, fexofenadine was shown to be effective over placebo in doses ranging from 60 to 240 mg, with little side effects. Likewise, loratadine at a dose of 10 mg per day has been shown to be more effective than placebo, and was similar in efficacy to hydroxyzine but without the side effects. Cetirizine is an active metabolite of hydroxyzine and does not require metabolic transformation. In studies by Charlesworth and others, cetirizine may result in a decrease in the influx of eosinophils at the site of the allergic reaction. This antiinflammatory effect may have an advantage in the treatment of the autoimmune type of urticaria, although this effect was observed with higher doses of 20 mg, which may result in some sedation.

C. Tricyclics

Nighttime control of urticarial itching can sometimes be enhanced by adding a tricyclic antihistamine such as doxepin in doses ranging from 10 to 50 mg, depending on the patient's tolerance of side effects. Doxepin has both H1- and H2-antihistamine receptor blocking effects and may have a therapeutic effect on anxiety and depression, both of which have the potential to aggravate the urticaria. Nevertheless, great caution should be used when treating older patients because of the soporific side effects and the increased risk for potentially hazardous falls.

D. H2-Antihistamines

The use of H2-antihistamines is controversial but some authorities feel that they offer some benefit. Certainly, cutaneous blood vessels possess H2-receptors and the specific blockade of these receptors in conjunction with H1-antagonists is more effective in the suppression of experimental histamine-induced whealing than H1-receptor antagonists alone. There are some controlled studies that suggest benefit by adding H2-antihistamines, and there are other studies that suggest there is no added benefit. Certainly, the benefit from adding an H2-antihistamine to an H1-antihistamine is small, but this may offer some benefit in selected patients.

E. Leukotriene modifiers

There are several anecdotal reports that leukotriene antagonists may have some benefit in selected patients with chronic idiopathic urticaria. To date, there are no double-blinded control studies using leukotriene receptor antagonists in the treatment of urticaria, and it is difficult to speculate on their place in the treatment. Because the eosinophil may play a role in some patients with urticaria, and leukotrienes are the major product of arachidonic acid metabolism in eosinophils, leukotriene antagonists may offer some clinical benefit. Furthermore, leukotrienes are released by other cells involved in the pathophysiology of urticaria and have been shown to be increased in blood samples during physical urticaria provocation testing.

F. Corticosteroids

Great caution should be exercised with the use of systemic corticosteroids in the long-term management of urticaria. Twenty percent of patients with chronic idiopathic urticaria will continue to have urticaria for more than 10 years and the long-term side effects of systemic corticosteroids may far outweigh the short-term benefit. In extraordinary circumstances, short-term use of corticosteroids may achieve some degree of control in order to allow the patient to attend an important social event "hive free." Far too often, the patient presses the physician to prescribe systemic corticosteroids or goes to the emergency department where they are given a "steroid shot" and then sent home. The patient realizes the short-term benefit but he or she is blinded to the potential long-term side effects. Ultimately, the physician has the responsibility to limit the use systemic steroids in chronic urticaria to very specific and narrow indications.

Urticarial vasculitis is unique among the urticarial syndromes and may not respond to antihistamines. Some of these patients may require a brief course of corticosteroids to control intermittent exacerbations of cutaneous or extracutaneous disease.

G. Various antiinflammatory therapies

A variety of alternatives to corticosteroids have been used in efforts to avoid corticosteroids, including indomethacin, colchicines, dapsone, and hydroxychloroquine. Although these drugs are generally considered to have fewer side effects than corticosteroids, each drug does have its own adverse risks and the therapeutic effectiveness may be inconsistent. In the severely affected patient with the autoimmune type of urticaria, cyclosporine has been shown to be effective, but one should be familiar with the potential for renal side effects and the development of hypertension. Other options for the autoimmune type of urticaria include intravenous gamma globulin infusion and plasmapheresis.

H. In summary, the treatment of urticaria can be quite challenging. The physician should set clear and realistic goals for the patient, and these goals may not include the complete abatement of the urticaria. The therapeutic goal should include diminishing the itching to the point where the patient can work and function socially with a minimal of inconvenience. The newer nonsedating antihistamines offer considerable benefit over the classical antihistamines without the central nervous system risks posed by the classical antihistamines, and are preferred.

VIII. Hereditary angioedema

HAE is an autosomal-dominant disorder caused by the absence of functional C1 esterase inhibitor. HAE is characterized by recurrent episodes of angioedema (without urticaria) precipitated spontaneously and variably after trauma. Multiple parts of the body may be involved, including and especially the face, extremities, and gastrointestinal tract. Edema of the bowel wall may result in crampy abdominal pain, constipation, vomiting, and abdominal rigidity. The most severe complication is laryngeal edema, which may result in asphyxiation and death.

Most cases of HAE manifest in childhood, but often worsen during adolescence. Because of the genetics of the disorder, a family history is positive in approximately 80% of patients. The severity and frequency of attacks vary greatly among patients. Only minor trauma is necessary to induce an attack, with common triggers including contact sports and dental work. Sometimes, an erythematous rash (erythema marginatum) may accompany attacks.

The diagnosis of HAE is made by examining patients' history and by evaluating complement levels. Patient will have low C4, C2, and antigenic or functional C1 esterase inhibitor levels. Patients with acquired forms of angioedema associated with C1 esterase inhibitor have decreased levels of C1. This is not the case in HAE.

Usually, patients with HAE respond to prophylactic therapy with androgens. This results in an increase in the levels of C1 esterase inhibitor. Patients taking chronic androgen therapy need to be observed for potential side effects.

Suggested Readings

Charlesworth EN. Urticaria and angioedema: a clinical spectrum. *Ann Allergy Asthma Immunol* 1997:76:484–493.

Charlesworth EN. The spectrum of urticaria. *Immunol Allergy Clin North Am* 1995; 15:641–657.

Cicardi M, Agostoni A. Hereditary angioedema. *N Eng J Med* 1996;334 1630–1624.

Grattan CEH, Wallington TB, Warin RP. A serological mediator in chronic idiopathic urticaria: a clinical immunological and histological evaluation. *Br J Dermatol* 1986; 114:583–590.

Greaves M. Chronic urticaria. *J Allergy Clin Immunol* 2000;105:644–672.

Hide M, Francis DM, Grattan CE, et al. Autoantibodies against the high affinity IgE receptor as a cause for histamine release in chronic urticaria. *N Engl J Med* 1993; 328:1599–1604.

Kennard CD. Evaluation and treatment of urticaria. *Immunol Allergy Clin North Am* 1995;15:785–801.

Wanderer AA, Bernstein IL, Goodman DL, et al. The diagnosis and management of urticaria: a practice parameter. Part I: Acute urticaria/angioedema. Part II: chronic urticaria/angioedema. *Ann Allergy Asthma Immunol* 2000;85:521–544.

10. ANAPHYLAXIS

Paul A. Greenberger

Systemic allergic reactions may occur to a wide variety of substances that are encountered in daily life. These reactions may occur rapidly without any prior warning and represent the most serious of medical emergencies. Despite recent advances in our understanding of allergic pathophysiology, the acute treatment has remained largely the same for many years.

Anaphylaxis is defined as an immediate generalized reaction that is mediated by the interaction of antigen with tissue-bound immunoglobulin E (IgE). Subsequent mediator release gives rise to a number of systemic manifestations including cutaneous, respiratory, cardiovascular, and gastrointestinal signs and symptoms. Anaphylactoid reactions may be clinically indistinguishable, but do not involve the participation of antigen-specific IgE. For the purposes of the foregoing discussion, the term anaphylaxis shall be used to denote a clinical syndrome with a variety of inciting etiologic agents and pathogenetic mechanisms.

I. Pathophysiology of generalized reactions
   A. Mechanisms
      A number of possible mechanisms enable exogenous agents to trigger immediate generalized reactions (Table 10.1).
      1. **Immunoglobulin E-mediated processes.** For many of the agents noted in this chapter, including antibiotics, foreign proteins, and foods, an IgE-mediated process has been defined or is likely. Notably, because immunologic sensitization must occur, reactions do not occur with first exposures. IgE antibodies may react directly with the foreign protein (e.g., insect venoms) or may bind to a hapten that is bound covalently to a carrier protein (e.g., penicillin major and minor determinants).
      2. **Complement system activation.** Reactions to blood and blood products are presumed to be associated with immune complex formation and subsequent complement activation. These reactions have been best defined in patients possessing IgG antibodies to IgA. These antibodies occur in approximately one-half of individuals lacking IgA (1 in 300 to 1 in 500 in general population), in individuals who have been transfused with blood products on multiple occasions, and rarely in otherwise normal individuals. The complexes of host IgG and donor IgA are thought to activate complement, generating anaphylatoxins C3a and C5a, which trigger histamine release.
      3. **Direct mast cell degranulation.** Commonly used medications that directly induce mast cell activation and degranulation include opiates and a variety of muscle relaxants. Systemic reactions may occur on the first exposure to such agents, because prior sensitization is not required.
      4. **Abnormalities of arachidonic acid metabolism.** Systemic reactions to aspirin and nonsteroidal antiinflammatory drugs (NSAIDs) may occur in as many as 1% of the population. The ability of aspirin and nonselective NSAIDs to induce anaphylaxis appears to be related to their potency in inhibiting prostaglandin synthesis. Approximately 10% of asthmatics develop bronchoconstriction after taking aspirin or nonselective NSAIDs. The reactions usually occur within 180 minutes of ingestion and are often associated with profuse rhinorrhea and flushing.
      5. **Unknown.** No precise mechanisms have been invoked to explain idiopathic or exercise-induced anaphylaxis.
   B. Mediators
      A large number of mediators have been identified in the urine and blood of persons experiencing anaphylactic reactions.

Table 10.1. Frequently reported causes of immediate generalized reactions

Causative agent	Mechanism
Foods	IgE mediated
Nuts	
Legumes (peanuts)	
Shellfish	
Egg whites	
Milk	
Pistachios, cashews	
Seeds (mustard)	
Insect venoms	IgE mediated
Wasps	
Hornets	
Honey bees	
Yellow jackets	
Fire ants	
Proteins or peptides	
Streptokinase	IgE mediated
Insulin	IgE mediated
Seminal plasma	Some IgE mediated
Allergen immunotherapy vaccines	IgE mediated
Latex	IgE mediated
Muscle relaxants	Mast cell activation (some IgE mediated)
Antibiotics	
Penicillins	IgE mediated
Cephalosporins	IgE mediated
Sulfamethoxazole	Some IgE mediated
Trimethoprim	Some IgE mediated
Fluoroquinolones	Unknown
Vancomycin	Mast cell activation
Diagnostic agents	
Radiocontrast media	Unknown
Gadolinium	Unknown
Fluorescein dye	Unknown
Procedure related	
Dialyzer membranes	Complements activation
Plasma (including platelet infusions)	Complement activation (some IgE mediated)
Intravenous immunoglobulin	Complement activation, IgG or IgE mediated
Miscellaneous	
Monoclonal or chimeric antibody	Likely IgE mediated
Aspirin, nonselective NSAIDs	Leukotriene D_4 production; suppression of prostaglandin E; mast cell activation
Angiotensin-converting enzyme inhibitors	Bradykinin potentiation
Exercise-induced anaphylaxis	Unknown
Exercise plus food-induced anaphylaxis	Unknown
Idiopathic anaphylaxis	Unknown

IgE, immunoglobulin E; NSAIDs, nonsteroidal antiinflammatory drugs.

1. **Histamine** is an important mast-cell-derived mediator that is released in large quantities during anaphylaxis. It promotes increases in vascular permeability, bronchial smooth muscle constriction, mucus secretion, and vascular smooth muscle relaxation. Although the first three effects are mediated primarily via the H1-histamine receptor, the vascular effects are promoted by both H1- and H2-receptors.

2. **Other mediators.** A number of other mediators have been postulated to participate in anaphylaxis. Although there is plentiful *in vitro* and animal model evidence to support their roles during systemic allergic reactions, data are generally lacking in humans. Some of these potentially important substances include: sulfidopeptide leukotrienes (LTC_4, LTD_4, LTE_4), which are potent mediators of bronchoconstriction and mucus secretion; calcitonin gene-related peptide (CGRP), which has potent vasodilating properties; and platelet-activating factor (PAF), which enhances the release of histamine and serotonin from platelets.

II. Etiologies

The most common causes of immediate generalized reactions are foods, medications, insect stings, and radiocontrast media, and a list of frequent causes is shown in Table 10.1. Although anaphylaxis caused by food, drugs, and insect stings is discussed at length in other chapters, the following list is a description of unique etiologies that are important to the practicing clinician.

A. **Exercise-induced anaphylaxis** represents a syndrome in which anaphylaxis follows vigorous exercise. Symptoms may range in severity from mild urticaria to severe laryngeal edema and hypotension. In some cases, ingestion of a food to which the patient is allergic (usually up to 6 hours before exercise) is required in order for exercise to elicit anaphylaxis. The most commonly implicated foods include celery and shrimp. Occasionally, however, any food eaten within 6 hours of exercise may contribute to an anaphylactic reaction. In most patients, the systemic reaction to exercise occurs on an intermittent basis despite participation in the same exercise routine.

B. **Idiopathic anaphylaxis** refers to patients who have no defined external cause for their anaphylactic episodes. Approximately half of patients with idiopathic anaphylaxis have other atopic conditions and some may have coexisting causes of anaphylaxis such as medications, foods, or exercise. The physiologic mechanism responsible for idiopathic anaphylaxis is not well defined.

C. **Radiocontrast media** (RCM) causes systemic reactions in approximately 1% to 10% of those initially exposed. Reexposure in those with a previous reaction carries a 17% to 35% risk of anaphylaxis if high-osmolality RCMs are used; the incidence of a repeat reaction is 4% with lower osmolality media. Reactions may be induced by injection into the systemic circulation as well as body cavities (e.g., urinary bladder). Patients typically develop flushing and urticaria within seconds to a few minutes of administration, which may progress to severe anaphylaxis with bronchoconstriction and hypotension. Because no accurate diagnostic tests are available, diagnosis is based solely upon the patient's history. Contrary to prior beliefs, RCM sensitivity is neither caused by "allergy" to iodine, nor can it be predicted by the presence of shellfish allergy. IgE is not involved in the pathogenesis of RCM sensitivity.

D. **Latex-induced anaphylaxis** is caused by IgE-mediated sensitivity to natural rubber latex proteins. Most often, patients with IgE-mediated allergy to latex experience localized urticaria/angioedema, rhinoconjunctivitis, and/or asthma; severe generalized reactions are unusual. Individuals at increased risk include patients with spina bifida (who have undergone multiple surgeries), rubber industry workers, and health care professionals. Irritant or allergic contact (type IV) dermatitis of the hands caused by latex gloves may also predispose patients to the development of IgE-mediated allergy to latex protein. Generally, occupational cases of latex allergy develop in patients who are atopic. Diagnosis may be currently confirmed with *in vitro tests* of antilatex IgE; standardized latex skin tests are in development.

E. **Undifferentiated somatoform idiopathic anaphylaxis** refers to patients whose symptoms suggest anaphylaxis but in whom objective evidence is lacking. Furthermore, there is a poor response to medications (prednisone, antihistamine, albuterol) that are usually successful in idiopathic anaphylaxis. Insight into the causes are typically absent, and often referral for psychologic or psychiatric consultation is met with refusal or hostility.

III. **Clinical manifestations**

A. **Symptoms and signs**

Systemic allergic reactions almost always occur within 3 hours of exposure to a putative causative agent, and in general, more severe reactions will occur more rapidly. Significant delays in the development of symptoms suggest a different disease entity (e.g., serum sickness).

1. **Skin.** Cutaneous tingling and warmth are very often the first symptoms of anaphylaxis, which may progress to symptoms of flushing, pruritus, urticaria, and/or angioedema. Skin symptoms have been estimated to occur in 70% of generalized systemic reactions. In mild generalized reactions, the skin may be the only end-organ involved.

2. **Upper airway.** Acute symptoms of rhinorrhea, nasal congestion, sneezing, and nasal and ocular pruritis may be seen during systemic reactions, particularly when patients suffer from concomitant allergic rhinitis. Upper airway angioedema may also occur and involve the uvula, tongue, pharynx, or larynx, which may be associated with sudden hoarseness, voice loss, dyspnea, or in severe cases respiratory arrest.

3. **Lower airway.** Involvement of the lungs usually results in bronchoconstriction and airway edema, causing symptoms of dyspnea, wheezing, or chest tightness. Pulmonary reactions may be particularly severe in patients with bronchial asthma.

4. **Gastrointestinal.** Abdominal symptoms are usually due to acute intestinal edema and smooth muscle spasm and may include acute abdominal pain, nausea, vomiting or diarrhea. Occasionally, frank rectal bleeding may occur due to intestinal ischemia or infarction.

5. **Cardiovascular.** Cardiac arrhythmias may be observed during generalized reactions, resulting in atrial or ventricular premature beats, atrial or ventricular arrhythmias, or cardiac ischemia and symptoms of palpitations, dizziness, or chest pain. Rarely, acute myocardial infarction may ensue, but this is most often seen when hypotension is present in patients with underlying coronary artery disease. Although administration of epinephrine has also been implicated as a cause of angina and myocardial infarction during anaphylaxis, such complications and cardiac arrest have occurred in the absence of epinephrine administration. Hypotension represents the most feared complication of anaphylaxis. Reductions in blood pressure may range in severity from mild, with symptoms of light-headedness, to severe, with loss of consciousness and full-scale cardiovascular collapse.

6. **Fatalities.** It has been estimated that there are approximately 1,500 anaphylactic deaths per year in the United States, most commonly caused by penicillin, Hymenoptera stings, and food allergy. Death due to anaphylaxis may occur in patients of any age, although the vast majority are older than 10 years. Asthma is a distinct risk factor for fatal anaphylaxis. Most often, the onset of fatal anaphylactic reactions begins within 20 minutes after exposure to the incriminated agent. The most frequent initial manifestation of a fatal anaphylactic event is acute respiratory distress or circulatory collapse occurring within a few minutes of exposure. In cases of fatal anaphylaxis, pathologic findings at autopsy most often reveal pulmonary abnormalities (congestion in 90%; pul-

monary edema and/or hemorrhage in 50%) and laryngeal swelling in one-third of patients.

B. Laboratory findings

Anaphylactic and anaphylactoid reactions are primarily diagnosed by the clinical presentation and response to treatment. However, when the diagnosis of anaphylaxis is uncertain, assays for mast cell mediators (i.e., tryptase and histamine) may be helpful.

1. **Serum tryptase.** Tryptase is a mediator released after mast cell activation, and serum concentrations of tryptase are elevated in patients with anaphylaxis and systemic mastocytosis. Because the serum half-life of tryptase is 2 to 6 hours, and the concentration usually peaks 1 to 2 hours after the start of a reaction, the optimal time for sampling is within 6 hours of the onset of anaphylaxis. Sampling up to 24 hours after the start of the reaction has clinical utility, because values greater than 10 ng per mL are suggestive of mast cell activation. Immediate freezing of the sample is critical, because the concentration may increase significantly if the sample remains at room temperature or warmer, potentially leading to an incorrect diagnosis. Beta-tryptase, which is stored in mast cell granules, may potentially be a more sensitive indicator of systemic allergic reactions and may more accurately distinguish between acute anaphylaxis and mastocytosis. More clinical investigation will be required before this test is used routinely in clinical practice.

2. **Urinary histamine and histamine metabolites.** Histamine and its metabolites (N-methylhistamine and N-methylimidazole acetic acid) may be elevated for several hours following anaphylaxis and may be accurately measured in 24 hour urine collections.

3. **Plasma histamine.** The half-life of histamine in plasma is on the order of 2 minutes, limiting the utility of these measurements for the confirmation of anaphylaxis.

4. **Routine laboratory tests**, such as the chemistry panel, complete blood count and differential, erythrocyte sedimentation rate, and urinalysis, are usually not helpful in confirming the diagnosis of anaphylaxis or in distinguishing a generalized systemic reaction from other acute illnesses. In selected circumstances, the serum glucose, fractionated creatine kinase, and arterial blood gas measurement may prove helpful in the differential diagnosis of anaphylaxis (see below).

IV. Differential diagnosis

A number of common conditions, particularly those that cause acute hypotension, loss of consciousness, dyspnea, or wheezing, need to be considered in patients presenting with acute anaphylaxis.

A. Vasovagal reactions often occur following phlebotomy or injections and occasionally during situations arousing extreme emotion. Patients usually present with acute pallor, diaphoresis, nausea, and hypotension. Skin and respiratory findings are notably absent and bradycardia is present, in contrast with the tachycardia of anaphylaxis.

B. Myocardial infarction may present with dyspnea and signs and symptoms of hypotension with minimal chest discomfort. Cutaneous and upper airway findings are absent. In these cases, the electrocardiogram and creatine kinase (myocardial bound) (CK-MB) concentration play a key role in diagnosis.

C. Insulin reactions due to hypoglycemia are characterized by weakness, pallor, diaphoresis, and loss of consciousness. However, cutaneous signs and respiratory symptoms are missing and blood pressure is usually maintained.

D. Pulmonary embolism may present with acute dyspnea, and in the case of a saddle embolism, severe hypotension. Again, skin and upper airway findings are absent. Evidence of a lower extremity deep venous thromboembolism is often present and will point to the correct diagnosis; an arterial blood gas showing a marked alveolar-oxygen gradient and ultimately radiographic imaging (spiral lung computer tomography [CT] or ventilation-perfusion [V/Q] scan) may be required to confirm the diagnosis.

E. In **acute hyperventilation**, paresthesias are common and there is no involvement of the skin nor any objective evidence of respiratory distress. Blood pressure is frequently elevated in these patients.

F. **Globus hystericus** presents with a feeling of fullness in the throat which is mistaken by the patients for swelling. The persistent and nonprogressive nature of the problem and normal throat examination, along with the absence of other signs and symptoms, helps confirm this diagnosis.

G. **Munchausen syndrome** may manifest as recurrent episodes of anaphylaxis. In these patients, anaphylactic symptoms may either be simulated or they intentionally and covertly self-administer an antigen (e.g., a food such as peanuts or drug such as penicillin) to which they are truly allergic; in either case, the patient repeatedly seeks medical attention. Recognition of such individuals is important, and appropriate psychiatric evaluation and treatment should be obtained, if possible.

H. **Mastocytosis** is a relatively rare disorder which most often presents with cutaneous collections of mast cells (urticaria pigmentosa). Occasionally, patients with mastocytosis may present with unexplained, recurrent episodes of flushing or anaphylaxis. Bone marrow biopsy is necessary to confirm the diagnosis of mastocytosis in these patients.

V. **Treatment**

Early and appropriate treatment of anaphylaxis is critical in ensuring a good outcome (Table 10.2). The longer initial therapy is delayed, the greater the incidence of fatality. Initial treatment should be directed to maintenance of an effective airway and circulatory system. Because anaphylaxis may progress rapidly, patients should be moved as soon as possible to an area in which severe symptoms (e.g., upper airway obstruction) can be treated appropriately. Principal modalities include the following:

A. **Epinephrine**, 1:1,000 concentration, should be administered by intramuscular injection at a dose of 0.01 mL per kg (maximum dose 0.3 mL). Epinephrine relaxes bronchial smooth muscle, supports vascular smooth muscle tone, and reduces on-going mast cell mediator release. A single injection may be sufficient to treat mild symptoms; however, it may be repeated every 20 minutes if necessary. For patients with cardiac disease or in the elderly, a reduced dose may be considered (0.1 to 0.2 mL, which can be repeated in 10 minutes). Clinicians should note that severe acute anaphylaxis always requires treatment with epinephrine.

B. **H1- and H2-antihistamines** may also be of clinical benefit in patients with moderate to severe symptoms. Drugs available as parenteral formulations include diphenhydramine (1 mg per kg) and cimetidine (4 mg per kg), which may both be given intravenously.

C. **Corticosteroids** should be given by the intravenous route (e.g., methylprednisolone, 125 mg) in repeated doses (every 4 to 6 hours) in patients with moderate to severe symptoms or in those who do not respond quickly to epinephrine.

D. **Inhaled beta-adrenergic agonists** may be given by metered-dose inhaler or nebulizer as an adjunctive treatment for acute bronchospasm. Because there is no salutary systemic effect, however, this is not a replacement for injected epinephrine.

E. **Fluids** should be given to patients with significant hypotension (systolic blood pressure less than 90 mm). Two intravenous access lines should be established and fluid infused as fast as possible to help reestablish a systolic blood pressure of greater than 90 mm.

F. **For refractory hypotension**, intravenous dopamine (400 mg in 500 mL of Dextrose 5% water) should be infused until the systolic blood increases to greater than 90 mm. If dopamine is not effective, intravenous levophed

Table 10.2. Treatment of anaphylaxis

Immediately give epinephrine 1:1,000, 0.3 mL in the deltoid muscle[a]

Stop intravenous infusion (radiographic contrast material, antibiotic, gamma globulin, etc.), or remove insect stinger

Record blood pressure and pulse; is CPR required? Consider calling for emergency medical services

Depending on severity, degree of response, and the individual patient
    Diphenhydramine 50 mg intravenously (slowly)
    Ranitidine 50 mg or cimetidine 300 mg intravenously (optional)
    Oxygen administration by mask or nasal
    Start intravenous line(s) and fluids
    Methylprednisolone 125 mg intravenously

Repeat epinephrine in 15–20 min if needed

Be prepared for intubation or hypotension

For systolic blood pressure <90 mm Hg
    Two intravenous catheters (no. 18 gauge needles or larger) with normal saline (lines wide open)
    Dopamine 400 mg (two ampules) in 500 mL of D5W, infuse until systolic blood pressure is 90 mm Hg, then titrate slowly. If ineffective, consider:
    Levophed 2 mg (one ampule) in 250 ml of D5W. Titrate after reaching systolic blood pressure of 90 mm Hg

For acute wheezing or dyspnea
    Epinephrine per above; if not effective, consider:
    Albuterol by nebulization (2.5 mg) or metered-dose inhaler, two puffs
    Supplemental oxygen, up to 100% by nasal cannula or mask

For acute stridor
    Epinephrine per above; if not effective, consider:
    Racemic epinephrine by nebulization
    Supplemental oxygen administration
    Intubation or tracheostomy for impending upper airway obstruction

[a] For some patients with cardiac disease or in the elderly, a reduced dose may be considered, i.e., 0.1–0.2 mL of 1:1,000 epinephrine. It can be repeated in 10 min. The pediatric dose is 0.01 mL/kg up to 0.3 mL.
CPR, cardiopulmonary resuscitation; D5W, Dextrose 5% water.

(2 mg in 250 mL of D5W) can be added and titrated until the systolic blood pressure is increased. Although these measures should be started in the emergency room, patients requiring these medications will require transfer to an intensive care unit setting for continued pressor therapy and sophisticated monitoring.

  G. **Supplemental oxygen** should be given to patients with dyspnea, wheezing, or stridor by nasal cannula or mask.

  H. **Inhaled albuterol**, given as a 2.5 mg dose by nebulizer or two puffs by metered-dose inhaler, is useful for treating bronchospasm that is refractory to epinephrine.

  I. **Intubation** may be necessary if upper airway obstruction compromises adequate ventilation. If intubation cannot be successfully performed due to obstructive laryngeal edema, tracheostomy should be performed without delay.

VI. **Prevention** of future episodes of anaphylaxis is a key component of long-term management (see Table 10.3).

  A. A thorough **medical history** of previous reactions to suspected antigens is critical before administering any medication (especially a parenteral medication).

Table 10.3. Suggestions to prevent anaphylaxis

Perform careful allergy history in all patients receiving drug therapy—ensure labeling of medical record

Give drugs orally, rather than by parenteral route, when possible

Follow-up appointment and instructions after treatment in the emergency department

Epinephrine self-injection kit should be prescribed to patients who are predisposed to anaphylaxis—instruction should be provided prior to discharge from the emergency department or before leaving office visit

Medic-Alert bracelet for patients who are predisposed to future systemic allergic reactions should be considered

Referral to allergist–immunologist for definitive diagnostic testing and treatment

Avoid test-challenges with incriminated foods or medications

For patients receiving allergy vaccine therapy, have patients wait minimum of 20 min after each injection

In patients with radiocontrast sensitivity, a prophylactic regimen prior to future use of lower osmolality radiocontrast media should be recommended

Self-discipline is needed for patients with exercise-induced anaphylaxis

---

B. **Careful follow-up** should be arranged at the time of acute treatment. An epinephrine self-injection kit should be provided to the patient, with careful instructions in how and when to use it. Identification information (Medic-Alert bracelet) should be ordered for the patient, and information regarding potential allergies noted in the patient's chart.

C. **Referral to an allergist–immunologist** should be made in most cases for definitive diagnostic testing and treatment. Test challenges with incriminated foods or medications should only be performed under the guidance of an allergist–immunologist.

D. For patients with **radiocontrast sensitivity**, the following regimen should be employed prior to future use of radiocontrast media:

1. Use of low-osmolality contrast media
2. Prednisone, 50 mg p.o., 13, 7, and 1 hour before the procedure
3. Benadryl, 50 mg p.o., 1 hour before the procedure
4. Albuterol, 4 mg p.o., 1 hour before the procedure (avoid in patients with histories of cardiac ischemia or arrhythmias)
5. Have emergency therapy available.

Selected Readings

Bochner BS, Lichtenstein LM. Anaphylaxis. *N Engl J Med* 1991;324:1785–1790.

Bock SA, Munoz-Furlong A, Sampson HA. Fatalities due to anaphylactic reactions to foods. *J Allergy Clin Immunol* 2001;107:191–193.

Bubak ME, Reed CE, Fransway AF, et al. Allergic reactions to latex among health-care workers. *Mayo Clin Proc* 1992;67:1075–1079.

Choy AC, Patterson R, Patterson DR, et al. Undifferentiated somatoform idiopathic anaphylaxis: non-organic symptoms mimicking idiopathic anaphylaxis. *J Allergy Clin Immunol* 1995;96:893–900.

Delage C, Irey NS. Anaphylactic deaths: A clinicopathologic study of 43 cases. *J Forensic Sci* 1972;17:525–40.

Ditto AM, Harris KE, Krasnick J, et al. Idiopathic anaphylaxis: a series of 335 cases. *Ann Allergy Asthma Immunol* 1996;77:285–291.

Greenberger PA, Miller M. Urine histamine during episodes of anaphylaxis. *J Allergy Clin Immunol* 1994;93:302.

James LP Jr, Austen KF. Fatal systemic anaphylaxis in man. *N Engl J Med* 1964;270:597–603.

Kay AB. Concepts of allergy and hypersensitivity. In: Kay AB, ed. *Allergy and allergic diseases*. Oxford: Blackwell Science, 1997:23–35.

Lin PY, Schwartz LB, Curry A, et al. Histamine and tryptase levels in patients with acute allergic reactions: An emergency department-based study. *J Allergy Clin Immunol* 2000;106:65–71.

Lin RY, Curry A, Pesola GR, et al. Improved outcomes in patients with acute allergic syndromes who are treated with combined H1 and H2 antagonists. *Ann Emerg Med* 2000;36:462–468.

Neugut AI, Ghatak AT, Miller RL. Anaphylaxis in the United States: an investigation into its epidemiology. *Arch Intern Med* 2001;161:15–21.

Schwartz LB, Metcalfe DD, Miller JS, et al. Tryptase levels as an indicator of mast-cell activation in systemic anaphylaxis and mastocytosis. *N Engl J Med* 1987; 316:1622–1626.

11. INSECT ALLERGY

David B. K. Golden

Insect bites and stings usually cause relatively mild, transient local inflammation. In sensitized individuals, allergic reactions may result in more severe local reactions as well as generalized systemic symptoms ranging from mild to fatal responses. Acute anaphylactic reactions can be abrupt in onset and are considered true medical emergencies. In the United States, almost 9 million people have had previous systemic reactions to stings, and as many as 50 million people are sensitized to insect venoms and have a risk of allergic reactions. Although anaphylaxis has been reported in a small number of cases from biting insects, it is the stinging insects that cause most systemic reactions and these will be the focus of this chapter.

Stinging Insect Allergy
I. Clinical manifestations
    A. Normal reactions to insect bites and stings generally cause localized itching, pain, burning, redness, and mild swelling. This normal reaction is caused by several components in the saliva (bites) or venom (stings) of the insects, including enzymatically active proteins and vasoactive amines (e.g., histamine and kinins). The reaction usually subsides in hours, although some individuals with sensitive skin describe more intense local reactions lasting several days.
    B. Large local reactions are usually late-phase allergic reactions causing severe swelling contiguous with the site of the sting; swelling distant from the site of the sting would be a sign of systemic reaction with angioedema. The abnormal swelling begins more than 6 hours after the sting, enlarging for 24 to 48 hours, and resolving slowly over 2 to 7 days. Such large local reactions cause induration and tense edema larger than 8 cm in diameter and can involve an entire limb. The intense local inflammation may cause the appearance of lymphangitic streaks toward the inguinal or axillary nodes, but this should not be mistaken for cellulitis when it appears in the first 24 to 48 hours. Infection at the site of the sting is quite uncommon and takes more than 48 hours to develop (usually after excoriation of the site). Large local reactions are not usually dangerous, but in the head and neck area they could cause delayed localized compression of the airway, especially in the case of a sting on the tongue or pharynx.
    C. Systemic reactions may cause any one or more of the signs and symptoms of anaphylaxis. Cutaneous signs occur in more than 80% of all cases, and are the only manifestation of the reaction in 15% of adults. Airway symptoms (throat tightness, dyspnea, cough, wheezing) are reported by 50% to 60% of adults and children, and circulatory symptoms (dizziness, syncope, hypotension, unconsciousness) occur in 30% of adults. Children have a higher frequency of isolated cutaneous reactions (60% of cases) and a lower frequency of vascular symptoms and anaphylactic shock (5%) compared to adults. Systemic reactions can become progressively more severe with each sting in some cases, but usually follow a more predictable and individual pattern in each patient. Anaphylaxis can be protracted or biphasic in more than 20% of cases, so medical observation is recommended for 6 hours. Occasionally, individuals are resistant to epinephrine, especially those taking a beta-blocker medication. Patients discharged from emergency care of anaphylaxis must receive instructions on the need for an epinephrine kit, an allergy consultation, and preventative treatment. It should be explained to all patients that self-administered epinephrine is not a substitute for emergency medical attention.
    D. Other unusual patterns of reactions have been reported including nephropathy, central and peripheral neurologic syndromes, idiopathic thrombocy-

topenic purpura, and rhabdomyolysis, but these responses are not im-munoglobulin E (IgE) mediated. Serum sickness reactions to stings are infrequent, but have been related to venom-specific IgE antibodies. There are also reports of allergic sting reactions being followed by months of chronic urticaria or cold urticaria.

II. Insect antigens

The most common insects causing systemic allergic reactions are of the order Hymenoptera (Table 11.1). There are three Hymenoptera families of importance: bees (honeybees, bumblebees) and vespids (yellow jackets, hornets, wasps) are best known. In recent years, fire ants (*Solenopsis* sp) have become a rapidly increasing public health hazard in the southeast and south-central United States, particularly on the Gulf Coast. For 50 years, whole body extracts were used for skin testing and immunotherapy, because it was believed that allergic sensitivity was related to an "intrinsic bee protein" present in the whole insect body as well as the venom. In the 1970s it was established that whole body extract tests and treatment were no more effective than placebo, whereas immunotherapy utilizing purified venom effectively prevented anaphylaxis in 98% of patients. Honeybee venom is immunochemically distinct, and the primary allergen is phospholipase A. The vespid venoms have a high degree of cross-reactivity and the same primary allergen, "antigen 5," is present in yellow jacket and hornet venoms. *Polistes* wasps are more distantly related to the other vespids, and only 50% of yellow jacket allergic patients have positive tests to wasp venom related to the cross-reactivity of the major allergen. Fire ant venoms are quite different in that they contain very little protein in an unusual suspension of alkaloid toxins that cause the characteristic painful vesicular eruption. The allergenic proteins in fire ant venoms are unique, except for one that shows limited cross-reactivity with vespid allergens. The diagnostic and therapeutic materials currently supplied by commercial laboratories are fire ant whole body extracts, but unlike the situation with the other Hymenoptera venoms, these fire ant extracts show reasonable allergenic activity for diagnostic skin testing and for preventive immunotherapy.

III. Epidemiology and natural history of reactions

A. Large local reactions occur with uncertain frequency, but are estimated to affect 10% of adults, because the size of the reaction is subject to exaggeration. Most patients (60% to 80%) with large local reactions have positive venom skin tests, but the limited data on the natural history of large local reactions in children and adults suggest a less than or equal to 10% risk of systemic reactions to subsequent stings.

B. Systemic reactions to insect stings can develop at any age, often following a number of uneventful stings. Systemic allergic reactions have been reported to occur in approximately 3% of adults and 1% of children. At least 50 fatal sting reactions occur each year in the United States and many other sting fatalities are believed to go unrecognized. In cases of unexplained sudden death in the summer, postmortem blood samples often show the presence of venom-specific IgE antibodies as well as an elevated level of serum tryptase, strongly suggesting the possibility of fatal insect sting anaphylaxis.

The risk of anaphylaxis to a subsequent sting varies according to the history and skin tests. The highest risk (60% to 70%) is in patients who have had recent and severe reactions. The chance of another systemic reaction declines gradually over time, down to 35% after 3 to 5 years, and 25% after 10 years. In some individuals the risk of anaphylaxis persists for decades even with no intervening stings. The lowest risk is in children with isolated diffuse urticaria, who have less than 10% risk of urticaria and less than 1% risk of anaphylaxis to subsequent stings.

C. IgE antibodies to Hymenoptera venoms are frequently found in the adult population. More than 20% of normal adults have positive skin tests or radioallergosorbent tests (RAST) to yellow jacket or honeybee venom, and these patients invariably report prior histories of stings. Half of those tests

Table 11.1. Characteristics of common stinging insects (Hymenoptera)[a]

Insect type	Appearance	Habitats	Sting characteristics	Venom characteristics
Honeybee	Hairy bodies with yellow and black markings	Domestic hives, hollow trees or caves (rural and suburban)	Barbed stinger; only insect to leave stinger; stings only if provoked	Hyaluronidase, phospholipase A, histamine, lecithinase; smooth muscle contractor
Wasp	Hairless body with narrow waist, black or brown markings	Trees, shrubs, eaves of houses (rural and suburban scavenger)	Often contaminated	Histamine, serotonin, hyaluronidase, lecithinase
Hornet	Short waist, truncated body, with sparse hair, dark band under eyes	Oval and pear-shaped nests in trees and above ground (rural scavenger)	Often contaminated	Histamine, serotinin, kinins, acetylcholine
Yellow jacket	Similar to hornet, with yellow markings but without dark band under eyes	Nests in ground and walls (rural scavenger)	Often contaminated, aggressive, most common cause of stings in most areas	Histamine, serotonin, kinins
Imported fire ant	Appearance of domestic ants but with well-developed posterior stinging apparatus	Nests in ground, primarily in Gulf Coast states (scavenger)	Bites and stings; produces multiple pustules for 3–8 days, with pain and burning	Cytotoxic and hemolytic alkaloids

[a] Generally, patients with honeybee sensitivity are not reactive to wasps, hornets, and yellow jackets. There is a 50% incidence of cross-reactivity among wasps, hornets, and yellow jackets.
Drawings of honeybee, wasp, hornet, and yellow jacket from *Insect allergy*, Spokane, WA: Hollister-Stier, Miles, 1978. Drawing of fire ant from Pap LF. Anaphylaxis—Preventable emergency. *Dermatol Allergy* 1980;3:45, with permission.

became negative after a few years, but almost 20% of those who were later stung had a systemic reaction. In untreated patients with systemic reactions to stings, venom skin tests may gradually become weaker over time but do not usually become negative during 5 to 10 years of follow-up. In patients receiving venom immunotherapy (VIT), venom-specific IgE increases in the first few months of initial therapy, returns to baseline after 1 year, and then declines steadily with time (even after an intercurrent sting or after venom therapy is discontinued). After 6 and 10 years of VIT, these patients become skin test negative in approximately 25% and 67% of cases, respectively.

D. Children have an estimated prevalence of systemic reactions to stings of at least 0.4% to 0.8%. The notion that children routinely outgrow insect sting allergy is probably due to the large number of children with isolated urticaria after a sting. In children with strictly cutaneous systemic reactions, the risk of anaphylaxis after a subsequent sting is less than 10%. However, children with histories of moderate or severe reactions who did not receive VIT experienced systemic reactions in 25% to 40% of cases when they were stung 5 to 20 years later. Children who received VIT had a much lower risk of developing systemic reactions 10 or more years after stopping treatment.

IV. Diagnosis

    A. History

    The patient's history of the reaction is most important in establishing a diagnosis of insect allergy. A thorough inquiry should include all of the details regarding the circumstances and location of the sting; the type, number, and location of the insect(s); the time course of the reaction; a description of the pattern and severity of all associated symptoms and signs; and the response to any treatment that was administered. The history should also include any previous stings that have occurred (especially in recent months), any atopic conditions, and all medications that were taken at the time of the sting. It may be difficult to distinguish historically between a large local swelling and angioedema, and between lightheadedness or dyspnea and anxiety or hyperventilation. It is also advisable to ask specifically about prior sting reactions during periodic health maintenance visits, because many patients will not volunteer this information.

    B. Venom skin tests

        1. Indications. Venom skin tests are best performed by specialists experienced with the technique and interpretation of the tests. Venom skin tests are recommended in patients with a history of systemic reaction to a sting, but not in those with large local reactions or in children with isolated diffuse urticaria.

        2. Testing materials and preparation. Commercial venom protein extracts are purified preparations of Hymenoptera venoms that have been standardized in order to maintain a consistent and reproducible response during skin testing and immunotherapy. There are five venoms available for testing: honeybee, yellow jacket, yellow hornet, white-faced hornet, and wasp venom. These products are supplied as lyophilized preparations and must be reconstituted with a special diluent containing 0.9% saline, 0.03% human serum albumin (HSA) (which stabilizes venom proteins and prevents their adsorption to the walls of the container), and 0.4% phenol. After reconstitution, the full-strength venom extract is diluted in a serial fashion to achieve the concentrations required for skin testing. Of note, the manufacturer's instructions concerning the storage of the lyophilized materials (do not freeze) and storage times before expiration should always be observed.

        Whole body extracts of Hymenoptera insects do not contain enough venom proteins for either accurate diagnosis or therapy of insect sting allergy. An important exception is the case of fire ant sensitivity, which can be tested and treated using whole body fire ant extracts.

3. **Methods.** The standard method for venom skin testing is the intradermal technique, beginning with an appropriately low concentration (0.001 µg per mL), and then increasing until a positive result is obtained or the highest concentration is achieved (1 µg per mL). Patients with a history of severe systemic reactions should be tested initially with a puncture technique using a venom concentration of 0.001 µg per mL before proceeding to the intradermal technique.

Sensitization to multiple venoms may be present even when there has only been a reaction to a single insect. Therefore, skin testing should be performed with a complete set of the five Hymenoptera venoms, a negative diluent (HSA–saline) control, and a positive histamine control. The preferred location for performing venom skin tests is on the flexor surface of the forearm.

4. **Interpretation** of venom skin tests is based upon the size of the wheal and erythema, and the presence of pseudopodia. Table 11.2 summarizes the recommended guidelines for skin test interpretation provided by major manufacturers. Reactions of 1+ or greater (larger than the negative control) at a concentration of 1 µg per mL or less of venom indicate the patient is venom-sensitive. The positive venom skin test confirms the allergic nature of the sting reaction and identifies the causative insect.

Skin test results in patients with a convincing history are usually clearly positive, but can be negative in up to 30% of patients. There are three situations in which skin tests may be negative: (i) In a patient with a strongly positive history in whom the sting has occurred in the remote past, and may represent a loss of sensitivity. (ii) During the refractory ("anergic") period for 3 to 6 weeks after a sting reaction. It is therefore reasonable to perform skin tests during this period if there is a seasonal need to begin immunotherapy as soon as possible. However, if the results are negative, the tests should be repeated in 4 to 6 weeks. (iii) Some cases of sting anaphylaxis have been said to be non-IgE mediated and may be related to subclinical mastocytosis or simply "toxic" mast cell hyperreleasability. There are reports of patients with sting reactions who had negative skin tests and experienced systemic reactions to subsequent stings. Most of these patients had a positive RAST, which suggests the importance of performing a serological test for venom-specific IgE antibodies in patients with a positive history and negative skin test.

There are many different patterns of venom skin test sensitivity. Skin tests are positive to all three of the common vespid skin test preparations (yellow jacket, yellow hornet, white-faced hornet) in 95% of vespid allergic patients. Notably, the degree of skin test sensitivity does not correlate reliably with the degree of sting reaction. The strongest skin tests often occur in patients who have had only large local reactions and

Table 11.2. Interpretation of venom skin test responses

| Grade | Mean diameters (cm) | |
	Wheal	Erythema
0	<0.5	<0.5
±	0.5–1.0	0.5–1.0
1+	0.5–1.0	1.1–2.0
2+	0.5–1.0	2.1–3.0
3+	1.0–1.5; pseudopodia	3.1–4.0
4+	>1.5; many pseudopodia	>4.0

have a very low risk of anaphylaxis, whereas some patients who have had abrupt and near-fatal anaphylactic shock show only weak skin test (or RAST) sensitivity. In fact, almost 25% of patients presenting for systemic allergic reactions to stings were skin test positive only at the 1.0 µg per mL concentration, demonstrating the importance of skin testing with the full diagnostic range of concentrations.

C. Radioallergosorbent test

The diagnosis of insect sting allergy by detection of allergen-specific IgE antibodies in serum (typically by RAST) is a method of high potential but variable performance. The test is often qualitative, poorly standardized, and is negative in at least 15% to 20% of skin-test-positive sting-allergy patients. As noted above, however, the RAST may be positive in some patients who have negative venom skin tests. When it is clearly elevated, the RAST result is diagnostic of insect sting allergy and may be used as grounds for starting VIT. RAST may also be used as an immunologic method for following patients on VIT to document possible changes in sensitivity.

D. Sting challenge

Because many patients with a positive history and skin tests do not react to subsequent stings, some European researchers have recommended that a deliberate sting challenge with a live insect should be performed as the diagnostic procedure of choice to determine the need for immunotherapy. Because of the risks and costs required by sting challenges, most allergists have judged this approach to be both unethical and impractical. Furthermore, sting challenge is not an accurate indicator of future risk of reaction, because patients with negative sting challenges experienced a 20% reaction rate following a second sting. This suggests that reactions following stings are not completely reproducible and depend upon multiple variables involving both the patient and the insect. Sting challenge is primarily useful as a research tool to investigate the allergic response to stings in relation to other variables and treatments.

V. Treatment

A. Acute reactions

1. Local reactions should be treated symptomatically, with initial cleansing and then ice or cold compresses for several hours after the sting. Oral antihistamines can help reduce the itching and local discomfort, as can a topical steroid cream or ointment. The late-phase allergic inflammatory reaction may require a brief course of oral corticosteroid (in adults, prednisone 40 to 60 mg initially and then reduced by 10 mg each day for 4 to 6 days). Local infection is uncommon and may occur many days after the sting, often because of excoriation. Severe allergic local reactions may show lymphangitic streaks toward the axillary or inguinal nodes, but this response is inflammatory in nature and not infectious, and does not indicate cellulitis when it presents within 2 days of the sting.

2. Systemic reactions should be treated in the same fashion as anaphylaxis due to any cause (see Chapter 10). Epinephrine injection is always the treatment of choice for acute anaphylaxis, with the possible exception of a patient with unstable cardiovascular disease. Intramuscular injection of epinephrine (in children 0.01 mg per kg, up to 0.3 mg total dose; 0.3 to 0.5 mg in adults) provides more rapid and more complete absorption than subcutaneous injection. Additional treatment is often necessary with intravenous fluids, oxygen, and other medications. Patients with anaphylaxis should be observed for 3 to 6 hours because 20% or more may develop delayed, prolonged, or biphasic anaphylaxis.

B. Prophylaxis

1. Avoidance measures. Patients who have had allergic reactions to stings should be counseled regarding basic avoidance measures, including avoidance of eating or drinking outdoors; drinking from a can; outdoor areas where there are food or trash receptacles; walking barefoot outdoors; gardening; and use of fragrances (see Table 11.3). Insect repellants do not seem to deter stinging insects.

2. Epinephrine for self-injection is a very important element in preparedness for potential episodes of anaphylaxis. Preloaded injectors are available commercially as the EpiPen and EpiPen Jr. (Dey Laboratories, Napa, CA) and the Ana-Kit (Hollister-Stier Laboratories, Spokane, WA). Patients need careful instruction and demonstration of the correct and safe use of the injector, when to use it (or not use it), and how to check for expiration or deterioration of the medication. Epinephrine injectors may be prescribed (if appropriate instructions are given) for patients who have had previous systemic or large local allergic reactions.

3. Allergy consultation is strongly recommended for patients who have had allergic reactions to stings. Those with systemic reactions will require detailed review of their history along with testing for venom sensitivity. Both systemic reactors and large local reactors will require lengthy discussion and counseling on the relative risk of reaction, strategies for avoidance, signs and symptoms to watch for, how to be prepared, prescription and instructions for use of epinephrine, and discussion of the indications, benefits, and risks of VIT.

4. Venom immunotherapy
   a. Indications for VIT require a history of previous systemic allergic reaction to a sting and evidence of a positive venom skin test (see Section IV on page 211). In adults and children with large local reactions, and children with strictly cutaneous systemic reactions, VIT is not required. However, some patients will still request treatment because of their fear of reaction and the impact upon their lifestyle; in such cases, improving the quality of life can be sufficient justification for treatment. There are limited data on adults with strictly cutaneous systemic reactions, but there are cases of progression in adults from urticaria alone to life-threatening anaphylaxis. In addition, some patients report reactions only with multiple or sequential stings, but not from isolated single stings. Therefore, because there is no test that accurately predicts which patients will progress to more severe reactions with single or mul-

Table 11.3. Patient information to limit the risk of insect stings

---

The risk increases in summer and with outdoor exposure

Exercise caution when doing yard work, handling garbage, picnicking, swimming, bicycling, riding in open-air vehicles, boating, camping, or other outdoor activity

Always wear shoes outdoors

Avoid loose-fitting clothing that may entrap insects. Insects are attracted to bright colors and floral patterns. Wear light-colored clothing; white, green, tan, and khaki.

Avoid scented perfumes, lotions, soaps, colognes, or hair preparations

Look for insects in vehicles before driving, and keep vehicle windows closed

Avoid rapid or jerking movement around insects. Remain still. Most insects will not sting unless provoked

All nests or hives in the vicinity of the home should be removed by a professional exterminator and not by the insect-sensitive patient

Insect repellents should not be depended on for protection. Immunotherapy does not lessen the need for other measures of prevention

Wear an identification tag or bracelet at all times

Have an emergency kit available at all times, especially if at greater risk. Instruct family members and companions in its use

Seek medical attention immediately after emergency treatment is given

tiple stings, it is recommended that adults with cutaneous systemic reactions and positive venom skin tests undergo VIT.

Fire ant immunotherapy is still at an early stage of development because the natural history of fire ant allergy is unclear. Ongoing trials suggest that fire ant whole body extract immunotherapy is reasonably safe and effective and should be employed in cases of significant systemic reactions. Current studies of fire ant immunotherapy are focused upon achieving more reliable clinical protection with improved safety.

b. Selection of venom extracts to be used for immunotherapy is entirely based upon venom skin test results. Therapy should include all venoms that demonstrate positive skin tests.

c. Immunotherapy schedule can follow any of several recommended schedules (see Tables 11.4 and 11.5). The common "modified rush" regimen is much more rapid than "traditional" regimens, achieving the maintenance dose after eight weekly injections rather than 4 to 6 months. With this regimen, adverse reactions are no more common than in traditional regimens of inhalant allergen therapy, and the mean venom-specific IgG antibody response is greater and more rapidly achieved. Rush regimens utilizing rapidly progressive doses over a period of just 2 to 3 days have also been reported to be very safe and highly effective.

d. Maintenance dose should be 100 µg of each of the venoms giving positive skin test. VIT is at least 98% effective in completely preventing systemic allergic reactions, but lower doses (less than 100 µg) may not provide complete protection in 15% to 20% of patients. The same dose has been recommended to children age 3 years and older.

e. Interval of maintenance injections should be every 4 weeks for at least 1 year. Most experts agree that the maintenance interval may then be increased to every 6 to 8 weeks during the next 1 to 2 years.

f. Monitoring venom immunotherapy
   (1) Venom-specific IgG is useful to determine whether VIT is producing a protective response. Venom-specific IgG can be quantitated 2 to 3 months after a maintenance dose has been reached and then after 2 to 3 years of treatment to determine whether the venom-specific IgG concentration is adequately maintained when injections are given less frequently (i.e., 6- to 8-week interval).
   (2) Venom skin tests and RAST may be repeated every 2 to 3 years to determine if and when there has been a significant decline in venom-specific IgE. Skin tests generally remain unchanged in the first 2 to 3 years, but may show a significant decline after 4 to 6 years. Less than 20% of patients become skin test negative after 5 years, but 50% to 60% become negative after 7 to 10 years.

g. Adverse reactions
VIT causes reactions no more frequently than inhalant allergen immunotherapy. Systemic reactions occur after immunotherapy injections in 10% to 15% of patients during the initial weeks of treatment, regardless of the regimen used. Most reactions are mild, and fewer than half require epinephrine. In the unusual case of recurrent systemic reactions to injections, therapy may be streamlined to a single venom and given in divided doses, 30 minutes apart. Large local reactions are common, occurring in up to 50% of patients, especially in the dose range of 20 to 50 µg. Unlike standard inhalant immunotherapy, there is a uniform target dose in VIT, so it is occasionally necessary to advance the dose in the face of moderately severe local reactions. Premedication with antihistamine is associated with fewer local and systemic reactions to injections, and fewer systemic reactions to strings.

Table 11.4. Representative treatment schedule
using Pharmalgen single venom preparation[a]

Week	Day	Dose No. per day at 0.5-h intervals	Concentration of venom to be used (μg/mL)	Volume for subcutaneous injection (mL)	Amount of venom injected (μg protein)
1	1	1	0.01	0.1	0.001
		2	0.1	0.1	0.01
		3	1.0	0.1	0.1
2	8	1	1.0	0.1	0.1
		2	1.0	0.5	0.5
		3	10	0.1	1.0
3	15	1	10	0.1	1
		2	10	0.5	5
		3	10	1.0	10
4	22	1	100	0.1	10
		2	100	0.2	20
5	29	1	100	0.2	20
		2	100	0.3	30
6	36	1	100	0.3	30
		2	100	0.3	30
7	43	1	100	0.4	40
		2	100	0.4	40
8	50	1	100	0.5	50
		2	100	0.5	50
9	57	1	100	1.0	100
Monthly[b]		1	100	1.0	100

[a] The following conditions for proceeding to next dose must be observed: (1) If a single dose results in more than a moderate local reaction (wheal >5.0 cm) within 0.5 h, an additional dose should not be given during that visit. Repeat the same dose at the next visit(s) until tolerated. (2) If a systemic manifestation of sensitivity occurs during or following a visit, or a single dose results in an excessive local reaction (wheal >10 cm) within 0.5 h, do not administer an additional dose during the visit, and reduce the total dosage for the next visit to half the total resulting in the reaction. (3) Delayed (24–48 h) local reactions <10 cm do not require a dose adjustment. For delayed local reactions >10 cm, hold dose at previous level.

For the mixed vespid preparation, the total venom protein concentration and the total amount of venom protein injected will be triple the amounts shown (300 μg maintenance), with no changes in injection volumes.

[b] If a patient on maintenance therapy is stung and has any systemic manifestation of sensitivity, the maintenance dosage should be increased to 200 μg for the relevant venom, using increments no greater than 50 μg.

From *Pharmalgen venom extract treatment schedule*. Wallingford, CT: Pharmacia Diagnostics, ALK America, Inc., 1995, with permission.

h. Discontinuing treatment
   (1) General. The product package insert, unchanged since its inception 22 years ago, states that therapy should be continued indefinitely. However, long-term follow-up studies of adults and children demonstrate that VIT can, in general, be stopped after 5 years, even in the presence of persistent positive skin tests. Observation of patients for 5 to 10 years after completing 5 to 8 years of venom treatment (mean 6 years) has shown a 10% risk of systemic symptoms each time he or she is stung, but only a 2% risk of a reaction requiring epinephrine treatment. Patients who show a higher frequency of significant systemic reactions include those who have had

Table 11.5. Representative treatment schedule
using Venomil single venom preparation[a]

Week number	Concentration of venom to be used (μg/mL)	Volume for subcutaneous injection (mL)	Amount of venom injected (μg protein)
1	1	0.05	0.05
2	1	0.10	0.1
3	1	0.20	0.2
4	1	0.40	0.4
5	10	0.05	0.5
6	10	0.10	1
7	10	0.20	2
8	10	0.40	4
9	100	0.05	5
10	100	0.10	10
11	100	0.20	20
12	100	0.40	40
13	100	0.60	60
14	100	0.80	80
15	100	1.00	100
16	100	1.00	100
18	100	1.00	100
21	100	1.00	100
Monthly	100	1.00	100

[a] Precaution regarding progression is similar to that in Table 11.4.
Multiple venom sensitivities are treated with individual single venom preparations given simultaneously at separate sites. (Except, if the patient has separate sensitivities to Yellow Jacket, Yellow Hornet, and White-Faced Hornet venoms concurrently, the patient can receive mixed vespid venom protein.) Patients with such sensitivities have an increased risk of systemic reactions.
From *Venomil hymenoptera treatment schedule.* Spokane, WA: Hollister-Stier, Miles, Inc., with permission.

a systemic reaction (to a sting or an injection) during the period of VIT and patients receiving honeybee VIT. Although studies differ on whether there is a higher reaction rate in patients with a history of very severe pretreatment sting reactions than in the patients who had milder reactions, experts agree that these patients are more prone to any reaction being more severe. Patients who had life-threatening reactions should be considered for indefinite treatment.

(2) Children. Insect allergy in children is said to have a more benign and transient course than in adults. Some surveys indicate up to 50% loss of sensitivity over a 10-year period in children and young adults. In a follow-up of the hundreds of children evaluated in the Johns Hopkins program 15 to 20 years ago, the frequency of systemic reaction to subsequent stings was significantly lower (4%) in those who had received a course of VIT than those who did not (15%). Among the untreated patients, the reaction rate was higher in those with a history of moderate-to-severe reactions (36%) than in patients who had had milder reactions (11%). These results suggest that children with mild systemic reactions do have a benign course. Those who have more severe reactions have a high residual risk up to 15 years later, which can be eliminated by a course of immunotherapy.

Biting insect allergy

Although stinging insects cause most insect-related systemic reactions, anaphylaxis has been reported in a small number of cases from biting insects. Allergic reactions to biting insects are more commonly manifest by large local swellings. There are also inhalant allergies (rhinitis and asthma) from the airborne allergens produced by certain insects, both indoors (e.g., cockroach) and outdoors (caddisfly and midge). Materials for testing are commercially available for some of these biting and inhalant insect allergens, but there are few studies of their diagnostic utility or predictive value.

Mosquito allergy is not uncommon and causes large local inflammatory reactions to the salivary antigens. Children with multiple such reactions are said to have "Skeeter syndrome." Like other large local reactions, antihistamines help the itching, but not the swelling. Oral prednisone is effective, but the reactions can be frequent and this could lead to significant steroid side effects. Commercial mosquito extracts are of uncertain value, and research is proceeding to improve the allergen vaccine to clinically reliable levels.

Triatoma (kissing bug) allergy may manifest as systemic reactions of variable severity. Characteristically, these insects are early morning feeders, and bites usually occur on exposed areas (e.g., arms and face) while the individual is sleeping. *Triatoma* live in warm climates, especially in the southwestern and southeastern United States, Texas, and the Gulf states. Rodents are common vectors. Allergy to these biting insects is uncommon, and anaphylactic reactions usually occur in individuals with repeated bites.

Treatment of allergic reactions to biting insects is directed to symptomatic management of the acute reaction and to avoidance precautions, as with Hymenoptera sensitivity. In the case of *Triatoma* allergy, immunotherapy using a salivary gland extract was demonstrated to be effective. However, no commercial extract is currently available.

Selected Readings

Golden DBK, Kagey-Sobotka A, Lichtenstein LM. Survey of patients after discontinuing venom immunotherapy. *J Allergy Clin Immunol* 2000;105:385–390.

Golden DBK. Stinging insect vaccines: Patient selection and administration of Hymenoptera venom immunotherapy. In: Lefford DK, Lockey RF, ed. Immunotherapy: a practical review and guide. *Immunol Allergy Clin North Am* 2000;20:553–570.

Golden DBK, Kagey-Sobotka A, Norman PS, et al. Insect allergy with negative venom skin test responses. *J Allergy Clin Immunol* 2001;107:897–901.

Portnoy JM, Moffitt JE, Golden DBK, et al. Stinging insect hypersensitivity: A practice parameter. *J Allergy Clin Immunol* 1999;103:963–980.

Yunginger JW. Insect allergy. In: Middleton E Jr, Reed CE, Ellis EF, et al., eds. *Allergy: principles and practice*, 5th ed. St. Louis: Mosby, 1998:1063–1072.

12. DRUG ALLERGY

Eric Macy, Michael H. Mellon, Michael Schatz, and Roy Patterson

Although the understanding of drug allergy is increasing, it remains a source of confusion for clinicians and patients. Much of the confusion is semantic. Allergy to an allergist means a reaction mediated through antigen-specific immunoglobulin E (IgE) and subsequent mediator release from mast cells and basophils. Thus, the spectrum of clinical symptoms possible in an allergic drug reaction is essentially limited to urticaria, angioedema, bronchospasm, hypotension, and other signs of anaphylaxis. Allergic reactions occur immediately when antigen cross-links IgE bound to mast cells. There can be a delay in onset of the reaction during which time the body is producing IgE, but when the IgE is already present and the antigen is introduced the reactions occur within minutes. Allergy to an immunologist can additionally include reactions mediated by antigen-specific antibody (non-IgE) or T cells. These reactions can have a much more protean set of manifestations, ranging from vasculitis to complement-mediated cell lysis to skin destruction. These reactions are generally slower to evolve and slower to resolve than IgE-mediated reactions in which people live or die within the first hour or so. Allergy as used in the *Physicians' Desk Reference* can mean any effect on cells or proteins potentially involved in immune responses, including, but not limited, to complement, cytokines, natural killer (NK) cells, mast cells, basophils, B cells, T cells, and macrophage/monocytic/dendritic cells. Allergy to the general population can also mean any adverse reaction, no matter what the mechanism. For the purposes of this chapter **allergic** will mean mediated by antigen-specific IgE; **immunologic** will be mediated by any antigen-specific immune response; and **pharmacologic** will be used to refer to drug effects on the cells or mediators involved in the immune system. The entire group will be referred to as **adverse drug reactions**.

I. **Classification of adverse drug reactions**
   A. **Non-drug-related reactions**
      1. **Psychogenic reactions**, such as vasovagal reactions to injections, can be manifested as anxiety, nausea, lethargy, or syncope.
      2. **Coincidental reactions**, caused by the disease under treatment, can be mistakenly attributed to a drug concurrently used (e.g., viral exanthemata in children treated with antibiotics).
   B. **Drug-related reactions**
      1. **Adverse reactions that can occur in all patients**
         a. **Side effects** are due to therapeutically undesirable but unavoidable pharmacologic actions of a drug occurring with normal drug dosages; side effects constitute the most frequent adverse drug reaction (e.g., tachycardia with epinephrine injection and sedation with classical antihistamines).
         b. **Overdose** refers to toxic pharmacologic effects of a drug that are directly related to the systemic or local concentration of the drug in the body (e.g., respiratory depression with sedatives). Overdose is one adverse effect that can be reduced by systems that double-check human action, e.g., physician prescriptions, pharmacist dispensing.
         c. **Secondary effects** are only indirectly related to the primary pharmacologic action of the drug (e.g., the release of microbial antigens and endotoxins after antibiotic treatment, such as the Jarisch-Herxheimer reaction seen in certain cases of syphilis treated with penicillin).
         d. **Drug interactions** can alter the normal physiology of the host and change the response to one or a number of drugs (e.g., enzyme induction by one drug causing altered metabolism of another drug). It is possible to dramatically reduce drug interaction problems

using computerized systems if patients have one source for their health care.

2. **Adverse reactions relating to patient susceptibility**

   a. **Intolerance** is the production of a characteristic pharmacologic effect by small dosages of a drug in certain persons. An example is excessive sedation with low doses of classical antihistamines or excessive cough with an angiotensin-converting enzyme (ACE) inhibitor.

   b. **Idiosyncrasy** is a qualitatively abnormal response to a drug that is different from its pharmacologic effects. It occurs only in susceptible patients and may or may not be predictable. Primaquine-induced hemolytic anemia in a patient known to be deficient in glucose-6-phosphate dehydrogenase and coumadin-induced skin necrosis in patients with known protein C deficiency are examples of predictable idiosyncratic reactions. Aplastic anemia with chloramphenicol is an example of an unpredictable idiosyncratic reaction. A partially predictable idiosyncratic reaction is angioedema amplification with ACE inhibitors.

   c. **Allergic, immunologic, and pharmacologic** reactions occur in selected patients with the production of specific antibodies, sensitized lymphocytes, and/or effects on immune system cells or immune system-generated biological response modifiers because of exposure to a drug or its metabolites. The general mechanisms of these adverse drug reactions are as follows:

      (1) **Allergic or immunoglobulin E-mediated reactions** involve the production of drug-specific IgE. The cross-linking of drug-specific IgE bound to mast cells or basophils and their subsequent degranulation mediates the clinical symptoms seen in drug allergy. There must be an adequate time of exposure to generate IgE, and typically the first exposure, if short, does not result in an allergic reaction. The clinical manifestations of allergic drug reactions (urticaria, angioedema, hypotension, bronchospasm, and/or other signs of anaphylaxis) often do not resemble known pharmacologic actions of the drug or the disease being treated. The three types of materials that can cause IgE-mediated reactions are antigenic proteins, typically greater than 5000 D in size, small molecules that function as haptens or have metabolic byproducts that can function as haptens, and bivalent small molecules such as certain neuromuscular blocking agents. Penicillins, which can function as haptens, are the class of drugs most commonly associated with allergic drug reactions.

      (2) **Pharmacologic activation or inactivation of immune-system-associated biologic response modifiers** occurs in the following examples: endotoxin contamination inducing interleukin 1 (IL-1) release, skin rashes associated with therapeutic uses of recombinant interleukin 2 (rIL-2), and flushing, fever, or urticaria associated with monoclonal antibody inactivation of tumor necrosis factor (TNF). Cytokine-mediated effects can result in general phenomena such as drug fever or very specific cell function defects such as hypogammaglobulinemia associated with phenytoin or carbamazepine.

      (3) **Antibody-mediated cytolytic reactions** occur in Coombs positive hemolytic anemias. The reaction proceeds when a drug such as penicillin causes the production of a penicillin-specific IgG or IgM, which then binds to penicillin haptenated to red blood cell surface proteins. Complement then binds to the antibody cross-linking the penicillin and lyses the red blood cell.

(4) **Immune complex reactions** occur when antigen-specific IgG binds with antigens and these antigen–antibody complexes are deposited in the kidney or joints. Examples include dextran- or methicillin-induced interstitial nephritis, serum sickness from xenoantisera or cefaclor, and drug-induced lupus. Immune complex reactions can result in a vasculitic appearance on pathologic exam.

(5) **T-cell-mediated delayed-type hypersensitivity** (DTH) is the mechanism of the classic poison oak reaction. The antigen binds to a skin protein and the T-cell arm of the immune system rejects the modified protein as it would a foreign tissue graft. Examples include contact sensitivity to adhesive tape, para-amino benzoic acid (PABA), and many other topical medications. Drug-specific T-cell clones have been identified that may contribute to maculopapular eruptions and help explain the high incidence of non-IgE-mediated rashes occurring in individuals receiving antibiotics during viral infections.

(6) **Cell-mediated cytotoxicity** reactions can occur from cancer treatment protocols that are directed at boosting endogenous immune reactions to tumor-specific cell proteins, such as through vaccines, *ex vivo* immune cell proliferation, or gene therapy.

(7) **Granulomatous reactions** include reactions to materials that cannot be cleared by the body, such as talc in the peritoneal cavity and bovine collagen under the skin.

   d. **Direct mast cell effects** are also called pseudoallergic or anaphylactoid reactions. Examples include reactions to intravenous (i.v.) contrast dye, hives with subcutaneous opiates, and hive amplification or asthma induced by nonsteroidal antiinflammatory drugs (NSAIDs).

II. Diagnosis of drug allergy

  A. History is the most important tool in evaluating drug allergy. Attention needs to be paid to exactly what drugs were taken, when they were started and stopped, what reactions occurred, and when the reactions started and stopped. Factors that influence reactions include age, genetic background, chemical properties of the drug, dose and duration of treatment, route of administration, and frequency of drug treatment. Relevant drugs usually have been taken within several weeks of the onset of the reaction. Demoly and coworkers have developed a useful drug hypersensitivity questionnaire.

  B. Diagnostic tests to confirm drug allergy are becoming more useful.

  Tryptase, which is a stable mast cell protein with a half-life of about 2 hours, is used to determine if mast cell degranulation was a part of the pathologic cause of the clinical manifestations seen. If a tryptase level (i.e., β-tryptase) is negative within 6 hours of the onset of the symptoms, it is very hard to implicate an IgE-mediated anaphylactic episode or a direct mast cell degranulation event. Tryptase can be measured postmortem and has been used to document anaphylactoid deaths in individuals using illegal opiates.

  Antigen-specific IgE can now be measured via a variety of *in vitro* test systems. A relatively limiting number of useful drug-specific tests are currently available, including native penicillin, penicilloyl-poly-lysine, latex, and egg for vaccines, but the list is growing. Flow cytometry has been used to measure IgG directed against cefotetan. Antigen-specific *in vitro* lymphocyte transformation tests may be useful in the future.

  Skin tests are still the most widely used tool to evaluate IgE-mediated reactions caused by potential haptens, such as penicillin metabolites, or intact protein allergy. Skin testing done on molecules that function as haptens must take into account potential reactive metabolites. If skin testing is to be done with an intact protein that has not been well studied, it can generally be safely done using the protocol worked out for honeybee venom, a well-characterized, highly purified, and antigenic protein. Most other materials would be less pure and less antigenic. One should start with 1 µg per mL of protein in a skin testing buffer via the prick–puncture technique. Diluent buffers are commercially available from companies that sell immunotherapy materials. Prick testing should always be done before any intradermal testing. The plain buffer should always be used as a negative control and a histamine-positive control. Prick testing with 1 µg per mL will typically result in potential systemic exposure of less than 1 ng of active allergen. Intradermal skin testing should be started with 0.01 µg per mL, followed by 0.1 µg per mL and them 1 µg per mL. Intradermal testing with 0.05 mL at 1 µg per mL will result in systemic exposure of less than 50 ng of protein. If the final therapeutic protein is of significantly greater concentration, additional intradermal skin tests should be done with 10-fold greater concentrations until the full-strength material is tested. Each test needs to be read at 20 minutes, thus the entire protocol can take several hours. A skin test should never be done with an intact protein allergen with an unknown concentration. Systemic reactions have occurred with latex glove extracts for which the protein concentrations were not quantitated prior to use. One typically starts parenteral protein desensitization regimens with 2-fold more protein than was used for the positive skin test and doubles the dose every 20 minutes until full therapeutic dose is achieved. The information cited above is not based on controlled studies. Skin testing with unproven agents may not have a predictive value for the diagnosis of drug allergies and should be done in the context of research.

Patch tests are used to determine DTH reactions.

Antinuclear antibodies (ANA), particularly antihistone, may be positive in drug-induced lupus (Table 12.1).

III. **Preventing allergic, immunologic, and pharmacologic adverse drug reactions**
Avoid agents associated with historical reactions. Not knowing history dooms one to repeat it. Computerized healthcare system-wide adverse drug event

Table 12.1. A comparison of drug-induced
and spontaneous systemic lupus erythematosus

Clinical and laboratory findings	Drug induced	Spontaneous
Clinical findings		
Age	Older	Younger
Sex	Often seen in males	More common in females
Renal involvement	Less common	More common
Central nervous system involvement	Less common	More common
Rash	Less common	More common
Anemia, thrombocytopenia, leukopenia	Less common	More common
Serositis	More common	Less common
Laboratory findings		
Antibodies to native (double-stranded) DNA	Rare	Often present
Antibody to histones	Primary antinucleoprotein antibody	One of several antinucleoprotein antibodies
Slow acetylators	More susceptible	Probably no increased incidence
Complement levels	Normal	Often reduced

surveillance has been shown to reduce these events. **Minimize overall drug exposure.** Individuals with a history of adverse reaction to antibiotics and who are penicillin skin-test-positive are anecdotally more likely to have adverse reactions with future unrelated antibiotics than individuals who are skin-test-negative. **Desensitization** can be used where an IgE-mediated reaction has been documented and the future use of the drug is essential. **Graded challenges and provocative dose testing** are commonly done in patients with histories of adverse reactions when there is no available predictive *in vitro* or skin test and there is a strong clinical indication for the drug. Patients with histories of toxic epidermal necrolysis (TEN) or Stevens-Johnson syndrome (SJS) are unique in that the risk of repeat adverse reaction is so great as to preclude any thought of rechallenge. No test adequately predicts these life-threatening types of reaction at present. Induction of true immunologic **tolerance** is the long-term, but still unrealized goal.

IV. **Management of allergic, immunologic, and pharmacologic adverse drug reactions**

Discontinuation of the responsible drug is the most important treatment in an ongoing drug reaction. Many patients experiencing an apparent drug reaction are taking multiple drugs and the causative drug may not be readily identifiable. The drug(s) that are most likely to be causing the reaction (based on the considerations previously discussed) and least essential for the patient's well being should be discontinued. The symptomatic treatment of anaphylaxis, urticaria, asthma, or contact dermatitis due to an adverse drug reaction is the same as the treatment when these conditions are the result of other causes. Aspirin and antihistamines often suffice in the treatment of serum sickness, but corticosteroids may be necessary. Local treatment of the pruritus associated with maculopapular eruptions is often sufficient, but oral antihistamines may be useful in addition.

The use of systemic corticosteroids, i.v. gamma globulin, or cyclosporin A is controversial when exfoliative dermatitis, TEN, or SJS is present. Stopping the offending medication and providing supportive care are the cornerstones of treatment. Pathologic exam of involved tissue in TEN and SJS has revealed features of graft versus host disease. Sulfa antibiotics, barbiturates, carbamazepine, and allopurinol have been reported as the most common causes of TEN. Sulfa antibiotics, chlormezanone, aminopenicillins, quinolones, and cephalosporins have been reported to have the highest rates of SJS, but in all cases the rates are less than 5 per 1 million users per week of exposure.

Supportive treatment of hematologic drug reactions may include transfusions, and the addition of corticosteroids may decrease red cell destruction in Coombs positive anemias. Corticosteroids may also be useful in hastening recovery from vasculitic, hepatic, renal, and pulmonary reactions. Certain patients with vasculitis related to drug reactions may require cytotoxic therapy in addition.

A. **Proteins used in health care**

1. **Human proteins include cytokines, hormones, antibodies, and other serum proteins**

   a. **Cytokines**

   IL-2 has been associated with a wide range of cutaneous reactions including erythema and pruritis in greater than 10% of individuals exposed to pharmacologic doses. Treatment is symptomatic.

   b. **Hormones**

   Insulin is the most widely used human hormone and serves as a good model for what to expect with reactions occurring with other protein hormones such as oxytocin, secretin, or adrenocorticotropic hormone (ACTH). **Local reactions** to insulin occur in 5% to 10% of patients and are usually mild, localized, and transient. The swelling, pruritus, and pain can occur and subside within an hour after insulin injection or may begin up to 24 hours afterward. Some patients exhibit a biphasic reaction, with an early reaction resolving in 1 hour followed by a later, more persistent reaction beginning after 4 to 6 hours. Local reactions occasionally progress to painful induration that persists for days. Local reactions generally develop within 2 weeks of the initiation of insulin therapy and usually resolve spontaneously within weeks. However, large local reactions, especially ones increasing in intensity, can precede a systemic reaction.

Systemic reactions to insulin are very uncommon. The most frequent clinical characteristic is generalized urticaria, although other features of anaphylaxis can be present. Systemic reactions usually occur soon after reinstitution of insulin therapy after a period, often years, without it. Lispro has also been used with success in individuals with systemic reactions to insulin.

Insulin **resistance** is rarely immunologic. It is most likely to occur within the first year of insulin therapy, usually develops over several weeks, and is usually temporary, lasting only several days to several months. Immunologic insulin resistance develops in some patients with insulin allergy within days of initiating insulin desensitization due to the production of increased amounts of anti-insulin IgG.

The causative **antigen** in apparent insulin allergy can be a **non-insulin** protein contaminant or possibly a nonprotein component such as protamine or zinc. However, skin test positivity and systemic reactions to highly purified human insulin occur, indicating the **insulin molecule itself** or closely related higher-molecular-weight polymers can induce IgE-mediated reactions. Almost all insulin now used is recombinant human insulin, which is less immunogenic than pork insulin. There are very rare patients who, by skin test titration, are more sensitive to human insulin than to pork insulin.

Because **local reactions** are usually mild and transient, no specific therapy is needed. For more troublesome or persistent reactions, the following sequential approach should be used: (i) administer **antihistamines**; (ii) divide the dose of insulin, using separate sites, until reactions disappear; and (iii) switch to purified pork insulin or synthetic human insulin without zinc. An increase in the intensity of local reactions demands **careful surveillance** for the onset of a systemic reaction. In insulin-dependent patients, discontinuation of insulin therapy because of local reactions is not advisable, both from the standpoint of optimal management of the diabetes and because interruption of therapy can increase the chances of a systemic reaction on subsequent readministration of insulin.

Treat systemic allergic reactions to insulin in the same manner as anaphylaxis (see Chapter 10). The occurrence of a systemic reaction dictates reassessment of the need for insulin. However, in most diabetic patients in whom insulin therapy is initiated, no substitute exists. If the patient is evaluated within 24 to 48 hours of the allergic reaction and if continued insulin therapy is essential, do not discontinue insulin therapy. In the hospital, with the patient under careful observation, the dose should be reduced to one-third or one-fourth of the original dose. The dose should be gradually increased over several days until a therapeutic dose is achieved. If there has been an interruption of insulin therapy for more than 48 hours, insulin skin testing and desensitization are indicated.

Insulin skin testing is used to determine the least reactive insulin for the patient (purified pork or synthetic human insulin) and the level of sensitivity. Fresh serial 10-fold dilutions of regular insulins should be prepared and serial intradermal tests should be performed starting at 0.000001 units per mL until positive reactions occur. To begin **desensitization**, the least reactive insulin should be used at a concentration one-tenth as strong as the most dilute preparation giving a positive test. A 30-minute wait between each subsequent dose is necessary. All desensitizations should be done in a hospital or clinical setting under direct observation with the ability to treat anaphylaxis. Regular insulin should be used initially and intermediate-acting or longer-acting preparations should be added only after the patient has tolerated full therapeutic doses of regular insulin. If a **local reaction** occurs, before the dose is increased, the same dose should be repeated until minimal or no reactions are present. If a **systemic reaction** occurs, the reaction should be treated and then the dose decreased by one-half and increased at smaller (2- to 5-fold) increments.

For patients with rapidly increasing insulin requirements, nonimmunologic causes should be ruled out. For immunologic insulin resistance persisting more than several days, switching to purified pork or synthetic human insulin may be the only therapy necessary. In other patients, switching to more concentrated (U-500 [500 units per mL]) or sulfated insulin preparations may be successful. When unstable diabetes or increasing insulin requirements complicate insulin resistance, corticosteroid therapy (initially to 60 mg of prednisone daily, 1 to 2 mg/kg/day in children) can be initiated. The clinician should watch for hypoglycemia at this time; it may occur as the insulin requirement falls rapidly. When insulin therapy has been stabilized, the prednisone can be converted to an alternate-day regimen, tapered, and possibly discontinued. The clinician should keep in mind that corticosteroids can increase blood glucose levels, so careful monitoring is essential.

c. **Antibodies**

Rare adverse reactions occur to IM administration of concentrated human disease specific antibodies such as RhoGAM or hepatitis B immune globulin. Acute febrile reactions probably secondary to immune complex formation are commonly reported with intravenous immunoglobulin (IVIg). Pretreatment with antiinflammatory medications and antihistamines, along with slowing the rate of infusion, adequately treats most of these reactions. Rare cases of IgE directed against contaminating IgA have been reported in IgA-deficient individuals receiving IVIg. These cases are best managed by using the preparations of IVIg that have the lowest amount of IgA.

d. **Other human serum proteins**

Materials such as ethylene-oxide-modified human albumin contaminating dialysis equipment sterilized with ethylene oxide have been associated with anaphylaxis. Anaphylactoid reactions to recombinant tissue plasminogen activator (rTPA) appear to be more common in individuals treated for stroke, up to 2%, compared to individuals treated for coronary disease, less than 0.02%. This difference is thought to be secondary to complement activation. This side effect can be treated promptly if care is taken to examine the oropharynx for edema 30 to 45 minutes after initiation of therapy in patients with presumed stroke. If edema is noted, prompt treatment with antihistamines is required. Individuals with acquired or hereditary angioedema secondary to reduced levels of functional C1 esterase inhibitor are at very high risk for this side effect.

2. **Humanized proteins (specifically humanized mouse monoclonal antibodies)**

Even though the frequency of IgE generation against these materials is orders of magnitude lower than that for native mouse monoclonal antibodies, reactions still occur in rare individuals. The anti-Her 2 receptor, trastuzumab (Herceptin) (which is active in breast cancer), is one of the most widely used product. By 2000, 15 deaths and 62 anaphylactoid reactions had been reported for trastuzumab. Another example of a similar mouse–human hybrid monoclonal antibody is the antitumor necrosis factor alpha, infliximab, used for rheumatoid arthritis.

3. Nonhuman proteins

Protein such as bovine serum albumin in cell culture material used in bone marrow culture or *in vitro* fertilization procedures has been documented to cause IgE-mediated allergy. Murine monoclonal antibodies have been associated with numerous IgE-mediated and other immunologic reactions. Chymopapain has been associated with IgE-mediated anaphylaxis, but could only be used for puncture skin testing because its effect as a proteolytic enzyme caused direct tissue damage when used intradermally.

a. Bacterial products

Streptokinase and asparaginase are two examples of therapeutic bacteria proteins. Allergy to one form of asparaginase has not been shown to adversely effect overall cancer therapy outcome.

b. Vaccines

The egg protein in vaccine raised in eggs, such as influenza, is a potential allergen, but only rarely causes a problem, even in egg-allergic individuals, because its level is so low in most modern vaccines. Hen egg allergen is heat labile, thus an individual who tolerates cooked eggs, but reacts to raw egg would be more likely to react to the raw egg in influenza vaccine. The full-strength vaccine itself can be used as the skin test reagent. Soluble diphtheria or tetanus toxoid can be used as a skin-testing reagent at full strength, although most older individuals with a history of "tetanus allergy" actually had serum sickness to equine tetanus antitoxin.

Hypersensitivity reactions to vaccines are rare and will usually occur soon after administration. The four types of allergic reactions considered to be related to vaccine constituents are listed in the following section.

(1) Allergic reactions to egg-related antigen (e.g., yellow fever and influenza vaccines). Patients with history of systemic reaction to egg ingestion may be skin tested with the vaccine and, if positive, given the vaccine in incremental dosing of subcutaneous injections of

  (a) 0.05 mL of 1:10 dilution
  (b) 0.05 mL of full strength
  (c) 0.10 mL of full strength
  (d) 0.15 mL of full strength
  (e) 0.20 mL of full strength

(2) Recent evidence suggests that influenza vaccine containing less than 1.2 μg per mL of egg protein can be given safely to egg-allergic children in a two-dose protocol—the first dose being one-tenth and the second dose being nine-tenths of the recommended dose for age. Measles, mumps, rubella (MMR); measles; and mumps vaccines contain insufficient amounts of egg protein currently to warrant prior skin testing before administration to egg-allergic children.

(3) Hypersensitivity reactions to mercury-containing preservatives (i.e., thimerosal) in vaccines such as diphtheria, tetanus, acellular pertussis (DtaP); *Haemophilus influenzae* type B (Hib) diphtheria, tetanus (DT, Td); and influenza. No live virus vaccines contain thimerosal.

(4) Antibiotic induced allergic reactions. Inactivated poliomyelitis vaccine (IPV) contains trace amounts of streptomycin, neomycin, and polymyxin B. Neomycin is also found in MMR and varicella vaccine. Neomycin may cause a delayed local reaction of erythematous pruritic papules and is not considered a contraindication for administration of these vaccines, unlike true anaphylactoid reactions.

(5) Hypersensitivity reactions to other vaccine components (e.g., gelatin in MMR and varicella vaccines) and to the infectious agent (e.g., tetanus) may require skin testing prior to administration of these vaccines or consideration of hyperimmuno-globulin (e.g., Hypertet), when available.

c. **Immunotherapy materials**

Immunotherapy (IMT) materials are thought to cause several deaths annually in the United States. Individuals need to be observed for at least 30 minutes after the injection. IMT should only be administered by individuals able to treat anaphylaxis.

d. **Latex allergy**

In the late 1980s, reports of severe, life-threatening, immediate-type allergic reactions after latex exposure appeared. These peaked in the early 1990s and have steadily decreased due to the reduction of natural rubber latex proteins in the healthcare environment. These reactions have occurred in nonmedical and medical settings, although the most severe have occurred in medical settings (e.g., intraoperative anaphylactic reactions, latex-cuffed barium enema catheters). High-risk groups for development of latex allergy include patients with spina bifida or urogenital abnormalities, and those who have had frequent surgical procedures, healthcare workers who regularly wear latex gloves, and workers employed in the manufacturing of rubber products.

All patients should be questioned about a history of latex allergy. Important clues include oral itching or swelling after dental examinations or blowing up balloons, local swelling or itching after vaginal or rectal examinations or after the use of condoms or diaphragms, and swelling or itching of hands after contact with latex. Any episode of unexplained anaphylaxis, particularly in a healthcare environment, could be from latex exposure. Some patients have milder generalized symptoms, such as increased nasal congestion and itching, similar to cat allergy. These high-risk patients should be offered commercially available *in vitro* enzyme-linked immunosorbent assay (ELISA) testing for latex allergy. All healthcare environments should strive to be as free of natural rubber latex protein as possible. Routine *in vitro* ELISA testing or skin testing for latex allergy is not recommended for persons with negative histories because of potential false-positive test results. It is much better to lower the overall exposure to latex to minimize sensitization and allergy in the whole population.

B. **Haptens**

1. **Beta-lactams**

Penicillins as a class are low molecular weight compounds that must covalently bind to tissue carrier proteins and form drug–protein conjugates, or haptens, to become immunogenic. Most reactions occur with parenteral administration, oral reactions are rarer, and healthcare workers are at a small risk for aerosolized beta-lactam-induced asthma if they are allergic. Topical exposures to penicillins are very sensitizing and oral penicillin can also cause T-cell-mediated skin reactions. Less than 10% of individuals with histories of "allergy" to penicillin are skin-test-positive. Skin testing to penicillin can also result in more appropriate antibiotic use, specifically less vancomycin, and may be safely done in advance of need.

Ninety-five percent of tissue-bound penicillin is found haptenated as benzylpenicilloyl and is thus termed the "major antigenic determinant."

The other 5% of tissue-bound metabolites are collectively termed the "minor antigenic determinants," a designation that refers only to their prevalence and not to their clinical or immunological significance. Three specific minor antigenic determinants have been identified that cover all clinically relevant penicillin core antigens. These minor determinant antigens are not immunologically cross-reactive and include benzylpenicillin, benzylpenicilloate, and benzylpenilloate. The major antigenic determinant is commercially available as a benzylpenicilloyl polylysine conjugate (Pre-Pen) to be used for prick and intradermal testing. Amoxicillin is used because it is the most common penicillin-class antibiotic and has an immunologically important side chain (Table 12.2). Skin tests to polyamines such as polylysine may result in false positives.

Alternative antibiotics should be used, if possible, in any patient with a positive history of a reaction to penicillin and especially with documented **skin test reactivity to penicillin major or minor determinant antigens**. Because all semisynthetic penicillins share the same highly reactive beta-lactam cores, patients with presumed or proved penicillin allergy should be considered allergic to the semisynthetic analogs of penicillin (e.g., ampicillin or amoxicillin). Significant clinical cross-reactivity between cephalosporins and penicillins is very rare. Antibodies to second- and third-generation cephalosporins are more often directed toward side-chain determinants that are not commonly shared among different beta-lactam drugs (Table 12.3). Standardized immunodiagnostic skin test reagents are not available to evaluate cephalosporin minor determinant sensitivity.

Three classes of antibiotics possess beta-lactam ring structures: the **monobactams, carbapenems**, and the **cephacarbams**. The cross-reactivity of the monobactams and carbapenems with penicillin has been well characterized. For example, in one study of 40 patients with positive allergic histories and positive skin tests to penicillin, almost 50% demonstrated reactivity to major and minor determinants of imipenem, a carbapenem. In contrast, there is no *in vitro* or clinical evidence of cross-reactivity between penicillin and aztreonam, the prototypical monobactam. Cross-reactivity between the cephacarbams and penicillin has not been determined.

In rare clinical situations, no suitable alternative antibiotic can be substituted for penicillin. In history-positive, skin-test-positive pa-

Table 12.2. Penicillin skin testing materials and concentrations

Reagent	Concentration	Source
Penicillin	0.01 molar	Benzylpenicillin sodium salt from www.sigma-aldrich.com, product no. 13752 or Na penicillin G for intravenous use
Pre-Pen	As supplied	Hollister Stier LLC
Penilloate	0.01 molar	Custom made by a university-level organic chemistry laboratory
Penicilloate	0.01 molar	Custom made by a university-level organic chemistry laboratory
Amoxicillin	0.01 molar	Amoxicillin from www.sigma-aldrich.com, product no. A8523
Control buffer		0.14 M NaCl and 0.02 M Trizma, pH to 7.4
Histamine control	1 mg/mL	Eli Lilly

Table 12.3. Beta-lactam antibiotics sharing side chains

Amoxicillin	Cefadroxil	Cefprozil[a,b]			
Cephalexin	Cephradine				
Ceftazidime	Aztreonam				
Cefamandole	Cefonicid				
Ampicillin	Cefaclor[b]	Cephradine	Cephalexin	Loracarbef	

[a] There have been 27 cases of serum sickness associated with cefprozil thru 1/97.
[b] Cefprozil and Cefaclor only differ by a single OH group on the relevant side chain.

tients, the risk of systemic or anaphylactic reactions is unacceptably high and penicillin cannot be administered without **desensitization**. Desensitization should be performed orally, because it is safer than parenteral desensitization. The outlined schedule (Table 12.4) begins by administering extremely small doses of antibiotic with a doubling of doses every 15 minutes. Full-dose oral therapy should be initiated immediately after completion of the schedule and must be continued without any lapses. If a dose is missed, repeat the desensitization. Adverse reactions, including pruritus, urticaria, and anaphylaxis are common, thereby mandating strict physician monitoring with continuous assessment of vital signs and cardiorespiratory status. An indwelling intravenous line must be in place for rapid administration of fluids and medications. Premedication, including H1-antihistamines or corticosteroids, has not been proven effective against systemic reactions induced by antigens (unlike radiocontrast material) and may mask the early signs of anaphylaxis. The development of systemic symptoms may

Table 12.4. Protocol for oral penicillin desensitization in patients with documented penicillin allergy

Time (min)	Concentration	Volume/ dose (mL)	Units of PCN/dose	Total (units of PCN)
0	10^2 units/mL[a]	0.5	50	50
15	10^2 units/mL	1.0	100	150
30	10^2 units/mL	2.0	200	350
45	10^2 units/mL	4.0	400	750
60	10^2 units/mL	8.0	800	1,550
75	10^3 units/mL	1.6	1,600	3,150
90	10^3 units/mL	3.2	3,200	6,350
105	10^3 units/mL	6.4	6,400	12,750
120	10^3 units/mL	12.5	12,500	25,250
135	10^4 units/mL	2.5	25,000	50,250
150	10^4 units/mL	5.0	50,000	100,250
165	10^4 units/mL	10.0	100,000	200,250
180	4×10^4 units/mL	5.0	200,000	400,250
195	4×10^4 units/mL	10.0	400,000	800,250
210	4×10^4 units/mL	20.0	800,000	1,600,250
225	Intravenous[b]		800,000	2,400,250

[a] Using Pen VK 125 mg/5 mL = 200,000 units/5 mL, or 40,000 units/mL; dilute 0.1 mL of "stock" into 40 mL for 100 units/mL. Dilute 1.0 mL of stock in 40 mL (final volume) for 1,000 units/mL and 10 mL of stock in 40 mL (final volume) for 10,000 units/mL.
[b] Penicillin G for intravenous use.
PCN, penicillin.

require repeating the previous dose or changing the incremental increases or dosage intervals. When possible, oral desensitization should be undertaken with the actual penicillin class antibiotic to be used. If future courses of penicillin are indicated, skin testing should be repeated and, if positive, desensitization must be repeated.

2. **Sulfonamides**

The diagnosis of sulfa allergy is evolving. IgE does not seem to be the predominate mechanism for sulfa reactions. There is no significant cross reaction with sulfa class antibiotics and other medications with sulfur moieties in them such as diuretics. Slow rechallenge or "desensitization" may be no better than full-dose rechallenge because there is about a 20% recurrence of the adverse reaction in either case.

C. **Bivalent small molecules**

Neuromuscular blockers are discussed in the Anesthesia reactions section (page 234).

V. **Management and treatment of materials associated with direct mast cell effects**

Intravenous contrast, NSAIDs, and **opiates** are three commonly used materials that are frequently associated with pharmacologic adverse drug reactions and all are mediated through their effects on mast cells, causing degranulation or amplification of ongoing degranulation. Fluorescein may cause adverse reactions via a similar mechanism.

A. **Intravenous contrast.** Adverse reactions occur in 5% to 8% of patients following administration of a radiocontrast medium (RCM). Serious reactions occur in 0.1% of patients, and the rate of fatal reactions is reported to be 1 in 40,000 to 1 in 50,000 procedures (a figure as high as 1 in 10,000 has been reported). The clinical manifestations can be classified by the type of the reaction (anaphylactoid, cardiopulmonary, miscellaneous) or the severity (minor, major). These reactions, except for renal failure, usually occur within 3 to 10 minutes after injection. Certain clinical conditions can increase the risk of certain types of contrast media reactions (Table 12.5). Although contrast media reactions can follow any route of exposure, they are most common with intravascular administration. RCM causes nonimmunologic mediator release in susceptible patients. Possible causes of the other reactions include direct chemotoxic effects, nonimmunologic complement activation, hemodynamic effects of the hypertonic solution, vagal stimulation, or other mechanisms. The majority of deaths following RCM are not associated with the clinical or pathologic features of anaphylaxis,

Table 12.5. Risk factors for contrast media reaction

Factor	Type of reaction
Age over 50 years	Cardiopulmonary
Preexisting cardiovascular disease	
Preexisting renal failure	Acute renal failure
Increased age	
Entities associated with potential renovascular impairment (diabetes, myeloma, hypertension, dehydration, hyperuricemia)	
Personal history of allergy, asthma	Mild or moderate anaphylactoid reaction (small increased risk)
History of prior anaphylactoid reaction to contrast media	Anaphylactoid reaction (large increased risk)

and autopsies often do not reveal the cause of death. Consequently, the cause of most fatal reactions to RCM is unknown.

Prevention of RCM reactions is difficult for several reasons. Because the reactions are nonimmunologic, sensitivity tests are not predictive. Furthermore, these reactions may occur on the first exposure to RCM. Preventive measures, however, can reduce the risk. In a patient with risk factors (Table 12.5), consider the feasibility of **alternative techniques** (such as radionuclide scanning or ultrasound) that may provide diagnostic information at less risk. The patient should be adequately **hydrated** to lessen the risk of acute renal failure in predisposed patients (although acute renal failure has occurred in adequately hydrated patients following contrast media studies). **Renal function** should be carefully monitored before and after the study in high-risk renal patients, so that supportive treatment of acute renal failure may be instituted as soon as possible. To reduce the risk of pulmonary edema in patients with cardiac disease, the clinician should **avoid sodium salts** of contrast media. **Electrocardiographic monitoring** should be used with cardiac patients during the procedure to allow early diagnosis and treatment of potentially fatal cardiac arrhythmias.

In terms of prevention of anaphylactoid reactions, if the RCM study is essential, the risk and probably the severity of a subsequent reaction can apparently be reduced by pretreatment with **antihistamines** and **corticosteroids**. Prednisone, 50 mg orally every 6 hours (1 mg/kg/dose for children), should be administered beginning 18 hours prior to the procedure, and **diphenhydramine**, 1.5 mg per kg intramuscularly (up to 50 mg) should be administered 30 minutes to 1 hour before the study. Whenever RCM is to be administered to a patient with a history of a prior reaction, the patient's informed consent should be obtained. Pretreatment can be given to patients with prior **miscellaneous** reactions, such as nausea, vomiting, or flushing, although these types of reactions may not significantly increase the risk of a subsequent adverse reaction. Lower osmolality contrast media should be used. **Remember:** Serious anaphylactoid RCM reactions may occur even with pretreatment. Therefore, the repeat test must be **essential** and the study must be performed under **careful observation**, with facilities and personnel immediately available to treat an adverse reaction. Pretreatment for the prevention of cardiopulmonary reactions, convulsions, or renal failure is not effective and **should not** be relied on to prevent these types of reactions.

The **treatment** of RCM reactions depends on the clinical manifestations. Minor miscellaneous-type reactions may require no treatment. Reactions mimicking IgE-mediated anaphylactic reactions should be treated as anaphylaxis (see Chapter 10). Standard therapy should be used for cardiac complications, convulsions, and renal failure following RCM administration. Delayed RCM reactions are more common with first exposure, previous reaction history, history of any allergy, and creatinine greater than 2 mg per dL.

B. **Nonsteroidal antiinflammatory drugs**

Aspirin is second to penicillins as a cause of adverse drug reactions. All of these reactions are mediated through the pharmacologic properties of aspirin, including nephrotoxicity related to salicylate abuse, hemolytic anemia in patients deficient in glucose-6-phosphate dehydrogenase, abnormal platelet function, gastrointestinal toxicity, hepatitis, and bone marrow suppression. The three syndromes of most interest to this review occur within 2 to 3 hours of aspirin ingestion: aspirin-sensitive asthma/rhinitis, urticaria/angioedema, and anaphylactoid reactions. The first two reactions are most common. The prevalence of aspirin-induced asthma (AIA) among asthmatics is much less than 10%. The prevalence of aspirin sensitivity by oral challenge in the subpopulation of asthma patients afflicted with nasal polyps and sinusitis increases to 30% to 40%. Females experience more adverse reactions than do males—as high as 2:1 in some studies. The genetics of aspirin sensitivity are not known, but a familial occurrence may exist.

1. Asthma/rhinitis
a. Pathogenesis

The pathogenesis of AIA remains undefined. An immunologic mechanism has not been proved in aspirin-sensitive asthmatic patients. The most attractive hypotheses relate to an imbalance of arachidonic acid metabolites. Prostaglandin synthesis inhibition (through inhibition of the cyclooxygenase (COX) pathway for arachidonic acid metabolism) is a function of aspirin, indomethacin, ibuprofen, and mefenamic acid. These seemingly unrelated compounds are all capable of provoking asthma in sensitive patients. The prostaglandin E series produces bronchodilation, whereas the prostaglandin F series causes bronchoconstriction. An imbalance between the effects of aspirin on the two series could cause asthma in susceptible patients. Alternatively, blockage of the COX pathway might increase the formation of products of the lipoxygenase pathway, particularly leukotrienes (LT) C, D, and E, which are also capable of causing bronchospasm, especially in aspirin-sensitive asthmatics. Recent studies of urinary LTE_4 before and after challenge in aspirin-sensitive asthmatics and the inhibitory effects of an LTD_4 antagonist on AIA support this hypothesis.

Another potential mechanism involves aspirin-induced nonimmunologic release of mediators from respiratory mast cells. The final explanation for aspirin idiosyncrasy may relate to the complex interactions between the respiratory mast cell, preformed mediators, prostaglandins, and leukotrienes (see also Chapter 6).

b. History

The typical aspirin-sensitive asthmatic patient begins with perennial rhinitis during young adulthood to middle age that can be exacerbated by aspirin intake. Subsequently, nasal polyps, hyperplastic and purulent sinusitis, peripheral eosinophilia, and asthma typically develop at variable intervals, leading to the classic "aspirin-triad" of asthma, nasal polyps, and aspirin idiosyncrasy. Aspirin-sensitive asthma can occur in patients without significant rhinitis, polyps, or sinusitis. Although nearly 50% of aspirin-sensitive asthmatics can have positive skin tests to common allergens, the asthma in such patients is usually triggered primarily by nonallergic or unidentifiable factors.

Acute AIA may be severe, prolonged, and occasionally fatal; is usually associated with profound nasal congestion, rhinorrhea, and/or ocular injection; and is occasionally associated with syncope. It should be treated vigorously, with therapy that includes the use of parenteral corticosteroids.

c. Diagnosis

The **history** and **physical findings** in aspirin-sensitive patients can be similar to such findings in other patients with asthma or rhinitis. A history of aspirin intolerance may or may not be elicited from the patient. Nasal polyps, commonly found in patients with the aspirin triad syndrome, are not distinctive for aspirin idiosyncrasy.

Laboratory and **radiographic studies** such as nasal and peripheral eosinophilia, sinus x-rays showing hyperplastic sinuses and polypoid changes, a prediabetic glucose tolerance test, and increased sensitivity to inhaled methacholine and histamine have all been observed in aspirin-sensitive patients, but are not specifically revealing. Skin tests with aspiryl–polylysine are not helpful in diagnosing AIA and **are not recommended** because of the danger of anaphylaxis and sensitization.

Oral challenge with aspirin is the only definitive way to diagnose current aspirin sensitivity. Such a challenge can identify reactive patients with no previous history of drug sensitivity. A protocol for aspirin challenge is described in Table 12.6. However, aspirin challenge is a potentially hazardous procedure and should generally be considered as an investigative tool to be performed only at centers with experienced personnel and intensive care units immediately accessible. In lieu of performing challenge testing, some allergists routinely advise asthmatic patients, especially those who are corticosteroid-dependent or who manifest nasal polyps, to avoid aspirin and other NSAIDs (Table 12.7).

d. Treatment

The patient must avoid all aspirin-containing drugs as well as other antiinflammatory drugs that work through inhibition of prostaglandin synthesis (Table 12.7). Patients should be cautioned to read labels routinely and to note that aspirin is also termed acetylsalicylic acid or salicylic acid acetate. Table 12.7 presents guidelines for drug use in the aspirin-sensitive patient. A recent report describes rofecoxib challenge in 65 aspirin-sensitive asthmatic patients in whom no reactions occurred. This suggests that this COX-2 inhibitor may be used safely in aspirin-sensitive asthmatic patients. However, until all of these agents have been studied in greater depth, alternative agents should probably be used (Table 12.7). Aggressive medical treatment of rhinitis, sinusitis, nasal polyps, and asthma, as outlined in Chapters 4 and 6, is mandatory. Inhaled and/or systemic corticosteroids are often needed to obtain control of symptoms. Either sinus surgery and/or polypectomies are necessary if sinusitis or nasal polyps are refractory to medical treatment. There is no evidence that these surgical procedures exacerbate asthma, and there is increasing evidence that control of coexisting rhinosinusitis in patients with asthma benefits the asthma. If aspirin or other NSAIDs are required for management of a concomitant disease in a patient with a history of aspirin sensitivity, oral aspirin challenge may be advisable. If the challenge is positive, aspirin desensitization may be considered. The potential therapeutic benefit of such aspirin desensitization for the asthma or rhinitis in aspirin-sensitive patients is still debatable. Leukotriene modifiers may be useful in these patients.

e. Prognosis

If aspirin idiosyncrasy is detected early and treated properly with appropriate preventive and therapeutic measures, it should have no worse a prognosis than other late-onset, non-IgE-mediated asthmatic syndromes. Aspirin avoidance has no apparent influence on the general course of aspirin-sensitive asthma other than to prevent aspirin-induced exacerbations.

Table 12.6. Protocol for 3-day oral aspirin challenge[a]

Time of day	Day 1	Day 2	Day 3
8:00 a.m.	Placebo	ASA, 3 mg or 30 mg[d]	ASA, 150 mg
11:00 a.m.	Placebo[b]	ASA, 60 mg	ASA, 325 mg
2:00 p.m.	Placebo[c]	ASA, 100 mg	ASA, 650 mg

[a] Subject must be symptom free. Challenge should be conducted in a hospital setting by experienced personnel equipped to treat anaphylactic or severe asthmatic reactions.
[b] May substitute tartrazine, 25 mg.
[c] May substitute tartrazine, 50 mg.
[d] Begin with 3 mg in more sensitive patients. Acetylsalicylic acid (ASA).
From Stevenson DD. Diagnosis, prevention, and treatment of adverse reactions to aspirin and nonsteroidal anti-inflammatory drugs. *J Allergy Clin Immunol* 1984;74:617, with permission.

Table 12.7. Pharmacotherapy in aspirin-sensitive patients

Drugs to be avoided	Permissible drugs[a]
Alclofenac	Acetaminophen
Azapropoxone	Choline magnesium trisalicylate
Diclofenac	Choline salicylate
Diflunisal	Chloroquine
Fenclofenac	Narcotics (e.g., codeine, meperidine)
Fenoprofen	Propoxyphene
Feprasone	Salicylamide
Flurbiprofen	Salsalate
Ibuprofen	Sodium salicylate
Indomethacin	
Ketoprofen	
Meclofenamate	
Mefenamic acid	
Naproxen	
Oxyphenbutazone	
Piroxicam	
Sulindac	
Tolmetin	
Zomepirac	

[a] Reactions in some patients have been reported.

2. **Urticaria and angioedema**

Urticaria and angioedema can be associated with aspirin ingestion through one of several distinct mechanisms. Aspirin and other NSAIDs may aggravate chronic urticaria in 14% to 35% of individuals. Patients with chronic urticaria should be advised to avoid aspirin and other NSAIDs. Aspirin and other prostaglandin synthetase inhibitors may precipitate urticaria in some patients without chronic urticaria. In some of these patients, rhinitis or asthma may occur along with the urticaria. Aspirin may occasionally induce urticaria on an immunologic basis. Aspirin anhydride (a contaminant of commercial acetylsalicylic acid) and the aspiryl hapten have been associated with IgE-mediated responses in some patients with aspirin-induced urticaria.

3. **Anaphylactoid reactions**

The incidence of anaphylactoid reactions to NSAIDs is not known. Women appear to be at higher risk. Urticaria and angioedema are the most common symptoms accompanied by laryngeal edema, rhinoconjunctivitis, hypotension, asthma, and/or abdominal pain. Patients with anaphylactoid reactions to NSAIDs exhibit a different clinical profile in relation to other NSAID reactors. Most patients appear to be otherwise normal; pyrazole derivatives are the most common specific drugs involved; and no cross-reactivity among NSAIDs that were not involved in the anaphylactoid reaction nor structurally related was found. The exact mechanism of these anaphylactoid reactions to NSAIDs is not known.

C. **Opiates**

Codeine can be used as a positive control for skin testing because it induces direct subcutaneous mast cell degranulation. Narcotics are often given with antihistamines to block the effects of histamine release, e.g., Dermerol and Vistaril.

VI. **Areas of special interest**

A. **Anesthesia reactions**

Anesthesia reactions may involve multiple mechanisms.

1. Local anesthetics

Adverse reactions following administration of local anesthetics can be classified as shown in Table 12.8. Although adverse reactions commonly occur, true local anesthetic (IgE-mediated) allergy appears to be extremely rare. Coincidental reactions or reactions due to the direct toxic effects of the local anesthetic are probably more frequent. Although the clinical manifestations of the prior reaction can help characterize it and better predict the present risk, many features, such as local swelling, hypotension, tachycardia, and syncope are seen in nonallergic reactions as well. Local anesthetics can be divided into two groups (Table 12.9): Group I contains the benzoic acid esters, and group II includes drugs with the amide structure. On the basis of contact dermatitis and patch test studies, it is believed that group I drugs cross-react with each other but do not cross-react with group II drugs. Although it has been thought that group II drugs do not cross-react with each other, recent patch test data has suggested that lidocaine, prilocaine, and mepivacaine (which share an amide structure) may cross-react with each other. Anecdotal clinical information suggests that reactions occur less frequently with group II drugs than with group I drugs. Adverse reactions and positive challenge tests have been reported in individuals who lack any IgE.

Avoidance of local anesthetic agents may be possible in patients with suspected "caine" allergy. However, avoidance in a patient undergoing a surgical or dental procedure for which a local anesthetic would suffice exposes the patient to increased pain (if no anesthetic is utilized) or increased risk (if general anesthesia is administered). Amiodarone is now recommended instead of lidocaine for certain types of cardiac arrhythmia. Avoidance of local anesthetics **may not** be in the patient's best interest, and the risk of not using the drug must be balanced against the risk of a subsequent reaction. Diphenhydramine can be used as a local anesthetic if the patient is truly intolerant of lidocaine or there is inadequate time to test. Delayed reactions can also occur and positive patch tests have been reported to local anesthetics.

It is reasonable to begin the process of identifying a safe local anesthetic for a patient with a history of a prior reaction with skin testing, also called **provocative dose testing** (Table 12.10). Skin test reactivity to paraben used as a preservative in lidocaine caused the only two positive reactions seen in more than 200 sequential lidocaine challenges done at the Kaiser Permanente San Diego Allergy office. Preservative-free lidocaine was clinically tolerated by both of these patients.

Table 12.8. Classification of adverse reactions
following local anesthetic administration

Reactions not due to local anesthetic agent
Psychomotor responses
Hyperventilation
Vasovagal syncope
Endogenous sympathetic stimulation
Operative trauma
Toxic responses in normal persons
Central nervous system effects
Cardiovascular effects
Local effects
Responses in susceptible persons
Idiosyncratic
Allergic

Table 12.9. Local anesthetic grouping

Group I: Benzoic acid esters	Group II: Other
Benzocaine	Bupivacaine
Butacaine	Dibucaine
Butethamine	Dyclonine
Chlorprocaine	Etidocaine
Cyclomethycaine	Lidocaine (Xylocaine)
Hexylcaine	Mepivacaine (Carbocaine)
Procaine (Novocaine)	Pramoxine
Proparacaine (Ophthaine)	Prilocaine (Citonest)
Propoxycaine	
Tetracaine (Pontocaine)	

From Schatz M, Fung DL. Anaphylactic and anaphylactoid reactions due to anesthetic agents. *Clin Rev Allergy* 1986;4:215, with permission.

The preparation used for skin testing should not contain a vasoconstrictor (which can mask a positive skin test). However, adverse reactions to vasoconstrictors (or the sulfites added to stabilize them) are not frequent or well documented enough to warrant the recommendation of avoiding vasoconstrictors in the preparations used for challenge or treatment. If the prick (puncture) and intradermal skin testing are negative, one can proceed to the incremental challenge (Table 12.10). If the history was of a delayed reaction, one can then confirm a negative reaction at 24 to 48 hours after the skin testing before proceeding to incremental challenge and at 24 to 48 hours after the incremental challenge before proceeding to clinical use. As always with incremen-

Table 12.10. Skin testing and incremental challenge in administration of local anesthetics

Step[a]	Route	Volume (mL)	Dilution
SKIN TESTING			
—	Puncture		$1:10^b$
1.	Puncture		Undiluted[c]
2.	Intradermal	0.02	$1:100$
SUBCUTANEOUS INCREMENTAL CHALLENGE			
—		0.5	Saline[d]
—		0.1	$1:100^b$
—		0.1	$1:10^b$
3.		0.1	Undiluted
4.		0.5	Undiluted
5.		1.0	Undiluted

[a] Administer at 20- to 30-min intervals.
[b] These steps may be considered for patients with histories of severe reactions consistent with IgE-mediated mechanisms.
[c] The concentration of an LA (usually 1%–2%) to be used for the procedure.
[d] A single-blind saline step may be inserted before LA injection for patients in whom the reaction is suspected to be due to the injection rather than the drug.
LA, local anesthetics; IgE, immunoglobulin E.
From Schatz M. Adverse reactions to local anesthetics. *Immunol Allergy Clin N Ampr* 1992;12:585, with permission.

tal challenges, it must be performed under careful observation and where facilities are available to treat adverse reactions. If incremental challenge is accomplished without adverse reaction, the risk of an adverse reaction to subsequent administration of that drug is apparently no greater than that for the general population.

2. **Anaphylactoid reactions during general anesthesia**
    a. **Clinical features.** Anaphylactoid reactions during general anesthesia occur in approximately 1:5,000 to 1:15,000 operations, with 4% to 6% of these reactions being fatal. They are most commonly attributed to either the induction agent or, more frequently, the muscle-relaxing agent (Table 12.11), although recent reports emphasize an important role for latex sensitivity, especially in children with spina bifida or congenital urologic abnormalities. The most common clinical features are cutaneous manifestations (erythema, urticaria, or angioedema), hypotension, bronchospasm, and abdominal symptoms. Reactions are reported to occur more commonly in women and in patients with a history of a prior reaction during general anesthesia. Data are conflicting regarding whether a history of atopy or asthma increases the risk.
    b. **Pathogenesis.** The agents listed in Table 12.11 are all capable of direct histamine release. Many reactions occur on first exposure, and increased plasma histamine has been reported during such reactions. Thus, exaggerated direct histamine release or increased target organ responsiveness to the histamine released in susceptible individuals may explain these reactions. However, recent studies support IgE-mediated mechanisms in many patients experiencing these adverse reactions, especially to muscle relaxants.
    c. **Diagnosis.** Skin testing with induction and muscle-relaxing agents has been recommended as a means of defining the responsible drug in patients experiencing an anaphylactoid reaction during general anesthesia and, potentially, as a method of defining safe agents for subsequent use (Table 12.11). Recently, radioimmunoassays for

Table 12.11. Concentrations of agents used in skin testing

Agents	Reagent concentration (mg/mL)	Minimal dilution/maximal concentration (μg/mL) for specific positive intradermal test[a]
Induction		
Thiopental	20	1:100/200
Thiamylal	10	1:100/100
Methohexitol	10	1:100/100
Muscle-relaxing		
Succinylcholine	10	1:100/100
Pancuronium	2	1:10/200
Vecuronium	4	1:10/400
Gallamine	20	1:100/200
Alcuronium	5	1:100/50
d-Tubocurarine	3	1:1,000/3
Afracurium	10	1:1,000/10

[a] Use volume of 0.02 mL. Consider preliminary prick testing or intradermal testing with one or two serial 10-fold dilutions of these maximum concentrations to reduce the chance of a systemic reaction. A wheal of $\geq$10 mm is considered positive.
From Birnbaum J, Vervolet D. Allergy to muscle relaxants. *Clin Rev Allergy* 1991;9:281, and Moscicki RA, et al. Anaphylaxis during induction of general anesthesia: subsequent evaluation and management. *J Allergy Clin Immunol* 1990;86:325, with permission.

specific serum IgE against induction and muscle-relaxing agents have been described, but their sensitivity, specificity, and predictive clinical value require further clinical study.

    d. Approach to patients. Anaphylactoid reactions during general anesthesia should be treated in the standard manner for treating anaphylaxis (see Chapter 10). The following approach is recommended for patients with histories of prior adverse reactions during general anesthesia who require subsequent surgery:

        (1) Use an alternative method of anesthesia if possible (inhalational, local, or spinal);

        (2) Obtain a complete list of all drugs used during the surgery associated with the prior reaction;

        (3) Skin test (or, if appropriate and available, use *in vitro* specific IgE tests) with relevant agents including latex;

        (4) Avoid as many drugs used during the prior surgery as possible, especially those producing a positive skin test; and

        (5) If general anesthesia is utilized, pretreat with antihistamines and corticosteroids using the protocol outlined previously for RCM.

B. Multiple drug sensitivity

The multiple drug allergy syndrome (or multiple antibiotic sensitivity syndrome) has been described in adults and children, and most commonly manifests as urticaria or other rashes after exposure to more than one class of antibiotics. However, whether or not this actually represents a distinct clinical syndrome remains to be determined. Patients with histories of penicillin allergy have been reported to be much more likely to experience immunopathological reactions to other classes of antibiotics than patients who did not report being penicillin allergic. However, Khoury and Warrington more recently found that the occurrence of multiple drug allergy was not significantly different among age- and sex-matched groups of the following patients:

        (1) Skin-test-positive penicillin allergic patients;

        (2) History-positive but skin-test-negative subjects; and

        (3) Control patients with vasomotor rhinitis.

Further prospective studies will be required to determine whether a distinct clinical syndrome of multiple drug sensitivity exists, and, if it does, the responsible mechanisms.

Selected Readings

Adkinson NF. Risk factors for drug allergy. *J Allergy Clin Immunol* 1984;74:567–72.

Arevalo JM, Lorente JA, Gonzalez-Herrada C, et al. Treatment of toxic epidermal necrolysis with cyclosporin A. *J Trauma Inj Infect Crit Care* 2000;48:473–478.

Bigby M, Jick S, Jick H, et al. Drug-induced cutaneous reactions. A report from the Boston collaborative drug surveillance program on 15438 consecutive inpatients, 1975 to 1982. *JAMA* 1986;256:3358–3363.

Bonfanti P, Pusterla L, Parazzini F, et al. The effectiveness of desensitization versus rechallenge treatment in HIV-positive patients with previous hypersensitivity to TMP-SMX: a randomized multicentric study. *Biomed Pharmacother* 2000;54:45–49.

Chen Z, Baur X, Kutscha-Lissberg F, et al. IgE-mediated anaphylactic reaction to imipenem. *Allergy* 2000;55:92–93.

Demoly P, Kropf R, Bircher A, et al. Drug hypersensitivity questionnaire. *Allergy* 1999;54:999–1003.

Drazen JM, Israel E, O'Byrne PM. Treatment of asthma with drugs modifying the leukotriene pathway. *N Engl J Med* 1999;340:197–206.

Edston E, van Hage-Hamsten M. Anaphylactoid shock-a common cause of death in heroin addicts? *Allergy* 1997;52:950–954.

Evans RS, Pestotnik SL, Classen DC, et al. Preventing adverse drug events in hospitalized patients. *Ann Pharmacother* 1994;28:523–527.

Fulcher DA, Katelaris CH. Anaphylactoid reactions to local anaesthetics despite IgE deficiency: A case report. *Asia Pac J Allergy Immunol* 1990;8:133–136.

Galletly DC, Treuren BC. Cutaneous sensitivity to atracurium and vecuronium in patients suffering anaphylactoid reactions to neuromuscular blockers. *Anesth Intens Care* 1985;13:305–310.

Garcia-Domingo MI, Aijotas-Reig J, Cistero-Bahima A, et al. Disseminated and recurrent sarcoid-like granulomatous panniculitis due to bovine collagen injection. *Invest Allergol Clin Immunol* 2000;10:107–109.

Garcia-Doval I, LeLeach L, Bocquet H, et al. Toxic epidermal necrolysis and Stevens-Johnson syndrome. Does early withdrawal of causative drugs decrease the risk of death? *Arch Dermatol* 2000;136:323–327.

Goss JE, Chambers CE, Heupler FA, et al. Systemic anaphylactoid reactions to iodinated contrast media during cardiac catheterization procedures: guidelines for prevention, diagnosis, and treatment. *Catheter Cardiovasc Diagn* 1995;34:99–104.

Grammer LC, Paterson BF, Roxe D, et al. IgE against ethylene oxide-altered human serum albumin in patients with anaphylactic reactions to dialysis. *J Allergy Clin Immunol* 1985;76:511–514.

Green, SM. What is the role of diphenhydramine in local anesthesia? *Acad Emerg Med* 1996;3:198–200.

Gruchalla RS. Approach to the patient with multiple antibiotic sensitivities. *Allergy Asthma Proc* 2000;21:39–44.

Gruchalla RS. Diagnosis of allergic reactions to sulfonamides. *Allergy* 1999;54[Suppl 58]:28–32.

Heckbert SR, Stryker WS, Coltin KL, et al. Serum sickness in children after antibiotic exposure: estimates of occurrence and morbidity in a health maintenance organization population. *Am J Epidemiol* 1990;132:336–342.

Hill MD, Barber PA, Takahashi J, et al. Anaphylactoid reactions and angioedema during alteplase treatment of acute stroke. *CMAJ* 2000;169:1281–1284.

Hosoya T, Yamaguchi K, Akutsu T, et al. Delayed adverse reactions to iodinated contrast media and their risk factors. *Radiat Med* 2000;18:39–45.

Humphreys F, Hunter JAA. The characteristics of urticaria in 390 patients. *Br J Dermatol* 1998;138:635–638.

James JM, Zeiger RS, Lester MR, et al. Safe administration of influenza vaccine to patients with egg allergy. *J Pediatr* 1998;133:624–628.

Jimenez I, Anton E, Picans I, et al. Occupational asthma specific to amoxicillin. *Allergy* 1998;53:104–105.

Kennel A, Bene MC, Hurault de Ligny B, et al. Serum anti-dextran antibodies in IgA nephropathy. *Clin Nephrol* 1995;43:216–220.

Khakoo GA, Lack G. Recommendations for using MMR vaccine in children allergic to eggs. *Br Med J* 2000;320:929–932.

Khoury L, Warrington R. The multiple drug allergy syndrome: A matched control retrospective study in patients allergic to penicillin. *J Allergy Clin Immunol* 1996;98: 462–464

Kumar D. Lispro analog for treatment of generalized allergy to human insulin. *Diabetes Care* 1997;20:1357–1359.

Kumar KL, Reuler JB. Drug fever. *West J Med* 1986;144:753–755.

Li JTC, Markus PJ, Osmon DR, et al. Reduction of vancomycin use in orthopedic patients with a history of antibiotic allergy. *Mayo Clin Proc* 2000;75:902–906.

Lynch JP, Renz CL, Laroche D, et al. Value of baseline levels in assessing tryptase release. *Inflamm Res* 2000;49:23–24.

Macy E, Bulpit K, Champlin RE, et al. Anaphylaxis to infusion of autologous bone marrow: An apparent reaction to self, mediated by IgE antibody to bovine serum albumin. *J Allergy Clin Immunol* 1989;83:871–875.

Macy E, Richter PK, Falkoff R, et al. Skin testing with penicilloate and penilloate prepared by an improved method: Amoxicillin oral challenge in patients with negative skin test responses to penicillin reagents. *J Allergy Clin Immunol* 1997;100:586–591.

Markham A, Lamb HM. Infliximab. A review of its use in the management of rheumatoid arthritis. *Drugs* 2000;59:1341–1359.

Matsui D, McLauchlin M, Rieder MJ. Predictive value of oral sulfonamide challenge for adverse reactions. *Pediatr Infect Dis J* 1997;16:1084–1085.

Moes GS, MacPherson BR. Cefotetan-induced hemolytic anemia. *Arch Pathol Lab Med* 2000;124:1344–1346.

Moneret-Vautrin DA, Gueant JL, Kamel L, et al. Anaphylaxis to muscle relaxants: cross-sensitivity studied by radioimmunoassays compared to intradermal tests in 34 cases. *J Allergy Clin Immunol* 1988;82:745–752.

Orasch CE, Helbling A, Zanni MP, et al. T-cell reaction to local anaesthetics: relationship to angioedema and urticaria after subcutaneous application—patch testing and LTT in patients with adverse reaction to local anaesthetics. *Clin Exper Allergy* 1999;29:1549–1554.

Ordoqui E, Zubeldia JM, Aranzabal A, et al. Serum tryptase levels in adverse drug reactions. *Allergy* 1997;52:1102–1105.

Panhans-Gross A, Gall H, Peter RU. Baboon syndrome after oral penicillin. *Contact Dermatitis* 1999;41:352–353.

Park J, Matsui D, Rieder MJ: Multiple antibiotic sensitivity in children. *Can J Clin Pharmacol* 2000;7:3841.

Parmiani G, Rodolfo M, Melani C. Immunological gene therapy with ex vivo gene-modified tumor cells: a critique and a reappraisal. *Human Gene Ther* 2000;11: 1269–1275.

Perez-Pimiento A, Gomez-Martinez M, Minguez-Mena A, et al. Aztreonam and ceftazidime: evidence of in vivo cross allergenicity. *Allergy* 1998;53:624–625.

Pichler WJ. Drug allergy: relationship between immunogenicity and clinical symptoms. *Allergy* 1999;54:5–7.

Pichler WJ, Yawalkar N. Pathophysiology of drug-elicited exanthems. *ACI Int* 2000; 12:166–70.

Quiralte J, Blanco C, Castillo R, et al. Anaphylactoid reactions due to nonsteroidal antiinflammatory drugs: clinical and cross-reactivity studies. *Ann Allergy Asthma Immunol* 1997;78:293–296.

Red Book 2000. American Academy of Pediatrics.

Romano A, Torres MJ, Quaratino D, et al. Diagnostic evaluation of delayed hypersensitivity to systemically administered drugs. *Allergy* 1999;54:23–27.

Roujeau JC, Kelly JP, Naldi L, et al. Medication use and the risk of Stevens-Johnson syndrome or toxic epidermal necrolysis. *N Engl J Med* 1995;333:1660–1667.

Sastre J, Quijano LD, Novalbos A, et al. Clinical cross-reactivity between amoxicillin and cephadroxil in patients allergic to amoxicillin and with good tolerance of penicillin. *Allergy* 1996;51:383–386.

Saxon A, Adelman DC, Patel A, et al. Imipenem cross-reactivity with penicillin in humans. *J Allergy Clin Immunol* 1988;82:213–217.

Schiller PI, Langauer Messmer S, Haefeli WE, et al. Angiotensin-converting enzyme inhibitor-induced angioedema: late onset, irregular course, and potential triggers. *Allergy* 1997;52:432–435.

Schwartz RA. Toxic epidermal necrolysis. *Cutis* 1997;59:123–128.

Seeger JD, Kong SX, Schumock GT. Characteristics associated with ability to prevent adverse drug reactions in hospitalized patients. *Pharmacotherapy* 1998;18: 1284–1289.

Stern RS. Improving the outcome of patients with toxic epidermal necrolysis and Stevens-Johnson syndrome. *Arch Dermatol* 2000;136:410–411.

Stevenson DD, Simon R. Lack of cross reactivity to rofecoxib in aspirin sensitive asthmatics. *J Allergy Clin Immunol* 2001;108:47–51.

Sullivan TJ, Ong RC, Gilliam LK. Studies of the multiple drug allergy syndrome. *J Allergy Clin Immunol* 1989;83:A393(abst).

Tan EM, Rubin RL. Autoallergic reactions induced by procainamide. *J Allergy Clin Immunol* 1984;74:631–634.

Van der Klauw MM, Wilson JHP, Stricker BHCh. Drug-associated anaphylaxis: 20 years of reporting in the Netherlands (1974–1994) and a review of the literature. *Clin Exper Allergy* 1996;26:1355–1363.

Van Ginneken EEM, van der Meer JWM, Netten PM. A man with a mysterious hypogammaglobulinaemia and skin rash. *Neth J Med* 1999;54:158–162.

Verhaar-Langereis MJ, Eagle KF, Keep PA, et al. Anaphylactic reaction to radio-immunotherapy despite plasmapheresis to remove anti-mouse antibodies. *J R Soc Med* 2000;93:75–76.

Warrington R: Multiple drug allergy syndrome. *Can J Clin Pharmacol* 2000;7:18–19.

Wedi B, Kapp A. Aspirin induced adverse skin reactions: new pathophysiological aspects. *Thorax* 2000;55:S70–S71.

Woo MH, Hak LJ, Storm MC, et al. Hypersensitivity or development of antibodies to asparaginase does not impact treatment outcome of childhood acute lymphoblastic leukemia. *J Clin Oncol* 2000;18:1525–1532.

Yawalker N, Pichler WJ. Pathogenesis of drug-induced exanthema. *Int Arch Allergy Immunol* 2001;124:336–338.

Zhao Z, Baldo BA, O'Brien RM, et al. Reaction with, and fine structure recognition of polyamines by human IgE antibodies. *Mol Immunol* 2000;37:233–240.

13. FOOD ALLERGY

A. Wesley Burks

Immunoglobulin E (IgE)-mediated hypersensitivity reactions account for the majority of well-documented food allergy reactions, but non-IgE-mediated immune mechanisms do cause some hypersensitivity disorders. A variety of gastrointestinal, cutaneous, respiratory, and generalized symptoms and syndromes have been associated with IgE-mediated food allergy. The diagnostic approach to adverse food reactions begins with a careful medical history and physical examination. Laboratory studies may then be utilized appropriately in the evaluation. Once the diagnosis of food allergy is established, the only proven therapy is the strict elimination of the food from the patient's diet. Studies in both children and adults indicate that symptomatic reactivity to food allergens is often lost over time, except possibly for peanuts, tree nuts, and seafood.

    I. Incidence. We now know that food allergy occurs in 6% to 8% of children and 1% to 2% of adults. Significant scientific studies in the last several years have increased the understanding and treatment of these allergic reactions. Up to 15% of the general population believe that they may be allergic to some food. Several well-controlled studies have revealed that the vast majority of food-allergic reactions present in the first year of life.

    II. Definitions. A variety of terms have been used to characterize adverse reactions to foods. The American Academy of Allergy, Asthma and Immunology and the National Institute of Allergy and Infectious Diseases at National Institutes of Health (NIH) have defined several terms in an attempt to standardize the literature. An **adverse food reaction** is a generic term referring to any untoward reaction after the ingestion of a food. Adverse food reactions may be secondary to **food allergy (hypersensitivity)** or **food intolerance.** A food allergy reaction is presumed to be the result of an abnormal immunologic response following the ingestion of a food, whereas a food intolerance is the result of nonimmunologic mechanisms.

    IgE-mediated hypersensitivity reactions account for the majority of well-documented food allergy reactions, but non-IgE-mediated immune mechanisms do cause a variety of hypersensitivity disorders (Table 13.1). Food intolerances probably make up the majority of adverse food reactions. Examples of food intolerance include: (i) reactions from toxic contaminants (e.g., histamine in scombroid fish poisoning, toxins secreted by *Salmonella* or *Shigella*); (ii) pharmacologic reactions (e.g., to caffeine in coffee, tyramine in aged cheeses); (iii) metabolic reactions (e.g., lactase deficiency); and (iv) idiosyncratic and psychological reactions.

    III. Food allergens. Foods are composed of proteins, carbohydrates, and lipids. Primarily, the major food allergens are water-soluble glycoproteins that have molecular weights ranging between 10,000 and 60,000 D. Generally, the allergens are stable to treatment with heat, acid, and proteases. Other properties that may account for their allergenicity are not well understood.

    A minority of foods are responsible for the majority of documented food-allergic reactions. In children, these foods are milk, eggs, peanuts, fish, soybeans, wheat, and tree nuts (Table 13.2). In adults, the primary foods causing reactions are peanuts, tree nuts, fish, and shellfish.

    IV. Pathophysiology

        A. Immunoglobulin E. A variety of hypersensitivity responses to an ingested food antigen may result from the genetically predisposed patient's lack of development of oral tolerance or a breakdown of oral tolerance in their gastrointestinal tract. Although IgE-mediated reactions have been studied in great detail, some of these disorders may involve more than one immunologic mechanism. Either a failure to develop or a breakdown in oral tolerance

Table 13.1. Classification of hypersensitivities to food and other dietary products

IgE ──▶ Non-IgE		
Immediate gastrointestinal hypersensitivity Oral allergy syndrome Urticaria and angioedema Atopic dermatitis Rhinoconjunctivitis Asthma Anaphylaxis		
	Allergic eosinophilic esophagitis Allergic eosinophilic gastritis Allergic eosinophilic gastroenterocolitis	
		Dietary protein enterocolitis Dietary protein proctitis Dietary protein enteropathy Celiac disease

IgE, immunoglobulin E.

results in excessive production of food-specific IgE antibodies. These food-specific antibodies bind high-affinity Fcε I receptors on mast cells and basophils and low-affinity Fcε II receptors on macrophages, monocytes, lymphocytes, eosinophils, and platelets. After the food allergen reaches the food-specific antibodies on mast cells or basophils, mediators such as histamine, prostaglandins, and leukotrienes are released. These mediators then promote vasodilation, smooth muscle contraction, and mucus secretion, resulting in the symptoms of immediate hypersensitivity. The activated mast cells also may release various cytokines that play a part in the IgE-mediated late-phase response. With repeated ingestion of a specific food allergen, mononuclear cells are stimulated to secrete histamine-releasing factor (HRF). The "spontaneous" generation of HRF by the activated mononuclear cells *in vitro* has been associated with increased cutaneous irritability in children with atopic dermatitis. An increase in plasma histamine has been associated with IgE-mediated allergic symptoms after blinded food challenges. In IgE-mediated gastrointestinal reactions, endoscopic observation has revealed local vasodilation, edema, mucus secretion, and petechial hemorrhaging. Increased stool and serum prostaglandin E_2 (PGE_2) and PGF_2 have been seen after food challenges causing diarrhea.

B. Nonimmunoglobulin E. Although a variety of reports have discussed other immune mechanisms causing food-allergic reactions, the scientific

Table 13.2. Major food allergens in children and adults

Children	Adults
Milk Egg Peanuts Soybeans Wheat Fish Tree nuts	Peanuts Tree nuts Fish Shellfish

evidence supporting these mechanisms is limited. Type III (antigen–antibody complex-mediated) hypersensitivity reactions have been examined in several studies. Although IgE–food antigen complexes are seen more commonly in patients with food hypersensitivity, there is little support for food antigen–immune-complex-mediated disease. Type IV (cell-mediated) hypersensitivity has been discussed in several disorders in which the clinical symptoms do not appear until several hours after the ingestion of the suspected food. This type of immune response may contribute to some adverse food reactions (i.e., enterocolitis), but significant, supporting evidence of a specific cell-mediated hypersensitivity disorder is lacking.

V. Clinical manifestations

Immunoglobulin E

A variety of gastrointestinal, cutaneous, respiratory, and generalized symptoms and syndromes have been associated with IgE-mediated food allergy.

   A. The **oral allergy syndrome** is considered a form of contact urticaria confined almost exclusively to the oropharynx. Typical symptoms include pruritus and angioedema of the lips, tongue, palate, and throat. The symptoms generally resolve rather rapidly. The symptoms are often associated with the ingestion of various fruits and vegetables. Patients with allergic rhinitis secondary to ragweed may develop symptoms after ingestion of melons (e.g., watermelon, cantaloupe, honeydew) and bananas. Similarly, patients sensitive to birch pollen may develop oral symptoms after the ingestion of raw potatoes, carrots, celery, apples, and hazelnuts.

   B. Generalized **anaphylactic** reactions secondary to IgE-mediated sensitivity to foods are not rare. Patients may develop cutaneous, respiratory, and gastrointestinal symptoms, and cardiovascular symptoms including hypotension, vascular collapse, and cardiac dysrhythmias. Patients with fatal or near-fatal food-induced anaphylactic reactions have several clinical features in common, including the following: (i) asthma, (ii) accidental ingestion of the food allergen, (iii) previous allergic reactions to the incriminated food, and (iv) immediate symptoms with about one-half experiencing a quiescent period before a major respiratory collapse.

   C. **Gastrointestinal anaphylaxis** refers to IgE-mediated gastrointestinal symptoms (nausea, abdominal pain, abdominal cramping, vomiting, and/or diarrhea) that will often accompany symptoms in other target organs. Symptoms generally develop within minutes to 2 hours of ingesting the offending food. The frequent ingestion of a food allergen in patients with atopic dermatitis and food allergy appears to induce a state of partial desensitization of the gastrointestinal mast cells, which will manifest itself in less pronounced clinical symptoms. After the food is removed from the patient's diet, the symptoms may become significantly more evident after an ensuing food challenge.

   D. **Respiratory** and **ocular** symptoms are common manifestations of IgE-mediated reactions to foods. Symptoms may include periocular erythema, pruritus, and tearing; nasal congestion, pruritus, sneezing, and rhinorrhea; and coughing, voice changes, and wheezing. Isolated nasoocular symptoms are an uncommon manifestation of food hypersensitivity reactions. Although the ingestion of food allergens is rarely the main trigger factor of chronic asthma, preliminary evidence suggests that food antigens can provoke bronchial hyperreactivity. Inhalation of a food allergen from cooking or food processing may cause acute bronchospasm.

   E. The **skin** is a frequent target organ in IgE-mediated food hypersensitivity reactions. The ingestion of food allergens can lead either to immediate cutaneous symptoms or aggravate more chronic symptoms. Acute **urticaria** and **angioedema** are probably the most common cutaneous manifestation of food hypersensitivity reactions, generally appearing within minutes of ingestion of the food allergen. The foods commonly causing these reactions in children include eggs, milk, peanuts, and tree nuts. In adults, this list includes fish, shellfish, tree nuts, and peanuts. Food allergy causing **chronic urticaria** is a rare phenomenon occurring in only about 1% of patients with this disorder.

F. Atopic dermatitis is a chronic skin disorder that generally begins in early infancy and is characterized by typical distribution, extreme pruritus, chronically relapsing course, and association with asthma and allergic rhinitis. In well-controlled studies, about one-third of children with atopic dermatitis have food-allergic reactions.

G. Another gastrointestinal disorder, **allergic eosinophilic gastroenteropathy**, is characterized by infiltration of the gastric and/or intestinal walls with eosinophils, absence of vasculitis, and frequent peripheral eosinophilia. Patients with this disorder typically present with postprandial nausea and vomiting, abdominal pain, diarrhea, and weight loss in adults or failure to thrive in young infants. IgE-mediated food hypersensitivity reactions have been implicated in a subset of patients with this disorder. It may take up to 12 weeks after elimination of the responsible food allergen from the diet for symptoms to resolve.

Non-immunoglobulin E-mediated food hypersensitivity

H. Food-induced enterocolitis is a disorder generally beginning in young infants between 1 week and 3 months of age. These patients present with vomiting and diarrhea often secondary to the ingestion of cow's milk and/or soybean protein formulas. At times the symptoms do not occur until several hours after the ingestion of the protein source. Their stools generally contain occult blood, neutrophils, eosinophils, and are positive for reducing substances. Any examination for specific IgE (skin prick tests, radioallergosorbent test [RAST]) is generally negative. These patients typically become tolerant of the food by 12 to 24 months of age.

I. Food-induced colitis, like food-induced enterocolitis, generally presents in the first several months of life with similar symptoms. Appearance of blood in the stool with or without diarrhea is usually observed, but unlike the previous disorder, the patients are not generally as ill. Protein-specific IgE antibodies are typically not found and these patients typically become tolerant of the food by 12 to 24 months of age.

J. Malabsorption syndromes (excluding celiac disease) often present in the first several months of life with diarrhea (not infrequently steatorrhea) and poor weight gain. The presenting symptoms include protracted diarrhea, vomiting, failure to thrive, and carbohydrate malabsorption. This syndrome has been associated with the ingestion most commonly of cow's milk proteins, but is also associated with soybean, eggs, and wheat. Complete resolution of the symptoms may take 6 to 18 months of allergen avoidance.

K. Celiac disease is a more extensive enteropathy leading to malabsorption. Total villous atrophy and extensive cellular infiltrates are associated with sensitivity to gliadin, the alcohol-soluble portion of gluten found in wheat, oats, rye, and barley. The typical symptoms include diarrhea or frank steatorrhea, abdominal distention and flatulence, weight loss, and occasionally nausea and vomiting. IgA antibodies to gluten are present in more than 80% of adults and children with untreated celiac disease. The immunopathogenesis of the disorder remains unknown, although studies in animal models suggest that a type IV, cell-mediated mechanism is involved. Several antibody determinations have been tried for diagnosis and followup, including antigliadin antibodies. Once the diagnosis of celiac disease is established (which requires an intestinal biopsy), life-long elimination of gluten-containing foods is necessary. One strong reason for long-term elimination of gluten in the diet is that this will significantly decrease the possibility of intestinal lymphoid malignancy.

VI. Food intolerance

A. Metabolic, idiosyncratic, psychologic. Food intolerance includes toxic, pharmacologic and psychologic reactions, as well as metabolic reactions from enzyme deficiencies.

    1. Toxic reactions may result from naturally occurring toxic substances or from microbial or chemical contamination of foods. Adverse reactions to sulfites, monosodium glutamate, and aspartame have been reported, although they probably occur with very little frequency. Microbial contamination of foods may result in poisoning because of the action of the microbial toxin or the microbial infection. Some foods contain active pharmacologic agents that in susceptible patients may cause clinical symptoms (e.g., caffeine).

    2. The most common metabolic reactions to food are the result of disaccharidase deficiencies. Carbohydrate malabsorption leads to bloating, cramps, flatulence, and diarrhea. For example, **lactase deficiency**, not uncommonly observed after significant episodes of diarrhea, is secondary to the ingestion of foods containing lactose. The small intestine cannot absorb the lactose, a disaccharide, and bacteria in the large intestine ferment the lactose. This disorder is present in up to 80% of North American African Americans and 5% to 20% of Caucasians. Primary acquired lactase deficiency begins to present in school-aged children.

    3. Psychologic aversions to foods are not uncommon and can be associated with various symptoms including nausea, vomiting, diarrhea, and headaches. In addition, patients with anxiety and depression sometimes complain of "food allergy." The physician must remain cognizant of these food-aversion reactions and be aware of specific gastrointestinal illnesses such as hiatal hernia or peptic ulcer disease that may mimic these problems.

VII. Diagnosis

The diagnostic approach to adverse food reactions begins with a careful medical history and physical examination (Fig. 13.1). Laboratory studies may then be utilized appropriately in the evaluation. In specific acute reactions to foods, such as systemic anaphylaxis, the medical history is important in diagnosis, but in other less acute reactions, the medical history can be verified in less than 50% of reported food-allergic reactions.

A. In the evaluation of possible food allergy, important elements of the history include: (i) the food suspected in provoking the reaction, (ii) the quantity of the suspected food ingested, (iii) the length of time between ingestion of the food and the development of symptoms, (iv) a description of the symptoms provoked, (v) if similar symptoms developed on other occasions when the food was eaten, (vi) if other factors (e.g., exercise) are necessary, and (vii) the time since the last reaction to the food occurred. In chronic disorders the history may not be a reliable indicator of the offending food allergen.

B. A number of methods have been utilized in the evaluation of food-allergic reactions, including diet diaries, elimination diets, skin prick testing, RASTs, basophil histamine release, intestinal mast cell histamine release, intragastric provocation under endoscopy, intestinal biopsy after allergen feeding, and double-blind placebo-controlled food challenges (DBPCFC).

C. A **diet diary** is frequently used as an adjunct to the medical history by providing a chronological record of all foods ingested over a specified period of time. This method rarely detects an unrecognized association between a food and a patient's symptoms.

D. Elimination diets are utilized both in diagnosis and management of adverse food reactions. The success of these diets depends on the identification of the correct allergen(s), the ability of the patient to maintain a diet completely free of all forms of the food allergen, and the assumption that other factors are not necessary or do not provoke similar symptoms. Elimination diets are rarely diagnostic for food allergy, especially in chronic disorders such as atopic dermatitis or asthma. In general, an elimination diet should

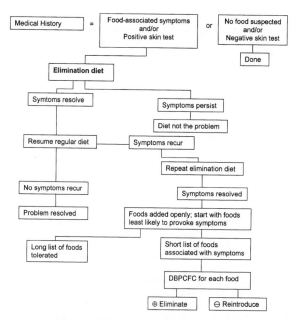

FIG. 13.1. Evaluation of adverse food reactions.

only be utilized either for a period of 1 or 2 weeks prior to a food challenge while eliminating only the foods suspected of causing the reactions.

E. **Allergy skin prick tests** are highly reproducible and often utilized to screen patients with suspected IgE-mediated food allergies. The glycerinated food extracts (1 : 10 or 1 : 20 w/v) and appropriate positive (histamine) and negative (saline) controls are applied epicutaneously by either the prick or puncture technique. A food allergen eliciting a wheal at least 3 mm or greater than the negative control is considered positive; anything else is considered negative. A **positive skin test** to a food indicates only the possibility that the patient has symptomatic reactivity to that specific food (overall the positive predictive accuracy is less than 50%). A **negative skin test** confirms the absence of an IgE-mediated reaction (overall negative predictive accuracy is greater than 95%). Both of these statements are justified if appropriate and good quality food extracts are utilized.

The **epicutaneous** (e.g., puncture or prick) skin test should be considered an excellent means of excluding IgE-mediated food allergies, but only "suggestive" of the actual presence of clinical food allergies. There are some minor exceptions, however, to this general statement, including: (i) IgE-mediated sensitivity to several fruits and vegetables (apples, oranges, bananas, pears, melons, potatoes, carrots, celery, etc.) is sometimes not detected with commercial-prepared extracts or reagents; this is thought to be the result of the lability of the responsible allergen in the food; (ii) children less than 1 year of age may have IgE-mediated food allergy without a positive skin test; (iii) children less than 2 years of age may have smaller wheals, possibly due to the lack of skin reactivity (uncommonly) and conversely (iv) a positive skin test to a food ingested in isolation which provokes a serious systemic anaphylactic reaction may be considered diagnostic.

An **intradermal skin test** is a more sensitive method when compared to the skin prick test, but it is much less specific when compared to a blinded food challenge. In one study, no patient who had a negative skin prick test, but a positive intradermal skin to a specific food had a positive DBPCFC to that food. In addition, intradermal skin testing has a greater risk of inducing a systemic reaction than does skin prick testing. Intradermal skin testing for foods has caused significant anaphylactic reactions in some patients (especially those patients who had intradermal skin tests only).

Skin testing may be done in any physician's office. However, referral to an allergist will be beneficial because they have the training and capability to interpret the skin test findings in light of the patient's history, and make an appropriate diagnosis and treatment plan.

F. **Radioallergosorbent tests.** RASTs and similar *in vitro* assays are used to identify food-specific IgE antibodies in the serum. Although frequently utilized to screen for IgE-mediated food reactions, these assays are generally considered slightly less specific than the skin prick tests. Highly positive levels of food-specific IgE antibodies determined by *in vitro* tests from high-quality laboratories can provide information similar to that of prick skin tests. Recent studies with the CAP-FEIA test (Pharmacia) have demonstrated that for some of the major food allergens, a better positive predictive accuracy can be achieved with the utilization of this test. These studies have shown that there may be better positive and negative predictive values for anticipating the outcome of an oral food challenge. For example, a level of greater than 15 kU_A/L of specific IgE to peanut has greater than 95% positive predictive accuracy of predicting a positive food challenge. For this test there are both positive and negative predictive values, which will aid in the diagnosis of patients with possible food-allergic reactions. Currently, the predictive values of CAP-FEIA results are limited to the major food allergens (milk, egg, peanuts, wheat, and soybeans).

G. **Basophil histamine release** assays specific for food allergens have been developed for diagnosis of food allergy, but in their present state they are not more predictive of clinical sensitivity than the skin prick test.

H. **Intestinal mast cell histamine release** is a research procedure where intestinal mast cells obtained from biopsy specimens are added to specific food antigens and a percentage histamine release is determined. The procedure correlates closely with symptoms of the gastrointestinal tract after challenge, but not with other symptoms provoked by challenge.

I. The **double-blind placebo-controlled food challenge.** DBPCFC has been labeled as the "gold standard" for the diagnosis of food allergies. This technique has been used by many investigators and clinicians in the evaluation of both adults and children with suspected food-allergic reactions. If the blinded part of the procedure (e.g., administration of the suspect food in liquid or opaque capsules) is negative, the **open** part of the challenge must be completed to ensure that the challenge is negative and to confirm the safe ingestion of a normal amount of the food in its usually prepared state. Physicians who perform food challenges must be prepared to treat the clinical reactions caused by the food challenges. Allergists have a unique role in that they have received training and experience in conducting food challenges.

VIII. **Unproven diagnostic and therapeutic techniques.** Because of the lack of complete understanding about the basic immunopathologic mechanisms and the prevalence of individuals believing they have an adverse food reaction, numerous medical techniques have developed for the diagnosis and treatment of these problems. Disproven or unproven techniques include cytotoxicity testing, provocative and neutralization treatment, autogeneous urine immunization, IgG subclass diagnosis of food allergy, and food immune complexes.

Tests for IgG or IgG4 to a specific food or specific food immune complexes have been proposed for use in the diagnosis of food-allergic reactions, but there is little evidence to support their use. Development of food-specific IgG and IgG4 is a normal immune response to food ingestion. Similarly, immune complex formation is a normal event in the course of an immune response and allows antigen elimination. Masking and addiction, rotary diets, and fasting, are all various techniques of dietary manipulation that have shown to have no role in the diagnosis or treatment of food-allergic diseases.

IX. Practical approach to diagnosis. The diagnosis of food allergy continues to be a clinical exercise that includes a careful history, the search for specific IgE (e.g., skin prick tests) if an IgE-mediated disorder is suspected, an appropriate period of elimination of the suspected food, and challenge with the food in question.

A. For patients with **suspected IgE-mediated food allergy**, the initial step is an elimination diet for 1 to 2 weeks consisting of all foods suspected by the history or skin prick testing. If no improvement is noted, it is not likely that food allergy is involved. Because atopic dermatitis and chronic asthma are multifactorial in nature, the elimination of the food allergen may not appear to change significantly the course of the disease. Open or single-blind challenges are useful in a clinical setting to screen suspected food allergens. Presumptive diagnosis of food allergy based only on skin prick tests is no longer acceptable. Of those children allergic to foods, almost 80% are allergic to only **one or two** foods.

B. For patients with suspected food-allergic reactions that are not thought to be IgE mediated, a careful medical history and an elimination diet of the suspected food for a period of 1 to 2 weeks (except in some gastrointestinal disorders for which a period of up to 12 weeks may be necessary) should be done before a food challenge is conducted.

For patients with food-induced enterocolitis or colitis, the symptoms provoked by food challenge (often done openly rather by DBPCFC) include vomiting and diarrhea, but dehydration and hypotension may occur. The symptoms may not occur until 1 to 6 hours after the ingestion of the food. In addition to the clinical symptoms, the patient's absolute polymorphonuclear leukocyte (PMN) count may increase to 3,500 cells/mm^3 at 4 to 6 hours after the challenge and the patients' stools will have increased PMNs and eosinophils.

X. Therapy. Once the diagnosis of food allergy is established, the only proven therapy is the strict elimination of the food from the patient's diet. Elimination diets may lead to malnutrition and/or eating disorders, especially if they include a large number of foods and/or are utilized for extended periods of time. Studies have shown that symptomatic food sensitivity generally is lost over time, except for sensitivity to peanuts, tree nuts, and seafood. Symptomatic food sensitivity is usually very specific, so patients rarely react to more than one member of a botanical family or animal species (Table 13.3).

A. Several **medications** have been used in an attempt to protect patients with food hypersensitivity, including oral cromolyn, H1- and H2-antihistamines,

Table 13.3. Food allergen cross-reactivity

	Specific IgE to multiple members of the family	Clinical reactivity
Milk	Common	Common
Legumes	Common	Uncommon
Wheat	Common	Uncommon
Fish	Common	Uncommon
Crustacea–mollusks	Common	???
Tree nuts	Common	Uncommon
Egg–chicken	Occasional	Rare
Milk–beef	Occasional	Uncommon

IgE, immunoglobulin E.

ketotifen, corticosteroids, and prostaglandin synthetase inhibitors. Some of these medications may modify food allergy symptoms, but overall they have minimal efficacy or unacceptable side effects. The use of **epinephrine** is vitally important in acute anaphylaxis.

B. Recent blinded, placebo-controlled studies of **rush immunotherapy** for the treatment of peanut hypersensitivity demonstrated efficacy in a small number of patients. However, the adverse reaction rates were significant and preclude general clinical application at this time. Newer types of vaccines for immunotherapy being developed include B- and T-cell epitopes, peptides, anti-IgE, and complementary DNA (cDNA) vaccines.

C. Patient education and support are essential for food-allergic patients. In particular, older children (and their parents) and adults prone to anaphylaxis must be informed in a direct but sympathetic way that these reactions are potentially fatal. When eating away from home, food-sensitive individuals should feel comfortable to request information about the contents of prepared foods. For the school-aged child, the American Academy of Pediatrics Committee of School Health has recommended that schools be equipped to treat anaphylaxis in allergic students. Children over the age of 7 years can usually be taught to inject themselves with epinephrine. The physician must be willing to explain and, with the parents, help instruct school personnel about these issues.

In the home, consider the need to eliminate the incriminated allergen, or if this is not practical, place warning stickers on foods with the offending antigens. A variety of groups can help provide support, advocacy, and education, including the Food Allergy Network (10400 Easton Place, Suite 107, Fairfax, VA 22030; www.foodallergy.org), the National Allergy and Asthma Network (3554 Chain Bridge Road, Suite 200, Fairfax, VA 22030), and the Asthma and Allergy Foundation of America (1125 15th Street, NW, Suite 502, Washington, DC 20005).

XI. Natural history. Food hypersensitivity is most common in the first several years of life. In one study 80% of children developed their reactions in the first year of life. The average length of time until the food could be tolerated was 1 year. In the group of patients studied with atopic dermatitis and food hypersensitivity, those placed on an appropriate elimination diet experienced a significantly greater improvement in their rash when compared with a similar group of patients who did not have food allergy or who did not adhere to the strict elimination diet. After 1 to 2 years of complete avoidance of the offending food allergen, approximately one-third of symptomatic food reactions were lost. The probability of developing tolerance with specific food avoidance varies with different allergens; patients commonly became tolerant of soybeans, whereas development of tolerance to peanuts was rare. Overall, patients with allergies to peanut, tree nut, fish, and shellfish rarely lose their clinical sensitivity. Skin prick tests or RAST results do not predict which individuals will lose their clinical sensitivity. It is generally thought that non-IgE-mediated food hypersensitivities in infants and young children (other than celiac disease) are outgrown, but there are few studies to document this.

XII. Prophylaxis. The possible prophylaxis of food allergy has been debated for a number of years. Recent studies suggest that in a group of infants at "high risk" for the development of allergic disease, maternal (peanuts during the last trimester) and infant avoidance of major allergenic foods (cow's milk, eggs, and peanuts in the first year of life) results in at least a decreased prevalence of atopic dermatitis. Nursing mothers who do not restrict their diet from such foods allow these food proteins to be ingested by the infants. For such diets to be used for both mothers and infants, these families should be in this "high risk" group; the diets should not necessarily be utilized for the general population. The general consensus would now be for patients in significantly at-risk families to avoid milk for 12 months, eggs for 12 to 15 months, and peanuts for 3 years.

XIII. Conclusions. After the diagnosis of food hypersensitivity is established, the only proven therapy is strict elimination of the offending allergen. It is important to remember that prescribing an elimination diet is like prescribing a medication; both can have positive effects and unwarranted side effects. Elimination diets may lead to malnutrition and/or eating disorders, especially if they include a large number of foods and/or are utilized for extended periods. Patients and parents should be taught and given educational material to help them detect potential sources of hidden food allergens by appropriately reading food labels. Education of the patient and family is vital to the success of the elimination diet. Families should be given instructional material to help them remember what foods contain the allergen they are to avoid. It is often difficult to determine what foods will contain an allergen without careful reading of the label. Studies in both children and adults indicate that symptomatic reactivity to food allergens is often lost over time, except possibly for peanuts, nuts, and seafood.

Symptomatic reactivity to food allergens is generally very specific. Patients rarely react to more than one member of a botanical family or animal species. Notably, initiation of an elimination diet totally excluding only foods identified to provoke food-allergic reactions will result in symptomatic improvement. This treatment generally will lead to resolution of the food allergy within a few years and is unlikely to induce malnutrition or other eating disorders.

Conditions That Mimic Food Allergies

I. **Vomiting** is particularly common in infants and children and is often attributed to food allergy. Vomiting is a symptom, not a diagnosis, and its cause may lie outside the gastrointestinal tract. It is important to determine whether or not the vomiting is associated with other gastrointestinal symptoms, such as abdominal distention or diarrhea. The differential diagnosis of vomiting is outlined in Table 13.4.

A. **Gastroesophageal reflux** (due to a lax lower esophageal sphincter) is the most common cause of vomiting in an otherwise healthy infant. The onset of vomiting is in the first month of life and may consist of spitting or be projectile. By 1 year of age, 80% of infants recover without therapy. This isolated vomiting, usually after meals and without diarrhea, is rarely due to allergy. **Multiple formula changes are not indicated** and may convince the parents that there is something intrinsically wrong with their child.

1. If the vomiting is troublesome, if weight gain is inadequate, or if complications such as recurrent pulmonary infections or apnea occur, the child must be evaluated in detail. An upper gastrointestinal series may demonstrate reflux and exclude distal outlet obstruction. Failure to demonstrate gastroesophageal reflux by x-ray does not exclude reflux. If necessary, esophageal manometry, pH studies, and radioisotope studies can be performed.

2. The **treatment** of esophageal reflux in infants consists of frequent small feedings (2 to 3 oz. every 3 hours), maintaining the upright position 24 hours a day, and antacids, 2 to 5 mL, 1 hour after each feeding. Additional drug therapy includes metoclopramide, which enhances gastric emptying. Only those infants who do not improve after months of intensive medical therapy and have systemic effects from the reflux should be considered possible candidates for surgery. Appropriate therapy of esophageal reflux in adults consists of H2-antagonists, proton pump inhibitors, elimination of exacerbating factors (e.g., alcohol, caffeine) and raising the head of the bed.

II. **Diarrhea**, a frequently encountered problem, is similarly often ascribed to food hypersensitivity and treated by multiple dietary manipulations without regard to the cause of the diarrhea or the specific dietary component causing symptoms. Unfortunately, these manipulations often result in a diet insufficient to meet caloric requirements. This can perpetuate the diarrhea, causing decreased pancreatic enzyme synthesis and intestinal mucosal function. Weight loss and increasing diarrhea result in increased malnutrition, thus setting up a vicious cycle. In young children, especially infants under 4 months of age, hypocaloric diets should be avoided for periods longer than 48 hours. If

Table 13.4. Causes of vomiting

Gastrointestinal
  Gastroesophageal reflux
  Obstruction
  Pyloric stenosis, antral web
  Malrotation, superior mesenteric artery syndrome
  Peptic ulcer disease
  Hepatitis
  Pancreatitis
  Infections: acute gastroenteritis (usually occurs with diarrhea)
  Motility disturbances
  Idiopathic pseudoobstruction
  Ileus from trauma, Addison disease
  Hypokalemia, hypothyroidism
  Acute gastric dilatation (trauma, body cast)
Psychogenic
  Psychogenic vomiting
  Anorexia nervosa, rumination
Extraintestinal
  Metabolic
    Reye syndrome
    Metabolic acidosis, uremia, lead poisoning
    Disorders of fat oxidation
    Carnitine deficiency
  Toxic
    Ingestion, drug toxicity (e.g., theophylline)
  Infectious
    Meningitis, encephalopathy
  Increased intracranial pressure
    Trauma, tumor, hydrocephalus, pseudotumor cerebri

---

the diarrhea becomes chronic and persistent (greater than 50 gm of stool/day in children, 100 gm/day in adults), or if it is impossible to achieve adequate caloric intake, a more detailed evaluation should follow, keeping in mind the differential diagnostic possibilities (Table 13.5).

  A. The **history** in a child with diarrhea should include the following items.
  1. The **temporal sequence** of abnormal stools, failure to thrive, and caloric intake.
  2. The temporal relationship to the **introduction of cereals** suggests the diagnosis of celiac disease.
  3. **Changes in feedings**, especially formulas, and correlation of protein and carbohydrate content with symptoms. High-carbohydrate fluids often cause diarrhea. Sorbitol-containing gums and candies as well as apples, pears, and peaches can cause an osmotic diarrhea.
  4. Previously normal stools followed by persistent abnormal stools after acute gastrointestinal infection.
  5. Abdominal pain or distention.
  6. Emotional disturbances.
  7. Physical and emotional environment (e.g., failure to thrive on a maternal deprivation basis).
  B. In the **physical examination**, particular attention should be paid to weight and height, general well being, irritability, and wasting of the buttocks. Other clues to chronic malabsorption include a protuberant abdomen (best viewed in profile with the patient standing), pallor, reddish tinge to the hair, clubbing of the digits, or edema.

Table 13.5. Differential diagnosis of diarrhea

Infections
 Viral (rotavirus, adenovirus, enterovirus), *Salmonella*, *Shigella*, *Amoeba*, *Yersinia*, *Campylobacter*, *Giardia*, *Cryptosporidia*
Chronic Inflammation
 Crohn disease, ulcerative colitis, tuberculosis, histoplasmosis
Abnormality of anatomy or motility
 Surgical short gut, malrotation, intestinal obstruction, Hirschsprung disease, chronic constipation (overflow diarrhea), idiopathic intestinal pseudoobstruction
Inadequate pancreatic function
 Cystic fibrosis, Schwachman-Diamond syndrome, malnutrition, lipase deficiency
Alteration of the enterohepatic bile salt circulation
 Metabolic immaturity of the liver (prematurity), cholestatic liver disease, ileal resection, Crohn disease, bacterial overgrowth of the small bowel ("blind loop")
Abnormality of the intestinal mucosa
 Celiac disease, immune deficiencies, postgastroenteritis changes, drug toxicity, cow's milk or soy protein intolerance
 Primary and secondary disaccharidase deficiencies, monosaccharide intolerance
Miscellaneous
 Irritable bowel syndrome, chronic nonspecific diarrhea
 Endocrine: hypoparathyroidism, hyperthyroidism, neuroblastoma

---

1. Because patients may have biases and misconceptions regarding normal stool characteristics, the physician must examine the stool. The following stool characteristics are helpful.
   a. **Pale color** suggests malabsorption or liver disease.
   b. **Mucous stools** suggest infection, colitis, or irritable bowel syndrome, though this type of stool is often a normal variant.
   c. **Bloody stools** suggest colitis or acute infection (e.g., *Shigella*, *Salmonella*, *Yersinia*, *Campylobacter*, enterohemorrhagic *Escherichia coli*).
   d. A **high liquid content** suggests sugar intolerance, bacterial overgrowth of the small intestine, bile salt malabsorption, or neuroblastoma.
   e. **Oiliness** (steatorrhea) suggests fat malabsorption (e.g., pancreatic insufficiency or celiac disease).
   f. Vegetable matter and meat fibers are of little diagnostic significance.
C. **Laboratory studies**
   1. A **stool culture** for common pathogens (e.g., *Salmonella* and *Shigella*), as well as rarer pathogens (e.g., *Yersinia* and *Campylobacter*)
   2. Stool analysis for **occult blood**
   3. **Complete blood and reticulocyte count.** Chronic intestinal disorders may lead to occult blood loss and malabsorption of iron, folate, or vitamin B12.
   4. The **erythrocyte sedimentation rate** is frequently elevated in inflammatory bowel disease.
   5. Examination of the stool for *Giardia lamblia*, *Cryptosporidium*, and *Entamoeba histolytica* and other endemic parasites
   6. **Sweat chloride determination.** Cystic fibrosis is a frequent cause of poor weight gain and abnormal stools in young children.
   7. **Fecal fat determinations.** If the stool volume is excessive and greasy, fecal fat content should be measured. A 72-hour fecal fat quantitation is more reliable than intermittent, randomly obtained fecal smears. Normal children excrete 5 to 10 g of fat per day; adults excrete

less than 5 g per day. These amounts represent less than 5% to 10% of dietary fat ingested during the study.

8. The watery portion of the stool should be examined for **reducing substances. Lactose intolerance** is shown by the presence of reducing substances in the aqueous portion of the stool in a patient on a lactose-containing diet. Two drops of stool and 10 drops of water are placed in a test tube and a Clinitest tablet is added. The color is read against the chart provided; a reading greater than 0.5% is significant. Sucrose (found in soy formula, juices) is not a reducing substance. To test for sucrose, the stool is hydrolyzed with an equal volume of 0.1 N HCl. The Clinitest procedure is then performed again. Determination of breath hydrogen after a test dose of the suspected sugar confirms malabsorption.

9. **Intestinal biopsy.** This invasive procedure may be necessary to elucidate the exact cause of diarrhea in complex cases. At the time of the biopsy, duodenal fluid is obtained for pancreatic lipase and trypsin determinations, for Gram stains and bacterial cultures, and for microscopic and immunoassay examination for *Giardia* and other parasites. Disaccharidase activity can be measured on mucosal specimens.

D. Table 13.5 lists the conditions to be considered in the differential diagnosis of diarrhea. Several points are worth noting. The most common causes of fatty stools are cystic fibrosis, celiac disease, and postinfectious steatorrhea. The most frequent causes of runny, liquid stools are acute infections, carbohydrate intolerance, and chronic nonspecific diarrhea (irritable bowel syndrome).

1. **Cystic fibrosis** should be suspected in any infant with abnormal stools and poor weight gain. Respiratory symptoms are not always evident. The diagnosis should be confirmed with a sweat chloride determination.

2. **Celiac disease** is a permanent intolerance to gluten and is characterized by diarrhea and poor nutrition. Malabsorption and histologic abnormalities of the jejunal mucosa are present. Improvement, determined by clinical observation and biopsy, occurs when gluten is removed from the diet. Reintroduction of gluten results in a relapse that is observable clinically and histologically. Serum reticulin and endomysial antibodies are useful screening tests. The correct diagnosis is crucial, because therapy is lifelong, and a gluten-free diet is difficult to follow; **a gluten-free diet should never be prescribed until the diagnosis of celiac disease has been confirmed by intestinal biopsy.**

3. **Postinfectious steatorrhea** occurs transiently following an acute insult, usually a viral infection, and is usually self-limited; if abnormal stools and weight loss persist, consider a medium-chain triglyceride formula (e.g., Pregestimil).

4. **Carbohydrate intolerance** frequently causes watery stools. The intolerance can be either primary or secondary. Primary lactose intolerance is commonly seen in African Americans, Asians, and those of Mediterranean ancestry. Secondary lactose or sucrose intolerance occurs following an acute injury to the intestine. Diagnosis is by demonstration of reducing substances in the stool. The treatment is to remove the offending sugar from the diet.

5. A frequent cause of loose stools in toddlers is the **irritable bowel syndrome.** Although the exact cause is unknown, it is harmless and self-limited, disappearing by age 3 to 4 years. The child has an average of four stools per day, ranging from two to seven per day. Growth is normal in these children if the diet is adequate, thus excluding malabsorption. Complex elimination diets are not indicated. Frequently, a history of excessive carbohydrate intake (juices, punches) is obtained. The child should be placed on a regular diet. A frequent cause of morbidity in these children is multiple dietary manipulations, leading to decreased caloric intake and weight loss.

Selected Readings

Anderson JA, Sogn DD, eds. Adverse reactions to foods. American Academy of Allergy and Immunology Committee on Adverse Reactions to Foods and the National Institute of Allergy and Infectious Disease, NIH Publication No. 84-2442. Washington, DC: U.S. Department of Health and Human Services, 1984.

Bock SA. Natural history of severe reactions to foods in young children. *J Pediatr* 1985;107:676.

Bock SA. Patterns of food hypersensitivity during sixteen years of double-blind, placebo-controlled food challenges. *J Pediatr* 1990;117:561.

Bock SA. Prospective appraisal of complaints of adverse reactions to foods in children during the first 3 years of life. *Pediatrics* 1987;79:683.

Burks AW, Sampson HA. Diagnostic approaches to the patient with suspected food allergies. *J Pediatr* 1992;121:S64.

Bush RK, Taylor SL. Adverse reactions to food and drug additives. In: Middleton E Jr, Reed CE, Ellis EF, et al., eds. *Allergy: principles and practice*, 4th ed. St. Louis: Mosby–Year Book, 1998:1183–1198.

Crowe SE, Perdue MH. Gastrointestinal food hypersensitivity basic mechanisms of pathophysiology. *Gastroenterology* 1992;103:1075.

Jenkins HR, et al. Food allergy: The major cause of infantile colitis. *Arch Dis Child* 1984;59:326.

Metcalfe DD, Sampson HA, Simon RA. *Food allergy: adverse reactions to foods and food additives.* Cambridge: Blackwell, 1997.

Sampson HA. Food allergy. *J Allergy Clin Immunol* 1989;84:1062.

Sampson HA, Mendelson L, Rosen JP. Fatal and near-fatal anaphylactic reactions to food in children and adolescents. *N Engl J Med* 1992;327:380.

Sampson HA. Adverse reactions to foods. In: Middleton E Jr, Reed CE, Ellis EF, et al., eds. *Allergy: principles and practice,* 4th ed. St. Louis: Mosby–Year Book, 1998:1162.

Terr AI. Unconventional theories and unproven methods in allergy. In: Middleton E Jr, Reed CE, Ellis EF, et al., eds. *Allergy: principles and practice,* 4th ed. St. Louis: Mosby–Year Book, 1998:1235.

Yunginger JW. Lethal food allergy in children. *N Engl J Med* 1992;327:421.

Zeiger RS. Secondary prevention of allergic disease: an adjunct to primary prevention. *Pediatr Allergy Immunol* 1995;6:127.

14. RHEUMATIC DISEASES

Julian L. Ambrus, Jr., Alan Baer, and Kathleen M. O'Neil

The clinical immunologist is often called to evaluate and manage patients with diseases that also fall under the purview of rheumatologists. The distinction between the clinical immunologist and rheumatologist is blurred in many parts of the country. It is more common, however, for the rheumatologist to manage patients with osteoarthritis and crystalline-induced arthritis than the clinical immunologist. The clinical immunologist may see more patients with systemic autoimmune diseases, such as systemic lupus erythematosus (SLE). Patients with multisystem disorders are often referred to clinical immunologists for the evaluation of possible vasculitides, granulomatous disorders, or genetically determined fever syndromes. Granulomatous disorders, such as sarcoidosis and granulomatous hepatitis, are covered in other sections of this manual.

This section will outline the diagnosis and management of patients with rheumatic diseases. It will discuss both adult and pediatric patients. It will focus on those disorders for which the clinical immunologist is often consulted.

I. Evaluation of the patient with arthritis

Inflammatory, structural, and psychogenic describe three broad categories of joint disorders that must be differentiated in the evaluation of a patient with joint pain or arthritis. In the first, inflammation is a major component, present both in the synovium and the synovial fluid. Examples include rheumatoid arthritis (RA) and SLE. In the second, mechanical or structural derangements of the joint are prominent. Examples include osteoarthritis and traumatic arthritis. These two types of joint disorders may occur together in the same joint. Inflammatory joint disorders often lead to structural derangement of the joint and similarly, structural joint problems often have an associated, albeit minor, inflammatory component. In psychogenic joint disorders, no definite organic etiology for the joint complaints can be identified.

A. Symptoms of joint disease

1. **Pain.** Pain in small distal joints tends to be more accurately localized than pain in larger, more proximal joints. Thus pain arising from the hip joint may be felt in the groin or buttock, over the greater trochanter, in the anterior portion of the thigh, or entirely in the knee. Pain that is diffuse, variable, poorly described, or unrelated to anatomic structures may be secondary to depression or other psychiatric disorders. Pain that occurs during usage, particularly if it worsens during use and quickly improves on resting, is typical of structural/mechanical joint disease. Pain that is present at rest and is worse at the beginning rather than at the end of usage is suggestive of inflammatory joint disease. Patients with advanced degenerative joint disease of the hips, spine, or knees may also have pain at night.

2. **Swelling of joints.** Patients may complain of joint swelling that is not evident on physical exam. It is important to determine whether the swelling is visible to others and whether the swelling conforms to an anatomically discrete area such as a particular joint or bursa. Normal collections of fat over the medial aspects of the elbow or knee and lateral aspect of the ankle may be misinterpreted as joint swelling.

3. **Limitation of motion.** This symptom is often related in the context of difficulties that patients may experience with their activities of daily living. Such difficulties can be screened for by asking, "Can you dress yourself completely without any difficulty?" and "Can you walk up and down stairs without any difficulty?" Restriction of joint motion may also be manifest as a gait disturbance.

4. **Stiffness.** Stiffness is the sensation of tightness perceived by the patient attempting to move his or her joints after a period of inactivity. The stiffness typically "wears off." Stiffness of the joints (especially the hands, feet) present on arising in the morning and lasting 1 hour or more is an important symptom of inflammatory joint disease. In osteoarthritis, brief periods of stiffness (e.g., 15 minutes) may be present on arising in the morning or during the day after resting an hour or more.

5. **Weakness.** A loss of muscular strength related to disuse may occur in the setting of arthritis and may result in decreased grip strength, difficulty in arising from a chair, or difficulty going up or down stairs.

6. **Fatigue.** Fatigue is a common complaint among patients with musculo-skeletal disease, yet it is an imprecise term. It implies exhaustion and depletion of energy. Fatigue occurring in association with inflammatory arthritides is usually noted in the afternoon or early evening and may be prominent even when the patient has not been active physically. In psychogenic disorders, fatigue is often noted on arising in the morning and is related to anxiety, muscular tension, and poor sleep.

B. **Signs of joint disease**

1. **Inflammatory joint disease.** The most reliable signs of an inflammatory arthritis are **synovial hypertrophy** and/or **joint effusion**. The normal synovial membrane is too thin to palpate. The thickened synovial membrane has a "doughy" or "boggy" consistency on palpation and is appreciated best at the joint line or joint margin. Joint effusions are usually indicative of inflammation in the joint, albeit sometimes low grade. They may also be a result of trauma, bleeding into the joint, and severe anasarca.

The normal joint is not tender to palpation. In examining the small joints, the examiner should be able to exert sufficient force to the joint to blanch her or his own thumbnail and not cause pain. In examining larger joints, one should be able to apply the weight of one's body to one's thumb or palm as one examines the spine, sacroiliac joints, or anterior hip. **Joint tenderness** is a sensitive sign of joint pathology, but is not specific for inflammatory joint disease. The absence of joint tenderness is thus a useful test to exclude joint pathology. The presence of joint tenderness in the absence of other joint abnormalities must be interpreted in the context of the patient's emotional state. The examiner should check whether the patient is also tender in adjacent areas away from the joint. Joint tenderness that is localized, rather than generalized, may indicate problems with specific intraarticular structures (e.g., tenderness of the medial joint line of the knee in medial meniscal tears).

Pain felt at the **extremes of motion of a joint** is also a useful test for the detection of joint disease. Overlying **warmth** and **erythema** are specific signs of inflammation in or about the joint, but may be absent in less acute cases of arthritis. Warmth is best appreciated using the back of the hand as a thermometer and comparing the temperature of the skin above, over, and below the joint.

2. **Structural joint disease.** Damage to the joint, resulting from inflammatory joint disease, trauma, or osteoarthritis, results in a variety of joint findings. **Crepitus** is a palpable or audible grating sensation produced during motion of the joint. It occurs when roughened articular or extraarticular surfaces are rubbed together. It is not abnormal for joints to make a coarse crackle with motion, usually due to tendons snapping over bony prominences. When crepitus is felt as a fine vibratory sensation throughout the available range of movement of the joint, it is clinically significant and represents grating of roughened cartilages against one another, bone rubbing against bone, or fibrinous inflammation of the synovium. **Bony overgrowth** of the joints, resulting from the formation of osteophytes, is a common finding in osteoarthritis. Those located at the distal interphalangeal (DIP) joints are called

Heberden nodes; those at the proximal interphalangeal joints are Bouchard nodes.

Joint deformities are of several types. (i) Restriction in the range of normal movements; e.g., flexion deformities of the elbow, hip, and knee: If a flexion deformity is irreversible, it is termed a joint contracture. (ii) Malalignment of the articulating bones, e.g., ulnar deviation of the fingers or "knock-knee" (genu valgum). Such a deformity may not be fixed, in which case it is referred to as instability. Instability of a lower-extremity joint may become apparent only with weight bearing. (iii) Alteration in the relationship of the two articulating surfaces: **Subluxation** implies that some contact between the articulating surfaces is still maintained. **Dislocation** implies complete loss of contact.

C. **Approach to the differential diagnosis of arthritis**

The many forms of arthritis are differentiated by integrating historical features, findings on musculoskeletal exam, and the results of ancillary studies. **Historical features** include (i) **host factors**, such as age, sex, family history, and social history; (ii) the **pattern of joint involvement**, including the number of joints involved as well as the symmetry and distribution of affected joints; and (iii) **extraarticular manifestations**. Involvement of the same joints on each side of the body (symmetric arthritis) is typical of RA and many other arthritides. An asymmetric polyarthritis characterizes psoriatic arthritis, Reiter disease, and Lyme arthritis. Certain arthritides affect certain joints and spare others. An example is the DIP joint of the fingers, which is affected in psoriatic arthritis, gout, and osteoarthritis and spared in RA. Weight loss, fatigue, and malaise suggest an underlying systemic disorder; these symptoms would not be expected in patients with osteoarthritis. The pattern of extraarticular manifestations often serves to characterize a specific form of arthritis. There are a number of rheumatic diseases in which the physical examination of the skin, but not the joints, indicates the specific diagnosis. Thus the morphology of a "rash" associated with arthritis is key. Examples include SLE, psoriatic arthritis, Reiter disease, erythema nodosum, Lyme disease, scleroderma, dermatomyositis (DM), Still disease, Henoch-Schönlein purpura (HSP), rubella, and serum sickness. **Involvement of the aortic root** is an occasional feature of the seronegative spondyloarthropathies, such as ankylosing spondylitis and reactive arthritis. Involvement of the **eye** in rheumatic diseases includes episcleritis and scleritis (e.g., RA), iritis (e.g., ankylosing spondylitis), iridocyclitis (juvenile RA), and conjunctivitis (e.g., reactive arthritis).

1. **Laboratory testing**

The value of laboratory studies is secondary to that of a careful history and physical examination in establishing a diagnosis. The results of many tests may be misleading if ordered for an individual in whom there is little evidence for the diagnosis being sought. Tests that are used to evaluate rheumatic diseases are often positive in the normal population; therefore, in random individuals, tests such as the antinuclear antibody (ANA), rheumatoid factor (RF), and serum urate, will have a high false-positive rate. The sensitivity and specificity of the tests used to evaluate rheumatic diseases should be known. Tests such as the ANA and erythrocyte sedimentation rate (ESR) are sensitive for disease but lack specificity. Thus, a negative ANA test virtually excludes a diagnosis of SLE. A normal ESR is useful in excluding the presence of an inflammatory disorder. Tests that have great specificity, such as the anti-double-stranded (ds)DNA and anti-Smith (anti-Sm) antibodies for SLE, suffer from a lack of sensitivity and thus can only be used to confirm a diagnosis in a fraction of the patients affected with SLE. The use of tests with relatively poor sensitivity and specificity (e.g., serum urate, RF) can be very misleading in the evaluation of patients with rheumatic complaints.

2. Synovial fluid analysis

The synovial fluid analysis will permit differentiation of inflammatory versus noninflammatory arthritides. The most important test in this regard is the synovial fluid white blood cell count (WBC), which is less than 200 per mm^3 in normal joints, between 200 and 2,000 per mm^3 in noninflammatory effusions, and greater than 2,000 per mm^3 in inflammatory arthritides. An inflammatory effusion is also characterized by poor viscosity and the formation of a poor mucin clot when dilute acetic acid is added to the joint fluid. The synovial fluid analysis may constitute the definitive test in the diagnosis of certain forms of joint disease, such as septic arthritis and crystal-induced synovitis. A joint may be affected by more than one process; thus, septic arthritis and gout or pseudogout may coexist in the same joint, and the finding of one does not exclude the occasional presence of the other.

In **septic arthritis**, the synovial fluid white cell count is usually 50,000 to 200,000 per mm^3 with greater than 90% polymorphonuclear leukocytes. Early in the course of septic arthritis or in patients with disseminated gonococcal infection, the synovial fluid WBC may be lower. The definitive test is a Gram stain of the synovial fluid (preferably performed on a concentrated sediment of centrifuged synovial fluid) and a synovial fluid culture. In **gout or pseudogout**, the synovial fluid WBC ranges from 2,000 to 100,000 per mm^3. With the use of polarized light microscopy, urate crystals are seen as needle-shaped with strong negative birefringence. Calcium pyrophosphate dihydrate (CPPD) crystals are seen as rhomboid-shaped with weak positive birefringence. A selenium quartz filter is used to determine the direction that polarized light rotates when passing through these crystals. Urate crystals appear yellow and CPPD crystals appear blue when their long axes are aligned parallel to that of the filter. In **traumatic arthritis**, the synovial fluid WBC is usually in the range of 50 to 2,000 per mm^3. Hemorrhage is common. The presence of fat globules should be sought by centrifuging the synovial fluid and looking for the development of a fat layer on top of the specimen. The presence of fat globules within the synovial fluid should raise the suspicion of a fracture adjacent to the joint.

3. X-rays of joints

The radiographic appearance of the joints is often quite distinctive for various forms of arthritis. However, these characteristic changes may not be apparent early in the course of the joint disease. The changes seen in osteoarthritis and those seen in RA are markedly different. In osteoarthritis, the changes include subchondral bony sclerosis, segmental joint space narrowing, marginal osteophyte formation, and cyst formation. Periarticular demineralization is not seen in osteoarthritis. In contrast, one of the earliest radiographic manifestations of RA is periarticular demineralization. Involvement of the articular cartilage is reflected by joint space narrowing, which, in contrast to osteoarthritis, is virtually always uniform or nonsegmental. Bony erosions become evident as the disease progresses. These erosions are most evident at the margins of the joints, corresponding to those parts of the bone within the joint that are not covered by articular cartilage. Bony erosions are not specific for RA; they are also seen, for example, in chronic gouty arthritis, psoriatic arthritis, and chronic forms of reactive arthritis.

4. Synovial biopsy

In the majority of rheumatic diseases, an accurate diagnosis can be established without synovial biopsy. However, in certain conditions, the histopathologic findings in the synovium are either pathognomonic or highly specific. The synovial biopsy may be of particular value in the assessment of a chronic inflammatory monoarthritis, in which histopathology and synovial tissue culture may help to differentiate the various granulomatous synovitides (e.g., tuberculous, fungal, sarcoidosis). The biopsy is also useful in the diagnosis of amyloidosis, synovial tumors, ochronosis, hemachromatosis, and multicentric reticulohistiocytosis.

D. Diagnosis of systemic rheumatic diseases

In many systemic rheumatic diseases, the diagnosis is established on the basis of a characteristic pattern of organ involvement and laboratory abnormalities. For many rheumatic diseases, specific tests either do not exist or are too insensitive to aid in the routine evaluation of patients with rheumatic complaints. Criteria have been established by the American College of Rheumatology (ACR) for the purpose of defining certain diseases, most notably RA and SLE. These criteria have been established primarily for epidemiologic surveys (in which the incidence and prevalence of the various rheumatic diseases are defined in a given population) and for the purpose of ensuring uniformity in what is classified as RA, SLE, etc. These criteria may not be helpful in early stages of these rheumatic diseases.

A diagnosis may not be attainable when a patient first presents with rheumatic complaints. The features that allow specific diagnoses to be established are often not evident on first exam and take time to develop or become apparent. Fortunately, many patients with the new onset of rheumatic complaints have a self-limited problem, which resolves spontaneously, often without a specific diagnosis ever being made. Thus, time and patience are important in approaching the patient with rheumatic disease. This necessity often runs counter to the expectation of the patient that a diagnosis should be achievable from the "start," so it is essential that the problem be discussed with the patient.

Clearly, there are some rheumatologic conditions in which a specific diagnosis should be sought promptly. These include a condition that is severe and involves a single joint or at most a few joints (e.g., septic arthritis, gout), a condition that is associated with a major systemic illness (as evidenced by fever, prominent weight loss, and evidence of multiple organ involvement), a condition that is associated with significant trauma (e.g., fracture, ligament disruption), and a condition that is associated with a significant neurologic problem such as nerve root compression or peripheral nerve entrapment.

II. Osteoarthritis

Osteoarthritis is a slowly progressive articular disorder that generally occurs late in life and principally affects the hands and large weight-bearing joints. The disease appears to stem from defects in the articular cartilage of unknown cause, and is associated secondarily with changes in the subchondral bone and synovium. It is the most common form of arthritis and is evident radiographically in 60% of the population 65 years and older.

A. Classification. Osteoarthritis is usually classified into primary (idiopathic) and secondary forms. Primary osteoarthritis occurs in the absence of any antecedent joint injury, inflammatory joint disease, or systemic disease associated with the development of osteoarthritis. Primary osteoarthritis is further characterized as localized or generalized. It is localized when only one or two joint groups are affected; for example, one or both knees and the DIP joints of the hands. When three or more joint groups are involved, the disease is generalized. The category of primary osteoarthritis also includes the syndromes of erosive osteoarthritis and diffuse idiopathic skeletal hyperostosis. In secondary osteoarthritis, the affected joint(s) has been affected by previous trauma or by previous episodes of inflammatory joint disease, such as RA, gout, or septic arthritis. Certain metabolic disorders are also associated with the development of secondary osteoarthritis, including hemachromatosis, hyperparathyroidism, and ochronosis. Other forms of secondary osteoarthritis occur in patients who have had a congenital (e.g., osteopetrosis, bone dysplasias), developmental (e.g., Legg-Calvé-Perthes disease, slipped femoral capital epiphysis), or acquired (e.g., Paget disease, acromegaly, or aseptic necrosis) disorder of cartilage or bone; patients with hemophiliac arthropathy; and patients with a neuropathic (Charcot disease) arthropathy.

B. **Clinical features.** In primary osteoarthritis, the joints that are typically involved include the distal interphalangeal joints of the fingers, the first carpometacarpal joint, the first metatarsophalangeal (MTP) joint, the hips, the knees, the cervical spine, and the lumbar spine. Involvement of the metacarpophalangeal joints, the wrists, the elbows, the shoulders, and the ankles should always suggest a secondary form of osteoarthritis. Patients with osteoarthritis have deep aching pain in the joint, which may be poorly localized in more proximal joints, such as the hip. Early in the disease, the pain is noted primarily with joint use, but as the disease advances, pain is noticed with minimal joint motion and eventually at rest. The patient also notices stiffness localized to the involved joint. This stiffness, usually 15 to 30 minutes in duration, is most notable on awakening in the morning and after inactivity during the day. The patient may notice crepitus of the joint as well as a limitation of joint motion. The latter may interfere with activities of daily living, such as climbing stairs or getting in and out of a car. In addition, the patient may notice that his or her weight-bearing joints "give way," a possible result of loose bodies in the joint that occasionally slip between the opposing articular surfaces. On examination, the involved joint may be tender on palpation and painful with passive motion. In more advanced cases, crepitus may be palpated and sometimes heard with joint motion. The joint is enlarged as a primary result of bony proliferation with osteophyte formation. If there is an associated element of inflammation, there may be some synovial proliferation and the presence of an effusion. Limitation of joint motion is observed as a result of incongruity of the joint surface, muscle spasm and contracture, and mechanical block related to osteophytes or the presence of loose bodies. Late in the disease there may be deformity and subluxation of the joint.

Osteoarthritis of the hand is characterized typically by a firm bony nodular enlargement of the distal (Heberden nodes) and proximal interphalangeal joints (Bouchard nodes). This type of "nodal" osteoarthritis is 10 times more common in women than in men and demonstrates a strong hereditary tendency. The nodes develop slowly and are not usually painful. However, on occasion they may present acutely with inflammation, and in these instances the possible presence of gout or pseudogout should be considered. Gelatinous cysts may sometimes develop on the dorsal aspects of the DIP joints. In those cases where there is a prominent inflammatory component in the osteoarthritic joints of the hand, the term "erosive osteoarthritis" is often applied. Patients with this disease are most commonly postmenopausal women who have attacks of mild to moderately painful synovitis involving the distal and proximal interphalangeal joints of the hand. Eventual joint deformity and sometimes ankylosis results. The acute flares of inflammation may occur periodically over a number of years, after which the joints become essentially pain-free. Restriction of motion of the carpometacarpal joints, leading to atrophy of the thenar eminences, is also a common finding in osteoarthritis of the hand. Involvement of the metacarpophalangeal joints is more commonly seen in osteoarthritis affecting the male hand. In every case of metacarpophalangeal joint involvement, one should exclude the possibility of a secondary form of osteoarthritis, especially calcium pyrophosphate deposition disease. Hemachromatosis may present initially with osteoarthritis affecting the metacarpophalangeal joints.

C. **Laboratory tests.** The synovial fluid in osteoarthritis is typically viscous and demonstrates a mild leukocytosis with less than 2,000 white blood cells per mm^3. The synovial fluid cells are predominantly mononuclear.

D. **Radiographs.** The radiographic abnormalities in osteoarthritis include localized loss of joint space, subchondral bony sclerosis and cyst formation, osteophytes, bony collapse, and intraarticular osseous bodies. In erosive osteoarthritis of the hands, there are erosions both at the articular margins and within the articulating surface, and collapse of the subchondral plate.

E. Therapy. Therapy of osteoarthritis has the dual objectives of reducing pain and improving function. The management of osteoarthritis is most effective when it is multifaceted and should thus include physical measures, medications, and occasionally surgery.

   1. Physical measures. The patient should be advised to limit aggravating factors such as strenuous exercise, stair climbing, prolonged sitting, or tasks that involve repetitive motion. If the patient is obese, he or she should lose weight. The patient should be prescribed an exercise program that includes range of motion and flexibility exercise, muscle conditioning, and aerobic cardiovascular exercise. Local heat and massage may be used to relieve muscle spasm surrounding the joint. Walking aids such as a cane or crutch and orthotic devices, such as braces and splints, may be used to decrease the weight bearing on an affected joint and to stabilize an unstable joint. Lateral wedged insoles are helpful for patients with medial tibiofemoral osteoarthritis. Assistive devices may be prescribed by an occupational therapist to help the patient in activities of daily living. These might include raised toilet seats, dressing sticks for putting on socks and hose, and wall bars for getting in and out of the bathtub.

   2. Medications. Antiinflammatory medication is commonly prescribed for patients with osteoarthritis, but this should be done with caution. Because nonsteroidal antiinflammatory drugs (NSAIDs) may induce gastrointestinal bleeding, especially in elderly patients, they should only be used chronically in patients with more symptomatic osteoarthritis. Thus, many patients with mild forms of osteoarthritis may have relief of joint pain with simple analgesics such as acetaminophen (in doses up to 4 g per day), propoxyphene/acetaminophen (Darvocet, one capsule q.i.d.) or tramadol (50 to 100 mg q.i.d.). Such patients may also benefit from the mild analgesic effects of glucosamine and chondroitin sulfate, and topical analgesics (such as capsaicin, applied to the symptomatic joint four times a day). NSAIDs should only be used after a careful assessment of the risk factors for upper gastrointestinal or renal toxicity. All NSAIDs may produce reversible renal failure, an effect most commonly observed in patients with intrinsic renal disease who are 65 years or older, have hypertension or congestive heart failure (CHF), or are taking diuretics or angiotensin-converting enzyme inhibitors. Cyclooxygenase 2 (COX-2)-specific inhibitors, such as rofecoxib or celecoxib, are associated with a reduced risk of gastrointestinal toxicity and are thus the NSAIDs of first choice in patients older than 65 years, those with a history of peptic ulcer disease or previous upper gastrointestinal bleeding, and those taking anticoagulants or oral corticosteroids. The concomitant use of low-dose aspirin (325 mg or less) may negate the gastrointestinal safety of selective COX-2 inhibitors. The gastrointestinal toxicity of nonselective NSAIDs may be reduced if they are taken in the lowest effective dose and concomitantly with gastroprotective agents, such as misoprostol (200 μg t.i.d.), omeprazole (20 mg q.d.), or famotidine (40 mg b.i.d.). Certain NSAIDs, such as indomethacin, piroxicam, and mefenamic acid, should be avoided for long-term use in osteoarthritis, because they have been found in epidemiologic studies to be associated with a higher incidence of adverse gastrointestinal events. In patients with symptomatic effusions, intraarticular steroids may be instilled in the affected joint. Intraarticular hyaluronic acid (viscosupplementation therapy) has also been shown to provide pain relief of symptomatic knee osteoarthritis for periods up to 3 months. Two preparations are available, hylan G-F 20 (Synvisc, given intraarticularly once a week for 3 consecutive weeks) and sodium hyaluronate (Hyalgan, given intraarticularly, once a week for 5 weeks).

   3. Surgery. Surgery should be considered for patients with severe pain or a deformity that causes severe disability. The surgical procedures include osteotomy (to redistribute joint forces), removal of loose bodies, and joint arthroplasty.

III. Bacterial arthritis

Acute bacterial arthritis is a medical emergency that requires early recognition and prompt initiation of antibiotic therapy and joint drainage in order to prevent joint damage. Bacterial arthritis is usually acquired hematogenously. Less often, joints may become infected by direct inoculation (e.g., contaminated corticosteroid injections into joints) or contiguous spread (e.g., from an adjacent bone or soft-tissue infection). Certain factors increase the risk of developing a septic joint in the setting of bacteremia. These include (i) **impaired host defenses** related to serious chronic illnesses (e.g., cancer, cirrhosis, diabetes), use of immunosuppressive drugs, hypogammaglobulinemia, inherited defects of phagocyte function, or complement deficiencies; and (ii) the **presence of joint pathology** such as is seen in RA and other forms of chronic arthritis, as well as after prosthetic joint surgery. Among adults with bacterial arthritis, approximately half are over the age of 60 years, and most have had a previous abnormality of the affected joint. Intravenous drug users are also prone to bacterial arthritis related to recurrent bacteremia as well as impaired host defenses; the infection has a predilection for the sternoclavicular, sacroiliac, and other axial joints.

A. **Responsible organisms.** In adults, *Staphylococcus aureus* is the most common organism, accounting for more than 60% of cases of nongonococcal bacterial arthritis. Various species of streptococci and Gram-negative organisms each account for 15% to 20% of cases. The most common Gram-negative organisms are *Escherichia coli*, *Pseudomonas aeruginosa*, and *Serratia marcescens*. Among intravenous drug users, bacterial arthritis is most often caused by methicillin-resistant *S. aureus* or a Gram-negative organism, especially *P. aeruginosa*. In prosthetic joints, infections developing during the first year following surgery are often a result of the surgery and are caused by *S. aureus* (50%) and mixed flora (33%). Late infections are usually blood-borne.

B. **Clinical features.** Nongonococcal bacterial arthritis is usually monoarticular. The knee is most commonly affected, but the shoulder, ankle, wrist, hip, interphalangeal, and wrist joints are also commonly involved. Systemic signs usually include low-grade fever (uncommon to be over 38.9°C). Shaking chills are unusual. Only 50% of patients have a peripheral leukocytosis, but most have an increased sedimentation rate. Infections of prosthetic joints may cause increased pain, but symptoms in the affected joint may be minimal. Less than 50% of patients are febrile and only 10% of patients have a peripheral leukocytosis.

C. **Diagnostic tests.** The diagnosis is established by synovial fluid analysis and **culture**. Typically, synovial effusions in bacterial arthritis are thick, purulent, and have a WBC greater than 50,000 per mm^3 with greater than 90% polymorphonuclear leukocytes. Only 40% to 50% of patients have a synovial fluid WBC greater than 100,000 per mm^3. A Gram stain of the synovial fluid should be done, preferably on concentrated sediment of centrifuged synovial fluid. A low synovial fluid glucose is seen in about 50% of patients with septic joints, but may also occur in RA. Polarizing microscopy of the fluid should be done, because a crystalline synovitis can cause a marked synovial fluid leukocytosis and simulate joint sepsis. However, identification of crystals does not exclude bacterial arthritis. The joint fluid culture is positive in 85% to 95% of cases of nongonococcal bacterial arthritis. Joint fluid cultures may be negative if the patient has received prior antibiotic treatment.

Because most cases of bacterial arthritis arise from hematogenous spread, a primary source for infection should be sought, such as the urine (especially in Gram-negative bacterial arthritis), the sputum (e.g., pneumococcal arthritis), and the skin (e.g., staphylococcal arthritis). Blood cultures are positive in approximately 50% of patients with nongonococcal bacterial arthritis and in 20% of patients with gonococcal arthritis. Potential sources of bacteremia should be cultured and may provide the only positive microbial identification, especially in disseminated gonococcal infection.

X-ray evaluation of bacterial arthritis is not generally helpful, but should be performed to exclude adjacent osteomyelitis and to serve as a baseline for follow-up studies to help in determining long-term prognosis. The earliest radiographic finding in bacterial arthritis is a synovial effusion and adjacent soft tissue swelling. If the infection persists, joint space narrowing and later subchondral bone erosions are seen.

Other diagnostic tests that may be performed include radionuclide imaging of the musculoskeletal system to look for unsuspected sites of infection or to help differentiate overlying cellulitis from bacterial arthritis or osteomyelitis. It is not, however, routinely necessary to do this for bacterial arthritis. If a diagnosis of bacterial arthritis is suspected, but the synovial fluid is unobtainable or sterile, a synovial biopsy should be considered. This is particularly useful in tuberculous or fungal arthritis.

D. Gonococcal arthritis. Gonococcal arthritis affects primarily young, healthy adults. Disseminated gonococcal infection (DGI) is more common in females, probably because they constitute the largest reservoir of asymptomatic and untreated gonococcal infection. The primary focus of infection is a genital source, but rectal and pharyngeal sites must also be considered. Dissemination of the infection usually occurs around menses, during pregnancy, or in the postpartum period. Patients with disseminated gonococcal infection usually present with a 3- to 5-day acute febrile illness characterized by fleeting polyarthralgias, dermatitis (usually small maculopapular or vesiculopustular lesions on the trunk or extremities), and tenosynovitis (characteristically involving the extensor tendons of the fingers or toes). Less commonly, DGI may present with an acute septic monoarthritis with especial involvement of the knees or wrists.

The diagnosis of DGI depends on a high clinical suspicion and positive cultures. Unfortunately, joint fluid cultures are positive in only 25% and blood cultures are positive in 10% to 20% of affected patients. Blood and synovial fluid cultures are almost never simultaneously positive. Cultures should be obtained from the cervix, rectum, and pharynx, as well as from the blood and synovial fluid. Thayer-Martin medium should be used for all mucosal samples, whereas chocolate agar should be used for blood and synovial fluid cultures. Genitourinary cultures are positive in 80% of patients with disseminated gonococcal infection. In the absence of positive cultures, a therapeutic trial of antibiotics is usually justified. The response to ceftriaxone (1 g intramuscularly [i.m.] or intravenously [i.v.] q.d.) is rapid. This parenteral drug should be continued until signs and symptoms resolve and then followed by daily cefuroxime, 500 mg orally twice daily or amoxicillin/clavulanate 500 mg orally three times daily for 7 days.

E. Treatment of bacterial arthritis. The components of treatment are appropriate antibiotic therapy, adequate drainage, and articular rest. The initial choice of antibiotics should be guided by the Gram stain of the synovial fluid and the clinical situation, as illustrated in Table 14.1.

The final choice of antibiotics is dictated by the culture results. A 2-week course of parenteral antibiotics is usually recommended for the treatment of uncomplicated bacterial arthritis in a normal host. A substantially longer duration of parenteral antibiotic therapy may be needed for infections that are slow to sterilize, are related to a resistant organism, or are associated with underlying bone destruction.

Joint drainage can generally be accomplished by repeated needle aspiration and should be continued until the effusion is minimal. Synovial fluid WBCs and cultures should be followed serially to monitor efficacy of therapy. Drainage can also be achieved surgically; this method has not been shown to be superior to repeated percutaneous needle aspiration. However, arthroscopy or surgical drainage is recommended if the joint is inaccessible

Table 14.1. Initial antibiotic treatment of suspected
bacterial arthritis, based on Gram stain results

Gram-positive cocci	Nafcillin (preferred), cefazolin, **or** vancomycin (if methicillin-resistant *S. aureus* is suspected)
Gram-negative cocci	Third-generation cephalosporin (e.g., cefotaxime, ceftizoxime, ceftriaxone). Alternatives include spectinomycin if DGI is suspected, and amoxicillin/clavulanate if *Hemophilus influenza* is suspected
Gram-negative bacilli	Third-generation cephalosporin **or** carbapenem **or** aztreonam **or** quinolone
Negative Gram stain	Nafcillin **and** third-generation cephalosporin (use alternatives above for patients with penicillin allergy)
Serious underlying disease, joint prosthesis, following joint procedure or surgery	Vancomycin **and** amikacin **or** antipseudomonal penicillin **or** antipseudomonal third/fourth generation cephalosporin **or** carbapenem **or** quinolone

DGI, disseminated gonococcol infection.
Table prepared with the assistance of Dr. Thomas Russo, Division of Infectious Diseases, SUNY at Buffalo.

to needle drainage (e.g., the hips) or cannot be adequately drained due to loculations, severe deformity, or reluctance of the patient to undergo repeated aspirations. Surgical drainage should also be considered if the organism is resistant to antibiotics or if there has been no clinical response in 3 to 5 days. The acute pyogenic joint should be immobilized in an optimal functional position with the use of a splint or brace. Passive range of motion should be started as soon as possible. Once the pain subsides, active range of motion exercises should be done.

IV. **Lyme arthritis**

Lyme disease is caused by the tick-borne spirochete *Borrelia burgdorferi*. The multisystem illness occurs in stages and can mimic other diseases. The diagnosis is based upon the presence of a characteristic clinical picture and an elevated antibody response to the spirochete.

A. **Vector.** The spirochete is transmitted primarily by certain ixodid ticks. *Ixodes dammini* is the principal vector in the northeast and midwest United States, and *I. pacificus* is the vector in the west. Although the illness has been recognized in 47 states, most cases have occurred along the northeast coast between Massachusetts and Maryland, in the midwest in Wisconsin and Minnesota, and on the western coast of northern California and Oregon. Lyme borreliosis is widely disseminated throughout Europe where *I. ricinus* is the vector. Cases have also been noted in Scandinavia, China, Japan, and Australia.

B. **Clinical manifestations**

Stage 1. After an incubation period of 3 to 32 days, about 30% to 80% of exposed patients develop a characteristic skin lesion, erythema chronicum migrans (ECM), at the site of the tick bite, usually in the thigh, groin, or axilla. This lesion usually begins as a red macule or papule that expands slowly to form a large annular lesion, up to 20 cm or more in diameter, and often with a bright red outer border and partial central clearing. Because ixodid ticks are no larger than a freckle, 50% of patients do not remember the preceding tick bite.

Within days after the onset of the initial skin lesion, most affected patients develop secondary annular skin lesions. The rash is frequently accompanied by severe headache, mild neck stiffness, fever, chills, myalgias, polyarthralgias, and profound malaise and fatigue. These symptoms reflect hematogenous spread of the organism. Less common manifestations include generalized lymphadenopathy or splenomegaly, hepatitis, sore throat, nonproductive cough, testicular swelling, conjunctivitis, iritis, or panophthalmitis. The fatigue and lethargy are often constant, whereas the other signs and symptoms of early Lyme disease are typically intermittent and changing. Even in untreated patients, the early symptoms usually improve or disappear within several weeks.

Stage 2. Stage 2 occurs several weeks to months after the initial infection and is characterized by neurologic and cardiac manifestations. Symptoms of meningeal irritation may occur at the beginning of Lyme disease when erythema migrans is present. After several weeks, about 15% of untreated patients develop frank neurologic abnormalities, including meningitis, subtle encephalitic signs, cranial neuritis (including bilateral facial palsy), motor and sensory radiculoneuritis, plexitis, mononeuritis multiplex, or myelitis, alone or in various combinations. About 8% of untreated patients develop cardiac involvement within several weeks after the onset of illness. The most common abnormality is fluctuating degrees of atrioventricular block (first degree, Wenckebach, or complete heart block). Some patients have more diffuse cardiac involvement including electrocardiographic changes of acute myopericarditis, radionuclide evidence of left ventricular dysfunction, or rarely, cardiomegaly or pancarditis. The duration of cardiac involvement is usually only weeks, but severe involvement may be fatal. Migratory pain in joints, tendons, bursae, muscle, or bone may occur, typically lasting hours or several days in one or two locations at a time.

Stage 3. Stage 3 occurs 5 or more months after the onset of the disease. About 60% of untreated patients in the United States develop frank arthritis. The typical pattern is brief, intermittent attacks of monoarticular or oligoarticular arthritis in a few large joints, especially knees. Although the pattern varies, episodes of arthritis often become longer during the second or third year of illness, lasting months rather than weeks. In about 10% of these patients, chronic arthritis begins during this period and usually affects only one or both knees. The knee is typically more stiff than painful. Large effusions are common. Months to years later, sometimes following long periods of latent infection, chronic neurologic manifestations may develop, most commonly a subtle encephalopathy and sensory polyneuropathy.

C. Diagnostic testing. Two to 4 weeks after infection, most patients have a positive antibody test to *B. burgdorferi*, determined by ELISA. Antibody testing in Lyme disease is subject to false-negative results and, more often, false-positive results. Moreover, it is not standardized and different laboratories may get different results. Patients with past infection often remain seropositive. A small percentage of patients who are incompletely treated with antibiotics during the first several weeks of infection are seronegative later in the illness.

Western blotting is used routinely as a definitive test, when positive enzyme-linked immunosorbent assay (ELISA) results are questionable, because of a low pretest probability, cross-reactivity with other spirochetes, or indeterminate titers.

D. Treatment. Patients presenting with the rash of ECM who do not have neurologic or cardiac manifestations may be treated with doxycycline 100 mg p.o. b.i.d. or amoxicillin 500 mg t.i.d. for 10 days or azithromycin 500 mg/d for 1 week. Doxycycline is contraindicated in patients < 9 years of age. In stage 2 disease, patients with mild neurologic (Bell's palsy alone) or cardiac (first-degree AV block with a PR interval of less than 0.3 seconds) may be treated with oral regimens of doxycycline or amoxicillin for a period of 3 weeks. More severe cardiac or neurologic manifestations should be treated with intravenous antibiotics, including ceftriaxone, 2 g i.v. daily for 2 to 4 weeks or cefotaxime 2 g every 8 hours for 2 to 4 weeks. Most patients with Lyme arthritis and no neurologic manifestations respond to oral regimens of antibiotics, given for 4 to 6 weeks. These include amoxicillin 500 mg four times a day or doxycycline 100 mg twice daily. Some patients require intravenous treatment with ceftriaxone 2 g per day or cefotaxime, 3 g twice daily for 4 to

6 weeks. The response to antibiotic therapy may be slow. Patients with chronic arthritis who do not respond to either oral or intravenous antibiotic therapy may be treated with intraarticular steroids and NSAIDs. If there is no response within 6 to 12 months, arthroscopic synovectomy may be helpful.

V. The seronegative spondyloarthropathies and reactive arthritis

The spondyloarthropathies are a group of rheumatic diseases defined by the presence of an inflammatory arthritis of the spine. A seronegative peripheral inflammatory arthritis is a common feature and may be the predominant musculoskeletal manifestation in some of these diseases. Characteristic lesions occur in the skin, bowel, eyes, aortic root, and genital tract that may help to establish the diagnosis. Included in this group are ankylosing spondylitis, reactive arthritis/Reiter syndrome, psoriatic arthritis, late onset pauciarticular juvenile RA, and arthritis associated with inflammatory bowel disease. These diseases are strongly associated with the human leukocyte antigen (HLA)-B27 allele. A distinguishing feature of these disorders is the presence of an enthesopathy, a pathologic process in which inflammation is targeted at sites of ligamentous and tendinous attachment to bone. Periosteal new bone formation may develop at these sites, resulting in characteristic radiographic features, such as sacroiliitis, fluffy heel spurs, "whiskering" of the ischial tuberosities, and syndesmophytes.

A. Ankylosing spondylitis

Ankylosing spondylitis (AS) is a chronic inflammatory arthropathy that primarily affects the axial skeleton, often beginning in the sacroiliac joints and later involving the entire spine. Sacroiliitis is a hallmark of the disease. Involvement of peripheral joints, especially the hips, knees, and shoulders, may also occur.

1. **Epidemiology.** The prevalence in Caucasians is between 2 and 14 cases per 1,000 adult persons. AS affects men approximately three times more frequently than women. Approximately 2% of unrelated HLA-B27+ individuals and 10% to 20% of the first-degree relatives of HLA-B27+ AS patients have signs or symptoms of AS.

2. **Clinical features.** Symptoms of AS usually begin in late adolescence or early adulthood. A chronically stiff and/or aching back is the most common presenting symptom. The back pain of AS is distinguished from mechanical back pain by its insidious onset, duration of greater than 3 months, association with prominent stiffness in the morning and after periods of rest, and improvement with exercise. The back pain is often dull in character and difficult to localize. Early in the disease it may be felt deep within the buttocks, with referral towards the iliac crests, the greater trochanters, or down the proximal part of the posterior thighs. The pain may be unilateral and intermittent at first, but later becomes bilateral and persistent. In some patients there may be tenderness at sites of muscle, ligament, or tendon insertion, such as the iliac crests, tibial tubercles, the base of the heel, and the circumference of the patella. Involvement of the costovertebral joints and costosternal junctions can result in the misdiagnosis of atypical chest pain and fibromyalgia.

   In early stages of the disease, physical signs may be minimal. The cardinal finding which should be sought is limitation of motion of the lumbar spine, particularly with lateral flexion or extension. The Schober test is utilized to detect limitation of forward flexion of the lumbar spine. (A 10-cm distance is traced cephalad from the level of the fifth lumbar spinous process. This distance on the skin should normally increase by 5 cm as the patient flexes forward to the maximum.) Restriction of chest expansion to less than 2.5 cm is a reasonably specific physical finding, especially in a young individual, and may also be detected early in the disease course.

   Peripheral joint involvement eventually occurs in 25% of patients and may be the presenting feature in some. It typically involves the hips, shoulders, knees, ankles, and heels. Extraarticular manifestations include iritis (25% of patients), aortitis resulting in aortic insufficiency, cardiac conduction defects, and apical pulmonary fibrosis, resembling tuberculosis (TB). In 2% of patients, recurrent attacks of acute iritis are the initial manifestation of the disease. Late complications of the disease include restrictive lung disease, cauda equina syndrome, spinal stenosis, and spinal fractures.

3. **Diagnosis.** The diagnosis of AS requires radiologic evidence of bilateral sacroiliitis and a history of inflammatory back pain. Not all patients with AS have radiologic evidence of sacroiliitis when they first present with back pain. Sacroiliitis is the earliest radiographic feature before clinical involvement extends to the lumbar spine. Early sacroiliitis is often not recognized on x-ray. Ferguson views of the sacroiliac joints are needed for optimal detection of sacroiliitis on plain radiographs. The features of sacroiliitis include loss of definition at the margins of the lower two thirds of the joint, often with patchy reactive sclerosis favoring the iliac side. Widening of the joint may appear somewhat later, due to marginal decalcification. The changes are usually bilateral and relatively symmetric. A computed tomography (CT) scan of the pelvis may be more sensitive that plain radiographs in detecting early signs of sacroiliitis. A bone scan may show a nonspecific increase in uptake in the sacroiliac joints before x-ray changes of sacroiliitis.

Other radiographic features may also help in the diagnosis. The anterosuperior margin of the vertebral bodies are normally concave when viewed on lateral radiographs; in AS, these vertebral corners become squared and sclerosed because of an enthesitis at the site of insertion of the longitudinal ligament. Later, bony spurs (**syndesmophytes**) form, following the margin of the annulus fibrosis. These bone spurs can form a bridge between vertebrae, finally ankylosing them to form a "bamboo" spine. Some patients may have inflammation of the disks, with destruction of adjacent vertebral bodies that radiographically resembles infection or tuberculosis (Romulus lesion).

Testing for the HLA-B27 antigen is not necessary in an individual who has classic findings of AS. However, the test is useful in the evaluation of adults who have equivocal radiographic changes of sacroiliitis, or adolescents who normally have blurred sacroiliac joint margins. A positive result in a patient with a history of inflammatory back pain strongly supports the diagnosis. A negative test in a patient without radiographic evidence of sacroiliitis decreases its likelihood, especially in Caucasians. The test result must be interpreted in the context of the clinical setting. A positive test does not, by itself, establish the diagnosis of AS, nor does a negative test exclude the diagnosis.

4. **Treatment**
   a. **Drug therapy.** Daily use of an NSAID is the mainstay of therapy. This regimen serves to reduce pain and stiffness and allows the patient to exercise and maintain proper posture. In moderate to severe cases, indomethacin is most effective, in doses of 150 to 200 mg per day in divided doses. For patients who have side effects to indomethacin, diclofenac, naproxen, and tolmetin are useful alternatives. Celecoxib has also been shown to be as effective as a traditional NSAID in such patients. Sulfasalazine in daily divided doses of 2 to 3 g is effective in early disease, particularly when there is concomitant arthritis of peripheral joints. The use of corticosteroids is unwarranted. Refractory cases may be managed with methotrexate and tumor necrosis factor (TNF) inhibitors.
   b. **Physical therapy.** All patients need to receive formal instruction in exercises that stretch spinal ligaments, strengthen spinal extensor muscles, and preserve range of motion of the neck, shoulders, and hips. Deep breathing exercises serve to maintain chest expansion. Lying prone, either during sleep or as a daily exercise, can prevent postural deformity.

    c. **Patient education.** Patients should receive instruction as to maintenance of proper posture. They should be advised not to smoke. The website, www.spondylitis.org, is an excellent resource for patients.

B. Reactive arthritis and Reiter syndrome

Reactive arthritis and Reiter syndrome are synonymous terms for a form of spondyloarthritis that develops 1 to 4 weeks following an enteric or urogenital infection. The responsible organisms include *Salmonella*, *Yersinia*, *Campylobacter*, toxigenic *E. coli*, and *Chlamydia* species. The organism cannot be cultured from the joint; however, recent studies have demonstrated Chlamydia antigens and ribonuclear material in the synovium of some patients with sexually acquired reactive arthritis. Reactive arthritis usually follows a venereal infection in North America, the United Kingdom, and western Europe, and an enteric infection in other parts of the world. The triad of arthritis, urethritis, and conjunctivitis that classically defined Reiter syndrome is seen with a variable frequency that is dependent on the arthritogenic agent. Only one-third of patients with sexually acquired reactive arthritis demonstrate the Reiter triad.

Reactive arthritis is defined clinically as an asymmetric oligoarthritis, usually of the lower extremities, that is associated with at least one characteristic extraarticular feature (e.g., urethritis or cervicitis, diarrhea, inflammatory eye disease, or mucocutaneous disease—including balanitis, oral ulceration, or keratoderma). In most, but not all cases of reactive arthritis, an antecedent extraarticular infection can be identified. As in other forms of spondyloarthropathies, the majority of patients affected with reactive arthritis have inherited the HLA-B27 antigen. Approximately 75% to 80% of Caucasians with reactive arthritis/Reiter syndrome are HLA-B27$^+$. About 20% of B27$^+$ individuals develop reactive arthritis/Reiter syndrome following exposure to an arthritogenic agent.

1. **Incidence.** The incidence of reactive arthritis is approximately 4 to 5 cases per 100,000 persons. Sexually acquired reactive arthritis is more common in men (male to female ratio 10 : 1), whereas postenteric reactive arthritis has an equal sex distribution. Postenteric reactive arthritis develops in 2% to 6% of HLA-B27$^-$ and in 20% of B27$^+$ infected individuals.

2. **Clinical features. Urethritis**, present in less than one-third of patients, is generally the first symptom, preceding other symptoms by 1 or more weeks. Urethritis is most common in men, but prostatitis and/or epididymitis may also occur. Women may present with dysuria, vaginal discharge, or a mucopurulent cervical discharge. **Conjunctivitis**, often bilateral, may accompany or follow the urethritis by a few days. It may occur in only one-third of patients with sexually acquired reactive arthritis. Iritis eventually develops in 20% to 25% of patients with arthritis. **Arthritis** typically begins after the urethral and ocular inflammation has subsided, and generally runs a course of weeks to months. The arthritis is asymmetric, typically oligoarticular, with predominant involvement of the lower extremity (especially knees, ankles, MTP joints). The finding of back or heel pain, sausage digits, Achilles tendonitis, and genital inflammation lends strong support to the diagnosis in an individual presenting with lower extremity arthritis. The mean duration of an episode of arthritis is approximately 19 weeks. More than 50% of patients with reactive arthritis have multiple attacks. Patients who have chronic joint involvement usually have several attacks before the chronic phase begins; thus, a long follow-up is needed to demonstrate the chronic nature of the disease. About 20% to 25% have a relentless arthritis. Skin involvement includes circinate balanitis and keratoderma blennorrhagica (inflammatory hyperkeratotic lesions of the toes, nails, and soles of the feet) resembling pustular psoriasis. Reiter syndrome occurs with particular severity in individuals infected with human immunodeficiency virus (HIV). HLA-B27 is found in 60% to 70% of these affected individuals.

3. **Radiographic abnormalities** may develop in patients with chronic musculoskeletal involvement. These include erosions and periosteal proliferation at the margins of joints and at sites of tendon or ligament insertions. One-third of patients with reactive arthritis develop unilateral or asymmetric sacroiliitis.

4. **Therapy.** NSAIDs are the primary treatment. In some patients, indomethacin is more effective than other NSAIDs or salicylates, especially if there is spinal involvement. Refractory cases are also managed with sulfasalazine and, if necessary, methotrexate or azathioprine. In a placebo-controlled prospective trial, a 3-month course of limecycline (a tetracycline derivative) decreased the duration of *Chlamydia trachomatis* reactive arthritis when given early in the disease.

C. Psoriatic arthritis

Psoriatic arthritis is a seronegative inflammatory arthritis that affects approximately 5% to 7% of patients with psoriasis. The disease affects both sexes equally.

1. **Clinical features.** Several clinical patterns of this disease have been described, but many patients have overlapping features. A minority of patients have a symmetric polyarthritis resembling RA (and may represent the coincidence of seronegative RA and psoriasis). The majority has a distinctive form of arthritis that does not resemble RA. This predominant form of arthropathy in psoriatic patients is characterized by one or more of the features shown in Table 14.2.

In 15% of cases, psoriatic arthritis may precede the onset of psoriasis and is recognized in these cases by its distinctive articular manifestations and/or by a careful search for hidden skin or nail lesions. Patients with more severe skin disease are at higher risk for developing the arthritis. Nail involvement (pitting and/or onycholysis) is more common and more severe in psoriatic patients with arthritis and is the only clinical feature that may identify patients with psoriasis who are destined to develop arthritis.

Psoriasis and psoriatic arthritis may be exacerbated in the setting of HIV infection. Crippling deformities may develop in a short period of time in some HIV-associated psoriatic arthritis patients.

2. **Laboratory features.** By definition, RF should be absent; however, low titer RF is present in up to 15% of healthy individuals and should not exclude the diagnosis of psoriatic arthritis if the distinctive musculoskeletal features are present. A minority of patients are HLA-B27+, especially if axial distribution is present.

3. **Radiographic features** help to distinguish psoriatic arthritis from RA. These include the absence of juxtaarticular osteoporosis, rapid destruction of isolated joints, ankylosis, acroosteolyis, and "pencil-in-cup"

Table 14.2. Distinctive clinical features of psoriatic arthritis

---

Asymmetric involvement of peripheral joints

Tendency to involve a limited number of joints, often two to five ("oligoarthritis")

Involvement of the DIP joints, usually in association with nail disease

Tendency to **early** bony ankylosis

Dactylitis (swelling of whole digit with inflammation of both the DIP and PIP joints)

Enthesopathic manifestations, such as heel pain, Achilles tendonitis, radiographic periostitis

Sacroiliitis (20%) and spondylitis (40%)

Occasional progression to a severe and destructive form of disease (arthritis mutilans)

DIP, distal interphalangeal; PIP, proximal interphalangeal.

deformities resulting from fluffy periostitis and new bone formation at the base of the distal phalanx, and whittling of the tip of the proximal phalanx. The predilection for DIP joints, lack of symmetry, and limited number of involved joints also support this distinction.

4. **Therapy.** NSAID therapy may be sufficient for mild disease. Methotrexate is used commonly for patients who do not respond to NSAIDs alone. The regimen is identical to that used for RA, although monitoring for hepatic fibrosis and cirrhosis should be more stringent because patients with psoriasis have a higher baseline incidence of fibrosis. Disease-modifying antirheumatic drugs (DMARDs) such as gold and hydroxychloroquine are used, but have the potential of aggravating the skin disease. Vigorous therapy of the skin disease may help the peripheral arthritis, but is not usually beneficial for the spinal involvement. Methotrexate, cyclosporine, and TNF inhibitors are beneficial in patients with both skin and joint disease.

D. **Enteropathic arthritis**

Approximately 15% to 20% of patients with active inflammatory bowel disease develop an asymmetric arthritis, mainly of the lower extremity joints. The activity of the arthritis is closely related to that of the bowel disease. The peripheral arthritis is not associated with the HLA-B27 allele. An axial arthritis, resembling AS, may develop in patients with inflammatory bowel disease, particularly in HLA-B27+ individuals. This spinal arthritis is unrelated to the activity of the bowel disease and its clinical course is similar to that of idiopathic AS.

1. **Clinical features.** Enteropathic arthritis affects men and women equally and has its onset usually in the third to fifth decade. In most patients, the onset is abrupt and limited to one to three joints, often with an asymmetric and migratory pattern. Knees and ankles are most commonly affected. Attacks of peripheral joint disease usually last less than 2 months but can last more than a year, often paralleling the intensity of enterocolitis. The arthritis is recurrent and migratory and usually resolves without joint deformity. Arthritic episodes before the onset of bowel symptoms are unusual (10% of patients). Joint swelling, redness, and effusion can occur, but occasionally there are no objective findings. Patients with inflammatory bowel disease who have uveitis, recurrent oral ulcerations, pseudopolyps, or perianal involvement are 3 to 4 times more likely to have arthritis than patients lacking these symptoms. About 25% of patients with the spondylitic manifestations have symptoms before the onset of their bowel disease. In these patients, back pain symptoms frequently do not parallel the intensity of the enterocolitis.

2. **Laboratory features.** Elevated ESR, anemia, and leukocytosis are common, but RF and antinuclear antibodies are characteristically absent. Both marginal erosions and periostitis can be evident on x-rays, but serious bone damage and deformity are unusual. About 55% of these patients with spondylitis are positive for HLA-B27, but patients with peripheral arthritis maintain the normal Caucasian distribution of 8% HLA-B27 positivity.

3. **Treatment.** The peripheral joint disease improves when the bowel disease is treated with sulfasalazine, systemic corticosteroids, or surgery. However, the status of the bowel disease, not the arthritis, should govern therapeutic decisions. Low doses of prednisone, 15 to 20 mg per day, are often quite effective for the peripheral arthritis. NSAIDs have to be used with caution in patients with active inflammatory bowel disease. Patients with spondylitis should be treated as described for AS.

VI. **Rheumatoid arthritis**

Rheumatoid arthritis is a systemic inflammatory disease of unknown origin, the principal manifestation of which is chronic inflammation of multiple diarthrodial joints. The articular involvement is usually symmetric, additive in its presentation, and persistent over many years. It commonly results in joint deformity and progressive functional impairment. A variety of extra-articular manifestations may occur, including scleritis, pleural and/or pericardial inflammation, pulmonary fibrosis, vasculitis, and splenomegaly with neutropenia. The disease affects approximately 1% of the adult population; women are affected three times as often as men. It most commonly develops during the fourth and fifth decades of life.

A. **Clinical features.** The ACR criteria for the diagnosis of RA are shown in Table 14.3.

A diagnosis of RA can only be made when other causes of arthritis are excluded by an appropriate clinical and laboratory evaluation or by clinical observation over a period of weeks to months. Some patients may initially present with clinical features of RA and later develop manifestations of other connective tissue tissues, such as SLE, systemic vasculitis, or even psoriatic arthritis.

The **onset** of RA is most often insidious, with the gradual development of symmetric polyarthritis involving the small joints of the hands and feet. An acute, polyarticular onset over the course of several days is uncommon; in such patients, consideration should be given first to a viral etiology (e.g., parvovirus B19, prodrome of hepatitis B) or a serum sickness reaction. The disease may begin in one joint and only months later spread to involve others. In elderly patients, the presentation may initially be that of polymyalgia rheumatica, with pain and stiffness of the hips and shoulders, and only later include synovitis of more distal, smaller joints. Constitutional symptoms may include fatigue, weight loss, and low-grade fever. The presence of prominent Raynaud phenomenon in a patient presenting with polyarthritis usually indicates the presence of a connective tissue disease, such as SLE or scleroderma, and not RA. Certain extraarticular manifestations, such as anemia, carpal tunnel syndrome, rheumatoid nodules and lymphadenopathy, may occur at any time in the disease course. Others characteristically occur late in the disease course; these include vasculitis, leg ulcers, scleritis, pleural or pericardial effusions, diffuse interstitial pulmonary fibrosis, and Felty syndrome.

B. **Laboratory tests.** A positive RF is eventually found in 80% of patients with RA. RFs may be seen in other diseases, including SLE, hepatitis C infection, idiopathic interstitial lung disease, as well as in 10% of elderly healthy individuals. An elevated ESR or C-reactive protein suggests an inflammatory cause of musculoskeletal pain. As markers of inflammation, the ESR and C-reactive protein are useful in the initial evaluation of patients with joint

Table 14.3. 1987 Revised criteria for the classification of rheumatoid arthritis

---

A person can be classified as having RA if four or more of the following criteria are present at any time:

Morning stiffness in and around joints lasting at least 1 h before maximal improvement.

Soft-tissue swelling (arthritis) of three or more joint areas observed by a physician (areas are right or left of PIP joints, MCP joints, wrist, elbow, knee, ankle, and MTP joints)[a]

Swelling (arthritis) of the PIP, MCP, or wrist joints[a]

Symmetric arthritis[a]

Subcutaneous nodules

Positive test for RF

Radiographic erosions or periarticular osteopenia in hand or wrist joints

---

[a] Present for at least 6 weeks

RA, rheumatoid arthritis; PIP, proximal interphalangeal; MCP, metacarpophalangeal; RF, rheumatoid factor.

pain and in monitoring the general degree of inflammatory activity in patients with established RA. Anemia is common in patients with active RA. It is typically normochromic, normocytic, with normal marrow iron stores (anemia of chronic disease). Iron-deficiency anemia caused by gastrointestinal blood loss secondary to drug therapy is also common. Markers of iron-deficiency anemia in RA include serum ferritin levels of less than 60 μg per L and serum transferrin receptor levels of less than 2.3 mg per L.

C. **Radiographic studies.** Early in the disease, x-rays of affected joints may show only soft tissue swelling. Later changes include periarticular demineralization, narrowing of the joint spaces, and finally, erosions at the margins of the joints. Joint radiographs early in the disease course are most helpful in patients with persistent joint swelling, crepitus, deformity, or limited range of motion, because they may uncover erosions and thus indicate the need for more aggressive treatment, or they may reveal findings indicative of an alternative diagnosis, such as calcium pyrophosphate deposition (chondrocalcinosis), gout (erosions with overhanging edges), or psoriatic arthritis (periostitis at joint margins).

D. **Synovial fluid analysis.** Synovial fluid WBCs in joints affected by RA are in the inflammatory range (greater than 2,000 per mm^3) and may reach above 100,000 per mm^3 in occasional patients with acute flares resembling bacterial arthritis. Septic arthritis occurs in patients with RA and should always be suspected in patients presenting with one or more joints that are disproportionately symptomatic. In these patients, the joint fluid should be aspirated and cultured.

E. **Treatment**

1. **Principles.** The goals of treatment are (i) to reduce joint pain and swelling, thereby maintaining or improving the patient's functional capacity; and (ii) to prevent or arrest the development of joint damage and destruction. A variety of treatment modalities should be employed to achieve these goals, including antiinflammatory and disease-modifying medications, physical and occupational therapy, intraarticular corticosteroid injections, and joint surgery. Although a cure for RA does not exist, current therapeutic regimens have been associated with improved long-term outcomes and the arrest of the radiographic progression of the disease. It is currently believed that the best therapeutic outcomes are associated with the initiation of effective therapies early in the disease course, prior to the development of joint erosions, and the vigorous suppression of synovitis, using disease-modifying agents either alone or in combination. Because the disease course may be variable, with some patients having only a self-limited course and others having mild synovitis with limited articular involvement, it is necessary to identify those affected individuals with a poor prognosis who would be the most appropriate candidates for the early initiation of aggressive treatment. Markers of a progressive disease course include persistent inflammation of multiple joints, elevated titer of RF, early appearance of erosions, extraarticular features, and early impairment of functional capacity.

   A commonly used approach to the pharmacologic management of early RA is shown as an algorithm in Fig. 14.1.

2. **Nonsteroidal antiinflammatory agents.** NSAIDs have proven benefit in RA, serving to reduce joint pain and swelling. In patients with mild disease, the use of NSAIDs may suffice as the only antiinflammatory therapy. However, most patients will require additional therapy with DMARDs (see Disease-modifying antirheumatic drugs on page 274). In contrast to osteoarthritis, maximal doses of NSAIDs are used to treat RA. In the past, therapy with salicylates was often initiated first, because it was inexpensive, equally effective as NSAID therapy, and could be monitored with salicylate levels. This practice has largely been abandoned; compliance with four times a day dosing was poor, many generic NSAIDs now cost little more than extended-release forms of enteric-

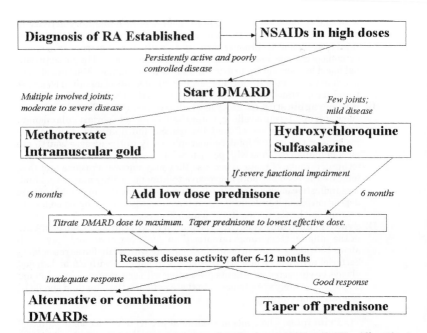

FIG. 14.1. Pharmacologic management of early rheumatoid arthritis. All patients are treated initially with nonsteroidal antiinflammatory drugs (NSAIDs) in antiinflammatory doses. If the disease is not adequately suppressed after an adequate trial lasting 3 or more weeks, disease-modifying antirheumatic drugs (DMARDs) are added. Low-dose prednisone is added if the patient has severe functional impairment. The choice of DMARD is dictated in part by the severity of the disease. In most patients, therapy is begun with one DMARD; others are introduced, either in lieu of or in combination with the initial DMARD, if the therapeutic response has been inadequate. Some rheumatologists initiate therapy with several DMARDs and then withdraw one or more as the disease becomes adequately suppressed.

coated aspirin, and achievement of a therapeutic salicylate level often required careful adjustment of the dose. There are more than 20 different NSAIDs. The NSAIDs are divided into two classes on the basis of their pharmacologic half-life. Those with a half-life of 12 hours or more are dosed once or twice daily and achieve steady-state levels within 3 to 7 days. Examples include naproxen, oxaprozin, nabumetone, sulindac, and piroxicam. NSAIDs with shorter half-lives, such as diclofenac, etodolac, ibuprofen, and indomethacin, must be given three or four times daily. The selective COX-2 inhibitors (celecoxib, rofecoxib) should be used in patients at risk of adverse gastrointestinal events, including the patients who are over the age of 65 years; have a history of peptic ulcer disease; are taking glucocorticoids, anticoagulants, or aspirin; or have a bleeding tendency.

3. **Disease-modifying antirheumatic drugs.** Therapy with DMARDs is appropriate for patients in whom the disease has proven over a period of observation to be unremitting, associated with the development of joint erosions or deformities, or unresponsive to NSAIDs alone. DMARD therapy requires a commitment from the patient and physician to regular clinic visits for drug administration over many months,

with repeated tests to detect potentially serious side effects. Prescription for these agents should not be renewed unless the patient has received appropriate laboratory monitoring for adverse effects. For women of childbearing potential, effective contraception is required during therapy with most DMARDs.

The choice of DMARD is dictated by a variety of factors, including severity of disease, comorbidities of the patient, expense, potential toxicity, and frequency of laboratory monitoring (see Table 14.4).

a. Disease-modifying antirheumatic drugs useful for patients with early or mild rheumatoid arthritis

(1) **Hydroxychloroquine** (Plaquenil) is an antimalarial drug that is used in either early RA, often before the introduction of more potent DMARDs, or in more aggressive RA, in combination with methotrexate and other DMARDs. The starting dose is 400 mg per day in two divided doses; the total dose should not exceed 5 to 7 mg/kg/day. The dose may be reduced to 200 mg per day after 6 months if a good response has been achieved. Common side effects include gastrointestinal symptoms (dyspepsia, diarrhea, and nausea), headache, rash, and blurred vision due to ciliary muscle dysfunction. These side effects may resolve by reducing the dose. **Retinal toxicity** may occur when the drug is used in a daily dose greater than 6.5 mg per kg, particularly in patients with abnormal hepatic or renal function or those over the age of 70 years. It is recommended that patients undergo ophthalmologic examinations every 6 months in order to allow for the early detection of retinal toxicity. Patients over the age of 40 years or those with previous eye disease should undergo an ophthalmologic evaluation prior to the initiation of therapy with hydroxychloroquine.

(2) **Sulfasalazine** (Azulfidine) may be used alone or in combination with hydroxychloroquine and/or methotrexate. It is a two-component drug, composed of sulfapyridine and 5-aminosalicylic acid; the sulfapyridine is absorbed systemically while most of the 5-aminosalicylic acid remains in the colon and is excreted in the feces. The drug is contraindicated in patients with a previous sulfa allergy. The starting dose is usually 500 mg twice a day; the dose is increased gradually to a total of 2 to 3 g in two divided doses. Common side effects include nausea, vomiting, diarrhea, and loss of appetite; these can be reduced by the use of the enteric-coated preparation and by introducing the drug at a low dose. Anemia, leukopenia, and thrombocytopenia may be observed in 1% to 5% of treated patients, particularly in the first 6 months of therapy. A complete blood count (CBC) should be monitored every 2 to 4 weeks for the first 3 months and then every 3 months.

(3) **Minocycline and other tetracyclines** have been shown to have measurable benefit in patients with RA and are most appropriate for those with mild disease. The benefit is thought related to the inhibition of synovial metalloproteinases and not to any antibacterial effect. The antirheumatic activity of minocycline appears to be augmented by the concomitant use of NSAIDs. For treatment of RA, the effective dose of minocycline is 100 mg twice a day and that of doxycycline is 100 once or twice a day. As with any tetracycline, the drug should not be used in pregnancy or in children under the age of 9 years. Patients taking minocycline should avoid sunlight because of the photosensitizing effects of the drug. Doxycycline is the preferred drug in patients with renal impairment.

Table 14.4. Comparative features of disease-modifying antirheumatic drugs used in the treatment of rheumatoid arthritis

Drug	Route of administration	Efficacy	Toxicity	Expense[a]	Special considerations
Hydroxychloroquine	Oral	+	+	+	Retinal toxicity
Methotrexate	Oral, s.c., or i.m.	+++	++	+	Teratogenicity, hepatotoxicity
Sulfasalazine	Oral	+	+	+	
Gold	Oral	+	+	++	Diarrhea
	Parenteral	++	++	+/++	Neutropenia, thrombocytopenia, proteinuria
Leflunomide	Oral	+++	++	+++	Teratogenicity
Cyclosporine	Oral	++	+++	+++	Nephrotoxicity
Etanercept	s.c.	++++	+	++++	Infection
Infliximab	i.v.	+++	++	++++	Infection, autoimmunity
Penicillamine	Oral	++	+++	+	Neutropenia, proteinuria
Azathioprine	Oral	++	++	+++	Infection, oncogenicity
Cyclophosphamide	Oral	+++	+++	+++	Oncogenicity, viral infection, sterility

[a] +, $50 or less/mo; ++, $50–$100/mo; +++, $100–$500/mo; ++++, $500 dollars or more/mo (prices apply to generic products, when available).
s.c., subcutaneous; i.m., intramuscular; i.v., intravenous.
From *Med Lett.* 2000;42 (July 10), with permission.

(4) **Auranofin** (Ridaura) is an oral gold preparation that is generally safer but less efficacious than parenteral gold. The daily dose is 6 mg, given either as 3 mg twice daily or 6 mg once daily. If there is no response after 3 months, the dose may be increased to 3 mg three times a day; the drug should be stopped if no benefit is observed after an additional 3 months. The most common side effects are diarrhea (more than 40% of treated patients), rash, and stomatitis, The less common occurrence of anemia, leukopenia, thrombocytopenia, and proteinuria mandate the monitoring a CBC and urinalysis every 8 weeks.

b. **Disease-modifying antirheumatic drugs commonly used for patients with moderate to severe disease**

(1) **Methotrexate** (Rheumatrex), a folic acid antagonist, is the most widely used DMARD for RA in the United States. Methotrexate is taken orally, subcutaneously, intramuscularly, or intravenously once a week. The usual starting dose is 7.5 to 10 mg weekly (tablets are 2.5 mg) at once or divided over 24 hours. The oral dose can be increased gradually to maximum doses of 20 mg per week. The administration of the drug by subcutaneous or intramuscular injection may improve its efficacy and/or reduce the occurrence of adverse gastrointestinal effects. This is the preferred route of administration when the dose is greater than 20 mg per week. Lower doses (2.5 to 5 mg) are used in elderly patients and individuals with renal impairment. Folic acid supplementation (1 mg per day) is used commonly to decrease the incidence of side effects. In patients with limited financial resources, the parenteral (injectable) form of the methotrexate (available in a 2-mL vial, 25 mg per mL) is inexpensive and can be administered i.m., subcutaneously (s.c.), or orally (diluted in water or fruit juice). Patients must be taught to draw up the correct amount of the drug (0.1 mL is equivalent to one 2.5-mg tablet) if they are to use the parenteral form. A baseline chest x-ray should be obtained prior to the initiation of methotrexate therapy.

Side effects of methotrexate include stomatitis, nausea, diarrhea, and mild alopecia; the incidence of these can be reduced with daily folic acid supplementation (1 mg). Uncommon but serious toxicities include pneumonitis, hepatic fibrosis, and myelosuppression. Methotrexate pneumonitis usually occurs within the first 2 years of therapy and is typically heralded by a 3- to 4-week period of shortness of breath, nonproductive cough, and fever. Patients who develop these symptoms should stop their methotrexate; the finding of new interstitial changes on chest x-ray and negative sputum cultures mandates permanent discontinuation of the drug. The ACR has formulated recommendations for monitoring methotrexate therapy for possible hepatotoxicity based on blood testing rather than on invasive liver biopsies. CBCs and liver enzyme tests should be obtained every 2 weeks for the first 2 months and checked at 8- to 12-week intervals in stable patients. Methotrexate should be stopped for 2 weeks before and 2 weeks after surgery to avoid interfering with healing or increasing the risk of infection. Myelosuppression induced by methotrexate occurs most commonly in patients with renal insufficiency, folate deficiency, and in those using concomitant folate antagonists such as trimethoprim (Table 14.5).

(2) **Leflunomide** (Arava) is an inhibitor of pyrimidine biosynthesis in activated lymphocytes; it has efficacy and safety comparable to that of methotrexate in the treatment of RA. Because

Table 14.5. American College of Rheumatology guidelines for monitoring
for hepatotoxicity in rheumatoid arthritis patients receiving methotrexate

---

Baseline
  Tests for all patients
    Liver blood tests (aspartate aminotransferase [AST], alanine aminotransferase
      [ALT], alkaline phosphatase, albumin, bilirubin), hepatitis B and C serologic
      studies
    Other standard tests, including complete blood cell count and serum creatinine
  Pretreatment liver biopsy (Menghini suction-type needle) only for patients with
    Prior excessive alcohol consumption
    Persistently abnormal baseline AST values
    Chronic hepatitis B or C infection
Monitor AST, ALT, albumin at 4- to 8-week intervals
Perform liver biopsy if
  Five of nine determinations of AST within a given 12-month interval (6 of 12 if
    tests are performed monthly) are abnormal (defined as an elevation above the
    upper limit of normal)
  There is a decrease in serum albumin below the normal range (in the setting of
    well-controlled RA)
If results of liver biopsy are
  Roenigk grade I, II, or IIIA, resume MTX and monitor as in B, C1, and C2 above
  Roenigk grade IIIB or IV, discontinue MTX
Discontinue MTX in patient with persistent liver test abnormalities (as defined in
  "Perform liver biopsy if") who refuses liver biopsy

RA, rheumatoid arthritis; MTX, methotrexate.
From Kremer JM, et al. *Arthritis Rheum* 1994;37:316–328, with permission.

of the long plasma half-life of the drug (15 to 18 days), loading doses of 100 mg per day for 3 days are given followed by
a daily dose of 20 mg in order to reach steady-state concentrations. Beneficial effects are observed as early as 4 weeks
following initial administration. Adverse events include gastrointestinal symptoms (especially diarrhea), allergic reactions,
alopecia, and elevated liver function tests. Reduction of the
dose to 10 mg a day often serves to minimize these side effects.
Aspartate aminotransferase (AST) and alanine aminotransferase (ALT) levels should be monitored regularly; if either
enzyme level is repeatedly greater than two times the upper
limit of normal, then the dosage should be reduced. Leflunomide is potentially teratogenic and is contraindicated in pregnant women or women of child-bearing potential who are not
using reliable contraception. Pregnancy must be excluded before the start of treatment. Prior to a planned conception, both
men and women taking the drug must discontinue it and take
cholestyramine (8 grams three times a day) for 11 days to bind
and eliminate the drug; women should then verify that plasma
levels of the metabolite are less than 0.02 mg per L.

(3) **Tumor necrosis factor inhibitors: Etanercept (Enbrel)
and infliximab (Remicade).** Two parenteral drugs that bind
to and block the activity of TNF are used to treat RA. TNF is
a cytokine that plays a central role in the perpetuation of inflammation in the rheumatoid synovium through its effects
on the recruitment of inflammatory cells, neoangiogenesis,
and joint destruction. Etanercept is a recombinant version
of the soluble human TNF receptor. Infliximab is a chimeric

human/mouse anti-TNF monoclonal antibody. Etanercept is given subcutaneously in doses of 25 mg twice a week. Clinical benefit is observed as early as 2 to 3 weeks. It is commonly given in combination with weekly methotrexate. Infliximab is given intravenously in doses of 3 mg per kg; treatment is initiated with doses at 0, 2, and 6 weeks and then continued with doses every 8 weeks thereafter. Injection-site reactions are common with etanercept, but generally do not mandate discontinuation of the drug. Adverse effects of infliximab include headache, infection, and infusion reactions (fever, urticaria, dyspnea, and hypotension). Serious infections, including tuberculosis, may occur with both etanercept and infliximab therapy; neither drug should be given to patients with active localized or chronic infections. Etanercept has been reported rarely to cause demyelination in the central nervous system (CNS) and should not be used in patients with multiple sclerosis.

c. **Disease-modifying antirheumatic drugs less commonly used for moderate to severe disease**

   (1) **Cyclosporine** is used in patients with refractory RA who have not responded to methotrexate. It can be used alone or with methotrexate. It is contraindicated in patients with renal insufficiency, uncontrolled hypertension, and malignancy. The initial dose is 2.5 mg/kg/day, taken twice daily as a divided oral dose. Onset of action generally occurs between 4 and 8 weeks. The dose may be increased by 0.5 to 0.75 mg/kg/day increments every 4 weeks to a maximum of 4 mg/kg/day, provided the serum creatinine has remained less than 30% above baseline. If there is no benefit after 16 weeks of therapy, the drug should be stopped. The principal adverse reactions of cyclosporine therapy are hypertension, renal dysfunction, headache, gastrointestinal disturbances, and hirsutism.

   (2) **Gold.** The use of parenteral gold has declined with the widespread use of methotrexate in RA. However, gold salts are occasionally quite effective in certain patients with RA. In the form of either gold sodium thiomalate (Myochrysine) or aurothioglucose (Solganal), they are given by deep intramuscular injection at weekly intervals. To test for idiosyncratic reactions, the dose is increased from 10 to 25 to 50 mg over the first 3 weeks. The dose of 50 mg a week is maintained until response or toxicity occurs. Responses with less than 3 months of treatment are unusual. If there is no benefit by the time a 1 g cumulative dose is reached, gold should be stopped. Once a response is achieved, it can often be maintained with 50 mg doses given at intervals gradually lengthened over several months from 2 to 4 weeks. Side effects include rash or stomatitis; bone marrow toxicity, manifested as thrombocytopenia followed by neutropenia and anemia; and renal toxicity, beginning as proteinuria. If gold is not discontinued, the hematologic and renal manifestations can be fatal. Before each injection, skin examination, a complete blood cell count with platelet counts, and urinalysis should be performed. If a rash appears, gold should be stopped. After the rash clears, gold can be restarted at a reduced dose. The occurrence of bone marrow and renal toxicity mandate permanent discontinuance. Eosinophilia is common but does not necessarily predict toxicity. Rarely, thrombocytopenia can occur months after gold is discontinued. About 1% to 3% of patients receiving gold sodium thiomalate injections experience an anaphylactic-like nitritoid reaction.

(3) **Penicillamine** is available as a tablet (Depen) or capsule (Cuprimine). As with gold, the onset of benefit may be delayed several months, the risk of toxicity is substantial, and one-third of patients may receive no benefit. The recommended adult regimen consists of 250 mg daily for 8 weeks, with the dose being increased by 125 mg per month to a maximum of 750 mg. Sites of serious toxicity include the bone marrow, kidneys, and gastrointestinal tract. Reduction or alteration of taste sensation is common but reversible when the drug is stopped. A complete blood cell count and urinalysis are used to check for thrombocytopenia, neutropenia, proteinuria, and hematuria; these are obtained every 2 weeks until a stable dose is achieved, then every 1 to 3 months. If any of these conditions occur, the drug must be discontinued. Penicillamine can induce a lupus-like illness, which reverses upon its discontinuation.

(4) **Azathioprine** (Imuran) is a purine analog immunosuppressive agent that is approved for use in RA. A dose of 1.0 to 2.5 mg/kg/day is effective in 70% of patients by 4 to 6 months of therapy. Side effects include gastrointestinal symptoms (20%), abnormal liver function tests (15%), and neutropenia/thrombocytopenia. Continuous use of azathioprine is limited because of an associated increased risk of developing an underlying lymphoproliferative malignancy (up to 10% after 20 years).

4. **Corticosteroids**
   a. **Systemic corticosteroids.** Although these agents are immediately effective in reducing joint pain and swelling, the dose necessary to maintain a remission is often associated with significant morbidity and rapid withdrawal frequently produces a flare. In patients with chronic joint inflammation, 5 to 10 mg of prednisone daily is a useful therapeutic adjunct, especially in elderly patients. Side effects still occur at this dose but are less pronounced. After improvement is noted, dose reductions of 1 mg per day every week should be attempted to find the minimum dose that maintains improvement. Doses greater than 15 mg of prednisone a day (or equivalent) should not be used chronically (longer than about 4 weeks) to control joint inflammation. There are instances in which systemic corticosteroids in high doses (40 to 60 mg of prednisone per day) for several weeks can be of benefit, especially in severe cases of vasculitis. Corticosteroids should be avoided unless absolutely necessary in diabetics and in patients with a history of gastric ulcers or severe osteoporosis.

   b. **Local injection of corticosteroids.** The injection of slow-release corticosteroid preparations into the synovial cavity of an inflamed joint can be beneficial. The major indication for local injection is when one joint produces a major share of the pain and disability. Septic arthritis must be excluded before injecting any joint with corticosteroids. Strict **aseptic technique** is advised. A 21- or 22-gauge needle is adequate for injection, although aspiration of large effusions may require an 18- to 20-gauge needle. After the effusion is removed, 0.3 mL of triamcinolone acetonide (Kenalog) 40 mg per mL (methylprednisolone [Depo-Medrol] or triamcinolone hexacetonide [Aristospan] are alternatives) for small joints (e.g., finger, wrist, or elbow), 1 mL for medium to large joints (ankle or shoulder), and 2 mL for the knee should be used. Dilution of the corticosteroid preparation with lidocaine, 1 mL or more, prior to injection, provides immediate yet temporary analgesia for the patient and facilitates dispersion of the corticosteroid throughout the joint space. Generally, injection of one medium or large joint at a time is the limit. The benefit may last from 2 days to several months. The same joint should not be injected more often than once in 2 months or four times in 1 year to minimize damage to cartilage. Cautioning the patient against the overuse of successfully treated joints may prevent joint damage.

5. **Physical and occupational therapy.** Rehabilitative measures are directed at the relief of pain, improvement of a patient's functional capacity, and prevention of joint deformity. The available modalities include the use of heat/cold and other pain-relieving measures, rest and splints (i.e., bed rest or local rest for joints with use of splints), and exercise. Assistive devices may also serve to improve a patient's functional capacity.

The application of either heat or cold to joints serves to relieve pain and to facilitate stretching. Heat can be applied simply in the form of a hot soak, warm towel, heating pad, light bulb, or paraffin bath, and is used more commonly than cold in the treatment of RA patients.

Rest is an effective modality for reducing joint inflammation. The spectrum of rest modalities ranges from brief naps, an orthotic device (e.g., wrist splints worn at night to reduce wrist synovitis), a cane to decrease weight bearing on an involved hip or knee, or complete bed rest. Bed rest causes deconditioning and promotes joint contractures, and thus should be limited to restorative rest periods of 30 minutes to 2 hours once or twice daily. Joint rest can also be facilitated by stressing joint protection techniques, in which patients are taught to carry out tasks with minimal joint stress (e.g., use of jar or bottle openers, use of shoulder strap rather than handle to carry a purse, etc.). Splints and braces are used to stabilize inflamed or biomechanically deranged joints and to maintain them in a functional position, thereby resting the joint and protecting it from excessive and potentially painful motion. Splints prescribed to correct or prevent deformity are probably of little benefit except in the postoperative period.

Exercise therapy in RA has various objectives, including preservation of joint motion, restoration of lost motion, strengthening of specific muscle groups and enhancement of endurance, and aerobic conditioning. Prescription of exercise in RA patients has to be individualized and depends on the goals to be accomplished and the status of the patient.

A variety of assistive devices are available to help patients with activities of daily living, including getting dressed, cooking, turning faucets on/off, etc. These are usually ordered by an occupational therapist.

6. **Joint surgery.** Joint surgery is an important component of the management of patients with advanced RA associated with joint destruction. Here the goals of surgery are relief of pain and restoration of joint motion and function. With the advent of joint replacement surgery—particularly of the knees and hips—these goals can be achieved routinely in most patients. Because the development of an infected prosthesis is a serious complication, it is important to carefully screen patients preoperatively for extraarticular infections (e.g., bladder, skin lesions).

Synovectomies have been advocated for years as a means to halt or retard the rheumatoid process before significant joint destruction occurs. The best evidence to date suggests that the results of surgical synovectomy are only transient because it is impossible to completely remove all diseased synovium. The recovery from an open synovectomy is often slow and may result in some loss of joint motion. Thus, synovectomies are considered only in patients in whom aggressive medical therapy has been unsuccessful in resolving a florid synovitis in an isolated joint in which advanced cartilage destruction has not yet occurred. One exception is dorsal synovectomy of the wrist, where timely operative intervention may prevent tendon rupture.

VII. Crystal-induced arthropathies

A variety of crystals may be found in articular tissue and their presence is often associated with arthritis. These include crystals of monosodium urate, CPPD, basic calcium phosphate (BCP), calcium oxalate, and cholesterol. The role of the crystal in the induction of the arthritic process may vary; for some crystal species, presence in the joint may be secondary and for others, it may be directly pathogenic. In gout, the role of crystal deposition is most clearly defined. Here, monosodium urate crystals are known to be phlogistic, their deposition precedes the development of arthritis, and their gradual removal with pharmacologic therapy (e.g., allopurinol) ameliorates the arthritis. In contrast, deposition of BCP or CPPD crystals is common in joints affected by osteoarthritis, but the role of the crystals in the induction of joint disease is uncertain.

A diagnosis of crystal-induced arthropathy is most accurately established by the demonstration of the crystal in the synovial fluid leucocytes or tissues of an affected joint. In an acute arthritis, such as gout or pseudogout, the crystals should be observed by polarized light microscopy to be within synovial fluid leucocytes. In a chronic arthritis, the finding of chondrocalcinosis on x-rays of the affected joint establishes the presence of the intraarticular deposition of calcium salts in the joint, most often calcium pyrophosphate. The demonstration of BCPs in the synovial fluid requires the use of Alizarin red staining of a wet preparation or the use of more specialized techniques, such as electron or atomic force microscopy. This is usually applied to the investigation of patients with a destructive arthritis of the shoulder or knee.

A. Gout

Gout is a disorder of purine metabolism in which hyperuricemia, sustained for many years, results in the gradual deposition of monosodium urate crystals in the articular cartilage, synovium, and periarticular connective tissue. Recurrent episodes of acute arthritis (acute gout) occur when monosodium urate crystals are either released from tissue deposits in the joint or are formed *de novo* in synovial fluid supersaturated with urate and incite an inflammatory response. If the hyperuricemia is left untreated, a destructive, chronic arthritis (tophaceous gout) may supervene, resulting from persistent inflammation and enlarging tophaceous deposits in the joint and adjacent bone.

1. **Hyperuricemia** is found in approximately 5% of the adult male and less than 1% of the adult female population of the United States. The development of hyperuricemia may be related to impairment of the renal excretion of uric acid, overproduction of uric acid, or both. Approximately 10% of patients with hyperuricemia are classified as overproducers of uric acid on the basis of the urinary excretion of more than 600 mg of uric acid per day on a purine-free diet. In the majority of individuals, the pathogenesis of these abnormalities has not yet been defined, although they are thought to have a genetic basis (so called "primary gout"). Specific inborn metabolic errors resulting in hyperuricemia have been identified in only a small minority of individuals. Secondary hyperuricemia may occur as a result of certain diseases or as a result of the use of certain drugs which are associated with increased nucleic acid turnover (psoriasis, blood dyscrasias), accelerated adenosine triphosphate (ATP) degradation (glycogen storage diseases, tissue hypoxia), or decreased renal excretion of urate (renal insufficiency, diuretics, lead nephropathy, etc.).

Only a minority of patients with hyperuricemia develop articular gout. The height of the serum urate level is the principal risk factor for the development of articular gout. In the Boston Normative Aging Study of healthy adult males with asymptomatic hyperuricemia, the cumulative incidence of gout after 5 years was only 22% in individuals with serum urate levels of 9 mg per dL or higher and only 3% in individuals with serum urate levels of less than 9 mg per dL. Additional risk factors for the development of gout include renal insufficiency, lead exposure, alcohol intake, hypertension, obesity, and excessive weight gain in young adulthood. Modification of several of these risk factors is possible and might serve to prevent the development of gout.

2. **Clinical features**

   a. **Acute gouty arthritis.** The first attack of gout in males usually occurs in the fourth, fifth, or sixth decade of life. The first attacks are most often monoarticular. Acute gout is predominantly a disease of the lower extremity, affecting in order of frequency the great toe, insteps, ankles, heels, and knees. Because the inflammation may also involve periarticular bursae and tendon sheaths, there is often widespread periarticular inflammation, resembling cellulitis. Post-inflammatory desquamation can occur. Attacks of acute gout typically **resolve completely**, after a period of time that may vary from hours to days to weeks, depending on the severity of the attack and its treatment. Some patients may never have a second attack. However, the majority will have a second attack within 6 months to 2 years of their first. The frequency of gouty attacks usually increases with time in untreated patients. Later attacks are often polyarticular and more severe.

   b. **Chronic tophaceous gout.** After many years (average 12 years) of gout and sustained hyperuricemia, a chronic arthritis may develop marked by chronic joint swelling and pain, joint destruction, and bony erosion. This stage, chronic tophaceous gout, is related to the increasing deposition of monosodium urate around joints—in the cartilage, synovial membranes, tendons, and soft tissues. Palpable tophi (i.e., deposits of monosodium urate) may be commonly found around the joints, on the ulnar surface of the forearm, in the olecranon bursa, or in the helix of the ear.

   In the absence of secondary causes of hyperuricemia, gout does not usually develop in women until 15 or more years after menopause. The use of diuretics is a particularly strong risk factor for the development of gout in elderly patients. The development of tophi in osteoarthritic interphalangeal joints is a distinctive presentation for gout among the elderly and may result in gout being misdiagnosed or unrecognized. Gout is also common in organ transplant recipients, as a result of several predisposing factors, including the common presence of renal insufficiency and treatment with drugs such as diuretics and cyclosporine, which elevate the serum urate level. Treatment of gout and hyperuricemia in these patients requires careful consideration of comorbidities and potential drug interactions.

3. **Diagnosis.** A definitive diagnosis of gout is established by aspiration of the affected joint and demonstration of intracellular urate crystals. During an attack of gout, uric acid levels often decline to the normal range. Thus, the finding of a normal serum urate level does not exclude a diagnosis of acute gout. In patients with a chronic arthritis (including patients labeled erroneously as having RA), tophaceous gout should be considered if there is a past history of acute gout or if examination reveals palpable nodules in the olecranon bursae, small soft nodules overlying Heberden nodes in the fingers, or several more acutely inflamed joints, marked by exquisite tenderness and erythema.

4. **Treatment of acute gouty arthritis**

   a. **Nonsteroidal antiinflammatory drugs.** Indomethacin is used most often, with a starting dose of 50 to 100 mg, followed by 25 to 50 mg four times a day. After symptoms resolve, the dose should be tapered over a period of several days. Other NSAIDs with a short half-life, such as ibuprofen or diclofenac, can also be used as long as they are used at their maximum recommended doses. In elderly patients, lower doses of NSAIDs are advisable, particularly in the presence of renal impairment. The COX-2 inhibitors, rofecoxib and celecoxib, are options for patients at risk of gastrointestinal ulceration or bleeding; however, their efficacy compared to the traditional NSAIDs has not been systematically evaluated in acute gout. NSAIDs should be used with caution in patients with CHF, hepatic cirrhosis, or renal insufficiency.

   b. Colchicine has been used for many years to treat acute gout, but its use should be restricted because it almost invariably causes significant abdominal cramps and diarrhea when given orally at therapeutic doses. The standard dose is 0.6 mg every hour until gout symptoms resolve or gastrointestinal symptoms develop. The maximum dose for an acute attack is 6 mg (10 tablets). It is most effective when given early in the evolution of the gouty attack.

   c. Corticosteroids are effective for elderly patients in whom NSAIDs and colchicine may be contraindicated or in patients who cannot take oral medications. These can be given as a single depot intramuscular injection of a long-acting crystalline preparation (e.g., triamcinolone acetonide, Kenalog, 60 to 80 mg) or as a short course of oral prednisone, initially 20 to 30 mg per day, and then tapered over a period of 7 to 10 days.

5. Management of intercritical gout. The symptom-free interval between episodes of acute gout is termed "intercritical gout." After the onset of gout, approximately three-fourths of patients will have a second episode of acute gout within 2 years. However, some patients may not have a subsequent episode of gouty arthritis for more than 10 years. The frequency of acute gout may be reduced by losing excess body weight, avoiding excessive alcohol intake, stopping the use of diuretic agents, and adhering to a diet restricted in purines. In patients with only mild hyperuricemia, this approach may provide adequate control of the gout. If a patient has repeated attacks of gout, particularly clustered in a short period of time, most physicians choose to initiate therapy to correct the patient's hyperuricemia. Once begun, such therapy is continued indefinitely and requires daily medication. Alternative approaches include expectant observation with treatment of each episode of acute gout or the use of a daily dose of colchicine ("prophylactic colchicine"). Colchicine 0.6 mg twice daily can significantly reduce the frequency of acute gout. The daily use of an NSAID may also be used for this purpose. In elderly patients, particularly those with renal impairment, the dose of prophylactic colchicine should be reduced to 0.6 mg once daily or every other day in order to avoid chronic toxicity.

6. Treatment of symptomatic hyperuricemia. A decision to treat hyperuricemia becomes a life-long commitment. There is no indication to treat asymptomatic hyperuricemia except in the rare individual with marked and persistent elevation of the serum urate level (e.g., greater than 12 to 13 mg/dL) or a marked increase in urinary uric acid excretion (greater than 1,100 mg per dL). Such patients are at high risk of developing a renal calculus. There is also some evidence that hyperuricemia may be nephrotoxic when this severe. Absolute indications for treating hyperuricemia in a patient with gout include the presence of tophi or x-ray evidence of bony erosion around the joints; evidence of renal damage or kidney stones; or the presence of severe hyperuricemia (e.g., levels greater than 12 to 13 mg per dL) or high levels of urinary uric acid excretion (e.g., greater than 1,000 mg per day).

   Drugs that act to lower the serum urate concentration should never be started during an acute attack of gout. Therapy for hyperuricemia should be started during an intercritical period when there are no signs of active inflammation. The initial treatment of hyperuricemia may be associated with an increased incidence of gout attacks. Accordingly, treatment of hyperuricemia should be started while the patient is taking colchicine 0.6 mg once or twice a day or a daily nonsteroidal antiinflammatory agent to reduce the frequency of gout attacks in this setting. The colchicine should be continued for 6 to 12 months after the last episode of gouty arthritis or until all visible tophi have disappeared. When treating hyperuricemia, the goal is to reduce the serum urate level to below 6 mg per dL.

Allopurinol. The majority of physicians use allopurinol to treat hyperuricemia, regardless of whether the patient is an overproducer or an underexcreter of urate. This is a choice dictated by the fact that allopurinol can be given once daily, does not pose a risk of precipitating renal stones, and has proven to be highly effective therapy for hyperuricemia. Allopurinol is clearly the drug of choice if the patient has renal impairment, tophi, or radiographic evidence of joint damage, or a history of renal stones. Adverse reactions to allopurinol do occur, the most common being the development of a skin rash. A life-threatening toxicity syndrome may occur rarely, particularly in patients with impaired renal function. The toxicity syndrome typically starts 2 to 3 weeks after the initiation of allopurinol and is marked by an erythematous desquamative rash, fever, hepatitis, eosinophilia, and worsening renal function. Allopurinol potentiates the cytotoxic effects of 6-mercaptopurine and azathioprine. When treating patients on these drugs, the dose of azathioprine or 6-mercaptopurine should be reduced by two-thirds and the dose of allopurinol started at 50 to 100 mg per day.

Uricosuric drugs may be used quite successfully in a gout patient who has no tophi, normal renal function, normal urinary uric acid excretion (less than 700 mg per day) and no history of renal stones. These drugs may also be used in gout patients allergic to allopurinol, provided their renal function is adequate (i.e., creatinine clearance of greater than 30 to 40 mL per min). The efficacy of uricosuric drugs is reduced or nullified in patients who are using concomitant salicylates. Probenecid and sulfinpyrazone are available in the United States and benzbromarone, a potent uricosuric agent, is also available in Europe; in contrast to probenicid and sulfinpyrazone, it can be an effective uricosuric agent in patients with mild renal insufficiency. The starting dose of probenicid is 250 mg twice daily. The daily dose is then increased by 500 mg every 2 to 3 weeks until the serum urate level is below 6 mg per dL. The usual maintenance dose is 500 mg twice a day; 40% of patients may require a daily dose of 1.5 g or more. The starting dose of sulfinpyrazone is 50 mg twice daily. The dose can then be increased by 50 to 100 mg every 2 to 3 weeks until the serum urate is less than 6 mg per dL. The usual maintenance dose is 300 to 400 mg per day in divided doses.

B. Calcium pyrophosphate crystal deposition disease
  1. **Diagnosis.** Two markers for calcium pyrophosphate crystal deposition disease are used in clinical practice. The first is the radiographic finding of chondrocalcinosis, resulting from calcification of fibrocartilage, hyaline cartilage, and occasionally periarticular structures. Chondrocalcinosis is usually, but not always, the result of deposition of CPPD crystals. The second marker is the identification of CPPD crystals within the synovial fluid of a patient with arthritis, using a polarizing microscope. In contrast to urate crystals, CPPD crystals are usually rhomboid in shape and have weakly positive birefringence. The finding of both of these markers, namely chondrocalcinosis and the presence of CPPD crystals within the synovial fluid, establishes a definite diagnosis of CPPD deposition disease in a given patient.
  2. **Etiology.** CPPD deposition disease is classified etiologically into three groups. The **sporadic** form is the most common. It is estimated that approximately 5% of the adult population has chondrocalcinosis. The frequency of chondrocalcinosis in the knees increases significantly with age, reaching as high as 30% in persons older than age 85 years. In addition to aging, a past history of joint trauma or a past history of

joint surgery predisposes to intraarticular CPPD deposition. A number of kindreds have been described worldwide who have a **hereditary** form of chondrocalcinosis. In these kindreds, the disease usually has an autosomal-dominant pattern of inheritance and penetrance is usually 100% by the age of 50. In members of these families, chondrocalcinosis is usually evident at a young age and is associated with the development of a florid form of osteoarthritis. CPPD deposition disease is also associated with certain **metabolic disorders**, including hyperparathyroidism, hypophospatasia, hemochromatosis, and gout.

3. **Clinical features.** There are **three clinical presentations** of CPPD deposition disease: incidental (asymptomatic), acute arthritis (pseudogout), and chronic arthritis (pyrophosphate arthropathy). Most commonly, CPPD deposition is clinically silent and is recognized as an **incidental finding** (namely, chondrocalcinosis) in the course of x-rays obtained for unrelated reasons. The development of an acute arthritis related to the presence of CPPD crystals within synovial fluid neutrophils is termed "**pseudogout**." Pseudogout occurs most commonly in the knee, with the wrist, ankle, elbow, and first MTP joint also being susceptible. The attack is most commonly monoarticular, but polyarticular involvement can occur. The attack of pseudogout may be accompanied by fever and other systemic signs, including confusion in the elderly. Attacks of pseudogout often occur following joint trauma and in hospitalized patients. The most common hospital settings are patients who have undergone orthopedic surgery (perhaps because such patients are more likely to have osteoarthritis and CPPD deposition) or who have suffered a stroke or myocardial infarction. Of particular interest is the observation that attacks of pseudogout are common immediately following surgical removal of a parathyroid adenoma for hyperparathyroidism. Thus, a decrease in the serum calcium level, related to removal of a parathyroid adenoma, major surgery or medical illness, and trauma appear to trigger attacks of pseudogout. The diagnosis of pseudogout is established by the finding of intracellular CPPD crystals in the synovial fluid of the acutely inflamed joint. Septic arthritis can occur in patients who are found to have intracellular CPPD crystals in the synovial fluid (i.e., concurrent pseudogout), and thus it is very important to exclude infection in patients with apparent pseudogout. Patients with CPPD deposition disease may develop a form of chronic osteoarthritis which is termed "**pyrophosphate arthropathy**." This is best characterized as an exuberant form of osteoarthritis, which has a predilection for joints not usually involved in uncomplicated osteoarthritis. Thus the patellofemoral compartment of the knee; the radiocarpal joint of the wrist; the metacarpophalangeal joints of the hands, elbow, and shoulder; and the talocalcaneonavicular joint of the ankle may be involved in pyrophosphate arthropathy. The radiographic findings tend to be quite dramatic, with joint space narrowing, large subchondral cysts, articular calcification, and subchondral sclerosis. In some patients, the joint destruction may be so severe as to resemble a Charcot joint, even if the patient does not have a neurologic deficit.

4. **Treatment.** Pseudogout is treated in one of several ways. If a large joint is involved, thorough needle aspiration is often sufficient. Instillation of a crystalline corticosteroid preparation into the joint provides rapid relief. Oral colchicine is not as effective as it is in the management of acute gout, and is attended by the usual gastrointestinal side effects. A course of a nonsteroidal antiinflammatory agent, such as indomethacin, is the mainstay of therapy for most attacks of pseudogout. Intravenous colchicine can be used in patients who cannot take oral medications (e.g., in the postoperative setting) and is effective.

Basic Calcium Phosphate Crystal Deposition Disease

The deposition of hydroxyapatite and other BCP crystals in periarticular structures, bursae, and tendons has been widely recognized. These crystals are responsible for the entities commonly known as "calcific periarthritis," affecting the shoulder and other joints. With the application of x-ray energy-dispersive techniques and electron microscopy to the analysis of synovial fluid, cartilage, and synovium, it has been recognized in the past two decades that BCP crystals may also be found within the joint. A particular association has been found with certain forms of destructive arthropathy affecting the shoulder or knee (Milwaukee shoulder/knee syndrome, cuff tear arthropathy of the shoulder). A role for these crystals in the pathogenesis of the destructive arthritis has been postulated. The Milwaukee shoulder syndrome affects predominantly elderly women, usually in the dominant shoulder. A shoulder effusion is common. On aspiration, the effusion may be blood-tinged; it is generally noninflammatory with low WBC and contains aggregates of BCP crystals, detectable by Alizarin red staining or electron microscopy. X-rays of the affected joint show upward subluxation of the humeral head and pseudoarticulation of the acromion process, indicative of a chronic rotator cuff tear. In addition, there is evidence of degenerative arthritis within the glenohumeral joint. Many of these patients have concomitant osteoarthritis of the knees, with frequent involvement of the lateral tibiofemoral compartments. Treatment of the Milwaukee shoulder syndrome is generally unsatisfactory. The use of NSAIDs, repeated shoulder aspirations, and decreased joint use are mainstays of therapy. Complete shoulder arthroplasties are effective for the relief of pain and recovery of some shoulder function.

VIII. Developmental and mechanical causes of chronic joint pain in childhood

    A. A number of developmental arthropathies may be seen in growing children, but these do not represent true joint inflammation or arthritis. Rather, they constitute diagnoses in the differential of juvenile arthritis and related conditions.

        1. Congenital hip dysplasia

            a. This disorder usually presents in the neonatal period as asymmetry of the gluteal folds, a foreshortened femur, or a click on Barlow or Ortolani maneuvers. In this condition, the acetabulum is shallow, ligamentous laxity is often present, and many infants with this condition were positioned in a breech position in utero. In infancy, it is treated with hip abduction of 45° to 60° using a splint.

            b. If not detected or treated in infancy, progressive instability and deformity of the hip may develop. In the walking child, the most common finding is limp. Other presenting findings are persistent foreshortening of the femur, and a hip adduction contracture. Bilateral dislocation can be difficult to detect because of the absence of asymmetry. The Trendelenburg test may be positive bilaterally, and the perineum may be widened. The diagnosis is confirmed by x-ray examination. Treatment most often requires surgical reduction of the dislocation.

        2. Legg-Calvé-Perthes disease

            a. Avascular necrosis of the femoral head occurs most commonly in boys between the ages of 3 and 12 years, with the peak at age 6. It may be associated with antecedent trauma, or in some cases with recurrent synovitis. Hereditary factors may play a role in the disease.

            b. Symptoms are constant or transient limp, anterolateral hip pain that may be referred to the anterior thigh, loss of rotation and hip abduction, and thigh and buttock muscle atrophy.

            c. Diagnosis is made radiographically. Plain radiographs show failure of epiphyseal growth with widening of the medial joint space. Metaphyseal bone density may be diminished. Crescent-shaped subchondral fractures of the femoral head, shortened femoral neck, and flattening and enlargement of the femoral head occur with progression of the disease. Technetium bone scan and magnetic resonance images are more sensitive indicators of early disease.

3. Slipped capital femoral epiphysis
   a. Acute or gradual development of hip pain with weight bearing in the preadolescent or early adolescent should raise the possibility of slipped capital femoral epiphysis. The pain is localized to the anterior and lateral groin, the thigh, or the knee. Range of motion causes pain, especially internal rotation and abduction. Flexion of the hip causes external rotation.
   b. Early radiographic findings consist of widening of the growth plate and mild osteopenia of the proximal femur. Most slips are posterior, so lateral views are essential.
   c. The femoral head loses vascular supply, and avascular necrosis is common. Degenerative arthritis of the hip may result from epiphyseal slip, even with optimal surgical treatment.
4. Toxic synovitis
   a. Limp with a shortened stance phase, groin or anterolateral thigh pain, spasm of the hip muscles, limitation of hip motion, or referred knee pain are the most common presenting signs and symptoms of toxic synovitis. It is most common in boys between the ages of 2 and 12 years. Careful exclusion of other pathologic processes is essential.
   b. Radiographs are usually normal, but may demonstrate a decrease in the definition of the soft tissue planes around the hip. CBC and ESR are usually normal. Arthrocentesis yields normal fluid, and cultures are sterile.
   c. Treatment consists of rest, with crutch walking if necessary. Resolution within 2 to 3 weeks is usual.
5. Excessive femoral anteversion
   a. Excessive femoral anteversion is frequent cause of postexertional knee and groin pain in children and adults. Knee pain is localized to the patella, particularly the superior pole. Occasional patellar tendonitis may occur, particularly after prolonged activity with repeated knee extension and hip flexion. Pain may be exaggerated by long periods of tight knee flexion, so children sleeping in the fetal position may describe morning pain that should not be confused with the true morning stiffness of arthritis.
   b. Normal internal rotation of the hip in the child is 50°. Children with excessive femoral anteversion are able to internally rotate their hips well beyond this. Internal rotation of the hip to 80° or more is associated with greater symptoms, and may predispose to early degenerative arthritis of the hip, especially when external rotation is limited to 15° or less. With time, external tibial torsion develops in many patients, correcting the intoeing seen with this disorder.
   c. Treatment using corrective shoes, twister cables, or orthoses is not successful. Corrective osteotomy is rarely indicated, and is reserved for children with greater than 80° of hip internal rotation.
6. Osgood-Schlatter disease
   a. Repeated microtrauma to the tibial tubercle in peripubertal children who are rapidly growing leads to either microtears in the quadriceps tendon at its insertion on the tibial tubercle, or a partial separation through the active growth plate, which in turn leads to painful enlargement of the tibial tubercle. The pain is worsened by activities involving strenuous and repeated knee extension, such as running and jumping. The condition is usually benign, and resolves with closure of the proximal tibial growth plate.
   b. Laboratory studies are rarely needed for diagnosis.
   c. Treatment includes gentle stretching, ice application to the tubercle after exercise, and limitation of activity to tolerance level. Uncommonly, avulsion of bony fragments from the tubercle may be necessary to relieve chronic pain.

7. Growing pains
   a. Intermittent pain in the muscles of the leg or thigh of a child between the ages of 3 and 12 years most commonly is due to "growing pains." The pain is deep in the limb, and does not localize to the joints. The pains occur in the late evening or after retiring, but are gone by morning, lasting several minutes to a few hours. They are more common in damp, cold weather, and often wake the child from sleep.
   b. Physical examination may demonstrate pronated feet or tight heel cords, but most often the exam is entirely normal. Laboratory studies and radiographs are normal when done.
   c. Treatment consists of massage, local heat (warm pajamas or blankets), and mild analgesics such as acetaminophen if necessary.
8. Hypermobile pes planus
   a. This common condition, in which the longitudinal arch disappears with standing, is asymptomatic except in severe cases. It is usually associated with ankle valgus, and symptoms usually occur following prolonged standing or walking. Medial ankle and medial or posterior knee pain are most common, related to the valgus position of the ankle. This is often associated with genu recurvatum, and in more extreme cases, with hyperlordosis of the lumbar spine.
   b. Radiographic examination is not required. Mild symptoms can be controlled with supportive shoes that have a one-eighth-inch medial heel wedge and arch support. More severe symptoms require formal shoe orthoses, but these are expensive, especially for the growing child.
9. Adolescent kyphosis
   a. Excessive rounding of the thoracic spine occurs in up to 5% of children in the United States. When postural in etiology, it is usually asymptomatic. If associated with vertebral end-plate irregularity, it is known as Scheuermann disease. This disorder is painful in approximately half of the affected individuals.
      (1) Postural kyphosis occurs equally in males and females. It is usually treated with exercises to correct lumbar hyperlordosis and thoracic hyperkyphosis. For curves up to 80°, exercise and orthoses may be helpful. For more extreme curves, corrective surgery may be required, but should not be performed until skeletal maturation is complete (thoracic vertebral growth plates typically fuse at age 17 years in females and 19 years in males).
      (2) Scheuermann disease is more common in males. It is identified radiographically by the presence of hyperkyphosis with greater than 5° of anterior wedging of two or more consecutive vertebrae. End-plate irregularity of the vertebral bodies and intervertebral disc space narrowing are common. Relative osteopenia or structural insufficiency of vertebral end plates related to rapid skeletal growth is believed to cause compression of the growing vertebral bodies.
IX. Infectious and postinfectious rheumatic syndromes of children
   A. Post-streptococcal rheumatic syndromes
      1. Rheumatic fever
         a. The classic post-streptococcal rheumatic syndrome is rheumatic fever (RF). Following invasive infection with group A streptococcus, most commonly pharyngitis, the systemic immune response to the organism may result in systemic inflammatory disease affecting joints, heart, skin, and basal ganglia.
         b. Clinical presentation. The first symptoms may include vague abdominal pain and/or epistaxis. Fever usually occurs 1 to 5 weeks following the primary pharyngitis. Arthritis involving large joints

and migrating from one to another over hours to a few days follows the onset of the fever. The joints are warm, often erythematosus, and exquisitely tender. Arthralgia may occur without findings of inflammation. Carditis may be manifest first by tachycardia, with new murmur, pericardial friction rub, and accompanying chest pain, and variable degrees of conduction block possible. Overt myocardial failure may produce dyspnea and orthopnea. Subcutaneous nodules (1 to 10 mm in diameter) may occur 2 to 8 weeks after the streptococcal infection, usually palpable along extensor surfaces, the scalp, spine, and scapulae. Erythema marginatum may occur in a minority of affected children, occurring for a few hours to days at a time, and recurring for several weeks. Chorea usually occurs late in the course (2 to 3 months after disease onset) and may be the presenting symptoms of the disease.

   c. **Diagnosis.** The diagnosis is made on clinical grounds, and supported by laboratory confirmation of an antecedent streptococcal infection. Prior microbiologic identification of group A streptococcal pharyngitis, or the presence of a systemic immune response to the agent (elevation of antistreptolysin O [ASO] or anti-DNAse B antibody titers) are important in confirming the trigger of the syndrome. Nonspecific indicators of the systemic inflammatory reaction common in RF include leukocytosis, increased ESR, and elevated serum C-reactive protein concentration. Cardiac involvement may be confirmed by conduction delay, ectopy, or low voltages on electrocardiogram (ECG), and valvular or myocardial involvement on echocardiography. Chest x-ray may indicate cardiomegaly, pulmonary venous congestion, or effusions. The characteristic pathologic finding is the Aschoff body in involved myocardium. The Jones criteria were developed and subsequently modified to assist in making a diagnosis of RF. The presence of two major, or one major with two minor criteria (when supported by evidence of antecedent streptococcal infection) make a diagnosis of true RF likely (see Table 14.6).

   d. **Treatment.** Antiinflammatory therapy using salicylates to attain a serum concentration between 15 and 20 mg per dL is recommended until the ESR returns to normal. In the presence of CHF, corticosteroids for 2 to 4 weeks should be employed. Inotropic support, diuretics, and other measures may be required in severe cardiac failure. Bed rest is indicated in CHF. Antimicrobial treatment for underlying group A streptococcal infection is indicated in all patients suspected of having acute RF. Penicillin or erythromycin (in penicillin-allergic individuals) is recommended for 10 days, followed by long-term prophylaxis to prevent further streptococcal infection and consequent RF episodes. Benzathine penicillin G 1.2 million units i.m. every 3 to 4 weeks, or oral penicillin 250 mg

Table 14.6. Modified Jones criteria (1992)

Major manifestations	Minor manifestations
Carditis	Fever
Arthritis	Arthralgia
Erythema marginatum	Prolonged PR interval on ECG
Subcutaneous nodules	High WBC, ESR, or CRP
Chorea	

ECG, electrocardiogram; WBC, white blood cell count; ESR, erythrocyte sedimentation rate; CRP, C-reactive protein.

twice daily is the preferred regimen, with sulfadiazine or sulfisoxazole (500 mg if the patient is less than 60 lb, 1,000 mg if the patient is greater than 60 lb) once daily in penicillin allergy. Individuals allergic to both agents may be treated with erythromycin 250 mg twice daily. Azithromycin or clarithromycin may be suitable alternatives. The recommended duration of prophylaxis is outlined in Table 14.7.

2. Post-streptococcal reactive arthritis

    a. A more persistent, nonmigratory arthritis may occur following a group A streptococcal pharyngitis, in the absence of sufficient clinical or laboratory findings to fulfill the Jones criteria. In these individuals, the response to salicylates or other nonsteroidal agents is less dramatic than in RF, and several months to a few years of therapy may be required.

    b. In some individuals with post-streptococcal reactive arthritis (PSRA), silent or delayed-onset carditis may be detected by echocardiography. If carditis is present, the patient should be treated for RF. There are no studies of the risk of carditis in PSRA, but because of scattered reports of carditis in PSRA, prophylaxis for 1 or 2 years is sometimes recommended.

B. Lyme disease

    1. Infection by *Borrelia burgdorferi*, a tick-borne spirochete, may cause a multisystem rheumatic syndrome involving joints, skin, nervous system, and heart. Like syphilis, it produces early, localized symptoms; early, disseminated disease (secondary); and late illness.

        a. The early, localized disease is characterized by an erythematosus skin lesion known as ECM, occurring at the site of the tick bite. The lesion begins as a macule or papule, and extends centrifugally over several days to a median diameter of 15 to 20 cm. Central clearing may occur. Systemic symptoms of malaise, fever, myalgia, arthralgia, headache, and stiff neck may accompany the rash. The systemic symptoms may be intermittent, resolving in a few weeks.

        b. Early, disseminated disease usually presents as multiple, smaller erythema migrans lesions, typically 3 to 5 weeks after the tick bite. Cranial nerve palsies, especially facial palsy, meningitis, and conjunctivitis may also occur, and fever, myalgia, arthralgia, headache, and malaise are common. Cardiac involvement is uncommonly encountered during this stage, presenting as variable conduction block.

        c. Late Lyme disease usually produces oligoarthritis involving large weight-bearing joints, particularly the knees. It may occur without prior evidence of early disease. A subacute encephalopathy and polyradiculoneuropathy may also be late manifestations of Lyme disease. Antimicrobial treatment of early manifestations prevents late disease.

    2. Diagnosis is made early if ECM is present. Culture of the advancing edge of the skin lesions may yield *B. burgdorferi*, but culture is not readily available. In the absence of erythema migrans, Lyme disease

Table 14.7. Duration of prophylaxis for persons who have had rheumatic fever

Clinical presentation	Duration of prophylaxis
Rheumatic fever without carditis	5 yr or until age 21 yr, whichever is longer
Rheumatic fever with carditis, but without residual valvular disease	10 yr or well into adulthood, whichever is longer
Rheumatic fever with residual valvular disease	At least 10 yr since last episode, and at least until age 40 yr

may be confirmed using serologic testing. Screening antibody testing employs ELISA technology, but may be negative early in the disease. Because some antigens of *B. burgdorferi* cross-react with antigens on other spirochetes, confirmation of positive ELISA results with Western blot is necessary.

3. Treatment of early localized disease in children 8 years of age or older is with doxycycline 100 mg twice daily for 14 to 21 days. Below the age of 8 years, amoxicillin 20 to 50 mg/kg/day for 14 to 21 days is used. With early, disseminated disease involving skin only, the same regimens are used. If isolated facial palsy is present, the duration of treatment is increased to 21 to 28 days, and arthritis is treated with the same oral regimen for 28 days. Persistent or recurrent arthritis, carditis, meningitis, or encephalitis requires treatment with parenteral medication. The usual regimens are ceftriaxone 75 to 100 mg per kg once daily (i.m. or i.v.) for 14 to 21 days, or penicillin 300,000 U/kg/day i.v. divided every 4 hours for 14 to 21 days (maximum 20,000,000 U/day).

C. Postinfectious arthritis

1. An acute, sterile inflammatory arthritis occurring after an infectious illness, at a site distant from the primary infection is referred to as postinfectious or reactive arthritis. The arthritis usually follows the primary infection by a period of 1 to 4 weeks, and the joint involvement is usually an asymmetric large joint oligoarthritis. The process is usually self-limiting, but may become chronic in a minority of cases. In some people, inflammation of conjunctivae, entheses (insertions), and mucosal surfaces occurs producing a condition known as Reiter syndrome (see Adult arthropathies on page 269). Association of Reiter syndrome, and to a lesser extent, other postinfectious reactive arthritis, with the class I major histocompatibility antigen HLA-B27 is well described.

2. A number of bacterial infections can cause reactive arthritis in addition to *Streptococcus* and *B. burgdorferi*. Brucellosis (which may also cause a septic monoarthritis) can produce aseptic spondylitis and oligoarthritis that is self-limiting. *Clostridium difficile* may cause reactive arthritis 1 to 3 weeks following colitis. It resolves within several weeks, and is seen more commonly in HLA-B27-antigen-positive individuals. Some strains of enterotoxin-producing *S. aureus* have caused large joint sterile oligoarthritis that is self-limiting. Enteric infection with Gram-negative bacterial pathogens such as *Yersinia* and *Shigella* species can be associated with a transient reactive arthritis. Similarly, intestinal parasites such as *Strongyloides stercoralis*, *Cryptosporidium*, and *Giardia lamblia* may induce a reactive arthritis, often accompanied by eosinophilia of peripheral blood and synovial fluid.

3. Postinfectious reactive arthritis usually responds to treatment with short courses of NSAIDs. Eradication of parasites from the intestinal tract may be required for resolution of the arthritis associated with parasite infestation. Most cases of reactive arthritis do not continue long enough to meet criteria for juvenile idiopathic arthritis (see Juvenile idiopathic arthritis on page 293).

4. Viral infection or immunization to some viral agents may be associated with transient synovitis. Rubella and varicella infections may cause reactive arthritis, and early rubella immunizations frequently resulted in short-lived polyarthritis, especially in adult women. The prodrome of hepatitis B virus causes a symmetrical polyarthritis and sometimes results in transient carpal tunnel syndrome from swelling of the wrist flexor tendon sheaths. Synovitis has been reported following immunization with current rubella vaccines (though much less frequently than with the early vaccines) and recombinant hepatitis B vaccine. Possible associations between reactive arthritis and administration of typhoid vaccine; bacilli bilié de Calmette-Guérin (BCG); influenza;

Campylobacter; and even the diphtheria, pertussis, and tetanus (DPT) vaccines have been reported, but such reactions appear to be rare and short-lived. Symptomatic treatment with NSAIDs suffices.

X. Juvenile idiopathic arthritis

Chronic arthritis in childhood (onset prior to the 16th birthday) occurs in approximately 0.1% of school-aged children, with a prevalence of 250,000 to 300,000 in the United States. The disease definition requires 6 weeks of arthritis symptoms. Subsets of the disease are defined by symptoms and the number of joints involved in the first 6 months of the illness. It is likely that improved understanding of the genetics and immunopathology of these disorders will lead to further refinement of the classification scheme in the future. The classification currently proposed by the European League Against Rheumatism (EULAR) is as follows.

A. Systemic onset juvenile arthritis

  1. Often called Still disease, symptoms of systemic illness predominate early in the disease. It affects approximately 10% of all children with juvenile idiopathic arthritis. Daily fever spikes, typically to 39 to 41°C are typically the presenting symptoms, and may last for weeks to months. Fever is often accompanied by an evanescent salmon-colored macular or maculopapular rash most prominent in warm areas of the body. Lymphadenopathy and hepatosplenomegaly are present in the majority of patients. Arthritis may occur with the fevers, but may not be present for months or even years after the onset of illness. Weight loss and cachexia may ensue. Most affected children will develop polyarthritis. Pleuritis and pericarditis may occur. Occasionally, a sterile peritonitis or meningoencephalitis may be seen.

  2. Laboratory findings are nonspecific, but may be severe. Leukocytosis, often with WBC as high as 50,000 to 100,000 cells/mm^3 is common, but the WBC may be normal. Thrombocytosis is typical, and may be severe. Anemia of chronic disease occurs after several weeks of fever, and may result in hemoglobin levels as low as 5 g per dL. ESR and CRP are often extremely high. Albumin may be low in the face of high total protein. Polyclonal hypergammaglobulinemia is common. Bacterial, fungal, and viral cultures are negative. Purified protein derivative (of tuberculin) (PPD) is negative, but cutaneous anergy may be seen. Because of high WBC and anemia in a child with generalized lymphadenopathy and fever of unknown etiology, many children with this disease require bone marrow examination to exclude the diagnosis of leukemia. The marrow is usually reactive, with no evidence of malignancy.

  3. Treatment of systemic onset juvenile arthritis is aimed at suppressing the systemic inflammation and controlling the joint disease.

    a. NSAIDs are the cornerstone of therapy, but with extreme systemic inflammation, hepatic enzyme elevation may be seen after initiation of NSAID therapy. This may require temporary discontinuation of the medication and use of corticosteroid for a short period of time. Once the systemic symptoms are controlled, NSAIDs are often required to control joint inflammation.

    b. Corticosteroids in low doses may be required for control of fever and systemic symptoms unresponsive to NSAIDs. Encephalitis and severe pleuritis or pericarditis may require glucocorticoids for control.

    c. Methotrexate in doses of 10 mg per M^2 body surface area/week to 1 mg/kg/week is often required for control of systemic symptoms and/or arthritis.

    d. Etanercept is effective in controlling systemic and joint symptoms in approximately 75% of individuals who respond poorly to NSAIDs, steroid, and methotrexate, or who have unacceptable toxicity from those medications. The drug is approved by the U.S. Food and Drug Administration (FDA) for juvenile polyarthritis.

    e. Other medications occasionally required for control of severe symptoms of this disease include cyclosporine, tacrolimus, azathioprine, and cyclophosphamide. No controlled trials of these medications in systemic juvenile arthritis have been published. Intravenous immunoglobulin at doses of 2 g per kg was efficacious in controlling fever in uncontrolled reports, but in a blind, placebo-controlled trial, efficacy could not be confirmed.

    f. The anemia of chronic disease usually responds poorly to oral iron supplementation, and may require parenteral iron therapy.

  4. Complications of systemic juvenile arthritis include a low risk of uveitis (approximately 5%), the anemia of chronic disease, and the possibility of cardiac tamponade from pericarditis or respiratory impairment from large pleural effusions. Long-term follow-up studies of juvenile arthritis reveal that up to 5% of those with systemic disease may die of suicide.

  5. Macrophage activation syndrome, which carries up to a 30% to 50% mortality, occurs in approximately 5% of children. It often follows infections, or changes in medication because of uncontrolled systemic inflammatory symptoms. The risk of developing this severe complication may be increased with the use of sulfasalazine, and thus this drug is relatively contraindicated in active systemic onset juvenile arthritis. Symptoms of macrophage activation syndrome include lethargy, tachycardia, respiratory distress, hypotension, and abdominal pain. Fever may be absent, but the child may appear to be developing a septic shock syndrome. ESR is often low, and this should be taken as an ominous sign in someone with Still disease who appears ill. Hepatic enzymes are typically elevated, and may rise precipitously. Hepatic gluconeogenesis may be impaired, and hyperammonemia may occur. Disseminated intravascular coagulation, shock, adult respiratory distress syndrome, myocardial failure, and renal failure occur in severe disease. This syndrome requires intensive care support and monitoring, and responds to high doses of parenteral glucocorticoid (up to 30 mg per kg daily for 3 to 5 days, maximum dose of 1 g daily) and cyclosporine at a dose of 2 to 5 mg/kg/day.

B. Juvenile oligoarthritis (pauciarticular juvenile arthritis)

  1. Oligoarthritis is defined as inflammation of fewer than 5 joints in the first 6 months of illness. Children with this form of arthritis typically have involvement of knees or ankles, and are usually younger than 8 years at the time of onset. The initial manifestations of this disease may be as young as the first year of life. Females outnumber males by a ratio of 7:1.

  2. The arthritis often resolves with antiinflammatory treatment within a few years, and seldom causes erosions. Bony overgrowth of the affected limbs may occur as a result of cytokine activity.

  3. Inflammation of the uveal tract of the eye, causing anterior and/or posterior uveitis, occurs in approximately 20% of children. The risk is highest in children with early-onset disease (below age 4 years), and if the ANA is positive. The inflammation is usually asymptomatic until vision is impaired by scar formation. Visual impairment may occur in up to 30% of affected children due to cataract formation, posterior synechiae, or band keratopathy. Slit lamp examination can identify early inflammation, and should be done every 4 months in the first 2 years, then every 6 years if no uveitis occurs. If the ANA is positive, screening exams should be done every 3 months.

  4. The arthritis is managed successfully with NSAIDs in approximately 65% to 75% of children. The NSAID medications approved by the FDA for pediatrics include aspirin (80 to 100 mg/kg/day divided q.i.d.), ibuprofen (30 to 40 mg/kg/day divided t.i.d. to q.i.d.), tolmetin (20 to 30 mg/kg/day divided t.i.d.), naproxen (10 to 20 mg/kg/day divided b.i.d.), and indomethacin (1 to 2 mg/kg/day divided q.i.d.). Sulfasalazine (30 to 40 mg/kg/day) is often effective in controlling joint inflammation in the majority of those with active arthritis despite adequate doses of

NSAID, but toxicity may limit its use. Intraarticular steroid injection can control monoarthritis effectively in many patients. Methotrexate (10 mg/M^2/week is usual starting dose) may be required occasionally.

C. Extended oligoarthritis

1. Children with fewer than five joints involved in the first 6 months who subsequently have inflammation of five or more joints are classified as having extended oligoarthritis. Often, they have three or four inflamed joints in the onset period, and upper extremity involvement may provide a clue that the child will follow a polyarticular course. Immunogenetically, these children have the same human leukocyte antigen DR4 (HLA-DR4) overrepresentation seen in children with polyarthritis. The risk of chronic progressive arthritis in adulthood is similar to that of children with RF-negative polyarthritis [see Polyarthritis (rheumatoid factor-negative) below]. Uveitis is uncommon, being seen in only about 5% of children with this form of juvenile arthritis.

2. Treatment is as for oligoarthritis (pages 294–295), but the majority will require treatment with a second or third medication, in addition to NSAID. Some children may respond to hydroxychloroquine (4 to 7 mg/kg/day, given q.i.d. or b.i.d.), and others may require methotrexate or TNF-α-blocking agents such as etanercept or infliximab (see etanercept in Systemic arthritis on page 293–294).

3. Slit lamp examinations should be performed every 6 months to screen for uveitis.

D. Polyarthritis (rheumatoid factor negative)

1. Childhood onset chronic arthritis affecting five or more joints in the first 6 months of the illness is considered polyarthritis. In the majority of children with polyarthritis, the RF is negative. In most children with RF-negative polyarthritis, the small joints of the hands and feet are involved. The arthritis tends to be symmetrical (involving similar joints on both side of the body. Inflammation of the cervical spine, temporomandibular joints (TMJs), and hips is also common. Age of onset varies widely, spanning the pediatric age groups.

2. As many as half of the children with this form of arthritis may be disease free at 10 years after onset. Nevertheless, chronic, progressive, erosive disease is seen in many of those who have persistent joint inflammation. Most require treatment with slower acting antirheumatic drugs.

3. Treatment of this disease begins with standard nonsteroidal drugs. Many patients will require the addition of sulfasalazine, hydroxychloroquine, methotrexate, or combinations of these because of inadequate response to single-agent therapy. TNF-α inhibitors, glucocorticoids, and immune suppressants such as cyclosporine, tacrolimus, azathioprine, and leflunomide may be required in severe persistent disease.

4. Complications of polyarthritis include growth failure and weight loss related to the chronic inflammation, erosion with subluxation of involved joints, and a variety of joint deformities. Micrognathia may be seen in children with severe TMJ arthritis, and limb asymmetry may be seen related to local growth perturbations. The anemia of chronic disease is common with severe disease, and other systemic signs of chronic inflammatory illness including hypoalbuminemia, thrombocytosis, and high CRP and ESR are frequently seen. Uveitis is uncommon in this subset of juvenile arthritis, occurring in approximately 5% of children. Screening for uveitis is recommended twice annually.

E. Polyarthritis (rheumatoid factor positive)

1. Polyarthritis with a positive RF is indistinguishable from RF-positive RA in adults. It has the same demographics, the same HLA associations, and the same extraarticular manifestations as RA, but because onset occurs in the peripubertal years (ages 9 to 16 years), the ultimate potential for chronic damage may be greater in children.

2. Prognosis is similar to that in adult onset RA, with a high percentage developing erosive disease, deformity, and disability.

3. Treatment is similar to that in RF-negative polyarthritis, but most pediatric rheumatologists will be more aggressive early in the disease because of the high potential for joint damage and subsequent disability.

4. Rheumatoid nodules may be seen in this form of juvenile-onset arthritis, and pulmonary disease, Felty syndrome, and other systemic manifestations of RA seen in adults may also occur in children with this disease, but often only after they have had the disease for several years.

F. Enthesitis-associated juvenile arthritis

1. Also known as the juvenile seronegative spondyloarthropathies, enthesitis-associated arthritis is an asymmetrical oligoarthritis or polyarthritis, often involving hips, sacroiliac joints, and/or spine. It is most common in the peripubertal child or adolescent. Tendonitis or plantar fasciitis may be present, sometime preceding true arthritis. Extraarticular manifestations include iridocyclitis, diarrhea, urethritis, genital lesions, and skin lesions. Poor growth or weight loss may suggest inflammatory bowel disease. This form of arthritis is more common in males. Some will develop AS (see Ankylosing spondylitis on page 267–268). In these individuals, progressive loss of spine and rib mobility may occur. Juvenile Reiter syndrome, in which enthesitis, arthritis, iridocyclitis, and mucosal lesions of the mouth, genitourinary, and gastrointestinal tracts, and sometimes associated with skin lesions such a palmoplantar pustulosis or keratoderma blennorrhogica, is another member of this group of disorders.

2. In Caucasian populations, approximately 90% of individuals with AS will have the class I major histocompatibility complex (MHC) antigen, HLA-B27. The prevalence of HLA-B27 is also high in the other enthesitis-associated arthropathies of childhood, though at lower frequency. Because HLA-B27 is present in 10% to 14% of the general population, its presence does not conclusively affirm, nor does its absence exclude the diagnosis. Diagnosis is made on clinical grounds. Radiographic demonstration of sacroiliitis strongly suggests that the older child with oligoarthritis has an enthesitis-associated arthritis. Reiter syndrome may be associated with an antecedent history of diarrheal illness or *Chlamydia* genital infection.

3. Initial evaluation should involve a careful history of bowel habits, because overt diarrhea may not yet be present in children with inflammatory bowel disease. Moreover, adolescents rarely complain of frequent stooling and urgency. The intestinal manifestations of the disease must be treated for successful control of joint inflammation in most patients. Urogenital symptoms including ulcers, discharge, hematuria, and dysuria should be sought, and risk of sexually transmitted disease questioned. An ESR out of proportion to the extent of the joint inflammation should suggest inflammatory bowel disease, and trigger study of the gastrointestinal tract.

4. Therapy should be initiated with NSAIDs; anecdotal reports suggest that indomethacin may be more effective in this family of disorders than other NSAIDs. No controlled comparison has been done. Individuals needing a second-line agent often respond to sulfasalazine at doses of 30 to 40 mg/kg/day in two to four divided doses. Serious toxic reactions to sulfasalazine include drug rash, Stevens-Johnson syndrome, agranulocytosis, marrow arrest, and hepatitis. Close monitoring of marrow and hepatic function is necessary. Physical therapy to maintain spine and thoracic mobility is important in the management of juvenile AS. One study of young adults with juvenile-onset AS suggests a high risk of aortic and cardiac valve disease at 10 years after diagnosis.

G. Juvenile psoriatic arthritis

1. Juvenile psoriatic arthritis often has onset in early childhood, with a mean age of onset of 6 years (4.5 years for girls, 10 years for boys). It

is more than twice as common in girls than boys. Arthritis may precede the onset of rash by several years. Skin psoriasis in family members should suggest this diagnosis in the child with arthritis, especially if DIP joints are involved. The most common pattern of arthritis is asymmetric polyarthritis of large and small joints. Dactylitis with tenosynovitis may cause diffuse digital swelling—the "sausage digit" of psoriatic arthritis. The skin overlying inflamed joints may have a red–violet color. Cervical spine involvement may occur. Nail pits may be early signs of dermal psoriasis. Some individuals develop erosive arthritis that may lead to deformations, particularly of the small joints of hands and feet.

2. Early radiographic changes are those of any inflammatory arthritis, but later in the disease, the pathognomonic "pencil-in-cup" erosions may be seen, where the proximal surface of the distal phalanges are splayed (the cup), and the distal portion of the proximal phalanx of the joint is narrowed to a point (the pencil).

3. Treatment with NSAIDs controls symptoms, but most children will require second-line agents to suppress signs of inflammation and progression of disease. Methotrexate not only suppresses joint disease, but also controls skin lesions; hepatic toxicity may be higher in adults with psoriasis than RA, so careful monitoring of liver function is required.

4. Eye inflammation identical to that of oligoarthritis may occur, and may be more resistant to treatment than in oligoarthritis, so recommendations for screening are the same as for children with juvenile oligoarthritis.

Systemic Autoimmune Diseases

XI. Systemic lupus erythematosus

SLE is a systemic autoimmune disease defined by clinical criteria. It has a strong female predominance and can occur at any age. The diagnosis is made when at least four of the following criteria are met.

1. Malar rash—this is an erythematous rash covering bilateral malar areas as well as the nasal bridge. It is generally photosensitive with telangiectasias and may leave scarring in discoid SLE. The differential diagnosis of photosensitive malar rashes includes rosacea (papular erythematous lesions that generally do not cross the nasal bridge), porphyria cutanea tarda (often blistering lesions involving multiple sun-exposed areas), actinic keratoses (may be flat and atrophic or lichenoid; often starts as a collection of telangiectatic capillaries), and solar urticaria.

2. Discoid rash—this is characterized by reddish scaly patches that occur in sun-exposed areas and tend to heal with atrophy, scarring, and pigmentary changes. The most commonly confused disease process is actinic keratoses.

3. Photosensitivity—generally applies to not only skin rash, but also flares of other disease manifestations, arthritis, constitutional symptoms, etc., on exposure to ultraviolet irradiation. The differential diagnosis includes bullous pemphigoid, lichen planus, rosacea, porphyria, and various drug reactions.

4. Oral ulcers—generally painless; often begin as red patches that break down to slit-like lesions. The differential diagnosis includes aphthous ulcers (generally painful), infections (especially viral, fungal, and syphilis), lichen planus, drug reactions, inflammatory bowel diseases, Behçet syndrome, Reiter syndrome, malignancies, and trauma.

5. Arthritis—must have synovial thickening or effusion with warmth and/or erythema; pain alone does not fulfill requirements for this diagnostic criterion

6. Serositis (pleuritis or pericarditis)—may be only pain on inspiration, but one would like to have an objective finding consistent with the diagnosis, such as demonstration of pleural or pericardial fluid. The differential diagnosis includes various infections, drug reactions, and other systemic disorders.

7. Renal disorder—although the official criteria list urinary abnormality or elevated serum creatinine as indicating renal disorder, this can be misleading, especially in patients with diabetes or hypertension or those taking medications that can alter renal function. Ideally, a kidney biopsy would document membranous and/or proliferative changes with positive immunofluorescence for immunoglobulin A (IgA), IgG, IgM, and C3. World Health Organisation (WHO) classification of SLE renal disease includes type I, normal; type II, mesangial; type III, focal proliferative; type IV, diffuse proliferative; type V, membranous; type VI, sclerotic.
8. Neurologic disorder—includes depression, psychosis, peripheral neuropathy, seizures, and strokes; however, this is the most difficult to use as a criterion because neurologic disorders, even in SLE patients, are often due to other causes, such as infections, drugs, atherosclerotic vascular disease, etc.
9. Hematologic disorder—the most common hematologic disorders in order of descending frequency are lymphopenia, anemia, thrombocytopenia, leukopenia. One must rule out other causes for these disorders, such as infections, drugs, tumors, and primary phospholipid antibody syndrome. Furthermore, for anemia to count as a criterion for diagnosis of SLE, it must be anemia secondary to Coombs-positive hemolysis, not secondary to blood loss or "chronic disease."
10. Immunologic disorder—(anti-dsDNA, anti-Sm, false-positive Venereal Disease Research Laboratory test [VDRL] or antiphospholipid antibody) most patients with SLE have autoantibodies in addition to an ANA. None of these are specific for SLE; the anti-Sm is specific for SLE when done by the Ouchterlony technique, but when done by ELISA, the test is so sensitive it can identify low titers in normals and in patients with other disorders.
11. Antinuclear antibodies (ANA)—now that the ANA is done with the Hep2 substrate, all patients with SLE have a positive ANA; 10% to 15% of the normal female population, especially women taking birth control pills, also has a positive ANA. Similar percentages of healthy children have a positive ANA, sometimes at high titer.

Other common manifestations of SLE that are not part of the diagnostic criteria include:

1. Alopecia—often patchy in nature
2. Livedo reticularis—occurs in the setting of antiphospholipid antibodies, thrombosis, Raynaud phenomenon, and/or true vasculitis
3. Raynaud syndrome—cold-induced vasospasm classically producing sequential blanching, then cyanosis, and erythema on rewarming. This occurs because of immune complex deposition in the endothelium of blood vessels and local complement activation. Antiphospholipid antibodies can also induce it via several mechanisms. All vessels can be involved with clinical manifestations occurring in the CNS (benign angiopathy of the CNS), heart (Prinzmetal angina), lungs (reversible hypoxemia), bowel (abdominal angina), and extremities.
4. Libman-Sacks endocarditis—occurs most commonly in the mitral values, more than the aortic valves, but is the most common cause of right-sided valvular heart lesions. It is seen most frequently in the setting of antiphospholipid antibodies.
5. Chronic interstitial pneumonitis—involves predominantly lymphocytic infiltration. This pneumonitis is slowly progressive but can lead to significant respiratory dysfunction. It is difficult to diagnose and is often missed until it is fairly advanced.

Autoantibodies Commonly Associated with Systemic Lupus Erythematosus

1. ANA—all patients are positive
2. Anti-dsDNA—occurs in 50% of patients; high titers often associated with renal disease; not specific; antinucleosome antibodies, currently under investigation, may be more specific

3. Anti-Sm—occurs in 15% to 20% of patients; seen predominantly in SLE; may be associated with CNS disease
4. Anti-nuclear ribonucleoprotein (anti-nRNP)—occurs in 25% to 30% of patients; seen commonly in patients with overlap syndromes including Raynaud, myositis, and scleroderma
5. Anti-Ro (Sjögren syndrome A [SS-A])—occurs in 25% of patients; commonly seen in patients with C2 deficiency; associated with photosensitivity, nephritis, vasculitis, pneumonitis, and Sjögren syndrome
6. Anti-La (Sjögren syndrome B [SS-B])—occurs in 15% to 20% of patients; associated with Sjögren syndrome and a lower incidence of renal disease
7. Antiribosomal P—occurs in 5% to 10% of patients; occurs predominantly in patients with SLE; associated with psychosis, depression, and rapidly proliferative glomerulonephritis
8. Antihistone—seen in a majority of SLE patients; when it occurs alone it suggests drug-induced SLE with predominantly arthritis and pleuritis
9. Antiphospholipid antibodies—(see Antiphospholipid antibody syndrome on pages 312–313); occur in 25% to 45% of patients with SLE; associated with thrombosis, thrombocytopenia, livedo reticularis, recurrent miscarriages, Libman-Sacks endocarditis, and stroke.

Principals of Management of Patients With SLE

A. Carefully define the extent and nature of organ involvement in each patient. In addition to history and physical exam, the initial evaluation should include:
   1. CBC with differential, urinalysis, electrolytes, blood urea nitrogen (BUN), creatinine, albumin, total protein, serum protein electrophoresis, ANA, ENA (anti-Ro, anti-La, anti-nRNP, anti-Sm), anti-dsDNA, complements C3 and C4
   2. Depending on the presenting complaints, chest x-ray, echocardiogram, and pulmonary function tests including carbon monoxide diffusion in the lung (DLCO) and magnetic resonance imaging (MRI) of head may also be warranted.
   3. Additional studies may be warranted depending upon symptoms and the results of the preliminary evaluation. Follow-up evaluations in each patient should determine which laboratory parameters correlate with disease activity in each individual patient.
B. Treat the clinical manifestations of each patient according to their organ involvement, not according to their serologies. Serologies can help distinguish active SLE from infections or other disease processes, but individual serologic tests vary with their utility in each patient.
C. Use the least toxic medication suitable to control particular organ manifestations, considering both acute and chronic medication use.
D. Use aggressive therapy with corticosteroids and cytotoxic drugs when major organ function is threatened, such as in systemic vasculitis or WHO class IV glomerulonephritis.
E. Meticulous general medical and surgical care to diagnose and treat all SLE and non-SLE problems, including infections, drug reactions, etc.
F. Therapies for particular organ involvement:
   1. Skin and mucosal manifestations
      Standard therapies—photoprotection, antimalarials (i.e., hydroxychloroquine 200 mg q.d. to b.i.d.), topical steroids
         Evolving therapies—dapsone (50 to 100 mg q.d.), thalidomide (100 to 400 mg q.d.), clofazimine, retinoids
   2. Serositis
      Standard therapies—NSAIDs (with attention to potential renal impairment), antimalarials, rarely low-dose steroids (i.e., prednisone 10 to 20 mg q.d.)

3. Arthralgias and constitutional symptoms
   Standard therapies—NSAIDs and antimalarials for musculoskeletal complaints, serotonin reuptake inhibitor antidepressants (i.e., amitriptyline 25 to 100 mg hs) for myalgia and depressive symptoms
   Evolving therapies—dehydroepiandrosterone (DHEA)
4. Myositis
   Standard therapies—high-dose corticosteroids (60 to 100 mg q.d.); if necessary, methotrexate (7.5 to 20 mg weekly) or azathioprine (50 to 200 mg q.d.)
5. Raynaud phenomenon
   Standard therapies—calcium channel blockers (i.e., nifedipine 10 to 20 mg t.i.d., or 30 to 60 mg extended release q.d.), α_1-adrenergic receptor antagonists (i.e., doxazosin 2 to 4 mg b.i.d.), nitrates (i.e., isosorbide mononitrate 30 mg q.d. to q.i.d.)
   Evolving therapies for refractory disease—intravenous prostaglandin E_1 PGE_1 (5 to 15 ng/kg/min for 5 to 7 days) or oral misoprostol (PGE_1 analogue, 100 to 200 µg q.i.d.)
6. Renal disease
   Standard therapies—WHO class I and II: nothing
   WHO class III or IV—prednisone (60 mg q.d. for 1 month then taper as tolerated; may stop prednisone in 4 to 6 months) and monthly i.v. cyclophosphamide (750 mg/M^2 initial dose; check WBC 10 to 14 days after infusion; aim for WBC 3,000 to 4,000 per mL; adjust dose up or down for next infusion depending upon WBC; generally given with mercaptoethanesulfonate (MESNA) at a dose of 20% of cytoxan dose, administered at the time of cytoxan infusion and then q4h for another 2 to 3 doses; generally 12 monthly infusions are given and then 3 additional infusions every 2 months; this will vary with the clinical response.)
   WHO class V—treat only if nephrotic; consider first high-dose, alternate-day or daily steroids; steroid failures should receive monthly i.v. cyclophosphamide; proteinuria often decreases with angiotensin-converting enzyme (ACE) inhibitor therapy.
   WHO class VI—dialysis and renal transplantation
   Evolving therapies—mycophenolate mofetil, 2'-chlorodeoxyadenosine, leflunomide, LJP 394
7. Hematologic disease
   Thrombocytopenia—corticosteroids (may require split-dose prednisone, 30 mg b.i.d. to q.i.d. initially if severe), intravenous Ig (i.e., sandoglobulin 0.4 to 1.0 g per kg infusion per day times 1 to 3), anti-D (i.e., anti-rho [D] 50 µg per kg single i.v. infusion), vinblastine, danazol, splenectomy
   Hemolytic anemia—steroids (may require split-dose prednisone, 30 mg b.i.d. to q.i.d. initially if severe), cyclophosphamide (either monthly i.v. infusions, as for WHO type IV nephritis, or daily oral cyclophosphamide given at a dose to maintain WBC between 3,000 and 4,000 per mL; generally requires 1 to 2 mg/kg/day), danazol, splenectomy
8. Interstitial pneumonitis
   Standard therapy—steroids (initially prednisone 40 to 60 mg q.d. then taper as tolerated); cyclophosphamide or azathioprine are sometimes required in addition
9. Systemic vasculitis with major organ involvement
   Standard therapy—steroids (initially 1 mg per kg for 1 month then taper as tolerated) and daily oral cyclophosphamide

Considerations In Pediatric Systemic Lupus Erythematosus
A. Prepubertal onset of SLE should prompt a search for congenital (genetic) risk factors
   1. Complement deficiencies. Children with congenital complement deficiency are at increased risk for SLE, and risk of complement deficiency may be as high as 30% to 50% in children with onset of disease prior

to puberty. Assessment should include 50% hemolyzing dose of complement (CH_{50}), with attention to specimen handling (transport on ice, maintain serum at $-70°C$ until assayed). Active SLE may deplete components, but CH_{50} should be measurable; results below 10% of normal suggest congenital complement deficiency. Complement deficiency may also cause recurrent infection with encapsulated bacteria, or disseminated bacterial infection (opsonic defect).

   2. IgA deficiency and common variable immunodeficiency. Selective deficiency of IgA and common variable immunodeficiency (CVID) can be associated with SLE, often presenting with rash, arthritis, and autoimmune cytopenias (hemolytic anemia ± thrombocytopenia). IgA deficiency-associated SLE rarely, if ever, causes nephritis or CNS disease, but the arthritis may be erosive, and the hematologic complications severe. Recurrent respiratory and skin infection may be present, and allergic symptoms are common.

B. Adolescent patients with SLE must be screened for the following depressive symptoms and signs and treated promptly: appetite disturbance, sleep disturbance, social withdrawal, and school problems. Denial of illness and noncompliance with medications are common.

   1. Noncompliance may signal CNS involvement, or adolescent defiance reaction.

   2. Glucocorticoid side effects of obesity, acne, and hirsutism are unacceptable to many adolescent female patients, and alteration of self-image may induce depressive symptoms.

C. Growth and development may be adversely affected by disease activity, and by medications used for therapy of SLE. Careful attention to nutritional needs of the growing child must include adequate supplementation of calcium and vitamin D, and avoidance of high-fat foods, while providing adequate nutrients for growth.

D. Prognosis of childhood-onset SLE is similar to that of adults if treated aggressively; poor outcome is associated with delay in treatment.

E. Neonatal systemic lupus erythematosus

   1. Neonatal SLE is the result of passive transfer of "autoantibody" from mother to the fetus via placental circulation. The fetus is affected but does not produce abnormal antibody.

   2. The mother may be asymptomatic, or may have SLE, Sjögren syndrome, or mixed connective tissue disease.

   3. Thrombocytopenia may lead to hemorrhage at birth or in the neonatal period. Hemolytic anemia and leukopenia may occur.

   4. Rash, which is often photosensitive, is detected in the first month of life. Rash is associated with SS-A (Ro) and SS-B (La) autoantibodies.

   5. Carditis with inflammation of the ventricular conducting system occurs early in gestation (15 to 20 weeks) leading to inflammation and subsequent destruction of the conducting fibers. Results in congenital heart block that requires permanent pacemaker placement. May cause hydrops fetalis and intrauterine demise of the fetus. Closely associated with SS-A antibody. Trials of antenatal steroid and intravenous immunoglobulin (IVIg) in SS-A-positive mothers with prior affected infants are in progress.

   6. Follow-up of affected infants suggests a possible increased risk of subsequent autoimmune disease in childhood and adolescence.

XII. Scleroderma

Scleroderma is a group of idiopathic disorders in which inflammation and fibrosis alter the collagen and other structural components in various organs, leading to different degrees of organ dysfunction. These disorders occur most commonly in women of Caucasian extraction, but can be seen in both sexes and all races worldwide. Both systemic and localized forms of scleroderma are recognized. Systemic scleroderma exists in many forms, including diffuse cutaneous scleroderma, limited cutaneous scleroderma, and scleroderma seen as part of overlap syndromes with other autoimmune (connective tissue) disease. Various localized forms of scleroderma are known, as well as syndromes with scleroderma-like features, such as eosinophilic fasciitis, eosinophilia myalgia syndrome, and toxic oil syndrome.

A. Systemic scleroderma

    1. Diffuse cutaneous scleroderma

        a. Skin involvement often begins with an edematous phase that is diffuse and not joint based. The edematous phase is generally, but not always, followed by an indurative phase of skin tightening. At the onset of the disease, distal digits are involved predominantly, but then spreading to the upper arms and legs, chest, abdomen, and face can occur rapidly. The peak of skin involvement tends to occur during the first 1 to 2 years of the disease. There is often some degree of spontaneous regression of the skin disease, occurring centripetally, after that time. The rate of spread and extent of skin disease generally correlate with internal organ involvement.

        b. Raynaud phenomenon may precede or occur concomitantly with skin changes. It occurs in a majority of patients (greater than 90%).

        c. Arthralgia and joint contractures occur in 90% of patients. Frank arthritis occurs in a much smaller percentage of patients.

        d. Esophageal dysmotility, due to involvement of the smooth muscle of the distal two-thirds of the esophagus, occurs in 60% of patients. Involvement of the small and large bowel, causing hypomotility, occurs in a smaller percentage of patients.

        e. Pulmonary involvement, which constitutes predominantly lymphocytic interstitial inflammation leading to fibrosis, occurs in 30% of patients. The presence of antibodies to topoisomerase I (Scl 70) are seen more frequently with this manifestation. Pulmonary hypertension generally occurs rarely late in the course of this type of pulmonary injury. Some patients with diffuse cutaneous scleroderma will develop primary pulmonary hypertension, without interstitial fibrosis, such as patients with limited cutaneous scleroderma.

        f. Cardiac involvement occurs in 10% of patients. Most commonly pericardial effusion is seen, but pericardial fibrosis, cardiomyopathy, and conduction defects, secondary to microvascular disease, occur infrequently.

        g. Renal crisis occurs in 15% to 20% of patients, but subclinical renal disease may occur in a much larger percentage of patients. Renal crisis is seen most commonly in patients with very rapid progression of skin changes. These patients often have antibodies to topoisomerase I and RNA polymerase III.

        h. Serologically, 95% of patients have ANA, 30% have antitopoisomerase 1 (Scl 70), and a smaller percentage have anti-RNA polymerase I and III or anti-U3 RNP.

        i. Pediatric patients have lower prevalence of disabling pulmonary and renal involvement, and thus have better outcome than do adult patients.

    2. Limited cutaneous scleroderma

        a. Skin involvement is generally restricted to face and distal hands and feet. It generally remains stable over several years and does not correlate with other organ involvement.

        b. Raynaud phenomenon occurs in greater than 95% of patients.

        c. Telangiectasia is prominent on the face, thorax, and extremities.

        d. Subcutaneous calcinosis is noted in 45% of patients.

        e. Esophageal dysmotility occurs in 80% of patients. Involvement of the small and large intestines occurs as well, but less frequently than in diffuse systemic scleroderma. Patients with small bowel involvement often express anti-Th antibodies.

        f. Pulmonary involvement is most commonly selective dysfunction of the pulmonary vasculature secondary to medial muscular hypertrophy and intimal fibrosis. Both reversible hypoxemia secondary to vascular spasm in the pulmonary vasculature and fixed pulmonary hypertension can be seen. This manifestation is associated with anticentromere and anti-Th antibodies. Interstitial fibrosis, like that seen in limited cutaneous scleroderma, can be seen in 25% of patients.

  g. Cardiac involvement is rare and generally is manifest as pericardial effusion.

  h. Renal disease is generally not seen in limited systemic disease.

  i. Serologically, 95% of patients have ANA, 25% to 50% have anticentromere antibodies, and a smaller percentage has anti-Th, anti-U1 RNP, or anti-PMScl antibodies. Anticentromere and anti-Scl 70 rarely coexist in the same patient.

3. Scleroderma overlap syndromes
Features of scleroderma can be seen in association with features of many other autoimmune disorders including Sjögren syndrome, SLE, dermatomyositis/polymyositis, RA, and primary biliary cirrhosis. The patients with scleroderma–myositis overlap often have antibodies to U1 RNP and/or PMScl (see pages 311–312).

B. Localized scleroderma

  1. Plaque morphea includes various subtypes:

  a. Morphea en plaque—superficial localized scleroderma restricted to the dermis and superficial panniculus

  b. Guttate morphea—multiple oval lesions with faint erythema, mild induration, and hypo- or hyperpigmentation; often found on the trunk

  c. Atrophoderma of Pasini and Pierini—asymptomatic hyperpigmented atrophic patches with well-demarcated borders generally found on the trunk

  d. Keloid morphea—isolated or confluent keloid-like nodules

  e. Lichen sclerosis et atrophicus—violaceous skin discoloration leading to shiny white plaques; tend to occur in anogenital area more often than trunk and extremities

  2. Generalized morphea—morphea including more than two anatomic sites

  3. Bullous morphea—tense subepidermal bullae in the presence of typical morphea or morphea profundus. Bullous morphea occurs on the extremities, trunk, face, and neck and may be superficial or deep. The condition is believed to be related to localized trauma.

  4. Linear morphea has several subtypes:

  a. Linear scleroderma—linear induration that usually affects the extremities and is unilateral in 95% of cases; may lead to deformities and limb atrophy. The disease process may involve not only the skin, but also underlying bone.

  b. Coup de sabre—unilateral involvement of face or scalp

  c. Progressive hemifacial atrophy—lesions in subcutaneous tissue, muscle, and bone cause hemiatrophy of the face; occasionally associated with seizures

  5. Deep morphea—involves the deep dermis, subcutaneous tissue, fascia, and/or superficial muscle in a diffuse rather than linear pattern. Deep morphea involves various subtypes:

  a. Subcutaneous morphea—rapid onset of symmetrical, ill-defined, hyperpigmented plaques

  b. Eosinophilic fasciitis—painful, peau d'orange appearance of extremities proximal to hands and feet; may be associated with various hematologic abnormalities including hemolytic anemic, thrombocytopenia, aplastic anemia, and leukemia. Peripheral eosinophilia are generally seen.

      c. Morphea profundus—diffuse, taut, deep sclerosis of skin; hyaliniza-
tion of panniculus and fascia; inflammatory infiltrate with lymphocytes and plasma cells

    6. Serologically, 50% of patients with morphea have ANA and 25% posi-
tive RFs; hypergammaglobulinemia is common.

C. Diseases with scleroderma-like features

    1. Toxic oil syndrome—1981 epidemic from adulterated rapeseed oil;
possible culprit 3-(N-phenylamino)-1,2-propanediol (PAP). Acute phase
symptoms are cough, chest tightness, fever, malaise, myalgias, arthralgias, pruritus, rash, eosinophilia, and diffuse infiltrates on chest x-ray.
Intermediate-phase symptoms are edema of skin and subcutaneous
tissue, alopecia, hyperpigmented papules, muscle cramps, and thromboembolism. Chromic phase symptoms are peripheral neuropathy, hepatomegaly, scleroderma-like skin changes, and pulmonary hypertension.

    2. Eosinophilia–myalgia syndrome—1989 epidemic from adulterated
L-tryptophan; possible culprits 3-(phenylamino) alanine (PAA) and 1,1′
-ethylide-nebis (L-tryptophan) (EBT). Acute phase symptoms are fever,
rash, dyspnea, arthralgias, myalgias, and eosinophilia. Chronic phase
symptoms are muscle cramps, subcutaneous edema followed by tense,
woody induration involving predominantly the upper and lower extremities. Peripheral neuropathy, neurocognitive abnormalities, restrictive cardiomyopathy, and cardiac conduction defects are seen in
a small percentage of patients.

    3. Chemicals associated with scleroderma-like skin lesions, occasionally
Raynaud, and/or pulmonary hypertension include silica, vinyl chloride, trichloroethylene, trichloroethane, benzene, xylene, methylene
chloride, toluene, perchlorethylene, metaphenylenediamine, bis
(4-amino-3-methyl-cyclohexyl) methane, bromocriptine, bleomycin,
and pentazocine.

    4. Graft versus host disease

    5. Porphyria cutanea tarda

    6. Amyloidosis

    7. Carcinoid syndrome

    8. Polyneuropathy, organomegaly, endocrinopathy, M protein, and skin
changes (POEMS)

    9. Premature aging (Werner syndrome)

    10. Diabetes—diabetic cheiroarthropathy

D. Treatment

The treatment of scleroderma is problematic because little is known about
drugs that influence the disease process. Because of the rarity of scleroderma, the variability of its presentations, and its tendency to regress
spontaneously, controlled clinical trials have been unable to establish the
unequivocal utility of any drug in these disorders.

    The only medication for which clinical trials more often support utility
than not is D-penicillamine, for the treatment of skin and possible other
internal organ manifestations of diffuse scleroderma. D-Penicillamine works
by interfering with the intermolecular cross-linking of collagen, as well as by
other poorly characterized immunosuppressive mechanisms. It must be
used early in the course of the disease, while inflammation is causing
fibrosis. The dose is increased from 250 to 750 mg b.i.d. gradually over
the course of 6 months. The 1,500-mg dose is then maintained for 12 to
18 months, barring the development of side effects. Side effects forcing discontinuation of D-penicillamine occur in 25% of patients. They include
skin rash, proteinuria, leukopenia, thrombocytopenia, glomerulonephritis,
myositis, pemphigus, and myasthenia gravis.

    For the management of lymphocytic interstitial pneumonitis, but not
other pulmonary manifestations of scleroderma, clinical trials have supported the utility of cyclophosphamide. Cyclophosphamide is used at 1 to
2 mg/kg/day. The CBC should be monitored weekly initially, and then at

least monthly, to ensure that the total WBC is maintained between 3,000 and 4,000 per mL. Patients must be encouraged to take the medication first thing in the morning, drink plenty of fluids during the day, and urinate before bedtime to avoid cystitis. Other complications include susceptibility to viral infections, sterility, and enhanced risk of malignancies.

Corticosteroids are generally used in low doses, 10 to 20 mg per day, for the management of acute inflammation, the edematous phase of the skin disease, and interstitial lung disease. High-dose steroids have been shown to be detrimental, whereas low-dose steroids are believed to be beneficial, without clinical trials to unequivocally support their utility. They are perhaps most useful in the limited forms of scleroderma, such as eosinophilic fasciitis. They should be used together with calcium, bisphosphonates, calcitonin, and/or vitamin D to prevent steroid-induced osteoporosis. Their use should be restricted as much as possible to reduce infection risk and various metabolic abnormalities including glucose intolerance.

Other medications believed to possibly impact on the inflammatory phase or early fibrosis, and which have failed clinical trials, include interferon gamma, cyclosporine A, methotrexate, relaxin, and dimethyl sulfoxide (DMSO).

Treatment of morphea has included a wide variety of drugs, none of which have been demonstrated to be useful in large numbers of patients. Some have shown benefit in individual cases, however, such as phenytoin, sulfasalazine, hydroxychloroquine, colchicine, and retinoids.

In the absence of drugs to reverse the disease process of scleroderma, the management of patients with these disorders involves supportive measures to control their organ dysfunction, along with very meticulous general medical and surgical care. These include:

1. Raynaud phenomenon—in addition to limiting cold exposure and avoiding vasoconstrictive agents, such as tobacco/nicotine, decongestants, and β-adrenergic blocking agents, patients can use calcium channel blockers (i.e., nifedipine 10 to 20 mg t.i.d.), α_1-adrenergic receptor antagonists (i.e., doxazosin 2 to 4 mg b.i.d.), and nitrates (i.e., isosorbide mononitrate 30 mg q.d. to q.i.d.). Severe Raynaud phenomena in the peripheral vessels can be managed with intravenous PGE_1 (5 to 15 ng/kg/min) and in the pulmonary vasculature with the prostacyclin analog Flolan (5 to 15 ng/kg/min).
2. Skin care—moisturizing creams, antihistamines for pruritus, and antibiotics for infections of digital ulcerations
3. Gastrointestinal tract—decreased motility can be improved with metoclopramide (10 to 20 mg q.i.d.), erythromycin (250 to 500 mg q.i.d.), and octreotide (50 μg S.Q. q.d.). Reflux esophagitis is treated by elevating the head of the bed, eating frequent small meals, and taking proton pump inhibitors (i.e., omeprazole 20 mg q.d. to b.i.d.), antacids, and H2-receptor antagonist antihistamines (i.e., ranitidine 150 mg b.i.d.).
4. Heart—pericarditis is usually managed with an NSAID (i.e., naproxen 500 mg b.i.d.), but occasionally requires low-dose prednisone (10 to 20 mg q.d.).
5. Kidney—hypertension, any renal disease, or diffuse cutaneous scleroderma and rapid skin changes should be treated with an ACE inhibitor (i.e., enalapril 2.5 to 20 mg b.i.d.). This has decreased the mortality of renal crisis from 50% to from 5% to 10%.

XIII. Sjögren syndrome

Sjögren syndrome may occur in isolation as a primary inflammatory disease, or more frequently may occur in association with other autoimmune diseases, such as RA, SLE and Hashimoto thyroiditis. It has a strong female predominance and tends to occur mostly in the fourth and fifth decades of life. The diagnosis of Sjögren syndrome requires meeting at least four of the following six criteria, as well as the exclusion of other consistent conditions:

1. Ocular symptoms—dry eyes
2. Oral symptoms—dry mouth
3. Ocular signs—Schirmer test with less than 5 mm tears in 5 minutes or Rose Bengal score greater than 4
4. Histopathologic features—minor salivary gland biopsy with focus score greater than 1 (at least 50 mononuclear cells infiltrating the salivary gland in a 4-mm^2 section of tissue)
5. Objective evidence of salivary gland dysfunction—salivary flow less than 1.5 mL in 15 minutes or abnormal salivary scintigraphy or parotid sialography
6. Autoantibodies—most patients have ANA. Other autoantibodies frequently present include anti-Ro (SS-A), anti-La (SS-B), and RF.
7. Causes of xerostomia and xerophthalmia to be excluded include: viral infections (mumps, influenza, cytomegalovirus (CMV), Epstein-Barr virus (EBV), coxsackievirus, hepatitis C, HIV, human T-cell lymphoma/leukemia virus (HTLV)-I and II, tuberculosis, sarcoidosis, amyloidosis, hyperlipoproteinemias, chronic pancreatitis, hepatic cirrhosis, diabetes, acromegaly, malnutrition, chronic sialoadenitis, senile atrophy, irradiation, cystic fibrosis, graft versus host disease, oral breathing (secondary to nasal polyps, deviated nasal septum, allergic rhinitis, etc.), psychogenic, dehydration, malignancies, and drugs (parasympatholytics, beta-blockers, etc.).

Other systemic manifestations are often seen with primary Sjögren syndrome, including the following:

1. Musculoskeletal—arthralgias (60%) and myalgias (25%), but rarely frank arthritis, unless the syndrome occurs in the setting of RA or SLE
2. Raynaud phenomenon—seen in 30% to 40% of patients with systemic manifestations
3. Pulmonary—seen in 5% to 10% of patients and include xerotrachea, lymphocytic interstitial pneumonitis, and pseudolymphoma
4. Gastrointestinal—seen in 10% of patients and include dysphagia, atrophic gastritis, and pancreatitis
5. Renal—seen in 10% to 15% of patients and generally consists of interstitial nephritis resulting in renal tubular defects; rarely, immune-complex-mediated glomerulonephritis
6. Nervous system—seen in 5% to 10% of patients and include peripheral neuropathies, cranial neuropathies, and diffuse CNS manifestations
7. Vasculitis—seen in 5% to 10% of patients with systemic manifestations; usually a leukocytoclastic vasculitis involving the skin and bowel. Other organ systems may also be involved. Vasculitis is often associated with elevated serum IgM and monoclonal IgM (especially in Caucasian patients), high titer RF, cryoglobulins, and positive anti-Ro antibodies.
8. Hematologic—leukopenia (20%), lymphadenopathy/splenomegaly (15% to 20%), malignant lymphoma (5% to 8%; generally derived from B-lymphocytes)

Treatment
The treatment of Sjögren syndrome depends upon the organ manifestations present. As with other autoimmune disorders, meticulous general medical and surgical care is essential. Because of the high incidence of non-Hodgkin lymphoma in primary Sjögren syndrome, lymphadenopathy and salivary gland enlargement must be evaluated thoroughly.

  A. Xerophthalmia
   1. No antiinflammatory or immunosuppressive drugs have demonstrated utility.
   2. Artificial tears are used during the day every 1 to 3 hours, and lubricating ointments are used at night.
   3. Plugging the nasolacrimal ducts with collagen to retain tears in the eyes can be used to treat patients with existing but diminished tearing.
  B. Xerostomia—no antiinflammatory or immunosuppressive drugs have demonstrated utility

1. Artificial saliva preparations are useful in some patients, but are not tolerated by most.
    a. Saliva substitutes are based upon carboxymethylcellulose, animal mucins, polyethylenoxide, linseed polysaccharide, polyacrylic acid, and/or xanthan gum.
    b. Highly mucoadhesive polymers, such as polyacrylic acid, are recommended in patients with low salivary flow rates.
    c. Saliva substitutes with moderate mucoadhesive properties and high elastic properties, such as xanthan gum, are recommended for patients with residual salivary flow.
2. Agents that stimulate flow of saliva have been helpful in some patients.
    a. Pilocarpine (5 to 10 mg t.i.d.) is a cholinergic agonist and is beneficial in many patients. Side effects, including sweating, chills, dizziness, rhinitis, and asthenia, often complicate its use. Slow-release preparations are better tolerated.
    b. Anethole trithione (25 mg t.i.d.) stimulates salivary gland secretions by unknown mechanisms and is better tolerated than pilocarpine. It acts synergistically with pilocarpine.
3. Oral hygiene must be strictly maintained. Foods containing sugars should be restricted. Teeth should be cleaned twice daily. Fluoride and possibly chlorhexidine rinses should be done weekly.
4. Oral candidiasis occurs frequently and can be treated with topical miconazole gel (2% gel applied q.i.d.), amphotericin B lozenges (10 mg q.i.d.), or oral fluconazole (100 to 400 mg q.d.).

C. Arthralgias and arthritis—usually adequately treated with NSAIDs. In refractory patients, hydroxychloroquine (200 mg q.d. to b.i.d.) may be useful.

D. Raynaud phenomenon—managed in the same manner as SLE (see pages 299–300).

E. Lymphocytic interstitial pneumonitis—no controlled trials are available to dictate therapy. This pneumonitis is generally managed with prednisone in low to moderate doses, depending on the degree of involvement; azathioprine, cyclosporine, and cyclophosphamide have all been utilized in refractory cases.

F. Gastrointestinal—managed symptomatically

G. Renal—rarely requires therapy; renal tubular acidosis may require sodium bicarbonate therapy (0.5 to 2 mmol per kg in four divided doses daily). Proliferative glomerulonephritis is generally managed in the same manner as proliferative glomerulonephritis in SLE (see Renal Disease on page 300).

H. Nervous system—peripheral and cranial nerve neuropathies are treated with corticosteroids in moderate to high doses initially (prednisone 40 to 60 mg q.d.) and then lower doses as tolerated. Refractory cases may require azathioprine or cyclophosphamide.

I. Systemic vasculitis—corticosteroids in moderate to high doses, often in combination with cyclophosphamide. Patients with predominantly IgM hypergammaglobulinemia may be treated with cyclophosphamide 750 mg/ M^2/month for 12 to 18 doses. Patients with predominantly IgG hypergammaglobulinemia should probably receive daily cyclophosphamide 1 to 2 mg per kg used to maintain the total WBC between 3,000 and 4,000 per mL for 12 to 18 months. Vasculitis restricted to the skin does not require therapy, but can be treated with hydroxychloroquine (200 mg q.d. to b.i.d.) for cosmetic reasons.

J. Hematologic—leukopenia generally does not require therapy. Lymphoma is treated by standard lymphoma protocols depending upon the type and distribution of the tumor.

XIV. Inflammatory myopathies
    The adult inflammatory myopathies consist of polymyositis (PM), DM, and inclusion-body myositis. In children, juvenile DM is most frequent, with PM occurring rarely. Each disorder has muscle weakness as a major symptom. Other disorders that may cause muscle weakness must be excluded: neuromuscular

disorders, such as genetic muscular dystrophies, Guillain-Barré syndrome, autoimmune polyneuropathies, porphyria, myasthenia gravis, Eaton-Lambert syndrome, myotonic dystrophies, and various familial periodic paralyses; endocrine and electrolyte disorders, such as hypokalemia, hyponatremia, hypomagnesemia, hypercalcemia, hypocalcemia, hypothyroidism, hyperthyroidism, Cushing syndrome, and Addison disease; metabolic myopathies, such as phosphofructokinase deficiency, acid maltase deficiency, and McArdle disease; disorders of lipid metabolism, such as carnitine deficiency and carnitine palmitoyl transferase deficiency; disorders of purine metabolism, such as myoadenylate deaminase deficiency; mitochondrial myopathies; toxic myopathies, such as those secondary to alcohol, hydroxychloroquine, cocaine, corticosteroids, penicillamine, 3-hydroxy-3-methylglutaryl coenzyme A (HMG CoA) reductase inhibitors, such as lovastatin, and zidovudine; infections, such as coxsackieviruses, influenza viruses, HIV, *Clostridium*, toxoplasmosis, trichinosis, cysticercosis; vasculitides, such as polyarteritis nodosa and giant cell arteritis (GCA); eosinophilia–myalgia syndrome; and various paraneoplastic syndromes. In children, the heritable muscular dystrophies and neuropathies are the predominant differential diagnoses.

A. PM is an inflammatory disease of skeletal muscle.

    1. Clinically, PM occurs predominantly in the fourth and fifth decades of life, has a female predominance, has an insidious onset over weeks to months, and results in various degrees of symmetrical limb–girdle muscle weakness. Associated symptoms may include fatigue, myalgia (which is often not severe), dysphagia, arthralgia, and cough or dyspnea, resulting from respiratory muscle involvement, pulmonary fibrosis, and occasionally myocarditis with CHF. Rarely, patients with acute myositis can develop renal failure from myoglobinuria.

    2. Electromyography (EMG) studies reveal nonspecific myopathic changes, including short, small, low-amplitude polyphasic motor unit potentials, fibrillation potentials, and high-frequency repetitive discharges.

    3. Laboratory studies reveal elevations in muscle-associated enzymes, creatine kinase, aldolase, lactate dehydrogenase (LDH) and transaminases (ALT/serum glutamate pyruvate transaminase [SGPT] and AST/serum glutamate oxaloacetate transaminase [SGOT]). Patients with interstitial pneumonitis, Raynaud phenomenon, and nonerosive arthritis often have antibodies to various transfer RNA (tRNA) synthetases, including Jo-1 (anti-histidyl tRNA synthetase). Patients with antibodies to signal recognition particle (SRP; not commercially available) have PM of very acute onset with profound weakness and often cardiac involvement; their disease often starts in the fall and they have a poor response to therapy. Various autoantibodies are seen with myositis/scleroderma overlap syndromes, including anti-PM Scl, anti-Ku, and anti-nRNP.

    4. Muscle biopsy reveals focal endomysial infiltration by mononuclear cells, especially CD8[+] T lymphocytes.

B. DM is an inflammatory disease of skeletal muscle associated with a photosensitive skin rash in the heliotrope (sun seeking) distribution, typically involving the eyelids, and a scaly dermatitis over the metacarpophalangeal and proximal interphalangeal joins of the hands (Gottron papules). Gottron sign may also involve the extensor surfaces of the knees, elbows, and medial malleoli. A maculopapular rash can involve the face, neck, and upper torso. Rarely, the skin rash can occur in the absence of the muscle disease, amyotrophic DM.

    1. Clinically, DM occurs predominantly in the fourth and fifth decades of life, has a female predominance, and exhibits a subacute to acute onset of symmetrical limb–girdle muscle weakness with characteristic skin rashes. It can be associated with fatigue, myalgias, dysphagia, and dyspnea due to respiratory muscle involvement and/or myocarditis. Five percent to 10% of patients have an associated malignancy that may precede, follow, or occur concurrently with the onset of DM. The most common malignancy is ovarian carcinoma, although hematologic, gastro-intestinal, nasopharyngeal, bladder, testicular, breast, lung, and skin (malignant melanoma) tumors have also been seen.

2. Electromyography in DM is indistinguishable from that in PM.

3. Laboratory studies reveal elevations in muscle-associated enzymes, creatine kinase, aldolase, LDH and transaminases (ALT/SGPT and AST/SGOT). Patients with anti-Mi-2 antibodies (not commercially available) have a syndrome of mild, acute-onset DM that is exquisitely sensitive to therapy. Rarely, patients may have antibodies to nRNP and symptoms overlap with SLE and/or scleroderma.

4. Muscle biopsy in DM is quite distinct from that in PM. Mononuclear cells, especially CD4+ T lymphocytes, are seen in a perivascular and interstitial distribution. Perifascicular myofiber atrophy is noted. Occasionally frank vasculitis is present, although this is more common in children than adults.

C. Inclusion-body myositis is a family of related muscle diseases characterized by vacuoles in the muscle fibers containing accumulations of β-amyloid precursor protein (β-APP), phosphorylated τ, and presenilin-1, all proteins that are also associated with Alzheimer disease. Both sporadic and hereditary forms of the disease have been characterized.

1. Sporadic inclusion-body myositis is a disease occurring predominantly in men over the age of 50 years, manifest by a slowly progressive course of both proximal and distal muscle weakness. Patients frequently develop respiratory muscle weakness and dysphagia. It is generally not associated with other systemic diseases, but may be seen with various malignancies. In addition to the characteristic vacuoles, muscle biopsies reveal varying degrees of mononuclear cell inflammation, with predominantly CD8+ T lymphocytes and macrophages.

2. Hereditary inclusion-body myopathies are generally distal as well as proximal myopathies. The conditions tend to onset in the third decade of life. Muscle biopsies generally do not reveal inflammatory cell infiltrates.

   a. The quadriceps-spared form maps to chromosome 9p1-q1 and occurs in Iranian Jews, Afghani Jews, Indians, Japanese, and Mexicans.

   b. The quadriceps-not-spared form occurs predominantly in French-Canadians and frequently includes CNS abnormalities.

   c. The autosomal dominant form has been seen in families of Swedish, Finnish, and Mexican descent.

D. Juvenile dermatomyositis

1. Definition. Juvenile dermatomyositis (JDM) is an inflammatory disease of skin and skeletal muscle with onset prior to the 16th birthday. It occurs in 1 in 10 million children, most commonly affecting school-aged children. As in adults, the diagnosis is made according to the criteria of Bohan and Peter, with four criteria indicative of probable JDM and five indicative of definite JDM.

   a. Symmetrical, proximal muscle weakness

   b. Abnormal levels of muscle-derived enzymes in serum (creatine kinase, aldolase, AST, ALT, LDH, and pyruvate kinase)

   c. Findings of myopathy on EMG (as described above for adult PM and DM)

   d. Muscle biopsy demonstrating endothelial swelling of small vessels in striated muscle with patchy atrophy of both types I and II muscle fibers. Compared to the biopsy findings in adult disease, JDM biopsies often demonstrate impressive lymphocytic vasculitis of small vessels in skeletal muscle. Immunofluorescence shows deposition of C5-9 complement proteins.

   e. Characteristic skin findings:

      (1) Periorbital edema

      (2) Heliotrope rash—eyelids, forehead, bridge of nose, malar eminences, chin; often violaceous

        (3) Eyelid telangiectasia

        (4) Photosensitivity—flares of myositis also may be triggered by sun

        (5) Gottron papules

        (6) Generalized macular rash—may have brawny nonpitting edema of extensor surfaces

        (7) Periungual telangiectasia—poor circulation may produce paronychia

        (8) Raynaud phenomenon

        (9) Livedo reticularis

        (10) Ischemic ulceration of fingertips, pressure points, sometimes eyelids

  2. Systemic manifestations—systemic vasculitis is far more common in JDM than in adult DM, accounting for significant morbidity and mortality

    a. Gastrointestinal tract—intestinal vasculitis leading to bowel edema and malabsorption (including poor absorption of medication), obstruction, ulceration, hemorrhage and perforation occurs in approximately 10% of children. Pneumatosis intestinalis may be seen. Pain and diarrhea are the most common gastrointestinal (GI) symptoms.

    b. Respiratory system—involvement of respiratory muscles may lead to hypoventilation with diminished forced vital capacity (FVC), hypercarbia, and hypoxemia. Less commonly (less than 10%), pulmonary vasculitis may lead to pulmonary infiltrates, diffusion defects, or pulmonary hemorrhage that can be fatal. Less vigorous vasculitis of the lung may produce interstitial fibrosis with ground-glass appearance on lung CT or x-ray.

    c. Cardiac disease—vasculitis of the myocardium may produce decreased ejection fraction with CHF, arrhythmias from vasculitis of the conduction system, or pericarditis. It is uncommon, occurring in fewer than 5% of patients, and is usually steroid responsive. If detected late, however, permanent damage to myocardium and conduction system may occur.

    d. Renal—steroid-sensitive nephritis with hematuria and proteinuria occurs uncommonly.

    e. Central nervous system—encephalopathy is rare. Ocular involvement with cotton wool spots and flame hemorrhages may be seen.

    f. Calcinosis—chronic vasculitis of muscle, skin, and subcutaneous fat (panniculitis) may produce saponification, leading to deposition of calcium in hypoperfused fatty tissues. Large nodules may form, which slowly are extruded through the skin, often leading to fistulous tracts that are prone to secondary infection and scarring. These may be disfiguring and impair gross motor function.

E. Treatment

  1. The treatment of PM and DM is essentially the same. Once the diagnosis has been firmly established, patients are started taking corticosteroids in high doses. Prednisone is given in a single daily dose of 60 to 100 mg. Calcium, bisphosphonates, and/or calcitonin or vitamin D are given to limit steroid-induced osteoporosis. After 1 month, patients will fall into one of two categories. (i) Steroid responders: These patients show improvement in muscle strength and decrease in muscle enzymes; for this group the prednisone is slowly tapered to maintain daily dosing for at least 12 months. After that time, patients are tapered to alternate day dosing schedules. Around 18 months after the onset of the disease, the prednisone dose should be in the range of 20 mg every other day, and a decision regarding a slow taper to no steroid medication can be made. (ii) Steroid nonresponders: These patients maintain significant muscle weakness despite prednisone 100 mg daily. An additional immunosuppressive agent is added, of which methotrexate

10 to 20 mg weekly along with daily folic acid 1 to 2 mg daily and aza-thioprine 100 to 200 mg daily are the most commonly used medica-tions. Less experience exists with cyclophosphamide, because of its greater toxicities, and mycophenolate mofetil. Cyclosporine A and FK506 have been used rarely with unclear efficacy. With the addition of a more potent immunosuppressive agent, corticosteroids are tapered to an alternate-day schedule more rapidly.

2. The treatment of the inclusion-body myositis syndromes is unknown. Patients may show limited benefit from moderate to high doses of corticosteroids, but it is unclear whether the minimal benefit achieved is worth the toxicity of the corticosteroids. Limited benefit from intra-venous immunoglobulin has been reported in a poorly controlled trial. No other treatment alternatives have shown significant promise.

3. The treatment of JDM has changed significantly during the past decade. Increasing evidence indicates that aggressive control of the vasculitic na-ture of the disease limits mortality and disability from complications, in-cluding permanent muscle atrophy, persistent myositis, calcinosis, and major organ system involvement.

   a. Mild disease may be successfully treated with oral corticosteroids in doses of 1 to 2 mg/kg/day prednisone or equivalent for up to 6 months, with tapering over an additional 12 to 18 months, em-ploying alternate-day regimens after 6 months. Many pediatric rheumatologists prefer intravenous pulse corticosteroid with rapid taper of oral steroid (see the section immediately following).

   b. Moderate disease is often treated with i.v. pulses of corticosteroids, usually starting with an induction phase using 30 mg/kg/day (to a maximum of 1 g per dose) three times over 3 to 5 days until enzymes return to normal, and strength improves. Pulses are repeated once or twice weekly until strength is near normal, and oral prednisone is below 0.25 mg/kg/day, then the frequency of infusions are de-creased over 1 to 2 years as prednisone is stopped, until all signs of disease are absent.

   c. Severe or steroid-resistant disease is treated with pulse steroid and methotrexate at doses ranging from 10 mg/M^2/week orally to 1 mg/kg/week i.v. or s.c. Cyclosporine at 2 to 4 mg/kg/day may be required in resistant disease, and some patients with more severe disease have required cyclophosphamide or other cytotoxic therapies.

XV. Overlap syndromes and undifferentiated connective tissue diseases
The concept of overlap syndromes and undifferentiated connective tissue dis-eases comes from the realization that many patients have features of one or more autoimmune ("connective tissue") diseases without meeting full criteria for any particular autoimmune disease, such as SLE or scleroderma. "Overlap syndromes" have supplanted an early syndrome, "mixed connective tissue dis-ease," because of the panoply of different overlaps that can occur.

The most common overlap syndromes involve Sjögren syndrome along with manifestations of some other systemic rheumatic disease, such as RA, SLE, scleroderma, PM, or primary biliary cirrhosis. Other overlap syndromes in-volve features of RA with SLE, scleroderma with SLE and PM, and sclero-derma with primary biliary cirrhosis. Patients will generally have a positive ANA, and frequently antibodies to nRNP. RFs may also be detectable. In some cases, more disease-selective autoantibodies, such as anti-Sm (SLE), anti-topoisomerase I (scleroderma), and anti-Jo-1 (PM) may be present. Over time, many patients will remain with their presenting clinical manifestations, whereas others may develop problems characteristic of a single autoimmune disease, such as SLE or scleroderma.

Patients with undifferentiated connective tissue diseases have serologies consistent with autoimmune disease, such as ANA and anti-nRNP, but only one or two clinical manifestations suggestive of an autoimmune disease, such as pleuropericarditis, interstitial pneumonitis, nondestructive polyarthritis, anemia, or Raynaud phenomenon. Many of these patients will never progress to a more complete systemic autoimmune disease, but some will eventually meet sufficient criteria for the diagnosis of SLE, RA, scleroderma, or PM/DM.

The management of patients with overlap syndromes and undifferentiated connective tissue diseases involves the same principles as the management of other systemic autoimmune diseases. First, do not give patients disease labels until they meet criteria. More importantly, do not treat patients based on their labels. Second, each patient should be managed with the least-toxic therapy available to control the existing clinical manifestations. For example, a patients with a positive ANA, mild hypergammaglobulinemia, and a nondestructive polyarthritis, whose x-rays did not show any periarticular osteopenia or erosions, and whose workup did not reveal an infectious or other cause for the polyarthritis, would be treated initially with hydroxychloroquine, because hydroxychloroquine is useful for the same problem in the setting of SLE, and is relatively benign. Finally, each patient should be given meticulous medical and surgical care. Each clinical problem should be evaluated with a complete differential diagnosis, including infectious, drug-related and other causes, as well as consideration of the problem as part of a more generalized autoimmune disease. Patients must be followed closely for the early detection of new problems as they arise.

XVI. Primary antiphospholipid antibody syndrome

The primary antiphospholipid antibody syndrome, or Hughes syndrome, is a group of disorders characterized by antibodies reacting to phospholipids, generally in association with various plasma proteins. The most common antibodies associated with clinical symptoms are antibodies to phosphatidyl serine and B2 glycoprotein 1, the protein that binds phosphatidyl serine, as well as many other lipids. Nonetheless, clinically relevant disease can be seen with antibodies to cardiolipin, phosphatidylcholine, phosphatidylinositol, phosphatidic acid, and phosphatidylethanolamine. Phosphatidylethanolamine is generally associated with high and low molecular weight kininogens, factor XI, and prekallikrein, rather than β_2 glycoprotein 1. IgG antibodies are generally pathogenic, although significant disease can also be seen with IgA or even IgM antiphospholipid antibodies occurring alone. Antiphospholipid antibodies are also seen frequently in association with SLE (15% to 40%). They were originally identified as the false-positive VDRL in SLE and as the "lupus anticoagulant." They can be seen less frequently with other autoimmune diseases, and transiently after various infections, including viral, bacterial, and fungal infections. In some instances, primary phospholipid antibody syndrome may be familial, although the mechanism of inheritance is currently unknown.

The clinical features of primary antiphospholipid antibody syndrome include:

1. Arterial occlusion—myocardial infarction, stroke, bowel ischemia, extremity gangrene, Addison disease, femoral head necrosis, thrombotic microangiopathy kidney, pulmonary hypertension, and multisystem thrombosis syndrome
2. Venous occlusion—peripheral, renal vein thrombosis, Budd-Chiari syndrome
3. Recurrent fetal loss—generally in the late second and third trimesters
4. Thrombocytopenia
5. Coombs-positive hemolytic anemia
6. Livedo reticularis with or without Raynaud phenomenon
7. Neurologic manifestations—migraine headaches, strokes, multiinfarct dementia, epilepsy, movement disorders, transverse myelopathy
8. Valvular heart disease—30% to 40% of patients have some valvular abnormalities that include valve degeneration and superimposed thrombus

Causes of death in primary phospholipid antibody syndrome include cardiac arrhythmias, strokes, liver failure, renal failure, pulmonary hypertension and cerebrovascular strokes. In the Italian registry, patients with antiphospholipid antibody syndrome had a high incidence of non-Hodgkin lymphoma.

Treatment of antiphospholipid antibody syndrome depends upon the clinical manifestations.

Patients who have never had thrombosis, but have Raynaud phenomenon, migraine headaches, or other symptoms suggestive of vascular spasm should receive aspirin 81 mg q.d., or clopidogrel (Plavix) 75 mg q.d., if they are aspirin sensitive. Patients should limit cold exposure and avoiding vasoconstrictive agents, such as tobacco/nicotine, decongestants, and β-adrenergic blocking agents. They should receive vasodilators, as needed, to eliminate their vaso-constrictive symptoms. These include calcium channel blockers (i.e., nifedipine, 10 to 20 mg t.i.d.), α_1-adrenergic receptor antagonists (i.e., doxazosin, 2 to 4 mg b.i.d.), and nitrates (i.e., isosorbide mononitrate 30 mg q.d. to q.i.d.). Severe vascular spasm in cerebral or peripheral vessels can be managed with intra-venous PGE_1 (5 to 15 ng/kg/min) and in the pulmonary vasculature with the prostacyclin analog epoprostenol (Flolan, 5 to 15 ng/kg/min).

Patients who have had venous or arterial thromboses require anticoagulation for life. Coumadin may be used. The international normalized ratio (INR) must be maintained in the 3 to 4 range for efficacy. In some patients, despite maintaining the INR in this range, thromboses continue to occur. This may be secondary to interference from the antiphospholipid antibodies with the INR test, so that the true level of anticoagulation is not known, or other factors may limit the efficacy of the drug. In that case, low molecular weight heparin is utilized. If enoxaparin is utilized, the starting dose is 1 mg per kg b.i.d. Higher doses may be required for patients who fail to respond to this dose.

Patients with thrombocytopenia are generally treated with corticosteroids, in the lowest effective dose. Severe thrombocytopenia may require high, split doses of corticosteroids (i.e., prednisone 60 mg b.i.d.), and/or the addition of intra-venous Ig (i.e., sandoglobulin 0.4 to 1.0 g per kg infusion per day times 1 to 3). On the basis of the experience with ITP, anti-D (i.e., anti-rho [D] 50 μg per kg single i.v. infusion), vinblastine, danazol, or splenectomy could also be tried if necessary. Hemolytic anemia, while rare in this disorder, may be treated in a similar manner.

Patients with "catastrophic" antiphospholipid antibody syndrome, in which diffuse thrombosis leads to multiorgan failure and often severe thrombocytope-nia, are treated with low molecular weight heparin, high, split-dose cortico-steroids, and IVIg. Plasmapheresis has been recommended, although its efficacy has never been tested.

Patients with recurrent fetal loss wishing to become pregnant are treated with aspirin 81 mg q.d. and low molecular weight heparin, which may be de-layed until the second trimester of pregnancy. Corticosteroids are generally not beneficial.

XVII. Primary vasculitides

The term "vasculitis" means simply inflammation of blood vessels. The most common vasculitides are due to known causes, drugs, and various infections. In addition, various other disorders including autoimmune diseases, such as SLE and Sjögren syndrome, and malignancies, such as chronic lymphocytic leukemia and multiple myeloma, are frequently associated with secondary forms of vasculitis. The diagnosis of a primary vasculitis requires a consistent clinical picture, histologic demonstration of inflammatory cells infiltrating blood vessel walls, and exclusion of all primary causes. No laboratory tests can be used alone to make a diagnosis of a primary vasculitis, although the pres-ence of certain serological markers, such as antibodies to proteinase 3 (cyto-plasmic antineutrophil cytoplasmic antibody [C-ANCA]), can be confirmatory for the diagnosis. The treatment of a vasculitis caused by a reaction to a drug is to stop the drug, whereas the management of vasculitis caused by an infec-tion is to treat the infection. The disorders discussed in this section are vas-culitides in which the etiologic agent is unknown.

A number of disorders can closely mimic primary vasculitides, but in fact be secondary to noninflammatory vascular compromise. These include athero-embolism, ergotism, neurofibromatosis, Ehlers-Danlos syndrome type IV, myxoma embolism, idiopathic arterial calcification, primary phospholipid antibody syndrome, and primary malignancies of blood vessels, such as angioendotheliomatosis. Atheroembolism is seen most commonly in the setting of patients with diffuse atherosclerosis who undergo invasive angiographic studies. The resulting cholesterol emboli can travel to any vascular beds, although the lower extremities are most commonly involved. Patients often develop livedo reticularis and may have low-grade fevers and areas of cyanosis. It is common for ESR to be elevated. Treatment with heparin may be helpful. Corticosteroids are generally avoided. Ergotamine, like phentolamine and pseudoephedrine, is a potent vasoconstrictor and can induce significant vascular compromise, especially in patients with Raynaud phenomenon or other predisposing factors for vascular spasm. The management of ergotism is to stop the drug and use vasodilating drugs if necessary. Neurofibromatosis, Ehlers-Danlos type IV, and Marfan syndrome all involve abnormalities of collagen that lead to weakening of vessel walls. Aneurysms may occur in blood vessels subjected to high pressures. Vascular rupture may cause major organ damage. The management consists of keeping the blood pressure low, anti-coagulation for areas of poor blood flow, and occasionally surgical correction of aneurysmal dilations. As noted above, primary antiphospholipid antibody syndrome leads to vascular compromise by causing vascular spasm, thromboses, and embolization from abnormal heart valves. The management consists of vasodilators and anticoagulation, not corticosteroids and other immunosuppressive agents, unless significant thrombocytopenia and/or hemolytic anemia are present. Atrial myxoma is a malignancy starting in the heart that metastasizes through the blood vessels, while malignant angioendotheliomatosis is a tumor of blood vessels. Both of these malignancies can cause vascular compromise mimicking small- and medium-sized vessel vasculitides. The management of these malignancies is largely surgical.

Vasculitides are classified according to the size of the blood vessels involved, as well as by specific syndromes with characteristic patterns of organ involvement. Vasculitides involving predominantly large vessels include GCA and Takayasu arteritis. Small- and medium-sized vessels are involved in polyarteritis nodosa, Churg-Strauss syndrome (CSS), microscopic polyarteritis (MPA), Kawasaki disease, Wegener granulomatosis, relapsing polychondritis, Behçet syndrome, Goodpasture disease (GD), HSP, thromboangiitis obliterans, Cogan syndrome, erythema elevatum diutinum (EED), and primary angiitis of the CNS.

A. Giant cell arteritis

GCA or temporal arteritis is a disorder that usually initiates in the sixth or seventh decades of life with a gradual onset. It starts with constitutional symptoms, raising the spectrum of a wide variety of diseases including chronic infections and malignancies. It involves predominantly the external branches of the carotid arteries, although all large vessels may be involved, especially the subclavian, axillary, and renal arteries. It is usually identified when temporal tenderness and unilateral more often than bilateral severe headaches dominate the clinical picture. Rarely, visual symptoms, especially transient and/or permanent partial visual loss can be the presenting manifestation. The existence of visual loss constitutes a medical emergency that must be treated immediately with high-dose corticosteroids. Some improvement in vision is generally the norm after treatment, although partial visual deficits may remain.

1. The ACR criteria to distinguish giant cell arteritis from other types of vasculitis are:
   a. Age of onset greater than 50 years
   b. New headache—generally localized pain
   c. Temporal artery abnormality—temporal artery is tender to touch and may exhibit decreased pulsation
   d. Elevated ESR
   e. Abnormal temporal artery biopsy—vasculitis with predominance of mononuclear cells; multinucleated giant cells are seen in 20% of biopsies

2. Additional clinical symptoms include:
   a. Anorexia, weight loss—seen in 50% to 60% of patients
   b. Fatigue, weakness—seen in 40% to 50% of patients
   c. Low-grade fevers—seen in 30% to 40% of patients
   d. Polymyalgia rheumatica—aching and morning stiffness lasting at least 30 minutes in the proximal portions of the extremities and torso; seen in about 50% of patients
   e. Jaw claudication—seen in 40% to 50% of patients; due to involvement of the submandibular artery
   f. Transient or permanent visual symptoms—seen in 15% of patients; seen as an optic neuritis with or without hemorrhages. Visual symptoms are due to involvement of the ophthalmic or posterior ciliary arteries.
   g. Dysphagia/tongue claudication—seen in 5% to 10% of patients
   h. Extremity claudication—5% to 10% of patients; subclavian and axillary artery involvement is common
   i. Peripheral synovitis or tenosynovitis—20% to 25% of patients; may have distal extremity swelling. This condition occasionally mimics RA.
   j. Neurologic manifestations—5% to 10% of patients; include peripheral neuropathies, and cerebral ischemic events secondary to extracranial involvement of the vertebral and carotid arteries. Primary intracranial vascular involvement is very unusual.
   k. Cardiac involvement—rare; includes pericarditis, coronary artery vasculitis, and aortic dissection
   l. Hearing impairment, vertigo, nystagmus (rare)
   m. Renal involvement—rare; usually not clinically significant, although microscopic hematuria can be seen
3. Diagnosis is made by a consistent clinical picture, generally elevated ESR (often in range of 100 mm per hour) and positive temporal artery biopsy.
   a. Adequate tissue must be obtained (15 mm section) for the biopsy. In some cases bilateral biopsies are necessary before a diagnosis is made.
   b. Fluorescein angiography can be used as an adjunct to make the diagnosis. Patients demonstrate delayed fluorescein dye appearance and choroidal filling.
4. Treatment
   a. Initial therapy consists of single daily dose corticosteroids, such as prednisone 1 to 2 mg per kg q.d.
   b. After 4 weeks, a gradual steroid taper can be initiated, assuming that clinical symptoms improve and ESR decreases significantly.
   c. Patients usually require daily steroids for 1 to 2 years.
   d. It is very unusual for patients to require a second agent, such as methotrexate or cyclophosphamide, to control their disease.
   e. Because long-term corticosteroids are utilized, steps must be taken to prevent steroid-induced osteoporosis. These include daily calcium intake of 1500 mg, a bisphosphonate (i.e., alendronate 10 mg q.d. or 70 mg every week) or calcitonin (200 µg nasal spray q.d.), and vitamin D (50,000 U three times per week or 800 U daily if the 24-hour urinary calcium is less than 150 mg) or thiazide (50 mg q.d. if the 24-hour urinary calcium is greater than 300 mg).
B. Takayasu arteritis
   Takayasu arteritis is a vasculitis involving predominantly the aorta and the large vessels branching from it. It is the most common cause of renovascular hypertension in Asia, especially Japan and India. It is rare in North America. The disease is seen mostly in women (female-to-male ratio is 9:1) in the second and third decade of life. It generally begins with constitutional symptoms that may be present for several months before symptoms

secondary to vascular compromise ensue. Pathologically, it produces a granulomatous vasculitis involving the intima, media, and adventitia of the great vessels. It must be distinguished from syphilitic aortitis, and other infectious arteritides of the great vessels, which involves primarily the vasa vasorum of the aorta, rather than the aorta itself. The natural course of the disease is the formation of ectatic and stenotic vessels, even after inflammation has been completely controlled. Surgical correction of abnormal vessels is inevitably required. Medical therapy alone is almost never adequate.

1. The following ACR criteria to distinguish Takayasu arteritis from other forms of vasculitis:
   a. Age at disease onset less than 40 years
   b. Claudication of extremities—generally worse in the upper extremities
   c. Decreased brachial artery pressure—the pressure may be decreased in one or both brachial arteries
   d. Blood pressure difference greater than 10 mm Hg in systolic blood pressure between the two arms
   e. Bruits over the subclavian arteries and/or aorta
   f. Arteriographic abnormalities—these include narrowing, occlusion or ectasia of the aorta, its primary branches, and/or the large arteries in the proximal upper and lower extremities; changes are generally focal and segmental

2. Additional clinical findings include:
   a. Anorexia, weight loss—seen in 30% of patients
   b. Low-grade fever—seen in 30% of patients
   c. Myalgias/arthralgias—seen in 50% of patients
   d. Synovitis—seen in 25% of patients; often large joint and asymmetric; 1% to 2% have an inflammatory arthritis consistent with RA
   e. Headache—seen in 50% to 75% of patients; may be diffuse or migrainous in character
   f. Hypertension—seen in 10% to 60% of patients
   g. Syncope/postural dizziness—seen in 30% to 40% of patients
   h. Ischemic chest pain—seen in 20% to 45% of patients
   i. Visual blurring or deficit—seen in 15% of patients; secondary to ischemic retinopathy
   j. Skin involvement—seen in 2% to 15% of patients; includes erythema nodosum, pyoderma gangrenosum, livedo reticularis, small vessel granulomatous vasculitis, and panniculitis
   k. Pleuritic chest pains and/or dyspnea—seen in 10% to 60% of patients; secondary to pulmonary arterial involvement
   l. Glomerulonephritis—seen in 1% to 5% of patients
   m. Inflammatory myocarditis—seen in 5% to 50% of patients; may result in chronic cardiomyopathy
   n. Other autoimmune diseases, including autoimmune hepatitis, inflammatory bowel disease, Sjögren syndrome—seen in 1% to 2% of patients

3. Classification of subtypes of Takayasu arteritis used in Asian surgical literature:
   a. Type I—involvement of aorta alone
   b. Type II—involvement of aortic arch and its branches
   c. Type III—involvement of predominantly the abdominal aorta and renal arteries
   d. Type IV—combination of type II and type III

4. Treatment
   a. Medical—medical therapy is rarely definitive in Takayasu arteritis, but several measures can be used to improve patients symptomatically:
      (1) Corticosteroids—prednisone is used in the range of 30 to 60 mg q.d. for at least 1 month; a slow taper, including use of alter-

nate day dosing, is then initiated as tolerated. The expected outcome is resolution of constitutional symptoms, musculoskeletal symptoms, and lowering of the ESR. These benefits of corticosteroids must be weighed against their side effects; in this case in particular, their inhibition of wound healing. If surgery is imminent, corticosteroids may have to be avoided or used only for a very short period of time.

(2) As many as 30% to 50% of patients will not respond to corticosteroids alone, especially in North America. Both cyclophosphamide (1 to 2 mg/kg/day used to maintain a total WBC 3,000 to 4,000 per mL) and methotrexate (10 to 20 mg weekly) have been used in this setting. The risk–benefit ratio of these therapies is unknown in this disease.

(3) NSAIDs can be used for musculoskeletal complaints.

(4) Aspirin 81 mg q.d. or clopidogrel 75 mg q.d. should be utilized to prevent thrombosis because of vast areas of abnormal blood flow. In the setting of severe CHF or cerebrovascular compromise, full-dose anticoagulation with heparin or warfarin may have to be considered.

(5) Hypertension and CHF must be controlled with vasodilators and diuretics as needed; agents causing vasoconstriction should be avoided.

b. Surgical—most patients with Takayasu arteritis will eventually require surgical therapy. The optimal timing for surgical therapy is when inflammation has been controlled. Angioplasty has generally not been helpful because of the nature of the inflammation, but can be used as a temporizing measure. The surgical techniques utilized are beyond the scope of this manual, but generally involve vascular bypass and/or grafting. The indications for surgery include:

(1) Renovascular hypertension

(2) Severe extremity ischemia

(3) Cerebrovascular insufficiency

(4) Dilated ascending aorta, especially if aortic insufficiency is present

(5) Aortic aneurysms

C. Classical polyarteritis nodosa

Classic polyarteritis nodosa (PAN) is a disease of medium-sized muscular arteries that involves most major organs except the lungs. It only rarely involves the CNS primarily, although hypertension and secondary infection, often related to therapy, may result in CNS injury. The disease has a slight male predominance and tends to occur in the fourth and fifth decades of life. It may have an acute or subacute presentation, with the first clinical manifestation being abdominal pains or peripheral neuropathy. Occasionally, bowel perforation is the presenting manifestation. The histopathology consists of neutrophilic infiltration of the intima and media of medium-sized muscular arteries, allowing the formation of aneurysms involving the adventitia. This creates the classic "berry aneurysms" identified by angiography in the hepatic, celiac, and renal circulation of patients with PAN. The venous system is not primarily involved. In some cases, PAN is caused by hepatitis B. The disease occurs in the acute stages of hepatitis B, when viral antigenemia is at the highest levels, but only in susceptible ethnic populations, such as the Alaskan Eskimos. Rapid diagnosis and therapy is essential.

1. The ACR criteria to distinguish PAN from other forms of vasculitis include:

a. Weight loss greater than 4 kg—this is due to abdominal involvement that occurs in more than 50% of patients. Acute cholecystitis occurs in 15% of patients and bowel rupture in 5% to 15% of patients.

    b. Livedo reticularis—acute livedo reticularis suggests ischemia occurring at the level of arterioles. Chronic livedo reticularis may be seen with venous or lymphatic obstruction. Livedo reticularis occurs only in 10% to 15% of patients with PAN. The most common skin lesion in PAN is palpable purpura from leukocytoclastic vasculitis; urticaria and nodular lesions can also be seen. A rare form of PAN, cutaneous PAN, involves only the skin.

    c. Testicular pain—occurs in only about 5% of patients with PAN, although autopsy studies have shown testicular vasculitis in 35% of patients with PAN

    d. Myalgias or muscle weakness—occur in 50% to 75% of patients and may be first symptoms. Myalgias may be severe; muscle weakness is usually minimal.

    e. Neuropathy—occurs in 50% to 60% of patients; generally mononeuritis multiplex, although it may be so extensive as to appear diffuse and symmetrical

    f. Diastolic blood pressure greater than 90 mm Hg—due to renal involvement that occurs in 50% to 60% of patients. Most commonly, PAN involves the renal arteries, the arcuate arteries, and arterioles, but not the capillaries. Urinalysis will show mild hematuria with or without proteinuria; renal angiograms show multiple berry aneurysms in the distal vessels. Kidney biopsies are often avoided because of their propensity to bleed. Glomeruli generally show only ischemic changes including mild mesangial expansion.

    g. Elevated BUN/creatinine—also secondary to renal involvement. Renal dysfunction requiring dialysis is very unusual.

    h. Hepatitis B virus—seen in 15% to 20% of patients; common in Alaskan Eskimos and rare in Chinese

    i. Arteriographic abnormalities—saccular berry aneurysms in the renal circulation are seen in 60% to 70% of patients; if hepatic and mesenteric circulations are included, 80% to 95% of patients will have vascular narrowings and berry aneurysms. The differential diagnosis of aneurysms includes drug abuse (cocaine), atrial myxoma, thrombotic thrombocytopenic purpura, endocarditis, neurofibromatosis, fibromuscular dysplasia, pseudoxanthoma elasticum, and Ehlers-Danlos syndrome.

    j. Biopsy of medium-sized artery containing PMN—arteries, but not veins are directly involved. The predominant inflammatory cell is the neutrophil, emphasizing the generally acute nature of this disease. The most common biopsy sites are muscle and nerve.

2. Additional clinical manifestations include:

    a. Cardiac involvement—occurs in 10% to 20% of patients; most commonly, CHF secondary to renovascular hypertension is noted. In addition, pericarditis, coronary vasculitis, and conduction abnormalities may be seen.

    b. Eye involvement—rare; includes hypertensive changes, retinal vasculitis, iritis, uveitis, and episcleritis

    c. Stroke syndromes—occur in 10% of patients; generally secondary to hypertension, uremia, or other extracranial vascular involvement. Intracranial vascular involvement can be seen very rarely.

3. Diagnosis—PAN is diagnosed by a consistent clinical picture, angiograms showing saccular aneurysms and intermittent areas of vascular narrowing, and biopsy of nerve, muscle, bowel and/or skin demonstrating medium-sized muscular artery vasculitis. The presence of potential drugs, infections, or malignancies that could induce vasculitis must be excluded. A search for hepatitis B and C must be part of the workup. Other laboratory studies are useful in determining the extent of organ involvement (i.e., CBC, creatine phosphokinase [CPK], aldolase, transaminases, and urinalysis). Many patients with PAN will have a positive perinuclear antineutrophil cytoplasmic antibody (P-ANCA) directed toward myeloperoxidase (MPO). The P-ANCA or anti-MPO test is not specific for PAN, and cannot be used to make a diagnosis of PAN in the absence of clinical, angiographic, and histological proof of a systemic disorder involving medium-sized muscular arteries.

4. Management
   a. Make diagnosis, document extent of organ involvement, and rule out other consistent disorders as soon as possible.
   b. Prescribe prednisone 1 mg/kg/day for 1 month, then taper to 1 mg per kg every other day over the second month, then taper off over the next several months as tolerated.
   c. Prescribe cyclophosphamide 1 to 2 mg per kg daily with the dose adjusted to maintain the total WBC between 3,000 and 4,000 per mL, maintained for 12 months after remission achieved. Azathioprine has been used in patients unable to tolerate cyclophosphamide.
   d. Treat causative infection if known—hepatitis B can be treated with lamivudine, vidarabine, and/or interferon-alpha
   e. Meticulous general medical and surgical care

D. Churg-Strauss syndrome
CSS is a rare systemic vasculitis involving venules and arterioles with granulomatous inflammation. It occurs with a slight male predominance in the fourth and fifth decades of life. Patients usually have an atopic history and present with the acute or subacute development of poorly controlled asthma requiring systemic corticosteroid therapy, along with evidence of other organ involvement, such as skin rash, paranasal sinus abnormalities, abdominal pain, peripheral neuropathy, and hematuria. Fleeting pulmonary infiltrates are present on chest x-ray. It is generally associated with a peripheral eosinophilia. Treatment includes high dose oral corticosteroids plus or minus cyclophosphamide (see Chapter 7 for a more comprehensive discussion).

E. Microscopic polyarteritis
MPA is a nongranulomatous vasculitis involving arterioles and capillaries. It is more closely related to Wegener granulomatosis than to PAN, despite its name. It differs from Wegener granulomatosis predominantly in the nature of the lung disease. The lung in Wegener granulomatosis has granulomatous arteriolitis and venulitis, whereas MPA has nongranulomatous capillaritis and arteriolitis. MPA occurs predominantly in the fourth and fifth decades of life with a slight male predominance. A typical presentation of MPA is a patient with fever, myalgias, and malaise lasting 4 to 6 weeks, followed by the rapid onset of glomerulonephritis with or without pulmonary hemorrhage or peripheral neuropathy.

1. Clinical manifestations
   a. Renal involvement—seen in 95% to 100% of patients. The renal disease is usually a pauciimmune, diffuse proliferative, crescentic glomerulonephritis; this lesion will destroy a normal kidney in 2 to 3 months if untreated. Sixty percent of patients will have secondary hypertension.
   b. Myalgias and arthralgia—occur in 50% to 60% of patients and can be quite severe. Frank arthritis is unusual.
   c. Skin involvement—occurs in 40% to 50% of patients; most commonly as palpable purpura that reveal leukocytoclastic vasculitis on skin biopsy. Ulcerations may occur; occasionally nodular skin lesions are present that reveal arteriolar vasculitis on skin biopsy.
   d. Lung involvement—occurs in most patients; respiratory hemorrhage occurs in 30% to 40% of patients. Fleeting pulmonary infiltrates or evidence of alveolar hemorrhage may be seen of chest x-ray and CT; biopsy shows nongranulomatous, predominantly neutrophilic capillaritis and arteriolitis.
   e. Nervous system involvement—occurs in 10% to 15% of patients. Peripheral neuropathy with mononeuritis multiplex is the most

common finding. Rare descriptions exist of CNS involvement, few of which were documented by biopsy, include seizures, monoplegias, optic atrophy, sensorineural hearing loss, subarachnoid hemorrhage, and pseudobulbar palsy.

f. Cardiac involvement—occurs in 10% to 20% of patients. Coronary vasculitis and pericarditis have been noted.

g. Gastrointestinal involvement—very rare, in contrast to PAN and CSS

2. Diagnosis—depends upon a consistent clinical picture, demonstration of pauciimmune crescentic glomerulonephritis in the kidney, and generally nongranulomatous capillaritis in another organ. Laboratory studies will reveal evidence of organ involvement, as well as positive P-ANCA (anti-MPO) in 70% to 85% of patients.

3. Management

    a. Early diagnosis is critical; untreated MPA has a very high mortality at 3 to 6 months.

    b. Prescribe prednisone 1 mg per kg per day for 1 month, then taper to 1 mg per kg every other day over the second month, then taper off over the next several months as tolerated.

    c. Prescribe cyclophosphamide 1 to 2 mg/kg/day with the dose adjusted to maintain the total WBC between 3,000 and 4,000 per mL. Maintain the dosage for 12 months after remission is achieved.

    d. Meticulous general medical and surgical care

F. Kawasaki disease (infantile polyarteritis)

Kawasaki disease is a syndrome of infants and young children that tends to occur in the winter and spring in cyclic epidemics and cluster in families. It is very common in Japan and unusual in the United States, where it is mostly seen in children of Asian descent. Various infectious agents have been implicated, including parainfluenza, mycoplasma, *Yersinia*, *Rickettsia*, *Streptococcus,* and *Staphylococcus*. It generally presents with high spiking fevers, skin rash, conjunctivitis, oral mucosal lesions, lymphadenopathy, and myocarditis with or without pericarditis. Diagnosis is based on meeting clinical criteria.

1. Clinical criteria for diagnosis

    a. Fever lasting longer than 5 days—spikes often to 400°F

    b. Presence of four of five of the following

        (1) Bilateral nonexudative conjunctival injection

        (2) Injected of fissured lips; injected pharynx; and/or "strawberry tongue"

        (3) Erythema of the palms and soles; edema of the hands and feet; and/or periungual desquamation—desquamation generally occurs after 2 weeks of the illness

        (4) Polymorphous exanthem—involves the trunk and proximal extremities early in the course of the disease. Macules, papules, and urticaria can be seen. Plaque-like perineal eruption is seen in 65% of patients during the first week.

        (5) Acute nonsuppurative cervical lymphadenopathy—occurs in 50% of patients; more common in older children

    c. Illness not explained by any other disease process

2. Other clinical manifestations

    a. Myocarditis with or without pericarditis—seen in 50% of patients during the first 3 weeks of the illness; may lead to ventricular dysfunction and last several months after the resolution of the acute illness

    b. Coronary artery aneurysms—occur in 15% to 25% of patients as part of the late stages of the illness; thrombosis in an aneurysm can lead to acute myocardial infarction and death. The condition frequently returns to normal with treatment.

    c. Cardiac valvular abnormalities—aortic regurgitation occurs in 5% of patients and mitral regurgitation in 25% of patients; generally resolve quickly with therapy

    d. Cardiac conduction abnormalities—frequent but generally transient

    e. Urethritis with sterile pyuria—frequent

    f. Aseptic meningitis—occurs in a minority of patients

    g. Hydrops of gallbladder—rare

    h. Hepatitis—common, but may also be related to therapy

    i. Abdominal pain, diarrhea, and vomiting—occur in a variable number of patients

    j. Pulmonary infiltrates—tend to resolve spontaneously after the acute phase of the illness

    k. Anterior uveitis—rare

3. Diagnosis—based on meeting clinical criteria. Laboratory studies are nonspecific and generally reveal leukocytosis, thrombocytosis, and elevated ESR. Biopsies are generally not helpful in making the diagnosis.

    a. The term "atypical Kawasaki disease" is used to denote patients with coronary artery involvement, but few other signs or symptoms.

4. Management

    a. Identify a pattern of organ involvement, including EKG and echocardiogram to evaluate possible cardiac disease.

    b. Aspirin given in four divided doses at a total dose of 80 to 100 mg per kg for 14 days to maintain serum salicylate levels at 20 to 25 mg/dL. Aspirin is then continued for 2 months at a single daily dose of 3 to 5 mg per kg, if no coronary abnormalities are detected, or indefinitely if cardiac abnormalities are present.

    c. IVIg is given in a single dose of 2 g per kg, generally infused over 12 hours; if patients cannot tolerate the fluid load, IVIg is given on four consecutive days at 400 mg per kg infused over 2 to 4 hours.

    d. Steroids are contraindicated because they lead to a higher rate of coronary artery rupture.

    e. Coronary artery aneurysms with thrombosis are managed with acute fibrinolytic therapy, chronic anticoagulation, and rarely coronary artery bypass surgery.

G. Wegener granulomatosis

Wegener granulomatosis is a granulomatous vasculitis of small arteries and veins that involves predominantly the upper airways, lungs, and kidneys. It involves both sexes equally and has a peak incidence in the fourth decade of life, although it can be seen at all ages. It often presents with symptoms referable to the upper airways, such as sinusitis not responding to antibiotic therapy, hearing loss, and bleeding from nasal ulcerations. Low-grade fever, arthralgias, and other constitutional symptoms may also be present. Rash, eye involvement, peripheral neuropathy, and rarely cardiac involvement can be seen. Preliminary evaluations reveal fleeting infiltrates on chest x-ray and urinary abnormalities, such as hematuria and proteinuria. Rapid institution of cyclophosphamide therapy is necessary for the preservation of major organs. Patients with upper and lower airway disease, but no renal disease, have been given the label "limited Wegener granulomatosis." This designation appears to be given to a wide variety of inflammatory disorders of the airways, many of which have little relationship to systemic Wegener granulomatosis. Less aggressive therapy is generally required for the management of patients with these disorders (see Chapter 7 for a more comprehensive discussion).

H. Relapsing polychondritis

Relapsing polychondritis is a very rare inflammatory disorder of hyaline and elastic cartilage that is often associated with vasculitis and antibodies to type II collagen. It occurs equally in the sexes, although nasal and subglottic involvement is more common in women. It is a disease with peak onset in the fourth and fifth decades of life that consists of acute episodes of inflammation involving the cartilage of the ears and nose, as well as variably other structures. It is characterized by recurrent bouts of disease that are often exquisitely sensitive to treatment with corticosteroids. Involvement of the lower airways is the most life-threatening manifestation of the disease. It may occur alone, but in 40% of cases occurs in association with another disease process, including RA, SLE, Sjögren syndrome, seronegative spondyloarthropathies, myelodysplastic syndromes, Behçet disease, Hodgkin disease, dermatitis herpetiformis, primary biliary cirrhosis, thymoma, and retroperitoneal fibrosis.

1. Diagnosis depends upon meeting three or more of the following criteria, or one or more criteria with histological proof of chondritis, or chondritis in two or more locations with a response to corticosteroids and/or dapsone:

   a. Recurrent chondritis of both auricles—occurs in 40% of patients at presentation, but in 80% to 90% of patients overall; violaceous and erythematous swelling of the pinna is noted. The disease may result in cauliflower deformity, and 30% of patients will experience hearing loss that may be secondary to eustachian tube chondritis, serous otitis media, and/or vasculitis of the internal auditory artery.

   b. Nonerosive inflammatory arthritis—occurs in 30% of patients at presentation and 70% to 80% of patients overall. Intermittent, migratory involvement of knees, ankles, proximal interphalangeal joints, metacarpophalangeal joints, elbows, and feet occurs; erosive changes are rarely seen in small joints. Overlaps may be seen with RA and seronegative spondyloarthropathies.

   c. Chondritis of nasal cartilage—occurs in 25% of patients at presentation and 55% of patients overall; may lead to saddle-nose deformity

   d. Ocular inflammation including conjunctivitis, keratitis, scleritis, and uveitis—occurs in 50% of patients; these may be resistant to steroid therapy alone

   e. Cochlear and/or vestibular damage manifest by sensory–neural hearing loss, tinnitus and/or vertigo—occurs in 10% to 25% of patients; may be secondary to both chondritis and vasculitis

2. Other clinical manifestations include:

   a. Pulmonary involvement—occurs in 25% to 50% of patients; consists of laryngotracheal and/or bronchial chondritis; may result in hoarseness, cough, inspiratory stridor, dyspnea on exertion or lying down. This is a major cause of death secondary to collapse of the tracheobronchial tree and infection.

   b. Cardiovascular involvement—occurs in 10% of patients; includes aortitis, valvulitis of aortic and mitral valves, and conduction abnormalities

   c. Renal involvement—occurs in 25% of patients; frequently a focal proliferative glomerulonephritis, but a purely interstitial nephritis can also be seen. This may lead to chronic renal failure if not aggressively treated.

   d. Neurologic involvement—occurs in 5% to 15% of patients and is generally secondary to vasculitis; most commonly second, third, sixth, seventh, or eighth cranial neuropathies, mononeuritis multiplex, or diffuse sensorimotor neuropathies. Rarely, aseptic meningitis and small vessel CNS vasculitis have been seen.

   e. Skin involvement—occurs in 30% of patients; most commonly, palpable purpura or ulcerations with biopsies demonstrating leukocytoclastic vasculitis. Other lesions include urticaria, erythema multiforme, livedo reticularis, erythema nodosa, and EED.

3. Management

   a. Identify the extent of organ involvement and possible primary causes—should include urinalysis to evaluate renal involvement and CT scanning to evaluate the upper and lower airways. CBC and serum protein electrophoresis should be done to look for myeloproliferative and lymphoproliferative disorders, especially in elderly patients.

b. Auricular and nasal chondritis can be treated with NSAIDs (rarely work), dapsone (50 to 100 mg b.i.d.; frequently works), or corticosteroids (20 to 40 mg q.d. given for 2 to 4 weeks for relapses and tapered as tolerated). Steroid failures may require azathioprine, cyclophosphamide, or cyclosporine, although there are little data to suggest which is most appropriate; hydroxychloroquine, methotrexate, and Azulfidine are generally not helpful.

c. Renal manifestations are treated with prednisone and/or a cytotoxic agent, depending upon the severity of the lesion.

d. Pulmonary manifestations require corticosteroids, antibiotics for secondary infections, aggressive pulmonary toilet, and possibly tracheostomy and various surgical corrections (although these may be difficult because of the general weakness of all the tissues).

e. Cardiac manifestations may require corticosteroids and possibly surgical replacement of abnormal valves and graft placement for aortic aneurysms.

f. Vasculitis should generally be treated with corticosteroids initially at a dose of 60 mg q.d. for 4 weeks and then tapering as tolerated. Patients with corticosteroid failures should be given daily oral cyclophosphamide 1 to 2 mg per kg q.d. to maintain the total WBC between 3,000 and 4,000 per mL.

g. Additional therapy may be required for primary causes and other types of organ involvement.

I. Behçet disease and syndrome

Behçet disease is a disorder manifest predominantly by genital and oral ulcers, uveitis, skin lesions, and pathergy that is seen almost exclusively in residents and descendants of residents of silk road countries: Turkey, Iran, Iraq, China, Korea, and Japan. It is often familial. The predominant histopathology of involved organs is a venulitis with polymorphonuclear cell infiltration and various areas of thrombosis. Behçet syndrome, which contains some of the disease manifestations of Behçet disease, is seen in the rest of the world. It can usually be explained by some other primary disorder, such as inflammatory bowel disease, Reiter syndrome, reactive spondyloarthropathy, pustular acne, Stevens-Johnson syndrome, drug hypersensitivity reactions, SLE, Kawasaki disease, various infections (especially *Herpes simplex*), and rarely Munchausen syndrome. In high-risk areas, there is a slight male predominance and onset of major disease manifestations in the third and fourth decades of life.

1. Diagnostic criteria—various criteria have been proposed, they all include:

a. Oral ulcers—present in all patients; shallow aphthous ulcers with reddened borders and frequently a grayish membrane; they are exquisitely painful and found mainly on the buccal mucosa. The ulcers generally recur three to four times per year, but heal without scarring.

b. Genital ulcers—present in all patients; aphthous ulcers that are generally not painful; in males the lesions are on the prepuce and scrotum; in women the lesions are in the vulva, vagina, and cervix uteri. The genital ulcers generally resolve with scarring; perianal ulcers may be associated and lead to urogenital and anorectal fistulae.

c. Eye lesions—present in a majority of patients; posterior more often than anterior uveitis. Anterior uveitis is often associated with hypopyon; choroiditis, retinitis, optic neuritis, and retinal vasculitis occur less frequently. Eye lesions are often painless and may occur several years after the onset of oral and genital ulcers. Eye lesions are the leading cause of acquired blindness in Japan.

      d. Skin lesions—very common but quite variable; include acneiform eruption, erythema nodosum, pseudofolliculitis, nodules, and papules

      e. Pathergy test—seen only in Behçet disease; 20- to 22-gauge needle is used to penetrate avascular skin to a depth of 5 mm; 48 hours later, an erythematous pustule is noted. Biopsy reveals platelets, mononuclear cells, and thrombi.

2. Additional clinical manifestations include:

      a. Musculoskeletal involvement—most patients develop arthralgias, and a smaller percentage frank arthritis; frequently large joint, asymmetrical with preference for the knees and ankles. Sacroiliitis is seen rarely.

      b. Gastrointestinal involvement—seen in a minority of patients; in addition to oral ulcers, aphthous ulcers of the esophagus, cecum, and terminal ileum are seen. Hepatitis, cholecystitis, and pancreatitis are less common.

      c. Hypercoagulable state—seen in a minority of patients, but often devastating; in many cases antiphospholipid antibodies are noted. This state may result in superficial thrombophlebitis, large vein thromboses including Budd-Chiari syndrome, arterial occlusions, aneurysms, and dissections; these have a very high mortality.

      d. Neurologic involvement—rare CNS disease includes patchy demyelination, cortical and cerebellar atrophy with brainstem predilection, pseudotumor cerebri, aseptic meningitis, dural sinus thrombosis, and various stroke syndromes.

      e. Lung involvement—seen in 5% to 20% of patients, mostly in Behçet disease. Vasculitis may lead to pulmonary aneurysms and hemorrhage. Thromboses may cause pulmonary embolization and secondary pulmonary hypertension.

      f. Heart involvement—rare; pericarditis, endocarditis, and myocarditis

      g. Renal involvement—rare; immune complex-mediated focal proliferative glomerulonephritis

      h. Secondary amyloidosis—very rare, mostly in Behçet disease

3. Management—Behçet disease generally follows a relapsing and remitting course that can be treated conservatively with symptomatic measures. Major organ involvement is generally treated aggressively with corticosteroids, cytotoxic agents, and anticoagulation, but the optimal therapy for these problems is poorly understood.

      a. Establish the degree of organ involvement.

      b. Topical therapies for oral and genital ulcers include corticosteroid ointments, azelastine hydrochloride, and topical tetracycline.

      c. Systemic therapies for oral and genital ulcers include colchicine 0.6 mg b.i.d., Rebamipide (chlorobenzylamine dihydro-oxoquinoline propanoic acid) 100 mg t.i.d., dapsone 100 mg b.i.d., and thalidomide 100 to 400 mg q.d. In severe recurrent ulcers, azathioprine 100 to 200 mg q.d. may be necessary.

      d. Treat arthritis initially with a NSAIDs; NSAID failures should receive sulfasalazine 1.5 g b.i.d. Low-dose daily or alternate-day corticosteroids may be used as adjunct treatment; rarely, azathioprine is utilized.

      e. Eye involvement may respond to topical cyclosporine A and/or corticosteroids. Systemic therapies include cyclosporine 5 to 10 mg per kg q.d., tacrolimus 0.05 to 0.015 mg per kg q.d., azathioprine 100 to 200 mg q.d., and/or corticosteroids (i.e., prednisone 20 to 60 mg q.d.).

      f. Vascular compromise secondary to thrombosis should be treated with full-dose anticoagulation with coumadin (maintain international normalized ratio [INR] 3 to 4) or low molecular weight heparin (i.e., enoxaparin 1 mg per kg b.i.d.). All patients with phospholipid antibodies should receive aspirin 81 mg q.d. to prevent thrombosis.

   g. True vasculitis should be treated with corticosteroids and possibly cyclophosphamide in addition, either monthly (750 mg/M²) or daily (1 to 2 mg per kg adjusted to keep WBC between 3,000 and 4,000 per mL). Therapy depends upon the organs involved and the nature of the inflammation.

   h. Gastrointestinal ulcerations have been treated with sulfasalazine 1.5 g b.i.d., thalidomide 300 to 400 mg q.d., and/or corticosteroids. If thrombosis and/or vasculitis are present, they should be treated accordingly.

   i. Surgical intervention may be required for multiple problems including intestinal perforation, vascular aneurysms, endomyocardial fibrosis, cataracts, and unremitting arthritis (treated with synovectomy or arthroplasty).

J. Goodpasture disease

GD is a rare pulmonary–renal syndrome associated with antibodies to the α_3 domain of type IV collagen. Extrarenal manifestations including leukocytoclastic vasculitis of the skin, arthritis, peripheral neuropathy, and uveitis are more common in patients who also have antimyeloperoxidase ANCA. GD occurs with male predominance in the third and fourth decades of life, and with an equal sex ratio in the fifth and sixth decades of life. The most common presentation of GD is flu-like symptoms followed by the rapid onset of microscopic hematuria and proteinuria with pulmonary infiltrates. Respiratory hemorrhage is seen in 20% to 30% of patients. Untreated, GD results in the rapid onset of renal failure and occasionally respiratory failure. Treatment modalities include corticosteroids, cyclophosphamide, plasmapheresis, and cyclosporine. See Chapter 7 for a more comprehensive discussion.

K. Henoch-Schönlein purpura

HSP is a common small vessel vasculitis that frequently follows viral and bacterial infections of the upper and lower airways. It presents with purpuric skin rash, abdominal pain, and renal disease. It is associated with deposition of IgA containing immune complexes in the tissues. It is predominantly a disease of children, with the mean age being 5 years. An identical disorder occurs in adults, with the mean age being 50 years. In adults, HSP may occur as a response to tumor antigens.

   1. The following ACR criteria distinguish HSP from other forms of vasculitis:

   a. Palpable purpura—occurs in all patients. Purpura are noted predominantly in dependent areas and may be pruritic. Purpura start as small urticaria and evolve into macules that coalesce; they generally resolve within two weeks without scarring. Purpura are associated with edema and exist simultaneously at various stages of healing. Skin biopsies reveal leukocytoclastic vasculitis with deposition of IgA immune complexes in the skin.

   b. Age less than 20 years—most vasculitides, except HSP and Takayasu arteritis, peak in the fourth and fifth decades

   c. Bowel angina—occurs in 50% of patients. Abdominal pain with variable amounts of self-limited hemorrhage is characteristic of HSP. Functional obstruction, intussusception, massive hemorrhage, and prolonged ileus can occur infrequently. Bowel biopsy reveals small vessel vasculitis.

   d. Granulocytes in wall of arterioles/venules—a biopsy is frequently helpful to establish the diagnosis

   2. Additional clinical manifestations include:

   a. Renal disease—occurs in 50% of patients; generally mild and self-limited. Urinalysis reveals hematuria and/or proteinuria. On kidney biopsy, mild mesangial expansion is noted; in 4% to 15% of patients, a proliferative glomerulonephritis is noted that may lead to renal failure if untreated. Kidney biopsy is indicated for evaluation of possible proliferative glomerulonephritis if the 24-hour urinary protein is greater than 1 g, casts are noted in the urinalysis, serum creatinine increase by 50%, or hematuria and proteinuria persist more than 1 month after other organ systems have returned to normal.

   b. Musculoskeletal disease—diffuse myalgias and migratory arthralgias are seen in 70% of patients. In a small percentage of patients, a large joint asymmetrical arthritis may be present that favors the knees.

   c. Pulmonary disease—occurs in 5% of patients and manifests as pleuritis, pulmonary infiltrates, and/or hemoptysis

   d. Cardiac involvement—extremely rare; may be secondary to hypertension

   e. Central nervous system involvement—extremely rare; may be secondary to hypertension or infection

3. Treatment

   a. The majority of patients require only supportive care. Aspirin and NSAIDs should be avoided because of gastrointestinal bleeding.

   b. Prolonged or severe abdominal pain should be evaluated radiographically for obstruction, intussusception, or bowel infarction. Surgical consultation should be obtained. In the absence of a surgical indication, low-dose corticosteroids (10 to 20 mg prednisone daily) may be used; high-dose corticosteroids should be avoided. Factor XIII has been proposed as an alternative therapy.

   c. Treatment of renal disease is controversial. In the majority of patients, renal disease requires no treatment; however, if 24-hour urinary protein is greater than 1 g, a 50% increase in serum creatinine is noted, or casts are noted in the urine, kidney biopsy should be obtained and the patient started on prednisone 1 to 2 mg/kg/day. The histopathology dictates further therapy: If focal proliferative changes are noted, prednisone can be used alone for a total of 3 to 6 months; if diffuse proliferative changes with greater than 50% of glomeruli showing crescent formation, cyclophosphamide 1 to 2 mg/kg/day should be given in whatever dose will maintain the total WBC between 3,000 and 4,000 per mL. Cyclophosphamide should be maintained for 1 year after remission; prednisone should be used for 3 to 6 months. Some physicians advocate switching patients from cyclophosphamide to azathioprine to reduce potential side effects.

L. Thromboangiitis obliterans

Thromboangiitis obliterans (TO) or Buerger disease is a rare inflammatory, occlusive vascular disease seen only in male smokers in the fourth and fifth decades of life. The majority of patients are Asian or Israeli Ashkenazi Jews. It generally presents with a gradual onset of worsening claudication of the lower extremities and migratory thrombophlebitis. Laboratory studies do not suggest inflammation.

1. Clinical manifestations include:

   a. Lower extremity involvement—occurs in all patients. Claudication, thrombophlebitis, paresthesias, nonhealing ulcers, hyperhidrosis, and Raynaud syndrome are seen.

   b. Upper extremity involvement—occurs in 30% to 40% of patients. The same symptoms and signs occur as seen in lower extremity involvement.

   c. Other vascular disease—extremely rare; pulmonary, cardiac, and CNS involvement have been described

2. Diagnosis
   a. Consistent clinical picture in a male smoker
   b. Angiography—abrupt, symmetrical, segmental, and multifocal occlusions of distal medium and small arteries of the extremities. There may be significant collateral flow around occluded areas.
   c. Histopathology—generally obtained at amputations. Neutrophil or mononuclear cell infiltration of the cell wall with microabscess formation and thrombosis is seen. In the late stages inflammation is replaced by fibrosis and possible recanalization of thromboses.
3. Treatment
   a. Smoking cessation
   b. Local therapy for ulcers
   c. Bypass grafting; amputations if gangrene ensues

M. Cogan syndrome

Cogan syndrome is an unusual inflammatory disease of the eyes and vestibular-auditory system that includes a systemic vasculitis in a small percentage of cases. The sexes are equally involved and the peak onset is in the third decade of life.

1. Clinical manifestations include:
   a. Eye involvement—occurs in all patients; presents as sudden onset photophobia, eye pain and lacrimation. The most common lesions are interstitial keratitis with subepithelial peripheral corneal stromal infiltration; less commonly, patients may have episcleritis, scleritis, orbital pseudotumor, uveitis, conjunctivitis, papillitis, or retinal vasculitis.
   b. Audiovestibular involvement—occurs in all patients usually within 1 month of ocular symptoms, although either manifestation can precede the other. The syndrome presents as sudden onset unilateral or bilateral hearing loss that can lead to profound hearing deficits within 3 months; vertigo, nystagmus, nausea, and vomiting also occur.
   c. Vasculitis—occurs in 10% to 15% of patients; involves skin, kidney, muscle, heart, and aortic arch. Vasculitis may be preceded by high fevers and splenomegaly. Aortic arch involvement may be associated with valvulitis, pericarditis, and/or coronary vasculitis— the only life-threatening manifestations of the disease.
2. Diagnosis
   a. Consistent clinical picture
   b. Patients with vasculitic symptoms should have angiography, which reveals occlusions and diffuse and irregular stenoses in large and medium-sized arteries.
   c. Skin lesions should be biopsied to reveal transmural infiltration of medium and small blood vessels with mononuclear cells.
3. Treatment
   a. Identify the extent of organ involvement as soon as possible.
   b. Ocular involvement—generally control with topical or systemic corticosteroids (initially prednisone 40 to 60 mg daily). In rare cases, cyclophosphamide or cyclosporine have been used in steroid failures.
   c. Audiovestibular involvement—high-dose corticosteroids (prednisone 60 to 100 mg daily) should be instituted as soon as possible and maintained for at least 1 month. A slow taper may then be initiated. In rare cases, cyclophosphamide or cyclosporine have been used in steroid failures.
   d. Vasculitis—high-dose corticosteroids initially 1 mg/kg/day, then tapered after 4 weeks to 1 mg per kg every other day, and finally tapered off over the next 3 to 4 months; cyclophosphamide 1 to 2 mg/kg/day used to maintain the total WBC 3,000 to 4,000 per mL. Some investigators have noted a better response to cyclosporine (5 to 10 mg/kg/day in two divided doses) than to cyclophosphamide.

N. Erythema elevatum diutinum
EED is a rare chronic leukocytoclastic vasculitis limited to skin. The disease has two peaks of onset, in females during childhood and equally in the sexes during the sixth decade of life. In adults there is a strong association with myeloproliferative and lymphoproliferative diseases, especially IgA gammopathy.
  1. Clinical manifestations
     a. Skin lesions—purpura and papules that evolve to plaques and nodules and then either heal, leaving hypo- or hyperpigmented areas, or form xanthomas. Lesions occur symmetrically along extensor surfaces, especially overlying the hands, feet, elbows, and Achilles tendon.
     b. Musculoskeletal disease—most patients have diffuse arthralgias, without frank arthritis. Acroosteolysis has been described rarely.
  2. Diagnosis
     a. Consistent clinical picture
     b. Skin biopsy shows massive, often nodular infiltration of the upper dermis with neutrophils; capillaries and post-capillary venules contain infiltrating neutrophils, fibrin deposition, and extravasated erythrocytes. Immunofluorescence is only rarely positive for IgA and/or complement.
     c. Laboratory findings frequently reveal hypergammaglobulinemia predominantly of the IgA class.
  3. Treatment
     a. Dapsone 100 to 150 mg daily is the drug of choice. It induces remission in most patients. Dapsone cannot be given to patients with sulfa allergy or glucose-6-phosphate dehydrogenase deficiency. The methemoglobin level should be checked monthly and kept below 3%.
     b. Alternatives to dapsone include glucocorticoids (i.e., prednisone 30 to 40 mg daily) and sulfasalazine 1 to 3 g daily.

O. Primary angiitis of the central nervous system
Systemic vasculitides only rarely involve the CNS. Primary angiitis of the CNS (PACNS) is a vasculitis involving the CNS, but not other organs, which cannot be explained by infections, malignancies, or drug ingestions. It must also be distinguished from noninflammatory vascular diseases of the CNS, including Raynaud ("benign angiopathy of the CNS"), hypertensive encephalopathy, thrombosis, and embolus. The disease presents most commonly in the fifth and sixth decades of life. A typical patient develops a viral upper respiratory infection, which is then followed by 3 to 4 weeks of headache, weakness, and subtle confusion. The patient then has the sudden onset of a focal neurological deficit. Systemic symptoms are absent and laboratory studies are normal.
  1. Diagnosis
     a. Consistent clinical picture
     b. Cerebrospinal fluid generally reveals elevations in cell count and/ or protein.
     c. Definitive diagnosis is made by leptomeningeal and/or cortical biopsies that reveal lymphocytic and mononuclear cell infiltration of small veins and arterioles.
     d. Cerebral angiography or magnetic resonance angiography will reveal, in 40% to 60% of patients, vascular narrowing alternating with focal dilations, occlusions, and occasionally new anastomotic channels; "berry" aneurysms are only rarely seen, and more commonly are secondary to fibromuscular dysplasia.
  2. Treatment
     a. Prednisone 1 mg/kg/day for 1 month, then taper to 1 mg/kg every other day over the second month, then taper off over the next several months as tolerated

      b. Cyclophosphamide 1 to 2 mg/kg/day, with the dose adjusted to maintain the total WBC between 3,000 and 4,000 per mL and maintained for 12 months after remission is achieved

      c. Meticulous general medical and surgical care

XVIII. Miscellaneous disorders

  A. Fever syndromes

A number of syndromes associated with recurrent bouts of fever and inflammation of various organs have been identified and genetically characterized. They are rare disorders, but well recognized in certain ethnic groups. They must be considered in the differential diagnosis of recurrent fevers because identification will lead to appropriate therapy and prevent unnecessary interventions.

    1. Familial Mediterranean fever

Familial Mediterranean fever (FMF) typically consists of acute episodes of fever lasting 12 to 72 hours, accompanied by abdominal pain, chest pain, and/or joint pain. It usually presents before the age of 20 years in ethnic groups of Mediterranean origin. Menses, emotional stress, or strenuous physical activity may trigger these attacks. There is often no identifiable precipitating factor.

      a. The following are common clinical features:

        (1) Fever—occurs in 95% to 100% of patients and is often associated with chills. The degree of temperature elevation may vary with attacks.

        (2) Abdominal pain—occurs in 95% to 100% of patients and may be diffuse or localized. Patients have often been incorrectly diagnosed with appendicitis or other abdominal emergencies.

        (3) Chest pain—occurs in 50% of patients and is often unilateral. Pleural effusions or atelectasis on chest x-ray may be seen.

        (4) Joint pain—occurs in 50% to 75% of patients; often diffuse arthralgias with large joint asymmetrical arthritis (knee, ankle or hip); rarely sacroiliitis. Joint pain often resolves with fever, but can rarely become chronic.

        (5) Erysipelas-like erythema—occurs in 3% to 46% of patients. Usually, the 10- to 15-cm erythematous lesions are restricted to the lower extremities.

        (6) Laboratory manifestations—leukocytosis with left shift, elevated ESR, elevated acute phase proteins, transient proteinuria and/or hematuria

      b. Uncommon clinical manifestations include:

        (1) Scrotal inflammation

        (2) Protracted fever and myalgias lasting up to 1 month

        (3) Aseptic meningitis

        (4) Pericarditis

        (5) Vasculitis—often similar to HSP

        (6) Amyloidosis—occurs in 1% to 7% of patients. Deposition of serum amyloid A cleavage products is noted. Amyloidosis may infiltrate kidney, adrenals, intestine, spleen, liver, lungs, thyroid, heart, and testes. The most common finding is proteinuria with or without nephrotic syndrome.

      c. Diagnosis—depends upon a consistent clinical picture and demonstration of mutations in the MEFV gene, encoding the protein "pyrin"

      d. Treatment

        (1) Continuous daily treatment with colchicine 1. 2 to 1.8 mg daily

        (2) NSAIDs and/or corticosteroids may be required during acute, prolonged attacks.

        (3) Interferon has been proposed as a therapeutic option for patients not responding to conventional therapy.

2. Familial hibernian fever or tumor necrosis factor-receptor associated periodic syndrome (TRAPS)

Familial hibernian fever (FHF) or TRAPS is a syndrome occurring in patients of Irish descent and often beginning in childhood. It consists of recurrent attacks of fever, erythematous skin lesions, abdominal pain, chest pain, localized myalgias, and oligoarthralgias. Attacks usually last longer than 1 week, and may be overlapping.

a. Common manifestations of disease include:

(1) Fever—occurs in 100% of patients; may have varying degrees of temperature elevations

(2) Abdominal pain—occurs in 94% of patients; often diffuse, but may be localized

(3) Localized myalgias—occur in 94% of patients; some degree of muscle stiffness occurs in 75% of patients

(4) Conjunctival injection—occurs in 81% of patients; generally involves only conjunctiva and not uveal tract. Periorbital edema occurs in 62% of patients.

(5) Skin rash—occurs in 69% of patients; generally tender, erythematous, well-demarcated lesions that occur anywhere on the body

(6) Arthralgias—occur in 69% of patients; rarely frank arthritis (10% to 12% of patients); generally involves large joints asymmetrically, knees more often than hips, shoulders, elbows

(7) Chest pain—occurs in 62% of patients

(8) Testicular pain—occurs in 50% of patients

(9) Laboratory reveals elevated ESR and neutrophilia

b. Diagnosis—based on a consistent clinical picture and demonstration of mutations in the extracellular domain of the p55 TNF receptor I (TNF-RI); leukocytes show enhanced expression of TNF-RI, while the amount of soluble TNF-RI is significantly decreased

c. Treatment

(1) Current therapy consists of corticosteroids during acute flares (i.e., prednisone 20 to 40 mg daily)

(2) Theoretically, although untested in clinical trials, medications blocking TNF, such as etanercept (Enbrel) and Infliximab (Remicade), should be of benefit.

3. Dutch type periodic fever or hyperimmunoglobulin D syndrome

Dutch type periodic fever (DPF) or hyperimmunoglobulin D syndrome (HIDS) is a disorder usually starting in infancy that consists of recurrent febrile episodes lasting 3 to 7 days in association with chills, headache, arthralgias, abdominal pain, skin rashes, and lymphadenopathy. It is inherited in an autosomal-recessive manner, and is seen predominantly in people of French and Dutch extraction. It is generally associated with leukocytosis and elevated IgD. Trauma, stress, infections, or immunizations may precipitate febrile attacks.

a. Common manifestations include:

(1) Fever—occurs in 100% of patients; often over 400°C, but may decrease in severity as children get older; 75% of patients experience chills with fevers

(2) Abdominal pain—occurs in 72% of patients and may be confused with acute appendicitis. Abdominal pain may be associated vomiting and/or diarrhea, but generally does not involve serositis (as in FMF).

(3) Arthralgias—occur in 80% of patients and may persist after acute attacks are over. Arthralgias may include frank arthritis in 70% of patients. Symptoms generally involve the large joints of the lower extremities.

(4) Headache—occurs in 50% of patients; often diffuse and severe

      (5) Skin rash—occurs in 80% of patients; generally macular or maculopapular; rarely urticarial, purpuric, or EED. Rash may be accompanied by oral and/or genital ulcers.

      (6) Lymphadenopathy—occurs in 95% of patients; generally involves the cervical nodes, but may also involve axillary, inguinal, and intraabdominal nodes. Splenomegaly occurs in 50% of patients.

      (7) Laboratory tests reveal elevated IgD in 100% of patients; most patients have leukocytosis and elevated ESR; 15% of patients have microscopic hematuria that resolves after acute attacks. Most patients have elevated mevalonic acid in the urine during acute attacks.

   b. Diagnosis—consistent clinical picture and demonstration of one of three characteristic mutations in the mevalonate kinase gene (G to A at base 1129, A to C at base 59, or T to C at base 803)

   c. Treatment

      (1) No specific therapy is known. Drugs such as NSAIDs, colchicine, cyclosporine, and intravenous immunoglobulins have been shown not to be useful

      (2) Short-term use of corticosteroids may be helpful during acute attacks.

Selected Readings

Textbooks

Arthritis and allied conditions, 14th ed. Koopman WJ, ed. Baltimore: Williams and Wilkins, 2001.

Clinical immunology. Principles and practice, 1st ed. Rich RR, ed. St. Louis: Mosby, 1996.

Diagnosis of bone and joint disorders, 3rd ed. Resnick D, Niwayama G, eds. Philadelphia: WB Saunders, 1995.

Review Articles

OSTEOARTHRITIS

Deyle GD, Henderson NE, Matekel RL, et al. Effectiveness of manual physical therapy and exercise in osteoarthritis of the knee. A randomized, controlled trial. *Ann Intern Med* 2000;132:173.

Kraus VB. Pathogenesis and treatment of osteoarthritis. *Med Clin North Am* 1997;81:85.

Manek NJ, Lane NE. Osteoarthritis: current concepts in diagnosis and management. *Am Fam Physician* 2000;61:1795.

BACTERIAL ARTHRITIS

Mader JT, Shirtliff M, Calhoun JH. The host and the skeletal infection: classification and pathogenesis of acute bacterial bone and joint sepsis. *Baillieres Best Pract Res Clin Rheumatol* 1999;13:1.

Perry CR. Septic arthritis. *Am J Orthop* 1999;28:168.

Ratnaike RN. Whipple's disease. *Postgrad Med J* 2000;76:760.

LYME ARTHRITIS

Steere AC. Diagnosis and treatment of Lyme arthritis. *Med Clin North Am* 1997;81:179.

Terkeltaub RA. Lyme disease 2000. Emerging zoonoses complicate patient work-up and treatment. *Geriatrics* 2000;55:34.

CRYSTAL-INDUCED ARTHRITIS

Cheung HS. Calcium crystal effects on the cells of the joint: implications for pathogenesis of disease. *Curr Opin Rheumatol* 2000;12:223.

Rosenthal AK. Calcium crystal-associated arthritides. *Curr Opin Rheumatol* 1998; 10:273.

SERONEGATIVE SPONDYLOARTHROPATHIES

Amor B. Reiter's syndrome. Diagnosis and clinical features. *Rheum Dis Clin North Am* 1998;24:677.

Braun J, Bollow M, Sieper J. Radiologic diagnosis and pathology of the spondylo-arthropathies. *Rheum Dis Clin North Am* 1998;24:697.

deCastro JAL. The pathogenetic role of HLA-B27 in chronic arthritis. *Curr Opin Immunol* 1998;10:59.

Leirisalo-Repo M. Prognosis, course of disease, and treatment of the spondyloarthrop-athies. *Rheum Dis Clin North Am* 1998;24:737.

Ruzicka T. Psoriatic arthritis: new types, new treatments. *Arch Dermatol* 1996;132:215.

RHEUMATOID ARTHRITIS

Alarcon GS. Predictive factors in rheumatoid arthritis. *Am J Med* 1997;103:19.

Kwoh CK, Simms RW, Anderson LG, et al. Guidelines for the management of rheuma-toid arthritis. *Arthritis Rheum* 1996;39:713.

Matteson EL. Current treatment strategies for rheumatoid arthritis. *Mayo Clin Proc* 2000;75:69.

Simon LS, Yocum D. New and future drug therapies for rheumatoid arthritis. *Rheu-matology (Oxford)* 2000;39:36.

Smolen JS, Breedveld FC, Burmester GR, et al. Consensus statement on the initiation and continuation of tumour necrosis factor blocking therapies in rheumatoid arthri-tis. *Ann Rheum Dis* 2000;59:504.

Tugwell P. Pharmacoeconomics of drug therapy for rheumatoid arthritis. *Rheumatology (Oxford)* 2000;39:43.

JUVENILE IDIOPATHIC ARTHRITIS

Fink CW, Fernandez-Vina M, Stastny P. Clinical and genetic evidence that juvenile arthritis is not a single disease. *Pediatr Clin North Am* 1995;42:1155.

Giannini EH, Cawkwell GD. Drug treatment in children with juvenile rheumatoid arthritis: past, present and future. *Pediatr Clin North Am* 1995;42:1099.

Lovell DJ, Giannini EH, Reiff A, et al. Etanercept in children with polyarticular juve-nile rheumatoid arthritis. Pediatric Rheumatology Collaborative Study Group. *New Engl J Med* 2000;342:763.

Wallace CA, Levinson JE. Juvenile rheumatoid arthritis: outcome and treatment for the 1990s. *Rheum Dis Clin North Am* 1991;17:891.

PEDIATRIC SYSTEMIC LUPUS ERYTHEMATOSUS

Iqbal S, Sher M, Good RA, et al. Diversity in presenting manifestations of systemic lupus erythematosus in children. *J Pediatr* 1999;135:500.

Lehman TJA. A practical guide to systemic lupus erythematosus. *Pediatr Clin North Am* 1995;42:1223.

Lockshin MD. Therapy for systemic lupus erythematosus. *N Engl J Med* 1991;324:189.

Szer IS. Clincal development in the management of lupus in the neonate, child, and adolescent. *Curr Opin Rheumatol* 1998;10:431.

JUVENILE DERMATOMYOSITIS

Huang JL. Long-term prognosis of patients with juvenile dermatomyositis initially treated with intravenous methylprednisolone pulse therapy. *Clin Exp Rheumatol* 1999;17:621.

Pachman LM. Juvenile dermatomyositis: Pathophysiology and disease expression. *Pediatr Clin North Am* 1995;42:1071.

Pachman LM, Hayford JR, Chung A, et al. Juvenile dermatomyositis at diagnosis: clinical characteristics of 79 children. *J Rheumatol* 1998;26:1198.

Rider LG, Miller FW. Classification and treatment of the juvenile idiopathic inflam-matory myopathies. *Rheum Dis Clin North Am* 1997;23:619.

CHILDHOOD SCLERODERMA

Emery H. Pediatric scleroderma. *Semin Cutan Med Surg* 1998;17:41.

Foeldvari I, Zhavania M, Birdi N, et al. Favourable outcome in 135 children with juve-nile systemic sclerosis: results of a multi-national survey. *Rheumatology* 2000;39:556.

Uziel Y, Krafchik BR, Sliverman ED, et al. Localized scleroderma in childhood: a report of 30 cases. *Semin Arthritis Rheum* 1994;23:328.

Uziel Y, Miller ML, Laxer RM. Scleroderma in children. *Pediatr Clin North Am* 1995;42:1171.

VASCULITIS IN CHILDHOOD

American College of Rheumatology. 1990 criteria for the classification of vasculitis. *Arthritis Rheum* 1990;33:1065.

Athreya BH. Vasculitis in children. *Pediatr Clin North Am* 1995;42:1239.

Burns JC, Kushner HI, Bastian JF, et al. Kawasaki disease: a brief history. *Pediatrics* 2000;106:e27.

Saulsbury FT. Henoch-Schönlein purpura in children: report of 100 patients and review of the literature. *Medicine* 1999;78:395.

Von Vigier RO, Trummler SA, Laux-End R, et al. Pulmonary renal syndrome in childhood: a report of twenty-one cases and a review of the literature. *Pediatr Pulmonol* 2000;29:382.

POSTINFECTIOUS AND REACTIVE ARTHRITIS

Arnett FC. The seronegative spondyloarthropathies. *Bull Rheum Dis* 1987;37:1.

Burgos-Vargas R, Pacheco-Tena C, Vazquez-Mellado J. Juvenile-onset spondyloarthropathies. *Rheum Dis Clin North Am* 1997;23:569.

Hughes RA, Keat AC. Reiter's syndrome and reactive arthritis: a current view. *Semin Arthritis Rheum* 1994;24:190.

Taccetti G, Trapani S, Ermini M, et al. Reactive arthritis triggered by Yersinia enterocolitica: a review of 18 pediatric cases. *Clin Exp Rheumatol* 1994;12:681.

SYSTEMIC LUPUS ERYTHEMATOSUS

Calabrese L, Stern T. Neuropsychiatric manifestations of systemic lupus erythematosus. *Psychosomatics* 1995;36:344.

Gladman D. Prognosis and treatment of systemic lupus erythematosus. *Curr Opin Rheumatol* 1996;8:430.

Orens J, Martinez F, Lynch JR. Pleuropulmonary manifestations of systemic lupus erythematosus. *Rheum Dis Clin North Am* 1994;20:159.

SCLERODERMA

Kane GC, Varga J, Conant EF, et al. Lung involvement in systemic sclerosis (scleroderma): Relation to classification based on extent of skin involvement or autoantibody status. *Respir Med* 1996;90:223.

Peterson LS, Nelson AM, Su WPD. Classification of morphea (localized scleroderma). *Mayo Clin Proc* 1995;70:1068.

Smiley J. The many faces of scleroderma. *Am J Med Sc* 1992;304:319.

Uziel Y, Miller ML, Laxer RM. Scleroderma in children. *Pediatr Clin North Am* 1995;42:1171.

White B, Moore WC, Wigley FM, et al. Cyclophosphamide is associated with pulmonary function and survival benefit in patients with scleroderma and alveolitis. *Ann Intern Med* 2000;132:947.

SJÖGREN SYNDROME

Daniels TE. Evaluation, differential diagnosis, and treatment of xerostomia. *J Rheumatol Suppl* 2000;61:6.

Gannot G, Lancaster HE, Fox PC. Clinical course of primary Sjögren's syndrome: salivary, oral, and serologic aspects. *J Rheumatol* 2000;27:1905.

Jonsson R, Haga HJ, Gordon TP. Current concepts on diagnosis, autoantibodies and therapy in Sjögren's syndrome. *Scand J Rheumatol* 2000;29:341.

POLYMYOSITIS AND DERMATOMYOSITIS

Dalakas MC. Medical progress—polymyositis, dermatomyositis, and inclusion-body myositis. *N Engl J Med* 1991;325:1487.

Euwer RL, Sontheimer RD. Amyopathic dermatomyositis—a review. *J Invest Dermatol* 1993;100:S124.

Hausmanowa-Petrusewicz I, Kowalska-Oledzka E, Miller FW, et al. Clinical, serologic, and immunogenetic features in Polish patients with idiopathic inflammatory myopathies. *Arthritis Rheum* 1997;40:1257.

Mastaglia FL, Phillips BA, Zilko P. Treatment of inflammatory myopathies. *Muscle Nerve* 1997;20:651.

Pachman LM. Juvenile dermatomyositis (JDMS)—new clues to diagnosis and pathogenesis. *Clin Exp Rheumatol* 1994;12:S69.

ANTIPHOSPHOLIPID ANTIBODY SYNDROME

Asherson RA, Cervera R, Piette JC, et al. Catastrophic antiphospholipid syndrome: clinical and laboratory features of 50 patients. *Medicine* 1998;77:195.

Finazzi G. The Italian registry of antiphospholipid antibodies. *Haematologica* 1997; 82:101.

Rand JH. Antiphospholipid antibody syndrome: New insights on thrombogenic mechanisms. *Am J Med Sci* 1998;316:142.

Sammaritano LR, Gharavi AE, Lockshin MD. Antiphospholipid antibody syndrome: immunologic and clinical aspects. *Semin Arthritis Rheum* 1990;20:81.

VASCULITIDES

Athreya BH. Vasculitis in children. *Pediatr Clin North Am* 1995;42:1239.

Balow JE. Renal vasculitis. *Curr Opin Nephrol Hypertens* 1993;2:231.

Bielory L, Conti J, Frohman L. Immunology grand rounds. Cogan's syndrome. *J Allergy Clin Immunol* 1990;85:808.

Blanco R, Martinez-Taboada VM, Rodriguez-Valverde V, et al. Henoch-Schönlein purpura in adulthood and childhood: Two different expressions of the same syndrome. *Arthritis Rheum* 1997;40:859.

Bosch T. Current status in extracorporeal immunomodulation: immune disorders. *Artif Organs* 1996;20:902.

Calabrese LH, Duna GF, Lie JT. Vasculitis in the central nervous system. *Arthritis Rheum* 1997;40:1189.

Cameron J. New horizons in renal vasculitis. *Klin Wochenschr* 1991;69:536.

Chen KR, Kawahara Y, Miyakawa S, et al. Cutaneous vasculitis in Behçet's disease: A clinical and histopathologic study of 20 patients. *J Am Acad Dermatol* 1997;36:689.

Csernok E, Gross WL. Primary vasculitides and vasculitis confined to skin: clinical features and new pathogenic aspects. *Arch Dermatol Res* 2000;292:427.

Davies L, Spies JM, Pollard JD, et al. Vasculitis confined to peripheral nerves. *Brain* 1996;119:1441.

Dean S, Saba S, Ramirez G. Systemic vasculitis in Goodpasture's syndrome. *South Med J* 1991;84:1387.

Duquesnoy B. Henoch-Schönlein purpura. *Baillieres Clin Rheumatol* 1991;5:253.

Fan P, Davis J, Somer T, et al. A clinical approach to systemic vasculitis. *Semin Arth Rheum* 1980;9:248.

Gaskin G, Clutterbuck E, Pusey C. Renal disease in the Churg-Strauss syndrome. Diagnosis, management, and outcome. *Contrib Nephrol* 1991;94:58.

Genereau T, Lortholary O, Guillevin L. Pathophysiology of viral vasculitis. *Pathol Biol* 1999;47:226.

Gonzalez-Gay MA, Garcia-Porrua C, Llorca J, et al. Visual manifestations of giant cell arteritis—trends and clinical spectrum in 161 patients. *Medicine* 2000;79:283.

Guillevin L, Durand-Gasselin B, Cevallos R, et al. Microscopic polyangitis—clinical and laboratory findings in eighty-five patients. *Arthritis Rheum* 1999;42:421.

Gur H, Tchakmakjian L, Eherenfeld M, et al. Polyarteritis nodosa: a report from Israel. *Am J Med Sci* 1999;317:238.

Hata A, Noda M, Moriwaki R, et al. Angiographic findings of Takayasu arteritis: new classification. *Int J Cardiol* 1996;54:S155.

Haynes B, Keiser-Kupfer M, Mason P, et al. Cogan's syndrome: studies in 13 patients, long-term follow-up, and review of the literature. *Medicine* 1980;59:426.

Hegab S, Al-Mutawa S. Immunopathogenesis of Behçet's disease. *Clin Immunol* 2000;96:174.

Hoffman GS. Takayasu arteritis: lessons from the American National Institutes of Health Experience. *Int J Cardiol* 1996;54:S99.

Hoffman GS, Kerr GS, Leavitt RY, et al. Wegener granulomatosis: an analysis of 158 patients [see comments]. *Ann Intern Med* 1992;116:488.

Hunder GG. Giant cell arteritis and polymyalgia rheumatica. *Med Clin North Am* 1997;81:195.

Jain S, Kumari S, Ganguly NK, et al. Current status of Takayasu arteritis in India. *Int J Cardiol* 1996;54:S111.

Jennette JC, Falk RJ. Medical progress: small-vessel vasculitis. *N Engl J Med* 1997; 337:1512.

Jover JA, Hernandez-Garcia C, Morado IC, et al. Combined treatment of giant-cell arteritis with methotrexate and prednisone—a randomized, double-blind, placebo-controlled trial. *Ann Intern Med* 2001;134:106.

Katz S, Gallin J, Hertz K, et al. Erythema elevatum diutinum: skin and systemic manifestations, immunologic studies, and successful treatment with dapsone. *Medicine* 1977;56:443.

Katz S, Borst M, Seekri I, et al. Surgical evaluation of Henoch-Schönlein purpura. Experience with 110 children. *Arch Surg* 1991;126:849.

Katzenstein ALA. Diagnostic features and differential diagnosis of Churg-Strauss syndrome in the lung—a review. *Am J Clin Pathol* 2000;114:767.

Kissel J, Mendell J. Vasculitic neuropathy. *Neurol Clin* 1992;10:761.

Klasa RJ, Abboud RT, Ballon HS, et al. Goodpasture's syndrome: recurrence after a five-year remission. Case report and review of the literature. *Am J Med* 1988;84:751.

Kobayashi M, Ito M, Nakagawa A, et al. Immunohistochemical analysis of arterial wall cellular infiltration in Buerger's disease (endarteritis obliterans). *J Vasc Surg* 1999;29:451.

Kone-Paut I, Yurdakul S, Bahabri SA, et al. Clinical features of Behçet's disease in children: an international collaborative study of 86 cases. *J Pediatr* 1998;132:721.

Lamprecht P, Gause A, Gross WL. Cryoglobulinemic vasculitis. *Arthritis Rheum* 1999; 42:2507.

Lanham J. Churg-Strauss syndrome. *Br J Hosp Med* 1992;47:667.

Lauque D, Cadranel J, Lazor R, et al. Microscopic polyangiitis with alveolar hemorrhage—a study of 29 cases and review of the literature. *Medicine* 2000;79:222.

Lee A, Nakagawa H, Nogita T, et al. Erythema elevatum diutinum: an ultrastructural case study. *J Cutan Pathol* 1989;16:211.

Leung D. Kawasaki disease. *Curr Opin Rheumatol* 1993;5:41.

Lie J. Systemic and isolated vasculitis. A rational approach to classification and pathologic diagnosis. *Pathol Annu* 1989;24:25.

Lie J. Cholesterol atheromatous embolism. The great masquerader revisited. *Pathol Annu* 1992;27:17.

Lie J. Vasculitis simulators and vasculitis look-alikes. *Curr Opin Rheum* 1992;4:47.

Martinez-Taboada VM, Blanco R, Garcia-Fuentes M, et al. Clinical features and outcome of 95 patients with hypersensitivity vasculitis. *Am J Med* 1997;102:186.

Mehregan D, Hall M, Gibson L. Urticarial vasculitis: a histopathologic and clinical review of 72 cases. *J Am Acad Dermatol* 1992;26:441.

Olin JW. Current concepts: thromboangiitis obliterans (Buerger's disease). *N Engl J Med* 2000;343:864.

Podder S, Shepherd RC. Cogan's syndrome: a rare systemic vasculitis. *Arch Dis Child* 1994;71:163.

Puechal X, Fiessinger JN, Kahan A, et al. Rheumatic manifestations in patients with thromboangiitis obliterans (Buerger's disease). *J Rheumatol* 1999;26:1764.

Rai A, Nast C, Adler S. Henoch-Schönlein purpura nephritis. *J Am Soc Nephrol* 1999; 10:2637.

Rottem M, Fauci AS, Hallahan CW, et al. Wegener granulomatosis in children and adolescents: clinical presentation and outcome. *J Pediatr* 1993;122:26.

Sakane T, Takeno M, Suzuki N, et al. Current concepts—Behçet's disease. *N Engl J Med* 1999;341:1284.

Saulsbury FT. Henoch-Schönlein purpura in children—report of 100 patients and review of the literature. *Medicine* 1999;78:395.

Savage C, Winearls C, Evans D, et al. Microscopic polyarteritis: presentation, pathology, and prognosis. *Q J Med* 1985;56:467.

Sharma BK, Jain S, Sagar S. Systemic manifestations of Takayasu arteritis: the expanding spectrum. *Int J Cardiol* 1996;54:S149.

Tohme A, El-Khoury I, Ghayad E. Behçet's disease: immunogenetic studies and therapeutic update. *Presse Med* 1999;28:1080.

Travers R, Allison D, Brettle R, et al. Polyarteritis nodosa: a clinical and angiographic analysis of 17 cases. *Semin Arthritis Rheum* 1979;8:184.

Wisnieski JJ. Urticarial vasculitis. *Curr Opin Rheumatol* 2000;12:24.

Yiannias J, El-Azhary R, Gibson L. Erythema elevatum diutinum: a clinical and histopathologic study of 13 patients. *J Am Acad Dermatol* 1992;26:38.

HEREDITARY FEVER SYNDROMES

Centola M, Aksentijevich I, Kastner DL. The hereditary periodic fever syndromes: molecular analysis of a new family of inflammatory diseases. *Hum Mol Genet* 1998;7:1581.

Frenkel J, Houten SM, Waterham HR, et al. Mevalonate kinase deficiency and Dutch type periodic fever. *Clin Exp Rheumatol* 2000;18:525.

Samuels J, Aksentijevich I, Torosyan Y, et al. Familial Mediterranean fever at the millennium: clinical spectrum, ancient mutations, and a survey of 100 Americans—referrals to the National Institutes of Health. *Medicine* 1998;77:268.

15. IMMUNOHEMATOLOGY

Lloyd E. Damon

Nearly all immune-mediated hematologic disorders are due to dysregulation of humoral immunity. Blood cells expressing surface or cytoplasmic antigens are the targets of these abnormal immunoglobulins, which may secondarily result in the activation, consumption, or inactivation of these cells.

I. **Blood cell antigens and agglutination**
  A. **Basic considerations.** An enormous number of antigens are present in blood components. Red cell blood groups contain close to 400 antigens; neutrophils and platelets share human leukocyte antigens (HLA) in addition to their own specific antigens; and plasma proteins are antigenically diverse. Aberrant immune reactivity to these antigens results in a wide variety of clinical disorders.
    1. **Agglutination** of red blood cells (RBCs) by antibody, a basic technique in immunohematology, has allowed definition of RBC antigens. The agglutination process is preceded by the coating of RBCs with antibody (**sensitization**), which is dependent on the concentrations of antigen and antibody as well as on the pH, temperature, and ionic strength of the reacting medium. Agglutination occurs when the **antibody** attached to the RBC overcomes the repelling force between two RBCs (caused by an ionic cloud of negative charges on the cell surface—the **zeta potential**). **Multimeric antibody** (e.g., immunoglobulin M [IgM], a large molecule with 10 binding sites) produces agglutination in a saline suspension. A monomeric antibody (e.g., IgG) cannot bridge the gap between two RBCs unless the zeta potential is reduced by suspending RBCs in a colloidal medium (i.e., bovine albumin) or by removing sialic acid residues from the RBC membrane with proteolytic enzymes (i.e., ficin, papain, bromelin, or trypsin). Agglutination also depends on **antigen availability** (number and location) on the RBC membrane. The common A and B antigens are glycoproteins on the RBC membrane, which easily bind anti-A or anti-B antibodies. However, many blood group antigens are proteins located within the RBC membrane. Enzyme treatment of the RBC can increase the accessibility of these antigens, notably the Rh antigens.
    2. The **antiglobulin test**, or **Coombs test**, is a practical application of the agglutination reaction.
      a. The **direct Coombs test** detects **antibody** or **complement** on the **RBC surface** in the following steps:
        (1) Antiglobulin serum (Coombs serum) is prepared by injecting human serum or purified human globulin into an animal (usually a rabbit). The antibody produced is purified to possess specificity against only one type of protein (e.g., anti-IgG or anticomplement).
        (2) Patient red cells are washed with saline to remove any trace amount of serum that could neutralize the antiglobulin and produce a false-negative result.
        (3) If antibody and/or complement is present on the RBC surface, the addition of antiglobulin serum will produce agglutination.
      b. The **indirect Coombs test detects antibody in the serum**. Patient serum is first incubated with a mixture of type O RBCs, and then the direct Coombs technique is used (as described in Direct Coombs test above)

   c. The following are diagnostic uses of the **direct antiglobulin** (Coombs) test:
     (1) Autoimmune hemolysis
     (2) Hemolytic disease of the newborn
     (3) Drug-induced hemolysis
     (4) Transfusion reactions
   d. The following are diagnostic uses of the **indirect antiglobulin** (Coombs) test:
     (1) Blood cross-matching
     (2) Alloantibody screening (including transfusion reactions)
     (3) RBC phenotyping (useful in genetic and forensic medicine, as well as to identify syngeneic twins for hematopoietic stem cell transplantation)
B. **Red cell antigens.** Antigens found on RBCs can be divided into two classes: **polysaccharide and protein antigens**. Polysaccharide antigens include the **ABO, MNSs, Ii, and P systems**; protein antigens include the **Rh, Kell, Kidd, and Duffy systems**.
   1. **Polysaccharide antigens** have the following characteristics:
     a. They usually elicit an IgM antibody response.
     b. They can stimulate **warm-reacting (37°C)** or **cold-reacting (4°C) antibodies**.
     c. They are responsible for isoantibodies, or **isoagglutinins**: type A blood has anti-B isoantibodies, type B blood has anti-A isoantibodies, type O blood has anti-A and anti-B isoantibodies, and type AB has neither.
     d. They can elicit antibodies causing **immediate** transfusion reactions.
   2. **Protein antigens** elicit primary **IgG warm antibodies** and, rarely, cold antibodies or isoantibodies. Transfusion reactions due to these antibodies are often of the **delayed** type.
C. **Platelet antigens.** Platelet antigens are primarily proteins that act either as receptors (platelet specific) or as integral components of the HLA system.
   1. **Glycoprotein antigens** are surface receptors involved in the following platelet actions:
     a. **Glycoprotein Ib/IX is the receptor for von Willebrand factor** (the ligand). Receptor–ligand binding results in platelet adhesion to endothelial surfaces.
     b. **Glycoprotein IIb/IIIa is the receptor for fibrinogen and collagen.** Receptor–ligand binding results in platelet–platelet aggregation.
   2. **Human leukocyte antigen proteins.** Platelets express both class I and II HLA antigens on their surface (see Chapter 16).
D. **Neutrophil antigens.** Neutrophils express both specific and shared antigens.
   1. **Neutrophil-specific antigens** are regulated at two independent genetic loci, called NA and NB.
   2. **Neutrophil-nonspecific antigens** include the HLA antigens and the 5b antigen (shared with red cells, lymphocytes, monocytes, eosinophils, platelets, spleen, and lymphoid tissues).
II. **Immunologic disorders of the erythrocyte**
A. The immune disorders of red cells result in **hemolysis**. Hemolysis is defined as shortened red cell survival (i.e., red cell life span less than 120 days). Hemolytic anemias result from an increased rate of RBC destruction due to either intracorpuscular defects or to extracorpuscular agents. Immune hemolysis is due to extracorpuscular agents (pathologic immunoglobulins) binding to red cell antigens (sensitization) resulting in early red cell destruction. **Isoimmune hemolysis** occurs when **alloantibodies** are the extracorpuscular agents. **Autoimmune hemolysis** occurs when **auto-**

antibodies are the extracorpuscular agents. **Other causes of hemolysis must be considered for effective diagnosis and management of a hemolytic disorder**, including: (i) congenital red cell membrane defects, (ii) secondary red cell membrane defects (mechanical red cell destruction, or **microangiopathy**), (iii) infections, (iv) congenital red cell metabolic and/or enzymatic defects, (v) hypersplenism, (vi) hemoglobinopathies, and (vii) thalassemias.

There are two major **mechanisms of red cell destruction** in the setting of immune hemolysis. The first is **cellular**, in which RBCs sensitized with IgG1 and IgG3 are susceptible to binding (via Fc receptors) and phagocytosis by macrophages within the reticuloendothelial system (spleen greater than liver). Partial phagocytosis results in the formation of **microspherocytes**, the hallmark morphologic feature of **extravascular hemolysis**. Complement fixed by immunoglobulin on the red cell surface, when converted to C3b, can result in binding (via the C3b receptor) and phagocytosis by macrophages. The strongest stimulus for phagocytosis occurs when IgG and C3b are both present on the red cell surface. Extravascular hemolysis is referred to as **warm** antibody-mediated hemolysis because the pathologic **IgG** binds its red cell antigens (usually Rh, but sometimes MNSs or glycophorin) most efficiently at 37°C.

The second mechanism of red cell destruction is **humoral**, in which **IgM** binds a red cell antigen (usually I or i). The pentameric structure of IgM has multiple C1-receptor binding sites in close proximity, thus favoring fixation of complement to the red cell surface. When the **membrane attack complex forms (C5 to C9)**, a transmembrane solute leak occurs; the red cell swells with water and lyses, thus RBC hemolysis is **intravascular**. Because IgM binding is most efficient at 4°C, this is also called **cold** antibody hemolysis. Rarely, IgG or IgA can cause this form of hemolysis. Table 15.1 compares the characteristics of warm and cold hemolysis.

The immune phenomena responsible for immune hemolysis are as follows:
1. Hapten (drugs)
2. Innocent bystander (infectious agents or drugs)
3. T-suppressor cell dysregulation (drugs)
4. Alterations in red cell antigens, which invoke a nonself immune response.
5. Red cell antigen similarity with nonself agents (infectious agents) invokes a nonself immune response.
6. Polyclonal or monoclonal B-cell dysregulation (usually associated with lymphoproliferative neoplasms, rheumatologic disorders, or idiopathic)

B. **Isoimmune major transfusion reactions.** The administration of ABO-incompatible blood results in an immediate, major transfusion reaction. The anti-A and anti-B isoagglutinins result in a cold-antibody, complement-mediated intravascular immune attack.

1. **Diagnosis.** The antibody–RBC reaction triggers the production of **anaphylatoxin** from activation of the complement system. There is intravascular hemolysis, resulting in the release of free hemoglobin into the plasma, the formation of methemalbumin (a brown pigment), and hemoglobinuria. Clinically, there is an acute onset of fever, chills, back pain, chest pain, shock, and renal failure. These symptoms can occur after a small amount of blood is infused. The majority of acute hemolytic reactions are due to ABO incompatibility resulting from **clerical error.** Thus, it is critical to label the cross-matched specimen properly and **check patient identification before blood is administered**.

A major transfusion reaction can be life threatening. Acute renal failure, disseminated intravascular coagulation, and cardiovascular collapse are complications of the intravascular hemolysis. The prognosis is related to the recipient's isoagglutinin titers and the volume of incompatible red cells infused.

Table 15.1. Characteristics of warm and cold autoimmune hemolytic anemias

	Warm (extravascular)	Cold (intravascular)
Primary Ig	IgG	IgM
RBC antigen	Rh	Ii
	MNSs,[a] glycophorin[a]	P in PCH[a]
Mediator of RBC destruction	Macrophage	Complement
Site of RBC destruction	Spleen > liver	Blood
DAT	IgG (+); C3 (±)	C3 (+)
IAT	IgG (+); C3 (±)	(−)
Associated illnesses	Idiopathic	Idiopathic
	Lymphoproliferative	Lymphoproliferative
	Disorders	Disorders
	Other neoplasms	Mycoplasma
	Rheumatic disorders	EBV
	Viral infections	Measles/mumps
	Drugs	Syphilis (PCH)
		Drugs
Treatment		
Corticosteroids	Yes	No
Folate	Yes	Yes
Splenectomy	Yes	No
Danazol	Yes	No
Cytotoxics	Yes	Yes
IVIg	Yes	No
Plasma exchange	Yes	Yes
Keep warm	No	Yes

[a] Rare causes of hemolysis.
Ig, immunoglobulin; Rh, rhesus factor; RBC, red blood cell; DAT, direct antiglobulin test; IAT, indirect antiglobulin test; EBV, Epstein-Barr virus; PCH, paroxysmal cold hemoglobulinuria; IVIg, intravenous immunoglobulin.

2. **Investigation of a transfusion reaction**
   a. When signs and symptoms of a transfusion reaction develop, **stop the transfusion immediately**.
   b. **Obtain a transfusion donor blood sample** (from the container) for **smear** and **culture** for bacteria. Similarly, culture a sample of blood from the **transfusion recipient** for bacteria.
   c. The unit of blood should not be discarded. Return the unit to the blood center with a sample of blood from the patient for a direct antiglobulin test, repeat ABO and Rh typing, repeat cross-matching, and screen for antibodies in the serum.
   d. Appropriate **blood chemistries** should be done to monitor renal function.

3. **Treatment of transfusion reactions**
   a. Treat **shock** with plasma expanders. Another unit of blood should be carefully cross-matched and transfused, with careful observation of the patient.
   b. With **acute intravascular hemolysis**, maintain an adequate urine output and consider **alkalinization** of the urine. (Hemoglobin is more soluble in alkaline than in acid urine.) Infusion of **mannitol** is recommended to maintain renal blood flow and glomerular filtration.

c. If **bacterial contamination** is highly suspected, **antimicrobials** should be initiated immediately.

d. Urticaria can be treated with **parenteral diphenhydramine**. As in the treatment of anaphylaxis, parenteral epinephrine and corticosteroids should be used if wheezing, laryngospasm, or hypotension is present (see Chapters 9 and 10).

C. **Alloimmune minor transfusion reactions.** Sensitization of red cells against foreign, minor, non-ABO red cell antigens results in an alloimmune response. The alloantibodies are IgG and result in a **delayed** extravascular hemolytic episode. Clinical hemolysis occurs 3 to 10 days after transfusion of the red cells. Symptoms are generally mild and include fatigue and dyspnea due to subacute anemia. Laboratory features show new anemia, microspherocytes on the blood smear, an elevated serum indirect bilirubin, and a low serum haptoglobin.

1. **Diagnosis.** Because this form of transfusion reaction is delayed, there is no offending blood sample remaining to examine for incompatibility as in an ABO-incompatible reaction. The recipient's blood should be sent to the laboratory to perform the indirect antiglobulin test on a wide array of standardized red cell antigens to screen for alloantibodies.

2. **Treatment.** This form of hemolysis is rarely severe enough to be life threatening; urine alkalinization and mannitol are rarely indicated. The hemolysis runs its course when the donor red cells are completely destroyed. Further red cell transfusions need to be red cells lacking the foreign antigen that invoked the alloimmune response.

D. **Autoimmune extravascular (warm) hemolysis.** Warm autoimmune hemolysis can be primary (55% of cases) or secondary to a lymphoproliferative neoplasm (20% have chronic lymphocytic leukemia, indolent non-Hodgkin lymphoma, Hodgkin disease, or other lymphoproliferative neoplasm), to drugs (20% of cases), or to rheumatologic disorders or viral infections (5% of cases). The clinical severity varies but can be **life threatening**. Mortality is less than 40% for patients with primary (idiopathic) disease; mortality in the secondary group reflects mostly the prognosis of the underlying disease.

1. **Clinical.** The onset of anemia is often insidious, with no associated symptoms unless there is an underlying disease. Severe hemolysis can occur causing fever, chills, nausea, vomiting, and pain in the abdomen, back, and chest. Jaundice can develop 24 hours later. Severe anemia can produce weakness, lethargy, and cardiac failure. The spleen may be palpable on physical examination.

2. **Diagnosis**

a. The complete blood count shows normochromic, normocytic anemia with increased polychromasia, nucleated red cells, spherocytes, and occasionally, fragmented red cells. Reticulocytosis is present, and if significant, can result in macrocytosis.

b. The urine may be positive for urobilinogen or blood (due to hemoglobinuria).

c. The **diagnostic test** is the direct antiglobulin test. Using specific antisera against immunoglobulin or complement, three patterns of red cell coating are identified: immunoglobulin alone (20% to 40%), immunoglobulin and complement (30% to 50%), and complement alone (30% to 50%). In 2% to 4% of patients with the clinical manifestations of autoimmune hemolytic anemia, the antiglobulin test may be negative. The **indirect antiglobulin test** is positive 60% of the time. By determining the reactivity pattern, it may help to exclude some diagnostic possibilities. For example, systemic lupus erythematosus as an associated illness is unlikely if RBCs are coated with IgG alone. **There is no correlation between the severity of the hemolysis and the degree of positivity of the antiglobulin test.**

    d. Antibody can be eluted from the surface of the RBC and tested for blood group specificity. If only IgG is involved, it usually reacts against antigen(s) of the Rh system. If the eluate contains a mixture of antibodies, specificity probably exists against multiple red cell antigens, making cross-matching for transfusion extremely difficult.

3. Therapy of autoimmune hemolytic anemia must be directed at correction of the underlying disease process, if present. In children, hemolysis is usually transient when secondary to viral infection. In all other cases, the natural course of the disease consists of periods of exacerbation resulting in severe anemia, which can be a medical emergency. The initial and chronic management of warm autoimmune hemolysis is as follows:

    a. Corticosteroids are the **drugs of choice**. Once the diagnosis of warm autoimmune hemolytic anemia is made, start prednisone, 1 to 2 mg/kg/day in divided doses. Higher doses of prednisone (4 to 6 mg/kg/day) for 3 to 5 days may be necessary for control of severe acute hemolysis. With improvement, reduce dosage slowly over a 3- to 4-month period to a dose that maintains remission. (Some patients require as small a dose of prednisone as 10 to 20 mg **every other day**, whereas others may require larger doses for prolonged periods). Two-thirds of patients respond to a full-dose, 3-week initial trial of corticosteroids.

    b. Splenectomy should be considered if the hemolysis is not responding to corticosteroids, or if high-dose corticosteroids (greater than 20 to 40 mg prednisone **daily**) are required to maintain a remission. There is no correlation between the antiglobulin reaction pattern and the response to splenectomy. Two-thirds of corticosteroid failures respond to splenectomy. Response means discontinuation or reduction of corticosteroids to low levels (prednisone, 5 to 10 mg per day or less).

    c. Cytotoxic agents should be considered when splenectomy fails to control hemolysis. **Cyclophosphamide**, 2 to 3 mg/kg/day orally, or **azathioprine**, 2.0 to 2.5 mg/kg/day orally, can be used alone or with corticosteroids. **White blood cell counts** should be monitored periodically.

    d. Transfusion with packed red cells should be given if hemolysis is rapid, resulting in severe anemia. Corticosteroids should be started simultaneously with the transfusion, because the benefits of blood transfusion are only transitory due to the subsequent destruction of transfused cells. It may be difficult to find compatible blood, especially with multiple transfusions, because alloantibodies are formed in addition to autoantibodies. This added sensitization can further complicate the cross-matching process.

    When transfusing such a patient, the blood bank should be notified that the patient has autoimmune hemolysis so that it can then release the "most compatible" blood rather than perfectly "compatible" blood. The latter is often not possible to obtain because the autoantibody interferes with the cross-matching indirect antiglobulin test.

    e. Folate. This vitamin, essential for erythropoiesis, is often depleted in the setting of chronic hemolysis. A dose of 1 mg per day is often adequate when hemolysis is controlled.

    f. Danazol, a semisynthetic androgen, results in hemolytic remission in up to two-thirds of corticosteroid failures. Its mode of action is unknown. The typical adult dose is 200 mg p.o. t.i.d.; responses usually take several months, ranging from 2 to 24 months.

    g. Cyclosporine (4 to 5 mg per kg p.o. b.i.d.) or **tacrolimus** (0.05 mg per kg p.o. b.i.d.) is showing promise in patients with warm autoimmune hemolysis refractory to other treatment modalities. These agents prevent T-cell activation, thus downregulating B-cell proliferation.

h. Rituximab is a chimeric murine–human monoclonal anti-CD20 antibody approved for use in relapsed or refractory low-grade non-Hodgkin lymphoma. Because of its specific anti-B-cell activity, it is now being explored in patients with refractory humoral autoimmune diseases and has shown activity in hemolysis. The lymphoma dose is 375 mg/m^2 intravenous once a week for 4 consecutive weeks.

i. Temporizing management. Exacerbations of warm autoimmune hemolysis are common. These can be managed as follows:

   (1) Corticosteroids. Reinitiation or an acute burst of corticosteroids will often control a hemolytic exacerbation.

   (2) Transfusion should be reserved for life- or organ-threatening anemia.

   (3) Intravenous gamma globulin (IVIg) (1 g per kg daily for 2 days) will sometimes quiet a hemolytic exacerbation. The mechanism of action is not entirely clear, but is likely related to blockade of the reticuloendothelial system and the passive infusion of antiidiotypic immunoglobulins.

   (4) Plasma exchange. Acute hemolytic episodes can be managed by large-volume plasma exchange. Removal of pathologic autoantibodies is the simplest explanation for response to this treatment, but other immune-modulatory events may be generated by plasma exchange. Generally, 1.5 to 2 plasma volumes (60 to 80 mL per kg) are removed and replaced with 5% albumin on an every-other-day schedule. This schedule allows the reequilibration of extravascular IgG into the intravascular compartment. Alternatively, **plasma immunoabsorption** can be performed, in which plasma is processed over a staphylococcal protein A column, which selectively depletes the plasma of IgG. This IgG-depleted plasma is then returned to the patient. The most important complication of immunoabsorption is an anaphylactic or anaphylactoid reaction, which primarily occurs in patients taking acetylcholine esterase inhibitors.

j. Table 15.2 outlines the chronic and temporizing management of warm and cold autoimmune hemolytic anemias.

Table 15.2. Treatment of autoimmune hemolysis: descending order of management

Warm	Cold
Chronic management	
Corticosteroids	Keep warm
Folate	Folate
Splenectomy	Cytotoxics
Danazol	
Cytotoxics	
Cyclosporine	
Rituximab	
Temporizing management	
Transfusions	Transfusions
Corticosteroids	Plasma exchange
Intravenous IgG	
Plasma exchange	

IgG, immunoglobulin G.

k. Other considerations

  (1) Secondary illnesses. When warm autoimmune hemolysis is due to lymphoproliferative malignancies or rheumatic diseases, then the treatment decisions must include therapy directed at these underlying diseases. Control of lymphoproliferative malignancies (i.e., chemotherapy) often results in remission of the hemolysis.

  (2) Hypercoagulable state. Patients with autoimmune hemolysis are often hypercoagulable. Because they have a higher incidence of thromboembolic disease than the general population, they should have thrombosis prophylaxis (e.g., heparin, antiembolism stockings) before and following elective surgery.

  (3) Gallstones. As with all chronic hemolytic disorders, patients with autoimmune hemolysis are prone to biliary pigment stones and choledocholithiasis.

  (4) Aplastic crises. Acute decreases in hemoglobin are not always hemolytic exacerbations. Viral infections (especially parvovirus) can suppress erythropoiesis and cause a rapid decrease in hemoglobin. The diagnosis is made by the documentation of an inappropriately normal or low reticulocyte count. Transfusions are necessary to support the patient through this transient illness. An infusion of intravenous gamma globulin (IVIg) may speed recovery of erythropoiesis if the aplastic crisis is due to parvovirus.

E. Cold autoimmune intravascular hemolysis. There are three major forms of cold autoimmune hemolysis. Over one-half of cases are primary (idiopathic), known as cold agglutinin disease. Just less than one-half are secondary to viral infections, infectious mononucleosis, malaria, mycoplasma pneumonia, or Waldenström macroglobulinemia (WM). The last form is termed paroxysmal cold hemoglobinuria.

  1. Cold agglutinins. Cold agglutinins, usually IgM or, rarely, a mixture of immunoglobulins, react optimally at lower temperature (4°C). They produce hemolysis by fixing complement to RBCs when the blood circulates to portions of the body exposed to cold ambient temperatures (the peripheral cutaneous microcirculation can normally reach 30°C). The thermal amplitude of the cold agglutinin determines whether the cold agglutinin causes clinical hemolysis. Cold agglutinins with wide thermal amplitudes stay bound to their red cell antigens as the blood returns to the warm core circulation. These warmer temperatures then facilitate complement fixation and red cell lysis. Cold agglutinins with narrow thermal amplitudes separate from their red cell antigens as the blood returns to the core circulation, thus complement is not then fixed. This latter scenario is typical of cold agglutinins associated with viral infections and mycoplasma pneumonia.

  a. Classification

    (1) More than half of the cases of cold agglutinin disease are classified as chronic idiopathic or chronic cold agglutinin disease. In this disorder, the cold antibody is monoclonal in origin, most often with κ light chains, has specificity against the I antigen of adult RBCs with titers greater than 1 : 1,000, and reacts over a wide temperature range, with substantial activity at 30° to 32°C (skin temperature).

    (2) Cold antibodies secondary to systemic disease are usually polyclonal, with low titers and a narrow thermal amplitude. IgM anti-I antibodies are associated with mycoplasma infection and some viral infections; anti-i antibodies are found in patients with infectious mononucleosis or lymphoreticular disease. Cold antibodies associated with WM macroglobulinemia or other lymphoproliferative neoplasms are monoclonal IgM molecules.

(3) Cold agglutinins can also be found in healthy persons. These antibodies are usually polyclonal, in low titers (less than 1:64), and have anti-I specificity.
   b. Cold agglutinins are not necessarily cryoglobulins. Cold agglutinins and cryoglobulins are often confused. Cold agglutinins are immunoglobulins that bind red cell antigens most efficiently at 4°C. Cryoglobulins are immunoglobulins that precipitate at low temperatures. Most cryoglobulins do not bind red cell antigens, although some do, and most cold agglutinins are not cryoglobulins. Cryoglobulins have the additional feature of being homo- or heterodymeric immunoglobulins.
2. Cold agglutinin disease. This condition is an idiopathic disorder primarily of elderly persons, more common in women than men. It produces a chronic hemolysis manifested by hemolytic exacerbations, especially when the patient is chilled.
   a. Clinical symptoms include a Raynaud-like phenomenon of the hands and feet (acrocyanosis, skin mottling, and numbness). The spleen may be enlarged. These symptoms are often worse in the winter, or during the summer if the patient is exposed to excessively cool air conditioning. Exacerbations of hemolysis result in typical intravascular hemolysis symptoms: fever, back pain, prostration, dyspnea, and red urine.
   b. Laboratory diagnosis
      (1) A complete blood count shows reduced hemoglobin and hematocrit, with polychromasia and rarely spherocytes on blood smear. If the blood smear was made at room temperature, RBC agglutination is seen. Agglutination is not present if the blood smear is made at 37°C. Erythrophagocytosis can occasionally be seen. Cold agglutinin disease should be suspected if a RBC count cannot be performed because of agglutination at room temperature.
      (2) The diagnostic test is to demonstrate the cold antibody in the serum. The direct Coombs test is often positive with anticomplement whether or not there is evidence of hemolysis. Collect blood in the following manner:
         (a) Draw blood into prewarmed syringes and into prewarmed tubes, and allow it to clot at 37°C.
         (b) Use an anticoagulant such as ethylenediaminetetraacetic acid (EDTA) to inhibit fixation of complement onto RBCs.
         (c) Titer the cold antibody at 4, 22, and 37°C to estimate the thermal amplitude of the reaction.
   c. Therapy. The chronic management of cold intravascular hemolysis is as follows:
      (1) Patients should avoid exposure to low temperatures. A warming coil should be used for transfusion of RBCs in patients whose antibodies show significant activity at low body temperatures.
      (2) Corticosteroids and splenectomy are not helpful (except in cases associated with lymphoproliferative neoplasms).
      (3) Cytotoxic agents, in particular, chlorambucil (2 to 4 mg per day) may be helpful. White blood cell counts should be monitored.
      (4) If blood transfusions are indicated because of severe anemia, the cross-matching should be done only after absorption of the cold antibody with the patient's own RBCs. This absorption allows detection of other alloantibodies. Blood warmers (37°C) should be used with these transfusions. The following precautions should be observed:

        (a) Do not allow an excessive length of tubing between the warmer and the intravenous needle to avoid repeat cooling of the blood.

        (b) The warmer should be well monitored because overheated RBCs are rapidly destroyed *in vivo* and can be lethal.

(5) Folate (1 mg per day) should be given because this vitamin is often depleted during chronic hemolysis.

(6) Rituximab is a chimeric murine–human monoclonal anti-CD20 antibody approved for use in relapsed or refractory low-grade non-Hodgkin lymphoma. Because of its specific anti-B-cell activity, it is now being explored in patients with refractory humoral autoimmune diseases and has shown activity in hemolysis. The lymphoma dose is 375 mg per m^2 intravenous once a week for 4 consecutive weeks.

(7) The **acute management** of exacerbations is as follows:

        (a) Keep the patient **warm**.

        (b) **Transfuse** as indicated.

        (c) **Therapeutic plasma exchange** can be used in extreme exacerbations to remove pathologic IgM and reduce ongoing hemolysis. About one and one-half to two plasma volumes (60 to 80 mL per kg) of plasma are removed every other day; protein and volume are replaced with 5% albumin. If for some reason it is necessary to replace with plasma, this plasma should be **decomplemented** because complement in fresh frozen plasma provokes further hemolysis *in vivo*. Finally, plasma exchange needs to be done in a room where the ambient temperature is as close to body temperature as reasonable. **The apheresis machine should be warmed up in the room** before beginning the procedure. The patient's blood running through a cold machine could induce more hemolysis. Because it is not easy for elderly patients to stay in warm rooms several hours at a time, they must be well hydrated.

        (d) See Table 15.2 for the chronic and acute management of cold intravascular hemolysis.

3. Secondary cold intravascular hemolysis. Cold intravascular hemolysis has been associated with a number of disease states, including **infection** (mycoplasma pneumonia, infectious mononucleosis, measles, mumps, and other viruses, trypanosomiasis, and malaria), **rheumatologic disorders** (rare), and **lymphoproliferative neoplasms** (indolent non-Hodgkin lymphoma, WM macroglobulinemia, and chronic lymphocytic leukemia), and Kaposi sarcoma.

    a. Therapy. The chronic and acute temporizing management of secondary cold intravascular hemolysis is the same as that for cold agglutinin disease except primary treatment of the associated illness is also necessary. **Many patients with these illnesses have cold agglutinins but do not hemolyze.**

4. Paroxysmal cold hemoglobinuria is a rare form of immunohemolytic anemia resulting from a biphasic reaction involving an IgG cold antibody, the **Donath-Landsteiner antibody**. In the first phase, IgG fixes complement onto the red cell at a low temperature. During the second phase, complement-mediated lysis occurs on rewarming of the cells to 37°C. The antibody has specificity against the P blood group antigen.

    a. Clinical presentation. This anemia, which is often associated with syphilis (particularly congenital syphilis), can also be a complication of viral infections such as measles, mumps, chickenpox, infectious mononucleosis, and "flu" syndromes. Exposure to cold produces pallor, hemoglobinuria, and other symptoms of hemolysis when the patient rewarms. The prognosis is good, because resolution is usually spontaneous. This disease rarely becomes chronic with intermittent episodes of hemolysis.

   b. Laboratory diagnosis is made by demonstrating the Donath-Landsteiner antibody. Mix patient serum with normal type O RBCs. Next, incubate the mixture at 4°C for 30 minutes (complement fixing) and then at 37°C for an additional 30 minutes (complement lysis). For a negative control, reverse the incubation conditions or use heat-inactivated serum (devoid of complement).

   c. Therapy. Patients should **avoid cold exposure**. Corticosteroids and splenectomy are not helpful. If blood transfusions are needed, use blood warmers. Treatment directed at the underlying associated illness is helpful (e.g., penicillin for syphilis).

F. Drug-mediated hemolytic anemias. Antibodies to drugs can interact with RBCs to produce hemolysis on an immune basis, accounting for approximately 20% of all cases of acquired immune hemolytic anemia.

  1. Four possible mechanisms have been proposed (Table 15.3):

    a. Immune complex (innocent bystander). Drug–antibody complexes attach to the RBC membrane **nonspecifically** and fix complement to produce hemolysis. The direct antiglobulin test is often positive for complement only; occasionally, IgG may be present. Antibodies in the serum may be demonstrated by incubating normal RBCs with the patient's serum in the **presence of complement and the suspected drug**. This immune complex mechanism is responsible for the majority of drug-induced hemolytic anemias (see Table 15.3). Small doses of a drug readministered after a latent period can produce acute intravascular hemolysis with hemoglobinemia, hemoglobinuria, and even renal failure.

    b. Hapten-type reactions (Gell and Coombs type II, cytotoxic antibody-mediated reactions [see Chapter 1]) result from a drug binding to the RBC membrane, becoming immunogenic, and stimulating antibody production (usually IgG). The direct antiglobulin

Table 15.3. Drugs commonly associated with hemolytic anemia

Immune complex (innocent bystander)
  Amino salicylic acid
  Chlorpromazine
  Isoniazid
  Phenacetin
  Quinidine
  Quinine
  Rifampin
  Stibophen
  Sulfonamides
  Thiazides

Hapten type
  Penicillin
  Cephalosporins
  Tetracycline

Aggregation of serum protein on red blood cell (RBC)
  Cephalosporins

Autoimmune type
  Levodopa
  Mefenamic acid
  Methyldopa

test is strongly positive for IgG. To demonstrate the antibody in the patient's serum, normal cells must be preincubated with the suspected drug before adding the patient's serum. A classic example of a hapten-type reaction is associated with high-dose penicillin therapy (greater than 10 million units per day). Although the direct antiglobulin test becomes positive in approximately 3% of these patients, hemolysis develops in only a few patients. The hemolysis produced is extravascular. The high titers of antipenicillin IgG present in these patients **do not correlate** with the presence or absence of IgE-mediated penicillin allergy (e.g., symptoms of urticaria, angioedema, or anaphylaxis).

   c. **Red blood cell membrane alteration with nonspecific adsorption** of aggregates of normal serum protein (IgG and complement) can produce a positive direct antiglobulin test. No reaction occurs if the patient's serum is mixed with normal RBCs. A variety of antibiotics, including the cephalosporins, can produce this reaction, although reports of hemolytic anemia are rare.

   d. An **autoimmune** type of reaction results when a drug stimulates production of antibodies (with Rh specificity), which then react with RBCs. These drugs appear to down-regulate a T-suppressor clone allowing the clonal expansion of a B-cell population that produces the offending IgG. The direct antiglobulin test is positive for IgG. Incubation of the patient's serum with normal RBCs **without a drug** leads to IgG coating of the RBCs (i.e., a positive indirect antiglobulin test). Drugs implicated in this reaction are alpha-methyldopa, levodopa, and mefenamic acid. The direct antiglobulin test becomes positive in approximately 15% of patients receiving alpha-methyldopa, but less than 1% of the patients will have hemolysis. The incidence of a positive direct antiglobulin test appears to be dose related. Anemia usually develops gradually after several months of treatment; intravascular hemolysis has not been reported.

2. **Therapy. The first and most important step in the treatment of any drug-mediated hemolytic reaction is to stop the offending drug.** In reactions of the immune complex type, prompt recovery occurs unless renal failure has developed. In autoimmune-type reactions, clinical recovery may take several weeks. The antiglobulin test can remain positive for 1 to 2 years.

G. **Neonatal immunohemolytic anemias.** There are two major forms of neonatal immune hemolysis invoked by the passage of maternal IgG into the fetal circulation: one is directed against Rh antigens (erythroblastosis fetalis) and the other is directed against A or B antigens.

   1. **Erythroblastosis fetalis.** Blood group incompatibility between mother and infant can produce hemolytic disease in the fetus and newborn infant. Severe anemia may lead to congestive heart failure in the fetus, resulting in **hydrops fetalis**. In all instances except ABO incompatibility, the mother must have been previously sensitized by the blood group antigen she lacks in order to produce specific antibody. During normal pregnancy, the amounts of fetal RBCs that enter the maternal circulation are insufficient to stimulate antibody production. However, during the third stage of labor, as much as 1 mL of fetal blood can enter the maternal circulation with resulting maternal immunization. Hemolytic disease of the newborn due to blood group incompatibility is unusual with the first pregnancy unless the mother has been previously transfused or sensitized as a result of abortion or amniocentesis. (In ABO incompatibility, in which anti-A and anti-B antibodies are naturally present, the first child can be affected by the placental transfer of these naturally occurring isoantibodies.) The most common cause of erythroblastosis is the D antigen of the Rh system (CDE/cde). Approximately

15% of white persons and 7% of black persons lack the D antigen and are termed Rh negative. Other antigens that may be implicated include c (rh or Rh4), E (rh or Rh3), Kell (K1), Duffy, and M, S, and U of the MNSs system.

a. Clinical presentation in the fetus. Hemolysis and anemia occur in the fetus and, in severe cases, lead to heart failure and hydropic stillbirth. Hyperbilirubinemia does not occur *in utero* because bilirubin is freely transported across the placenta into the maternal circulation. **In the newborn infant,** the major problem is hyperbilirubinemia, which can lead to kernicterus and brain damage. Hepatosplenomegaly can be present. The differential diagnosis includes neonatal hepatitis, infection, metabolic disorders, and hemorrhage.

b. Diagnosis

  (1) Early in the pregnancy, a prenatal maternal ABO and Rh blood type should be determined and the serum screened for unusual blood group antibodies. If the mother is Rh-negative, the probable Rh genotype of the father is determined. The anti-D titer in maternal serum should be monitored periodically to detect sensitization.

  (2) In sensitized mothers, amniocentesis and spectrophotometric analysis of amniotic fluid are more reliable means to assess the severity of the disease than the maternal anti-D titers.

  (3) At birth, the hemoglobin and serum bilirubin levels of the cord blood in a known case of blood group incompatibility should be immediately determined.

  (4) Perform the direct antiglobulin test with the infant's RBCs. If the antiglobulin test is positive, the specificity of the eluate from the infant's cells should be determined. If this specificity does not correspond to that of the maternal antibody, further evaluation of the cause of the positive direct antiglobulin test is necessary.

c. Prenatal therapy. Early, aggressive **prenatal** therapy can lead to decreased morbidity and mortality in the newborn infant. The following guidelines should be used:

  (1) When the titer of anti-D antibody exceeds 1:8 in the mother, amniocentesis is performed. The optical density of the amniotic fluid is measured at 450 μ as an indirect measure of bilirubin. This determination reflects the severity of hemolysis.

  (2) A high optical density (based on standard nomograms) of amniotic fluid in mid- to late gestation indicates severe hemolysis in the fetus. This is an indication to perform perumbilical cord vein blood sampling (PUBS) via ultrasound guidance. An umbilical vein hematocrit less than 18% should prompt the transfusion of type O Rh-negative RBCs into the umbilical vein (to be repeated at 2- to 3-week intervals as determined by repeat PUBS). The production of RBCs by the fetus may be partially or completely suppressed after repeated transfusions.

  (3) The fetus can be delivered by cesarean section when the gestation weight is estimated to be adequate (around 33 to 36 weeks).

  (4) Determine the infant's blood type and the direct antiglobulin test immediately after delivery. (A successful intrauterine transfusion may result in an Rh-negative typing in the infant.)

  (5) Infants with a positive direct antiglobulin test at birth will probably require subsequent exchange transfusions.

d. Postnatal therapy. Postnatally, hyperbilirubinemia must be treated with phototherapy, and if necessary, with exchange transfusions.

(1) **Phototherapy** (blue light that decomposes bilirubin to water-soluble products) can be used with caution as an **adjunct** to exchange transfusion (either before or after transfusion), but **should not be substituted for a complete diagnostic evaluation** of the cause of jaundice. During phototherapy, serum bilirubin monitoring is essential because the infant may not appear to be jaundiced, but can still have severe hemolysis. Protect the eyes of the infant with bandages to prevent retinal damage.

(2) **Exchange transfusions**
  (a) **Indications for exchange transfusion** after delivery include:
      (i) Hydrops of the neonate (congestive heart failure with anasarca). To correct the anemia, exchange of the patient's blood volume (equal to 0.5 to 1.0 blood volume) should be performed using packed RBCs.
      (ii) A bilirubin greater than 20 mg per dL for term infants and 12 to 16 mg per dL for premature infants. Twice the patient's blood volume should be exchanged with whole blood.

(3) **Packed red blood cell transfusions** may be necessary after intrauterine transfusions or exchange transfusions to correct anemia (hemoglobin less than 7 to 10 g per dL). Sometimes, anti-D-coated cells are slowly removed from the circulation, and 3 to 6 weeks after birth, a late anemia rather than hyperbilirubinemia may occur.

(4) **Passive immunization of the mother.** The incidence of Rh sensitization is markedly reduced if anti-D immunoglobulin (RhoGAM) is given to an Rh-negative mother. This is given at the end of the second trimester and again within 72 hours of delivery of an Rh-positive baby. Also, give RhoGAM following abortion or amniocentesis in which fetal cells can enter the maternal circulation. One ampule of anti-D (300 µg) is capable of "neutralizing" about 15 mL of blood containing D-positive cells. Higher doses are necessary if greater fetal–maternal bleeding is suspected and confirmed by staining for fetal RBCs in the mother's blood (Betke method).

2. **ABO incompatibility.** Hemolytic disease due to ABO incompatibility is usually seen in infants with blood-type A, B, or AB with blood-type O mothers who have naturally occurring isoagglutinins (anti-A and anti-B antibodies) in their serum. Prenatal diagnosis is not possible. A high maternal titer of anti-A or anti-B is not predictive of ABO hemolytic disease in the newborn.
  a. **Clinical picture.** The first pregnancy can be affected. In the full-term infant, severe anemia and hydrops fetalis are rare. In some infants, jaundice can develop on the first day of life, but hemolysis is not as severe as in Rh incompatibility. As is the case with Rh incompatibility, **other causes of hyperbilirubinemia must be excluded.**
  b. **Diagnosis**
      (1) The blood smear shows spherocytes and, occasionally, fragmented cells (ABO hemolytic disease may be difficult to differentiate from hereditary spherocytosis).
      (2) A direct antiglobulin test on the infant's RBCs is usually negative or weakly positive because of the small number of A or B antigenic sites on fetal RBCs and the relative insensitivity of the current manual method of performing the direct antiglobulin test. Eluates from the infant's RBCs react normally against adult A or B cells.

c. **Therapy** for ABO incompatibility is directed toward reduction of hyperbilirubinemia. The use of phototherapy, with close monitoring of bilirubin levels, has reduced the need for exchange transfusions, and the latter procedure is necessary in fewer than 1 in 3,000 infants with ABO incompatibility. Low-titer (of anti-A and anti-B) type O blood is used.

III. **Immunologic disorders of platelets.** Immune destruction of platelets can occur in a manner similar to that in immunohemolytic anemia, although less is known about the immunology of specific antiplatelet antibodies. Demonstration of antiplatelet antibodies is difficult. Methods of demonstrating platelet antibodies include agglutination, complement fixation, consumption of antiglobulin, platelet lysis, inhibition of clot retraction, release of platelet factor 3 or serotonin, and immunofluorescence. The complement fixation and antiglobulin consumption techniques usually give more consistent results than the other methods. Immune-mediated mechanisms are responsible for acute idiopathic thrombocytopenic purpura, chronic idiopathic thrombocytopenic purpura, isoimmune neonatal thrombocytopenia, and some forms of drug-induced thrombocytopenia.

A. **Acute immune thrombocytopenic purpura** is predominantly a disease in children between the ages of 2 and 6 years. The majority of children have a history of antecedent febrile illness, with or without a viral exanthem, days or weeks before the onset of purpura. Immunization with live virus vaccines can also be associated with acute immune thrombocytopenic purpura (ITP). The bleeding manifestations are usually cutaneous, with sudden onset of widespread petechiae and bruising. Epistaxis, hematuria, oozing from the gums, and gastrointestinal bleeding can occur, usually within the first week of illness. Intracranial bleeding is rare and is commonly associated with bleeding from mucosal surfaces. Mild splenomegaly (palpable spleen tip) is present in 5% to 10% of the children with acute ITP.

1. **Diagnosis.** Acute ITP is diagnosed by exclusion of other disorders.

a. The **complete blood count** is usually normal except for thrombocytopenia. Occasionally, mild eosinophilia or atypical lymphocytes are present.

b. **Bone marrow examination** shows no specific diagnostic features. The number of megakaryocytes may be normal or increased. Eosinophilic myeloid precursors may or may not be increased. With the typical history of onset of the illness and absence of abnormal white blood cells on the blood smear, the diagnosis of ITP can often be made on clinical grounds without a bone marrow examination. However, bone marrow examination may be appropriate to exclude other causes of thrombocytopenia, if treatment with corticosteroids or splenectomy is considered or if the diagnosis is not certain.

2. **Therapy**

a. **General treatment measures** for acute ITP include avoidance of trauma, especially to the head, and avoidance of intramuscular injections, which can cause painful hematomas or even blood loss. Drugs that inhibit platelet aggregation (e.g., salicylates and nonsteroidal antiinflammatory agents) should be withheld, and enemas, hard toothbrushes, and abrasive foods should be avoided.

b. **Bleeding is most severe during the first week.** During this time it may be necessary to observe the child in the hospital.

c. Corticosteroid therapy for acute ITP is controversial. There is no consensus of opinion as to the dose or duration of corticosteroid use. Corticosteroid treatment does not accelerate the rate of recovery or influence the prognosis. However, an increase in platelet count may be seen as a result of blocking the ability of the reticuloendothelial system to remove antibody-coated platelets. Generally, prednisone 1 to 2 mg/kg/day, is used in patients with bleeding from the mucosal surfaces because of the potential risk of intracranial hemorrhage. Another consideration to use prednisone is the activity of the child. It is impractical, if not impossible, to observe constantly an active youngster, and this may prompt the use of corticosteroids to acutely elevate the platelet count. It may be advisable to use low doses of corticosteroids, such as an alternate-day prednisone regimen, to minimize the side effects from prolonged corticosteroid treatment.

   d. The use of high-dose intravenous gamma globulin (1 gm/kg/day for 2 days) can be used in patients with acute ITP in whom corticosteroid therapy is contraindicated or in patients with chronic ITP who are unresponsive to corticosteroid therapy. The response to intravenous gamma globulin is variable.

   e. Platelet transfusion is rarely indicted—the survival of transfused platelets is very short.

   f. If there is persistent or increased mucosal bleeding, **emergency splenectomy** is recommended. The result is often satisfactory, with a return of normal platelet count in 1 to 3 days in the majority of patients.

   g. The child may return to normal activity when clinical signs of bleeding subside, even if the platelet count has not returned to normal. Body-contact sports, riding bicycles, or climbing heights should be avoided until the platelet count becomes normal.

   3. Prognosis. The disease is self-limiting in the majority of patients. About 50% of children with ITP recover within 4 weeks; 85% recover within 4 months. The remaining patients recover spontaneously within a year; in a few instances, after several years. Recovery is usually permanent, although the disease may recur in a small number of children following a viral infection or live virus vaccine. Patients with persistent thrombocytopenia for longer than a year are considered to have the chronic form of ITP.

B. Chronic immune thrombocytopenic purpura (ITP) is predominantly seen in adults and older children, with a slightly greater incidence in young women. The onset is insidious, and a history of antecedent infection is rarely obtained.

   1. The diagnosis of chronic ITP is made by exclusion of other causes of chronic isolated thrombocytopenia, such as thrombocytopenia associated with bone marrow disease, systemic lupus erythematosus, drug-induced thrombocytopenia, transfusion-associated purpura, or thrombocytopenia secondary to other miscellaneous causes including the human immunodeficiency virus (HIV). Bone marrow examination is sometimes necessary to exclude other causes of ITP.

   2. Therapy (chronic management)

      a. Corticosteroids are often given initially (prednisone, 1 to 2 mg/kg/day) with a response expected after 1 to 2 weeks. If there is no improvement after 3 to 4 weeks, splenectomy is the treatment of choice. **Splenectomy** results in improvement in 70% to 90% of patients and produces long-term adequate (greater than 50,000 per μL) platelet counts in two-thirds. No reliable method of predicting the response to splenectomy is available.

      b. Danazol, a semisynthetic androgen, can be tried in patients failing corticosteroids and splenectomy. The usual dose is 200 mg orally t.i.d. It is often several months before a response is seen. Some hematologists use danazol following primary corticosteroid failure in an attempt to avoid splenectomy.

      c. For splenectomy and danazol failures, correction of thrombocytopenia may be possible with corticosteroids or other **immunosuppressive treatment. Vincristine** can be given intravenously every 7 to 10 days at 0.025 to 0.03 mg per kg, with a maximal single dose of 2 mg. Alternatively, **vinblastine** (0.1 to 0.2 mg per kg) can be given as an intravenous bolus injection or infusion over 4 to 6 hours every 7 to 10 days. **Azathioprine** (2.0 to 2.5 mg/kg/day orally) can also be tried. These immunosuppressive measures should be tried if there is a contraindication for splenectomy in those patients failing corticosteroid therapy.

    d. A small number of ITP patients refractory to all of the above treatments have responded to twice daily oral **cyclosporine**. Doses (5 to 6 mg per kg b.i.d.) are adjusted to deliver therapeutic trough blood levels of 50 to 400 ng/mL.

    e. **Immunoabsorption** has been used to treat refractory ITP. Two liters of plasma are processed over a staphylococcal protein A column every other day for six treatments. Approximately one-half of otherwise refractory ITP patients (including HIV-infected patients) respond to this treatment, which can last 2 to 6 months. This suggests ongoing **secondary immune modulatory events** as a result of the apheresis procedure. The stimulation of antiidiotypic antibodies and uncoupling of immune complexes have been demonstrated following immunoabsorption. **Plasma exchange** (40 to 60 mL per kg) can also be performed (instead of immunoabsorption) every other day for six treatments. Five percent albumin is used as plasma replacement. It is not clear whether immunoabsorption is superior to plasma exchange as treatment for chronic ITP.

    f. **Rituximab** is an investigational treatment for chronic ITP. Rituximab is a chimeric murine–human monoclonal antibody directed against the B-cell-specific antigen, CD20. It is approved for use as therapy for relapsed or refractory low-grade non-Hodgkin lymphoma. Four weekly doses of intravenous Rituximab (375 mg/m^2/dose) results in no detectable circulating B cells for 6 months. Preliminary results suggest activity in refractory chronic ITP.

    g. For patients with refractory ITP with a **cyclic component** to their illness (fluctuating platelet counts), **lithium carbonate** (300 mg orally t.i.d.) sometimes dampens the fluctuations and increases low platelet counts.

3. Therapy (acute bleeding)

    a. The acute bleeding of ITP can sometimes be controlled by a burst of **corticosteroids**. Corticosteroids are believed to diminish bleeding acutely, before the platelet count rises, by tightening capillary junctions.

    b. **Intravenous immunoglobulin.** IVIg provides the fastest means of increasing the platelet count. A dose of 1 g per kg is given once a day for 2 consecutive days. The platelet count reliably rises in 24 to 48 hours and responses last a week or more in some patients. The response to IVIg is sometimes used as a **diagnostic test** in patients for whom the diagnosis of ITP is uncertain. IVIg is believed to work via reticuloendothelial blockade, the passive administration of antiidiotypic antibodies, and a shift toward accelerated clearance of pathologic autoantibodies over normal antibodies.

    c. **Platelet transfusions** can help the acute bleeding of chronic ITP. Allogeneic platelets are subject to the same pathologic immunoglobulins and consumptive forces as autologous platelets. These should be reserved for severe or life-threatening bleeding.

C. Isoimmune neonatal thrombocytopenia. Destruction of fetal platelets by maternal antibodies can occur in a manner similar to that in Rh incompatibility. The PlA1 (Zwa) platelet antigen accounts for the majority of the cases of isoimmune neonatal thrombocytopenia. In contrast to Rh incompatibility, firstborn infants are affected in approximately 50% of the cases. Bleeding manifestations, which start shortly after delivery, range from petechiae and bruises to gastrointestinal or intracranial hemorrhage.

1. **Diagnosis.** Serologic incompatibility between maternal serum and fetal or paternal platelets can be demonstrated with the techniques of platelet antibody detection (paternal platelets are more readily obtainable for study than those of the infant). Other causes of neonatal thrombocytopenia must be excluded: infection, hemangioma, congenital absence of megakaryocytes, maternal ITP, and maternal drug therapy (e.g., thiazides).

2. **Therapy.** The disease is self-limiting, with recovery of normal platelets within a few days or up to 2 months, when maternal antibodies disappear. If there is active bleeding, the following treatment should be considered:

   a. Random donor platelet transfusion may not be effective because the PlA1 antigen occurs in 98% of the population. **Administration of washed maternal platelets** is the treatment of choice to stop bleeding.

   b. **Exchange transfusion** may be performed to remove antibodies. This is followed by platelet transfusion. Potential complications of exchange transfusions are listed in Table 15.4.

   c. **Prednisone**, 1 mg/kg/day, may be tried to decrease the rate of platelet destruction.

D. **Drug-induced thrombocytopenia.** The immune complex mechanism is the most frequent cause of immune destruction of platelets (innocent bystander). The antibody in the patient's serum reacts with platelets only in the presence of the drug. Occasionally, the drug binds directly to platelets to form a primary antigen (hapten carrier), which then reacts with the antibody. Drugs associated with thrombocytopenia on an immune basis with a high degree of probability are listed in Table 15.5.

   1. **Clinical presentation.** Bleeding manifestations (petechiae, purpura, and bleeding from the gastrointestinal and urinary tracts) appear within days to weeks after beginning administration of the offending drug. The duration of symptoms depends on the rate of excretion of the drug. After the drug is stopped, the platelet count usually returns to normal in approximately 5 to 7 days. The one exception is ITP due to **gold**, in which platelet recovery takes months. Major bleeding occurs in 9% of individuals and fatal bleeding occurs in 0.8% of individuals.

   2. The **diagnosis** is often difficult to confirm by *in vitro* demonstration of specific antibodies against suspected drugs. The diagnosis is usually made by temporal correlation of drug administration and resulting thrombocytopenia and the resultant normalization of the platelet count following discontinuation of the drug.

Table 15.4. Complications of exchange transfusions

Bleeding
  Overheparinization of donor blood
  Thrombocytopenia
  Perforation of umbilical vein
Cardiac
  Heart failure due to hypervolemia or transfusion overload
  Cardiac arrest due to hyperkalemia, hypocalcemia, and/or citrate toxicity
Embolism and thrombosis
  Air emboli
  Portal vein thrombosis
Infection
  Bacterial sepsis
  Viral infections from donor blood
  Necrotizing enterocolitis

Table 15.5. Drugs associated with platelet destruction

Acetaminophen	Difluormethylornithine	Oxprenolol
Acetazolamide	Digitoxin	Oxyphenbutazone
Alprenolol	Ethambutol	Oxytetracycline
Amiodarone	Fluconazole	Phenylbutazone
Aminoglutethimide	Glibenclamide	Phenytoin
Aminosalicylic acid	Gold salts	Piperacillin
Amphotericin B	Haloperidol	Procainamide
Ampicillin	Heparin	Quinine
Amrinone	Hydantoins	Quinidine
Captopril	Ibuprofen	Ranitidine
Carbamazepine	Interferon-α	Rifampin
Cephalothin	Isoniazid	Sulfamethoxazole
Chlorothiazide	Levamisole	Sulfasalazine
Chlorpromazine	Levodopa	Sulfisoxazole
Chlorpropamide	Lithium	Sulindac
Chlorthalidone	Meclofenamate	Sulfonylureas
Cimetidine	Methicillin	Tamoxifen
Danazol	Methyldopa	Thiazide diuretics
Desferoxamine	Minoxidil	Thiothixene
Diaoxide	Nalidixic acid	Tolmetin
Diazepam	Naphazoline	Trimethoprim
Diclofenac	Nitroglycerine	Vanionycin
Diethylstilbesterol	Novobiocin	

3. Therapy

   a. Observe the general measures of the management of thrombocytopenia.

   b. **Stop all nonessential drugs.** Avoid related compounds and known antiplatelet medications.

   c. Platelet transfusions are minimally effective because transfused platelets are similarly affected. Platelet transfusions should be given in the setting of severe or life-threatening bleeding.

   d. It is essential to avoid reexposure to the drug.

   e. Corticosteroids and IVIg do not reliably help this problem, but can be considered in extreme cases.

E. Heparin-induced thrombocytopenia

Heparin-induced thrombocytopenia (HIT) is a limb- and life-threatening complication of heparin therapy. HIT occurs in 3% of patients receiving unfractionated heparin, making this the most common form of drug-induced thrombocytopenia. The major clinical consequence is thrombosis, not bleeding. There are two types of HIT: type I is nonimmune in nature and of no clinical significance. Type II is due to the development of antibodies directed against the complex of heparin and platelet factor 4 (PF4). PF4 is a chemokine derived from the α granules of platelets. The immune complex of Ig–heparin–PF4 is taken up by the platelet FcγRIIa receptor, resulting in platelet activation, consumption, and prothrombocytopenia. Activated platelets release more PF4 and prothrombotic platelet microparticles. PF4 attaches to endothelial cell heparan sulfate, to which the HIT antibody also binds. Thrombin generation is enhanced on the activated endothelial surface. The net result of this cascade of events is thrombosis. Thrombi are rich in platelets relative to fibrin, giving the gross description of the "white thrombus."

   ### 1. Clinical presentation

      a. **Heparin-induced thrombocytopenia type I.** This is a nonimmune thrombocytopenia that occurs in nearly 30% of patients receiving therapeutic doses of unfractionated or low molecular weight heparin. The thrombocytopenia occurs in the first four days of heparin use, is mild, and resolves with continued heparin administration. There are no clinical consequences of this phenomenon.

b. Heparin-induced thrombocytopenia type II. In patients with their first exposure to heparin, a decrease in platelet count tends to occur in the sixth to ninth day of heparin administration. The platelet nadir is modest (median 50,000 to 70,000 per µL) in contrast to other drug-induced thrombocytopenias in which the platelet nadir is severe (usually less than 20,000 per µL). In some patients, there is a significant (greater than 50%) decrease in platelet count, but not to a level below the lower limit of normal. HIT type II can occur with any dose of heparin (intravenous flushes, low-dose prophylaxis, or therapeutic doses), and is more common with porcine-derived than bovine-derived heparin and more common with unfractionated heparin than low molecular weight heparin.

The thrombocytopenia persists as long as heparin is continued. The major clinical consequence of HIT type II is thrombosis (the rate of venous to arterial thrombosis is 4 to 1). Venous thromboembolic complications include deep venous thrombosis, pulmonary embolism, warfarin (Coumadin)-associated venous limb gangrene, cerebral sinus thrombosis, and adrenal gland hemorrhagic infarction. Arterial thromoembolic complications include lower limb thromboses, stroke, transient ischemic attacks, acute coronary syndromes (including myocardial infarction), and thrombosis of other major arteries (aorta, mesenteric, renal, etc.). One-half of patients with HIT type II develop an adverse event, including death, new thrombosis, major hemorrhage, or limb amputation.

2. Diagnosis

The diagnosis of HIT type II is generally based on the timing of the onset of thrombocytopenia, the degree of thrombocytopenia, the absence of an alternative explanation, and/or the new onset in some cases of thromboembolism, as described above. A highly sensitive and specific confirmatory test is the ^{14}C–serotonin release assay (SRA). A positive test occurs when serum containing HIT antibodies is incubated with donor radiolabeled platelets in the presence of heparin, resulting in platelet activation and ^{14}C–serotonin release. A sensitive, but less specific test is enzyme-linked immunosorbent assay (ELISA) based and it detects the binding of HIT antibodies to a well containing a heparin–PF4 complex. Because a positive SRA and/or ELISA does not necessarily mean clinical thrombocytopenia and/or thrombosis, these are not practical screening tests. Their main importance is in confirming HIT in an individual who may need continued anticoagulation or may need heparin-based anticoagulation in the future.

3. Therapy

a. Stop the heparin! It takes an average of 4 days for the platelet count to return to normal.

b. Continue the warfarin. Most patients are taking heparin while awaiting therapeutic anticoagulation with warfarin. As proteins C and S (vitamin-K-dependent) decrease at about the same rate as factor VII, but before factors II, IX, and X, patients are paradoxically hypercoagulable during early warfarinization before factors II, IX, and X decrease. This, plus the hypercoagulability of HIT as previously described, means that another type of anticoagulation is needed early in the HIT type II syndrome.

c. Danaparoid sodium. Danaparoid sodium (Orgaran) is a low molecular weight glycosaminoglycan comprised of 84% low molecular weight heparan sulfate, 12% dermatan sulfate, and 4% chondroitin sulfate. It functions as an inhibitor of factor Xa mediated via antithrombin III. Only 6% of patients with HIT type II will cross-react with danaparoid. For most HIT type II indications, the dose is 1,250 anti-Xa units subcutaneous twice a day. Danaparoid can be used in patients with renal failure without dose adjustment. Danaparoid has been shown to decrease death, new thromboembolism, and limb amputation in the setting of HIT type II.

   d. Hirudin. Recombinant hirudin (Lepirudin, Refludan) is a direct thrombin (factor IIa) inhibitor. Because of predominant renal excretion, it must be used with caution in renal failure patients. For most HIT type II indications, the dose is 0.1 to 0.15 mg/kg/day of intravenous Lepirudin. The dose is adjusted to achieve an activated partial thromboplastin time (APTT) ratio of 1.5 to 3.0 compared to the baseline of aPTT. Forty percent of HIT patients develop an anti-Lepirudin antibody, which paradoxically enhances its anticoagulation effect and requires a 60% average decrease in dose. Lepirudin has been shown in HIT type II patients to decrease death, new thromboembolism, and limb amputation.

   e. Intravenous gamma globulin. Intravenous IgG presumably contains antiidiotypic HIT antibodies and speeds the recovery of the platelet count to normal. Intravenous IgG may be useful in facilitating recovery from HIT type II in conjunction with other anticoagulants such as danaparoid sodium or Lepirudin.

   f. Plasma exchange. Plasma exchange will acutely reduce HIT antibodies and cooperate with other anticoagulants such as Danaparoid Sodium or Lepirudin.

F. Post-transfusion purpura

1. **Clinical presentation.** Post-transfusion purpura (PTP) is a rare immunologic complication of **red cell transfusion therapy**. The clinical presentation is the sudden development of severe thrombocytopenia and mucocutaneous bleeding 7 to 10 days following a red cell transfusion. There is no specific diagnostic test except the temporal relationship between the transfusion and thrombocytopenia. PTP is much more common in multiparous women and patients who have been multiply transfused as opposed to nulliparous women or patients receiving a first transfusion. The pathophysiology resembles that of isoimmune neonatal thrombocytopenia. All PTP patients are lacking the platelet PlA1 antigen (now known to be a subcomponent of the glycoprotein IIb/IIIa complex). Exposure of these patients to red cells contaminated with PlA1-positive platelets results in an antibody response to this foreign antigen. The pathologic immunoglobulin presumably reacts with the remaining intact portion of the IIb/IIIa complex, leading to platelet consumption.

2. **Therapy**

   a. Platelet transfusions rarely help and the platelets must be PlA1-negative. Only 2% of the population is PlA1-negative.

   b. Corticosteroids (e.g., prednisone 1 to 2 mg/kg/day orally) may decrease bleeding and improve the platelet count.

   c. This illness generally runs its course when antigenic stimulation is removed.

   d. Further transfusions must be from PlA1-negative donors.

IV. Immunologic disorders of the neutrophil. Studies of immune destruction of the neutrophil have been few until recently, mainly because of the complexity and lack of reliability of methods for testing neutrophil antibodies. Leukocyte-agglutinating antibodies were originally observed in multiparous women and patients who had previously received multiple transfusions. From these observations evolved the identification of the HLA system and tissue-typing techniques. **Detection** of specific neutrophil antibodies is mainly by an agglutination technique, which is more tedious than RBC agglutination, requiring special attention to the method of cell separation, the type of medium used, the temperature of the reaction, and the physiologic state of the cell. Another method of detecting neutrophil antibodies is by testing the opsonic activity of the serum by macrophage ingestion of sensitized neutrophils.

A. **Isoimmune neonatal neutropenia** results from maternal antibodies directed against the infant's neutrophils and becomes apparent when an infection develops. Affected infants with mild neutropenia remain asymptomatic and undiagnosed. Firstborn infants can be affected.

1. **Diagnosis**

   a. The total **white blood cell count** may be normal, increased, or slightly decreased, and the neutrophil count is very low or absent. There is moderate monocytosis and occasionally an increase in eosinophils.

   b. The **bone marrow** is hypercellular, with maturation of the myeloid cells arrested at the metamyelocyte or band stage.

   c. Demonstration of the **specific antibody** (anti-NA1, anti-NA2, and anti-NB1) can be done in some medical centers and may be used to help establish the diagnosis of autoimmune neutropenia. This diagnosis is more often made by exclusion of other causes of neutropenia.

2. **Treatment.** The neutropenia usually lasts 2 to 17 weeks, with a mean duration of 7 weeks. Treatment is supportive, with prompt institution of antimicrobials when infection occurs. Corticosteroids are not helpful.

B. **Autoimmune neutropenia** is usually associated with another autoimmune disease, especially with autoimmune hemolytic anemia, immune thrombocytopenia, or both. Autoantibodies reactive with neutrophil-specific antigens NA2 and NB1 can often be demonstrated. Detection of these antibodies can elucidate some cases of idiopathic neutropenia as cases of isolated autoimmune neutropenia. The primary treatment is corticosteroids, with the subsequent treatment algorithm similar to that for extravascular autoimmune hemolytic anemia and ITP.

V. **Immunologic disorders of coagulation. Hemostasis** is maintained in two ways. The first is via a **cellular** system (platelets) and the second is via a **soluble protein** system (**coagulation**). Coagulopathic bleeding presents as hemorrhage in joints, along fascial planes, in soft tissues, in the retroperitoneum, and from the gastrointestinal tract.

Congenital disorders of coagulation result from the absence of a coagulation factor or the presence of a dysfunctional coagulation factor. **Acquired disorders** are related to decreased synthesis of coagulation factors due to systemic disease (e.g., liver disease) or through the use of anticoagulants (e.g., warfarin). On rare occasions, autoimmune antibodies (inhibitors) develop that find coagulation factors and either inactivate the factors or accelerate their clearance. Most acquired anticoagulants inhibit the activity of factor VIII (antihemophilic factor) and are characteristically IgG, although some are IgM or IgA antibodies. The cause of anticoagulant production is unclear.

A. **Factor VIII inhibitors**

1. **Clinical conditions.** The following clinical conditions are associated with circulating **factor VIII inhibitors**:

   a. An inhibitor to injected factor VIII develops in about 10% of patients with severe hemophilia. There is no correlation between the incidence of inhibitor and the degree of exposure to factor VIII. Factor VIII inhibitors are less commonly seen in patients with mild hemophilia than in patients with severe hemophilia. In the cases of severe hemophilia A, this represents **alloimmunization**. All other factor VIII inhibitors are **autoimmune** in nature.

   b. **Autoimmune disorders**, such as systemic lupus erythematosus, rheumatoid arthritis, ulcerative colitis, or regional enteritis, can lead patients to develop anticoagulants.

   c. Previously healthy **postpartum** women may demonstrate anticoagulants for days to several months after childbirth.

    d. Idiopathic anticoagulants can develop in otherwise healthy persons.

2. Diagnosis. The partial thromboplastin time (PTT) is markedly prolonged. The presence of a factor VIII inhibitor can be demonstrated by mixing the patient's plasma with normal plasma in varying concentrations, and measuring PTT and factor VIII functional activity. As a result of the mix, the PTT will remain prolonged and the factor VIII functional activity will be low. Strong inhibitors affect normal plasma immediately on mixing. For weaker inhibitors it is necessary to incubate the mixture of test plasma and normal plasma for 1 to 2 hours to demonstrate the inhibitor activity. (Incubation of normal plasma with saline, to determine spontaneous loss of factor VIII activity with time, is a necessary control). Quantification of the factor VIII inhibitor is reported in **Bethesda units**. One Bethesda unit is defined as the amount of inhibitor present in 1 mL of a patient's plasma that produces a residual factor VIII activity of 50%.

3. Therapy

    a. Treatment is directed at managing the underlying disease process if possible.

    b. In the event of **bleeding**, large quantities of **factor VIII concentrate** (10,000 to 40,000 units per day) can be given to overcome the antibody activity. An anamnestic response can be expected 2 to 4 days after reexposure to factor VIII, reaching a maximum within 2 weeks. Factor VIII concentrates work poorly in patients with Bethesda units greater than 5.

    c. In patients with high titers of inhibitors (greater than 5 Bethesda units), plasma **exchange** or **exchange transfusion** may be necessary to lower the titer of inhibitor, followed by large doses of factor VIII concentrate.

    d. Another approach to patients with factor VIII inhibitor is to administer **activated vitamin K-dependent factors** (prothrombin complex, 70 to 90 factor IX units per kg, repeat in 12 to 24 hours if indicated), bypassing the factor VIII-dependent steps in intrinsic coagulation. Thrombosis (disseminated intravascular coagulation) can be a complication of this type of treatment, especially in the presence of liver disease. An anamnestic increase in inhibitor can also occur secondary to contamination with factor VIII in this preparation.

    e. The use of corticosteroids is not useful in **hemophiliac patients** with allogeneic factor VIII inhibitor. Long-term treatment with corticosteroids or other immunosuppressive agents (especially cyclophosphamide 1.0 to 1.5 g per m^2 intravenously every 21 to 28 days) can be helpful in **nonhemophiliac patients**.

    f. Factor VIII inhibitors are often species specific. **Porcine factor VIII** preparations can be effective in securing hemostasis in the event of life-threatening bleeding in some patients. Anaphylaxis is expected with repeated use of these preparations.

    g. In some patients with factor VIII inhibitors, high-dose **IVIg** is associated with a rapid decrease in anti-factor VIII antibodies and long-term suppression of these antibodies. In others, IVIg and cyclophosphamide together are required to induce tolerance to the factors. In some of these patients, there is evidence that antiidiotypic antibodies in the IVIg manipulate the immune response.

    h. Recombinant activated factor VII (rVIIa) can be used in patients with an acquired factor VIII inhibitor and severe bleeding. rVIIa activates the common coagulation pathway by converting factor X to Xa, and avoids the need for factor X activation via factors IXa and VIIIa. The major complication of rVIIa is thrombosis.

    i. Generally, patients with acquired factor VIII inhibitors are severely ill and many die of bleeding. Treatment always involves a combination of coagulation factor replacement, plasma exchange, and immunosuppression (treatment options b through h).

   4. Prognosis. Even with aggressive therapy, one-half of patients with acquired (nonhemophiliac) factor VIII inhibitors will die of unmanageable hemorrhage. Idiopathic inhibitors occasionally spontaneously remit. The survival of hemophiliacs with the inhibitor is shorter than that of hemophiliacs without the inhibitor.

B. Factor V inhibitors. Acquired inhibitors to factor V are rare, yet are the next most common form of coagulation factor inhibitor after those to factor VIII.

   1. The following **clinical conditions** are associated with circulating **factor V inhibitors**:

    a. Early **postcardiovascular surgery** is seen most commonly in patients who have received streptomycin in the postoperative period. It is unclear if streptomycin is potentially causative or an epiphenomenon of reporting biases.

    b. Healthy elderly individuals (idiopathic)

   2. Diagnosis. The presence of a factor V inhibitor should be suspected when the prothrombin time (PT) is prolonged and a mixing study does not correct the PT. Not all patients with a factor V inhibitor bleed. A positive PT mixing test and a low factor V functional coagulant level make the diagnosis.

   3. Therapy

    a. Fresh frozen plasma can be given to a bleeding patient to try to deliver enough factor V to overcome the inhibitor. Because of the colloidal nature of plasma, giving enough volume to achieve this is difficult without the development of pulmonary edema.

    b. Platelet transfusions. Platelets are rich in factor V. Platelet transfusions can be tried in bleeding patients.

    c. Most factor V inhibitors spontaneously remit.

C. Other inhibitors. Other acquired coagulation inhibitors are extremely rare, including factor IX, factor XIII (due to isoniazid), factor X (due to the immunoglobulin light-chain of primary amyloidosis), and factor II (associated with the use of bovine thrombin during open heart surgery and leprosy).

D. Idiopathic thrombotic thrombocytopenic purpura (TTP) is a rare coagulopathic disorder only recently recognized as autoimmune in nature. Most of the clinical manifestations of the disease are a consequence of microvascular thrombosis. Once uniformly fatal, the mortality rate with modern therapy should be no greater than 10%.

   1. Clinical presentation. Patients present with the signs and symptoms of anemia and thrombocytopenia: fatigue, dyspnea on exertion, paleness, and purpuric (mucocutaneous) bleeding. Mucocutaneous petechiae are usually present. Unexplained fever is sometimes present. In classic TTP, there can be waxing and waning central nervous system abnormalities including altered level of consciousness, coma, personality change, blindness, paresis, aphasia, global amnesia, and/or seizures. Renal disturbances can be present, ranging from microhematuria or proteinuria to oliguric or anuric renal failure. Noncardiogenic pulmonary edema can occur with small fluid challenges, such as RBC transfusions.

   2. Pathophysiology. Idiopathic TTP is the consequence of the development of an inhibitor (autoantibody) to a blood metalloendopeptidase, the normal function of which is to cleave supra molecular weight von Willebrand factor (VWF) to high molecular weight VWF. The presence of the inhibitor results in the persistence of supra molecular weight VWF, which triggers a cascade of events including platelet activation, thrombocytopenia, and the formation of microvascular fibrin strands causing microvascular ischemia and the sheering of RBCs (schistocytes).

3. **Diagnosis.** The diagnosis of TTP is clinical and requires the combination of microangiopathic hemolysis (reticulocytosis plus schistocytes on the blood smear), thrombocytopenia, an elevated lactate dehydrogenase (LDH; often greater than 1,000 IU per L), and no alternate explanation. Disseminated intravascular coagulation (DIC) must be excluded by demonstrating normal coagulation tests and a normal or elevated fibrinogen. The blood smear shows schistocytes (obligatory), polychromasia, occasionally spherocytes, and low platelets. Other features of TTP, including fever, central nervous system abnormality, and/or renal disturbance, may or may not be present and are not necessary for the diagnosis. A confirmatory laboratory test that detects the presence of the VWF protease antibody is not readily available. Delays in the test result should not delay the clinical diagnosis of TTP or the initiation of therapy, because delays in therapy can prove fatal.

4. **Differential diagnosis.** Patients meeting the diagnostic criteria for TTP, with or without central nervous system abnormalities, but without significant renal disturbance are diagnosed as having "TTP." Patients with the signs and symptoms of TTP associated with significant renal disturbance are generally diagnosed as having hemolytic uremic syndrome (HUS). The differential diagnosis of microangiopathic hemolysis includes: TTP, HUS, DIC, pregnancy-induced microangiopathy (DIC, catastrophe of pregnancy, preeclampsia, eclampsia, hemolysis with elevated liver tests and low platelets [HELLP], and postpartum TTP), march hemoglobinuria (from walking or running too far), prosthetic cardiac valves, drugs (mitomycin C, cyclosporine A, tacrolimus, rapamycin, quinine, quinidine, and adenosine diphosphate [ADP]-receptor blockers [ticlopidine and clopidogrel]), familial microangiopathy (usually brought on by oral contraceptives or pregnancy), giant cavernous hemangiomas, and infections (viral dysentery, HIV, virotoxin producing *Escherichia coli*). Autoimmunity has only been established in idiopathic TTP.

5. **Therapy**
    a. **Plasma exchange.** The principle therapy for idiopathic TTP is therapeutic plasma exchange. Forty to 60 mL per kg of plasma is removed and exchanged on a daily basis with an equal volume of fresh frozen plasma or cryosupernatent plasma. Some studies suggest cryosupernatent plasma may be superior to fresh frozen plasma. Plasma exchange induces remissions by: (i) removing the inhibitor and supra molecular weight VWF; and (ii) replenishing the supra molecular weight VWF metalloprotease. Remission is achieved in 60% to 80% of patients with plasma exchange delivered daily for as long as 2 months or more. Although there are no uniform rules for stopping therapy, one algorithm is to continue plasma exchange until two exchanges beyond the achievement of platelet count and LDH normalization (provided a minimum of seven plasma exchanges have been performed).
    b. **Corticosteroids.** The use of corticosteroids in idiopathic TTP was controversial. However, mild cases of idiopathic TTP can remit with prednisone alone, and now that the presence of the metalloendopeptidase autoantibody is established, corticosteroids are a standard adjunct to plasma exchange. Prednisone at 1 to 2 mg/kg/day in divided doses is given until remission is achieved, then slowly tapered over 1 to 2 months.
    c. **Splenectomy.** Patients failing plasma exchange and corticosteroids often respond to splenectomy. It can take 1 week or more to see the hematologic response to splenectomy, so continued plasma exchange and corticosteroids following the procedure is warranted. Many hematologists add dextran 70, 1 L continuous i.v. per day, at the time of splenectomy until remission is achieved. Dextran 70 serves as a qualitative platelet inhibitor.

    d. Cytotoxic chemotherapy. Cytotoxic chemotherapy has been used in difficult cases of TTP with variable success. The most popular agents are **vincristine** 1.0 mg i.v. twice a week or 2.0 mg i.v. once a week, or azathioprine 2 mg/kg/day orally. **Cyclophosphamide** 1 g per m² i.v. once every 3 weeks can also be tried.

VI. Paraproteinemias/paraproteinurias are **monoclonal** immunoglobulins (or immunoglobulin light chains or heavy chains) produced by benign or malignant clonally expanded B cells. The diagnosis is established by a monoclonal spike on serum or urine protein electrophoresis, a monoclonal determination on serum, or urine immunofixation or immunoelectrophoresis (as when a spike is not detectable on protein electrophoresis (see Chapter 19). The differential diagnosis of a paraprotein is shown in Table 15.6. Two-thirds of paraproteins are benign in nature; the remainder are associated with malignant lymphoproliferative disorders. Because the clonal B-cell expansion is a random event in these disorders, the proportion of heavy and light chain classes which make up the paraproteins reflect the usual proportions seen in a normal gamma globulin pool (IgG 60%, IgA 10%, IgM 20%, IgD less than 1%, IgE rare, light chains only 7%, κ to λ ratio 2:1).

    A. Monoclonal gammopathy of uncertain significance (MGUS) is a common paraprotein disorder found in 1.0% to 1.5% of the normal population over age 50 years and in 3% of the normal population over age 70 years. There are no clinical symptoms, and the disorder infrequently progresses.

        1. Diagnosis. Common findings include: the presence of a serum or urine monoclonal immunoglobulin, less than 5% plasma cells in the bone marrow, normal serum calcium, and lack of lytic bone lesions. When in serum, the monoclonal immunoglobulin level is usually less than 3 g per dL. Mild anemia and/or hypogammaglobulinemia may be present.

        2. Therapy. No treatment is necessary except to observe these patients for the development of lymphoproliferative disorders. Long-term follow-up of these patients shows 47% die with (not of) MGUS, 19% are alive with MGUS, 16% develop multiple myeloma (MM), 10% have an increase in their serum paraprotein to greater than 3 g per dL without neoplastic conversion, 3% develop primary amyloidosis, 3% develop WM macroglobulinemia, and 2% develop other lymphoproliferative disorders. The actuarial risk of these patients developing a malignant lymphoproliferative disorder is 17% at 10 years and 33% at 20 years following diagnosis.

    B. Multiple myeloma (MM) is the most common form of plasma cell neoplasm. The neoplastic cells produce excessive amounts of monoclonal immunoglobulins and/or light chains.

        1. The **clinical symptoms** depend on the extent of disease. Back pain, rib pain, loss of height, osteopenia, and/or pathologic fractures occur commonly with skeletal involvement. Anemia is universal. The anion gap is low. Hypercalcemia, especially with extensive osteolytic bone lesions, is common. Impaired renal function can occur (especially with

Table 15.6. Etiologies of paraproteins

Etiology	Frequency of diagnosis
Monoclonal gammopathy of uncertain significance	63%
Multiple myeloma and variants	14%
Primary amyloidosis	9%
Indolent non-Hodgkin lymphoma	5%
Extramedullary or solitary bone plasmacytoma	4%
Chronic lymphocytic leukemia	3%
Waldenstrom macroglobulinemia	2%

light-chain disease). Advanced MM can result in leukopenia and thrombocytopenia. **Hyperviscosity** syndrome from the monoclonal immunoglobulin can produce visual disturbances, retinal hemorrhages, central ischemic neurologic disturbances, pulmonary edema, and a bleeding diathesis. Other disease complications include peripheral sensory neuropathy, recurrent bacterial infections, amyloid deposition, and autoimmune hyperlipidemia.

2. **Diagnosis**

   a. Serum monoclonal immunoglobulin greater than 3 g per dL

   b. Urine monoclonal light chain greater than 12 g per 24 hours

   c. Greater than 30% bone marrow plasma cells

   d. Normal (nonmyeloma) serum immunoglobulins are quantitatively low.

   e. Lytic bone lesions and/or diffuse osteopenia on skeletal x-ray series. The diagnosis of MM is not always straightforward. Not all of the above diagnostic criteria need be met to establish a diagnosis. For instance, a diagnosis of MM can still be established if the bone marrow demonstrates 10% to 30% plasma cells if other criteria are present.

3. **Therapy.** The treatment of MM is designed to prolong survival, prevent complications of the disease, and ameliorate symptoms. With conventional-dose chemotherapy, the median survival is only 3 years in patients with advanced disease. Prognosis is determined by the level of monoclonal paraprotein, presence of hypercalcemia, degree of anemia, presence of thrombocytopenia, the level of LDH or β_2 microglobulin, the presence of renal failure, and the type of monoclonal immunoglobulin produced (from best to worse prognosis, IgG, IgA, light chains only, IgD; patients whose monoclonal proteins include κ light chains do better than those including λ light chains). Bone marrow cytogenetics (karyotype) is also prognostic: chromosome 13 deletions or monosomy 7 or monosomy 5 confer a particularly poor prognosis.

   a. **Chemotherapy.** Many treatment regimens are available which utilize corticosteroids, melphalan, cyclophosphamide, vincristine, doxorubicin, nitrosoureas, chlorambucil, bleomycin, and etoposide.

   b. **Radiotherapy** can be administered to pathologic fractures, painful bony lesions, or extramedullary plasmacytomas to ameliorate symptoms.

   c. **Treatment of multiple myeloma complications,** such as renal failure, hypercalcemia, infections, neuropathy, endocrinopathy, and hyperviscosity, can be necessary.

   d. **Allogeneic hematopoietic stem cell transplantation.** Although MM is generally considered incurable, myeloablative therapy followed by allogeneic hematopoietic stem cell transplantation produces long-term disease-free survivals in 20% to 25% of patients (data from the International Bone Marrow Transplant Registry). A plateau to the survival curve suggests these patients are cured, presumably, the result of a graft versus myeloma effect. The treatment-related mortality is high, approaching 50%. This, plus the fact that only 25% to 30% of patients will have an HLA-matched sibling donor, makes this treatment only applicable to a small proportion of young (less than 60 years old) MM patients.

   e. **Autologous hematopoietic stem cell transplantation.** The standard approach to patients under age 70 years with advanced MM involves autologous stem cell transplantation (ASCT). A prospective, randomized trial has demonstrated superior overall survival for MM patients randomized to high-dose therapy and ASCT (greater than 5 years) compared to conventional-dose chemotherapy only (3 years). Patients generally receive three to four cycles of conventional-dose chemotherapy, then mobilization and cryopreservation of autologous peripheral blood stem cells using myeloid growth factors plus chemotherapy, and then high-dose chemotherapy (such as melphalan 200 mg per m² i.v.) and ASCT. The treatment-related mortality is low (less than 5%) but relapse is high, presumably due to a lack of graft versus myeloma effect. ASCT is not considered curative, but as many as 10% of patients are relapse-free 7 or more years after transplantation.

   f. Thalidomide. Up to one-fourth of patients with relapsed or refractory MM will respond to 100 to 800 mg per day of thalidomide. Thalidomide remissions last an average of more than a year. Thalidomide is believed to work through antiproliferative and anti-angiogenesis mechanisms. Dose-limiting toxicities include lethargy, reversible peripheral neuropathy, and constipation.

   g. Pamidronate. Pamidronate is a bisphosphonate given 90 mg intravenously once a month. Pamidronate corrects hypercalcemia and has been proven to reduce skeletal events (pathologic fractures, pain, narcotic use) in patients with advanced MM.

C. Waldenström macroglobulinemia (WM) is best characterized as a low-grade non-Hodgkin lymphoma with IgM gammopathy. The neoplastic cells differentiate out to the preplasma cell. When the serum IgM is greater than 3 g per dL, hyperviscosity and plasma volume expansion are common, and the disease is referred to as WM macroglobulinemia. When the serum IgM is less than 3 g per dL, this is generally called lymphoplasmacytic lymphoma. Spleen and bone marrow involvement with the monoclonal lymphoplasmacytic cells are universal. This disease, common in the sixth or seventh decade of life and with a slight male predominance, can present with fatigue and weakness. Raynaud phenomenon, cold urticaria, and cold hypersensitivity are major symptoms in those whose IgM paraprotein behaves as a cryoglobulin. In some patients a bleeding tendency can be related to abnormal platelet function or decreased levels of clotting factor. The hyperviscosity syndrome can be present. The lymph nodes are enlarged, as are the liver and spleen. Lytic bone lesions are notably absent.

   1. Diagnosis

   a. Anemia, usually due to hemodilution from plasma volume expansion, is a common finding.

   b. The direct antiglobulin test is negative.

   c. A serum and/or urine monoclonal IgM paraprotein is demonstrated by electrophoresis (usually greater than 3 g per dL in the serum).

   d. There may be an associated decrease in the levels of normal immunoglobulins. The activity of the macroglobulins in certain patients resembles that of cold agglutinin antibody or anti-IgG antibody (forming cryoprecipitable IgM–IgG complexes known as cryoglobulins).

   e. Bone marrow is greater than 30% involved with malignant plasmacytoid lymphocytes.

   f. Presentation differs from MM by lack of lytic bone lesions, the presence of lymphadenopathy and hepatosplenomegaly, and the lack of hypercalcemia.

   2. Therapy. The course of WM macroglobulinemia is variable, but usually with slow progression over years. Therapy is directed toward the amelioration of symptoms. **Plasma exchange** is commonly performed to quickly treat hyperviscosity symptoms by rapidly unloading IgM from the serum.

   a. Traditional **chemotherapy** resembles that for other non-Hodgkin lymphoma: chlorambucil plus prednisone, or cyclophosphamide/vincristine/prednisone. Because of the indolent nature of the disease, anthracyclines (such as doxorubicin) are reserved until later in the disease process due to the potential cardiac toxicity of these agents.

b. **Purine nucleoside analogues.** The purine nucleoside analogues, fludarabine and 2-chlorodeoxydenosine, are showing great promise in WM. They appear to produce greater response rates than alkylating agents with fewer side effects.

c. **Rituximab.** Rituximab is a chimeric monoclonal murine–human anti-CD20 antibody approved for use in relapsed or refractory low-grade non-Hodgkin lymphomas. The antibody produces cell death by antibody-directed cellular cytotoxicity, complement fixation, and induction of apoptosis. Rituximab is administered at 375 mg/ m²/dose for 4 weekly i.v. doses. It is showing a high level of activity in patients with relapsed or refractory WM.

D. **Heavy chain disease** is a very rare group of disorders in which a defective immunoglobulin heavy chain is synthesized (the C_H1 portion of the heavy chain is deleted, but the Fc portion is intact). The abnormal protein is monoclonal in origin. Four types of abnormal heavy chains have been identified: γ, α, μ, and δ. The abnormal protein reacts with antisera to the corresponding immunoglobulin, but not with antisera to κ or λ light chains. The clinical picture resembles that of malignant lymphoma, with lymphadenopathy and hepatosplenomegaly. The bone marrow is diffusely infiltrated by lymphocytes, plasma cells, eosinophils, and histiocytes. Surface immunoglobulin is not observed on the lymphocytes. The causes of these disorders are unknown.

1. **γ-Heavy-chain disease** is usually found in patients over 40 years of age, although it has been identified in a few patients between 12 and 40 years of age. Fever, lymphadenopathy, and anemia are common presenting features. The serum concentrations of normal immunoglobulins are usually decreased; the levels of abnormal serum paraproteins usually exceed 2 g per dL. There is no standard treatment for this disorder. The course of the disease is variable. Patients may survive for a few months to years. In the terminal phase, there is a marked increase in the number of plasma cells in the bone marrow, similar to plasma cell leukemia.

2. **α-Heavy-chain disease** is the most common form of heavy-chain disease, and is seen in persons less than 50 years of age. The peak incidence of the disease is in the second and third decades. The abdominal lymphoid tissue is commonly involved, with markedly enlarged mesenteric lymph nodes and infiltration of the intestinal mucosa by lymphocytes and plasma cells. Villous atrophy is present. Chronic diarrhea and malabsorption are common symptoms. Some patients respond to treatment regimens for malignant lymphoma, whereas others achieve complete remission with antimicrobials alone.

3. **μ-Heavy-chain disease** is rare. Nearly all affected patients have chronic lymphocytic leukemia. Lymph node enlargement is uncommon. Vacuolated plasma cells and mature lymphocytes are present in the bone marrow. Most patients excrete large amounts of κ light chains in the urine. The diagnosis is made by demonstrating the abnormal monoclonal protein by careful immunochemical studies including protein electrophoresis, immunoelectrophoresis, and/or immunofixation electrophoresis. The treatment is directed to the underlying disease, chronic lymphocytic leukemia.

4. **δ-Heavy-chain disease** is extremely rare. One patient presented with renal insufficiency, osteolytic lesions, and a bone marrow picture of myeloma. Electrophoresis demonstrated a paraprotein peak between the γ and β regions, reactive with anti-δ but not with anti-κ or anti-λ sera.

E. **Cryoglobulinemia.** Cryoglobulins are immunoglobulins that precipitate in the cold. To detect cryoglobulins, blood is drawn in a prewarmed syringe and allowed to clot at 37°C. The supernatant serum is then chilled to 4°C and examined for precipitation 3 days later. Normal serum contains up to 80 μg per mL of cryoglobulins; symptomatic patients with cryoglobulinemia have 500 to 5,000 μg per mL of cryoglobulins in their serum.

1. **Clinical presentation.** Patients with cryoglobulinemia suffer from the cryoactive properties of the excessively produced immunoglobulins. These result in Raynaud phenomenon, acrocyanosis, peripheral dry gangrene, and **vascular (palpable) purpura**. This purpura generally affects the lower extremities, especially the skin over the malleoli (which can ulcerate). Cold exposure brings on arthralgias, joint stiffness, and if the cryoglobulin functions also as a cold agglutinin with an appropriate thermal range, intravascular hemolysis occurs. Late complications include renal failure with nephrotic-range proteinuria, and hypertension. Kidney biopsy shows immunoglobulin and complement deposition beneath the glomerular basement membrane.

2. **Classification.** Table 15.7 shows the three types of cryoglobulinemia and their associated illnesses. Nearly half of patients with mixed cryoglobulinemia (types II or III) suffer from lymphoproliferative disorders and/or vasculitis.

3. **Therapy**
   a. **Avoid cold exposure.**
   b. Treat associated illnesses.
   c. Severe symptomatic disease can be temporarily ameliorated by **plasma exchange**. As with cold agglutinin hemolysis, plasma exchange must be in a room warmed to near body temperature to avoid exacerbating the cryoactive condition (see Therapy on page 345). The use of plasma exchange to treat the renal failure or nephrotic syndrome associated with cryoglobulinemia is controversial.
   d. **Cytotoxic therapy.** Cytotoxic agents including cyclophosphamide, chlorambucil, and/or corticosteroids are sometimes used to try to decrease cryoglobulin production.

F. **Monoclonal immunoglobulin deposition diseases** (MIDD) are a group of paraprotein disorders characterized by the deposition of monoclonal immunoglobulin components in tissue or blood vessels. There are two major types: **primary amyloid, and light chain or light and heavy chain deposition disease**.

   These two types of disorders are remarkably similar in their clinical behavior and natural history and differ primarily in the manner of Ig deposition. In primary amyloid, monoclonal κ or λ light chains deposit in tissue bound to a protein called the amyloid P-component. This produces positive staining and apple-green birefringence under polarizing light with Congo red and the demonstration of fibril formation by electron microscopy. In light chain and light and heavy chain deposition disease, κ and λ light chains (plus or minus heavy chain) deposit without binding the amyloid P-component. This produces nonfibrillar, amorphous depositions which are Congo red negative.

Table 15.7. Cryoglobulinemias

Type	Name	Ig type	Associated disorders
I	Single monoclonal	Variable	Multiple myeloma Waldenström macroglobulinemia Idiopathic
II	Mixed monoclonal	IgM, and IgG or IgA	Lymphoproliferative disorders Rheumatologic disorders Infections (especially hepatitis C)
III	Mixed polyclonal	IgM, and IgG or IgA	Lymphoproliferative disorders Rheumatologic disorders Infections (especially hepatitis C)

Ig, immunoglobulin.

1. **Primary amyloidosis.** Primary amyloidosis is a paraprotein disorder characterized by the deposition of monoclonal Ig light chains in tissues. This results in end-organ damage and shortened survival. Primary amyloidosis is not associated with any other illness except MM.

   a. **Clinical presentation.** Depending on the predominant site of light chain deposition, patients present with variable signs and symptoms. These can include weakness, fatigue, peripheral neuropathy, periorbital purpura, dyspnea, pedal edema, syncope, lightheadedness, hoarseness, and dysphagia. At presentation, 34% have hepatomegaly, 22% have macroglossia, and 4% have splenomegaly and lymphadenopathy. The median age of onset is 65 years. The organs involved with amyloid include the heart (35% have congestive heart failure), tongue (20%), gastrointestinal tract (manifested by dysphagia or malabsorption), kidneys (35% with nephrotic syndrome), nerves (17% with peripheral and autonomic neuropathy), bone marrow (30%), and autonomic nerves (orthostatic hypotension). The synchronous onset of bilateral carpal tunnel syndrome can be a presenting sign of primary amyloidosis.

   b. **Diagnosis.** Patients with the appropriate clinical presentation should be evaluated to establish a diagnosis of primary amyloidosis as follows:

      (1) **Protein electrophoresis.** Forty percent of patients have a monoclonal spike on serum protein electrophoresis; 68% have a monoclonal spike on serum immunoelectrophoresis; and 89% have a monoclonal spike on combined serum and urine protein electrophoresis. Of patients with a monoclonal spike, two-thirds have a full monoclonal immunoglobulin and one-third have light chains only (compared with MM, the κ-to-λ ratio is reversed 1:2).

      (2) **Biopsy** of the affected organ, including bone marrow, abdominal fat pad, rectum, kidney, carpal ligament, liver, skin, sural nerve, or heart confirms the diagnosis. Biopsy shows birefringent apple-green filaments with Congo red dye under polarizing light.

      (3) About 20% of patients meet the diagnostic criteria for MM as determined by bone marrow biopsy, skeletal survey, and elevated serum calcium; therefore, these tests are a necessary part of the diagnostic evaluation.

      (4) At presentation, 82% of patients have proteinuria, 50% to 60% have an elevated serum creatinine, and 50% have decreased IgG levels. Patients are usually not anemic unless they have concurrent MM.

   c. **Prognosis.** Primary amyloidosis is not curable. Because of heightened sensitivity to the disease and the establishment that MM chemotherapy prolongs survival, the overall median survival from diagnosis has increased from 12 to almost 30 months. Overall prognosis primarily reflects the predominant organ involved with amyloid as follows (from best to worst): peripheral nerves, carpal ligaments, kidney, autonomic nerves, and heart. Patients with amyloid-associated congestive heart failure and syncope only live an average of 3 months from diagnosis.

   d. **Therapy**

      (1) **Chemotherapy.** Two prospective, randomized trials demonstrate that oral melphalan and prednisone administered every 6 weeks improves survival in primary amyloidosis compared to colchicine alone (now considered a toxic placebo). **Amyloid patients most likely to respond and benefit from chemotherapy have as their predominant organ involvement kidney, peripheral nerves, or carpal ligaments.**

     (2) **Solid organ transplantation.** The transplantation of a failed amyloid-involved organ (e.g., kidney or heart) is now discouraged because amyloid tends to rapidly progress in other organs after the transplant.

     (3) **Autologous stem cell transplantation (ASCT).** The use of high-dose melphalan (140 to 200 mg/m² intravenous) followed by ASCT is currently an investigational form of treatment for primary amyloidosis. Although there is no proof yet that ASCT will improve survival compared to conventional-dose melphalan and prednisone, the hope is that it will, on the basis of the extrapolation of results of ASCT in MM (see Autologous hematopoietic stem cell transplantation on pages 363–364). Compared to MM, the treatment-related mortality is greater in primary amyloid patients undergoing ASCT (15% versus less than 5%). The treatment-related mortality approaches two-thirds in patients with symptomatic heart involvement, because of sudden death during ASCT.

  2. **Light chain, and light chain and heavy chain deposition disease** (LCDD and LHCDD, respectively) closely resemble primary amyloidosis in organ involvement, clinical presentation, diagnostic features (except the Congo red negative status), and prognosis. Notable differences compared to primary amyloidosis are that LCDD/LHCDD is more rare and that more patients with LCDD/LHCDD will meet the diagnostic criteria for MM (50% versus 20%). It is most appropriate to consider LCDD/LHCDD the same as primary amyloidosis and to not consider them differently simply on the basis of their differing pathologic features. The treatment approach for LCDD/LHCDD is the same as for primary amyloidosis.

VII. Immune-mediated suppression of hematopoiesis. After birth, the cellular elements of blood originate in the bone marrow. Certain immune disorders can act to suppress normal hematopoiesis, resulting in cytopenias. The two major disorders of this type are idiopathic aplastic anemia and pure red cell aplasia (PRCA).

  A. Idiopathic aplastic anemia. Aplastic anemia presents as **pancytopenia** on the complete blood count (neutropenia, anemia, and thrombocytopenia). Further analysis shows reticulocytopenia and either bone marrow aplasia or severe hypoplasia (less than 10% cellularity). **Idiopathic aplastic anemia** is a combination of an immune and clonal hematopoietic stem cell disorder. **Secondary aplastic anemia** results from bone marrow exposure to hematopoietic stem cell toxins such as ionizing radiation, cytotoxic chemotherapy, certain medications, and other organic or inorganic chemicals (such as benzene). Depending on the dose and duration of exposure, secondary aplastic anemia may or may not be reversible.

    Patients with **idiopathic aplastic anemia** have circulating T-suppressor clones that inhibit hematopoiesis *in vitro* and presumably *in vivo*. The latter is supported by the high response rate to immunosuppressive therapy, by the requirement for immunosuppressive therapy as conditioning for syngeneic hematopoietic stem cell transplant in order for engraftment to occur, and by autologous hematopoietic recovery after cyclophosphamide conditioning for allogeneic hematopoietic stem cell transplantation. Because growth of hematopoietic cells in culture from normal individuals can be suppressed by sera from patients with aplastic anemia, humoral autoimmunity may also play a role. Whether autoimmunity is responsible for initiating or maintaining (or both) the suppression of hematopoiesis is unclear. In some occasions, exposure to hepatitis viruses produces an autoimmune response to hematopoiesis. Like idiopathic aplastic anemia, hepatitis-associated aplastic anemia responds to immunosuppressive therapy. That immune dysfunction is not solely responsible for impaired hematopoiesis is evidenced by the fact that some patients responding to immunosuppressive therapy later develop **myelodysplasia, paroxysmal nocturnal hemoglobinuria,** or **acute myeloid leukemia**. These occurrences suggest the presence of an intrinsic clonal hematopoietic stem cell defect.

1. **Diagnosis.** Patients present to physicians because of symptoms and signs related to their pancytopenia. Common complaints are fatigue, dyspnea on exertion, fevers, and mucocutaneous bleeding. There is a reticulocytopenia with normal blood cell morphology. A significant toxin exposure history is usually absent. The bone marrow biopsy is less than 10% cellular and bone marrow cytogenetics (karyotype) are normal. Occasional pockets of preserved erythroid cells can be seen. Idiopathic aplastic anemia must be distinguished from **hypoplastic myelodysplasia** or **hypoplastic acute leukemia** based on careful examination of the bone marrow biopsy and cytogenetics.

2. **Therapy.** Without effective treatment, idiopathic aplastic anemia is associated with a 90% 1-year mortality. The following treatment options are available.

   a. **Allogeneic hematopoietic stem cell transplantation.** High-dose cyclophosphamide (200 mg per kg ideal body weight) plus antithymocyte globulin (ATG, 90 mg per kg) immunosuppression is followed by infusion of HLA-matched allogeneic hematopoietic stem cells as cyclophosphamide rescue. In adults, the donor hematopoietic stem cells must be a five of six or six of six HLA type match (HLA A, B, and DR loci) in order to be successful. More than one major locus mismatch results in an unacceptably high incidence of **graft versus host disease (GVHD)** (see Graft versus host disease on page 371). In children, HLA haplomatched transplants can sometimes be accomplished. The major complications of allogeneic hematopoietic stem cell transplant for aplastic anemia are graft rejection, GVHD, and prolonged immunosuppression. Current success rates are 80% to 90% in children, and 60% to 70% in adults. It is controversial whether it is advisable for adults over age 40 years with an HLA-matched sibling to undergo allogeneic hematopoietic stem cell transplantation or immunosuppression as first therapy. Hematopoietic stem cell transplantation eliminates the future occurrence of myelodysplasia and acute myeloid leukemia in these patients, presumably due to a graft versus hematopoiesis effect.

   b. **Immunosuppression** with **antithymocyte globulin** or **antilymphocyte globulin**. Approximately 60% of patients with severe aplastic anemia respond to ATG. Typical horse ATG (ATGAM) doses are 40 mg per kg for 5 days or 20 mg per kg for 8 days. Responses take up to 3 to 4 months to occur. About 50% of children respond to this therapy. Complications include opportunistic infections, reactions to foreign proteins, and serum sickness. The latter occurs 7 to 10 days after ATG administration and presents as fever, a serpiginous macular erythematous rash, and arthralgias. Immune complex nephritis rarely occurs. Serum sickness is treated with high-dose corticosteroids.

   c. **Combination therapy.** This involves **antilymphocyte globulin (ALG)** (or ATG) plus **cyclosporine**. This combination regimen produces a response rate of 70% in adults. These responses occur faster (1.5 to 3 months) compared with ALG alone. Cyclosporine is given orally beginning at the time of ALG infusions (0.75 mL/kg/day for 8 days) and continuing for up to 6 months post ALG. The dose of oral cyclosporine is 6 mg per kg b.i.d., adjusted for toxicity and to achieve through blood levels approximately 400 ng per mL. One advantage of combining ALG with cyclosporine is that the latter greatly ameliorates serum sickness.

    d. Transfusions. Red cell and platelet transfusions are needed to support patients through their therapies. All transfusions should be irradiated (3,000 cGy) to kill lymphocytes and prevent unwanted lymphocyte engraftment and transfusion-associated GVHD. Historically, transfusions were avoided in patients likely to undergo hematopoietic stem cell transplantation because exposure to blood products increased graft rejection. The addition of ATG to cyclophosphamide in the transplant conditioning regimen has greatly reduced graft rejection in transfused patients. Hence, there is no longer a need to avoid transfusions in patients likely to benefit from them.

    e. Androgens. Oxymetholone 0.5 to 1.0 mg per kg b.i.d. (maximum 200 mg per day) has been used historically to improve the anemia and sometimes the other cytopenias in patients with aplastic anemia. The overall response rate is low. This drug should not be used as alternate therapy to definitive treatments such as ATG, cyclosporine, or hematopoietic stem cell transplantation.

    f. Growth factors. The **myeloid growth factors** (granulocyte colony stimulating factor and granulocyte macrophage colony stimulating factor) and **erythropoietin** can be used as additive, supportive measures to the other more definitive treatments.

    g. In patients with aplastic anemia secondary to hematopoietic toxins, spontaneous recovery can occur depending on the exposure dose and duration. The only cure without spontaneous recovery is allogeneic hematopoietic stem cell transplantation. Immunosuppression alone does not work and is contraindicated.

B. Pure red cell aplasia. Like idiopathic aplastic anemia, the immune disorder associated with idiopathic PRCA is both humoral and cellular. Serum from patients with PRCA suppresses *in vitro* erythropoiesis of bone marrow from other individuals, suggesting that a serum factor (not yet identified) is responsible. T cells appear to be responsible for mediation of this serum factor.

    1. Clinical presentation. Patients generally present with symptoms of anemia: dyspnea on exertion, fatigue, and headaches. These patients rapidly develop red cell transfusion dependence. Because there are illnesses associated with PRCA, signs and symptoms of these other illnesses maybe dominant features of the clinical presentation. Associated illnesses are (i) thymoma (with or without myasthenia gravis), (ii) rheumatologic disorders, (iii) ulcerative colitis or Crohn disease, and (iv) chronic lymphocytic leukemia.

    2. Diagnosis. PRCA should be suspected when a new transfusion-dependent anemia develops that is not clearly explainable by other causes. The mean corpuscular volume is usually mildly elevated (100 to 105 fL) with normal red cell morphology on the blood smear. The white cells and platelets are usually normal. There is reticulocytopenia. The bone marrow biopsy shows near total absence of erythroid progenitors with no other marrow pathology and normal cytogenetics (karyotype).

    3. Therapy

        a. Corticosteroids. Half of the patients with PRCA taking 1 to 2 mg/kg/day of prednisone show improved erythropoiesis. The response can take several weeks to a few months to occur.

        b. Treat underlying illnesses. Some patients with an enlarged thymus on radiographic examination respond to **thymectomy**. Other patients without an enlarged thymus also respond to thymectomy. Treatment of associated rheumatologic disorders and ulcerative colitis or Crohn disease will often help the PRCA.

        c. Splenectomy does not help.

      d. Cytotoxic therapy. About 60% of patients respond to cyclophosphamide (50 mg per day orally) or azathioprine (1 to 2 mg/kg/day orally).

      e. Antithymocyte globulin or antilymphocyte globulin (see Combination therapy on page 369) produces remissions in many patients with idiopathic PRCA failing to respond to therapies a through d.

      f. Intravenous immunoglobulin G. There are case reports demonstrating some refractory PRCA patients responding to a course of IVIg (0.4 to 0.5 gm/kg/day for 5 consecutive days).

VIII. Graft versus host disease. GVHD is a life-threatening immune disorder that can produce aplastic anemia and other end-organ failure. It generally occurs when allogeneic (donor) lymphocytes engraft in an immunosuppressed patient (host). A normal immune response is activated when graft lymphocytes recognize the host as foreign. Activated T-cytotoxic (CD8) cells promote an attack on host organs expressing foreign antigens. Severe pancytopenia is the hallmark feature of this illness.

  A. Clinical presentation. GVHD presents with a classic macular, erythematous rash on the ear lobes, nape of the neck, upper chest and back, and palms. Oral mucosal ulcerations are common. Chronic ulcerations give a "cobblestone" appearance to the oral mucosa (with or without a lacy, white discoloration). Fevers are common. Early in the course, there is hyperbilirubinemia. Pancytopenia is uniformly present. Advanced cases demonstrate voluminous, watery diarrhea, which may become bloody as the GVHD progresses. Patients die from liver failure, complications of pancytopenia, and the complications of uncontrolled diarrhea (dehydration, metabolic derangement, malabsorption, and exsanguination). There are several clinical circumstances associated with the development of GVHD:

      1. Immunosuppressed recipients of unirradiated blood transfusions, such as cancer patients (especially Hodgkin disease), primary or secondary immunosuppressed patients, and organ transplant patients, are at risk. Patients with HIV disease do not appear to be at particularly high risk for GVHD.

      2. Normal (immunocompetent) recipients of a closely human leukocyte antigen-matched unirradiated blood transfusion. This situation is usually a coincidental occurrence. There are cases of recipients of blood donated by family members (children) acquiring GVHD because the blood was HLA-identical. In these cases, there were unknown shared haplotypes between spouses in the family. Thus, the children were homozygous for one parental haplotype.

      3. Solid organ transplant recipients. Especially in liver transplant patients, GVHD can occur when passenger lymphocytes in the donor organ happen to engraft. The HLA typing of the recipient and donor are usually identical or very closely matched. This is less likely to occur in renal or heart transplant recipients because those organs harbor very few lymphocytes.

      4. Allogeneic hematopoietic stem cell transplant recipients. This is an expected complication of hematopoietic stem cell transplantation. In this setting, GVHD is immunologically similar to solid organ transplant rejection, but in the opposite direction. Steps are taken to prevent GVHD from occurring in this form of transplant. These involve: (i) the transplantation of HLA-matched or minimally mismatched grafts; (ii) if significantly mismatched transplants are done, then T-cell depletion is performed on the graft prior to transplantation; (iii) an effort to use grafts from a donor of the same gender as the recipient whenever possible; and (iv) the use of GVHD prophylaxis with cyclosporine (or tacrolimus) plus intravenous methotrexate and/or corticosteroids. With such efforts, the incidence of mild GVHD is about 30% to 40% and the incidence of moderate to severe GVHD is

10% to 20%. When sibling donors are used, bone marrow suppression is less common with GVHD following hematopoietic stem cell transplants than with other forms of GVHD, because the hematopoiesis is technically autologous in the eyes of the engrafted immune system.

B. Diagnosis. Patients presenting with the appropriate signs and symptoms in the right circumstance should be suspected as having GVHD. Biopsies of skin, oral mucosa, liver, and gastrointestinal tract show lymphoid infiltrates, suggesting the diagnosis. Gastrointestinal tract cells are often undergoing programmed cell death (apoptosis). No biopsy result is specifically diagnostic. Except in the hematopoietic stem cell transplant setting, the bone marrow biopsy is aplastic. If enough lymphocytes can be obtained from a biopsy specimen (usually bone marrow) for HLA-typing, then infiltrating lymphocytes are found to be of donor origin, confirming a diagnosis of GVHD.

C. Therapy. The best therapy for GVHD is **prevention**. All susceptible patients (cancer patients receiving chemotherapy or radiation, congenital immunodeficiency patients, organ transplant patients, fetuses needing intrauterine transfusions, and normal recipients receiving blood from primary relatives) should receive only **irradiated** (3,000 cGy) blood transfusions. Immunosuppressed patients should avoid blood products from siblings whenever possible. If they are necessary, they must be irradiated. The management of ongoing GVHD is difficult. Most cases are **fatal** (84% mortality at a median of 21 days after onset) outside of the hematopoietic stem cell transplant setting. Because of GVHD prophylaxis measures in hematopoietic stem cell transplantation, death due to GVHD occurs less than 20% of the time. In addition, GVHD is associated with a graft versus leukemia (or hematopoietic malignancy) effect, resulting in a lower leukemia relapse rate.

1. In transfusion-related GVHD, **lymphocytotoxic** therapy has been tried with little success.

2. In the setting of **solid organ transplantation**, the treatment decisions are problematic because:

   a. **Increasing immunosuppression** (corticosteroids, cytotoxic agents, ATG, or the monoclonal antibody OKT3) to eliminate the engrafted lymphocytes is associated with increased opportunistic infections in patients already neutropenic from GVHD.

   b. **Decreasing immunosuppression** so the recipient might reject the donor lymphocytes may result in the transplanted organ being rejected as well.

3. In the setting of **allogeneic hematopoietic stem cell transplantation**, GVHD in the first 100 days (acute GVHD) is treated with a corticosteroid pulse. If this is not effective, then other immunosuppressive therapies can be tried (e.g., **ATG, OKT3, mycophenolic acid mofetil, or daclizumab**). After the first 100 days, chronic GVHD is treated with combinations of corticosteroids, mycophenolic acid mofetil, and cyclosporine. GVHD often resolves over time as immune tolerance develops between graft and host. There is a benefit to GVHD in the setting of allogeneic hematopoietic stem cell transplantation: Fewer leukemia patients relapse with their malignancy if they have GVHD, compared with those without GVHD, which is known as the **graft versus leukemia** effect.

Selected Readings

Anderson KC, Weinstein HJ. Transfusion-associated graft-versus-host disease. *N Engl J Med* 1990;323:315.

Attal M, Haroussear J-L, Stappa A-M, et al. A prospective, randomized trial of autologous bone marrow transplantation and chemotherapy in multiple myeloma. *N Engl J Med* 1996;335:91.

Bataille R, Harosseau J-L. Multiple myeloma. *N Engl J Med* 1997;336:1657.

Boxer LA. Immune neutropenias: clinical and biological implications. *Am J Pediatr Hematol Oncol* 1981;3:89.

Brouet J-C, et al. Biologic and clinical significance of cryoglobulins. A report of 86 cases. *Am J Med* 1974;57:775.

Buxbaum JN. Mechanisms of disease: monoclonal immunoglobulin deposition. Amyloidosis, light-chain deposition disease, and light and heavy chain deposition disease. *Hematol/Oncol Clin N Am* 1992;6:323.

Chaplin H Jr. Clinical usefulness of specific antiglobulin reagents in autoimmune hemolytic anemia. *Prog Hematol* 1974;8:25.

Dale DC. Immune and idiopathic neutropenia. *Curr Opin Hematol* 1998;5:33.

Frankel AH, et al. Type II essential mixed cryoglobulinemia: presentation, treatment and outcome in 13 patients. *Q J Med* 1992;82:101.

Frickhofen N, Kaltwasser JP, Schrezenmeier H, et al. Treatment of aplastic anemia with antilymphocyte globulin and methylprednisolone with or without cyclosporine. *N Engl J Med* 1991;324:1297.

Furlan M, Robles R, Galbusera M, et al. von Willeband factor-cleaving protease in thrombotic thrombocytopenic purpura and the hemolytic-uremic syndrome. *N Engl J Med* 1998;339:1578.

George JN, Raskob GE, Shoh SR, et al. Drug-induced thrombocytopenia: a systematic review of published case reports. *Ann Intern Med* 1998;129:886.

Greinacher A. Treatment of heparin-induced thrombocytopenia. *Thromb Haemost* 1999;82:457.

Grey HM, Kohler PF. Cryoimmunoglobulins. *Semin Hematol* 1973;10:87.

Hashmoto C. Autoimmune hemolytic anemia. *Clin Rev Allergy Immunol* 1998;16:285.

Kelton TG, et al., eds. *Blood transfusion: a conceptual approach.* New York: Churchill Livingstone, 1984.

Kyle RA. "Benign" monoclonal gammopathy—after 20 to 35 years of follow-up. *Mayo Clin Proc* 1993;68:26.

Kyle RA, Gertz MA, Greipp PR, et al. A trial of three regimens for primary amyloidosis: colchicine alone, melphalan and prednisone, oral melphalan, prednisone, and colchicine. *N Engl J Med* 1997;336:1201.

Kyle RA, Greipp PR. Amyloidosis (AL). Clinical and laboratory features in 229 cases. *Mayo Clin Proc* 1983;58:665.

McLaughlin P, Labanillas F, Grillo-Lopez AJ, et al. Rituximab chimeric anti-CD20 monoclonal antibody therapy for relapsed lymphoma: half of patients respond to a four-dose treatment program. *J Clin Oncol* 1998;10:2825.

Queenan JT, ed. *Modern management of the Rh problem*, 2nd ed. New York: Harper and Row, 1977.

Rock GA, Shumak KH, Buskard NA, et al. Comparison of plasma exchange with plasma infusion in the treatment of thrombotic thrombocytopenic pupura. *N Engl J Med* 1991;325:393.

Rosse WF. Autoimmune hemolytic anemia. *Hosp Pract* 1985;20:105.

Shapiro SS, Hultin M. Acquired inhibitors to the blood coagulation factors. *Semin Thromb Hemost* 1975;1:336.

Skinner M, Anderson JJ, Simms R, et al. Treatment of 100 patients with primary amyloidosis: a randomized trial of melphalan, prednisone, and colchicine versus colchicine only. *Am J Med* 1996;100:290.

Stroncek DF. Neutrophil antibodies. *Curr Opin Hematol* 1997;4:455.

Thrompson LE, Damon LE, Ries CA, et al. Thrombotic microantiopathies in the 1980s: clinical features, responses to treatment, and the impact of the HIV epidemic. *Blood* 1992;80:1890.

Tsai HM, Lian EC. Antibodies to von Willebrand factor-cleaving protease in acute thrombotic thrombocytopenic purpura. *N Engl J Med* 1998;339:1585.

Visentin GP. Heparin-induced thrombocytopenia: molecular pathogenesis. *Thromb Haemost* 1999;82:448.

Warkentin TE. Clinical presentation of heparin-induced thrombocytopenia. *Semin Hematol* 1998;35:9.

Winkelstein A, Kiss JE. Immunohematological disorders. *JAMA* 1997;278:1982.

Young N, Maciejewski J. The pathophysiology of acquired aplastic anemia. *N Engl J Med* 1997;36:1365.

16. TRANSPLANTATION IMMUNOLOGY: HISTOCOMPATIBILITY

Beth W. Colombe

Organ and tissue transplantation offers new hope to patients with life-threatening acute and chronic disease. In addition to the transplantation of kidney, heart, lung, liver, partial liver and lung, pancreas, and stem cells, the field of transplantation is expanding to include pancreatic islet cells, bowel, multiorgan transplants, limbs, tissue-engineered organs, and organs and tissues from nonhuman sources (xenotransplants).

The organs are obtained either from cadavers, or from living related or unrelated donors. The transplantation of tissue from a donor other than an identical (monozygotic) twin generally provokes a strong immune response by the recipient to various alloantigens present on the graft and its vasculature. The most widely studied of these immunogenic antigens are the molecules of the human leukocyte antigen (HLA) system. HLA antigens are also known as transplantation antigens or histocompatibility antigens because they are the primary targets of immune rejection processes in organ transplantation.

Successful transplantation relies upon the immunologic compatibility of recipients and their organ donors. This compatibility depends on both the extent of matching of the tissue types (HLA types) of donor and recipient, and the absence of any pre-existing antibody reactivity of the recipient with the donor. Both these factors influence the degree of immunosuppression required to prevent rejection of the graft by the recipient.

There are three basic tests performed to determine the histocompatibility of a patient and any potential donors:

1. **Human leukocyte typing** to ascertain the inherited HLA antigens. For both living and cadaveric organ donation, HLA typing is used to determine the extent of antigen matching of the donor HLA type with that of the patient. Within a family, typing can direct the choice of a donor toward the best matched relation. For cadaveric transplantation, the recipient's phenotype is registered with the national organ allocation network called The United Network for Organ Sharing (UNOS). All cadaver donors are also tissue typed and registered with UNOS. Under the mandate of a special UNOS program, when a cadaver donor kidney is found to have no mismatched HLA antigens with a particular patient (a "zero" antigen mismatch) the kidney will be sent to that specific patient.
2. **Cross-matching.** The cross-match test indicates the current status of histocompatibility between the patient and a specific donor by testing for the presence of recipient antibodies reactive to donor HLA. A donor that is reactive with the patient's current antibodies to HLA is generally considered to be incompatible and unacceptable for transplant.
3. **Antibody screening.** Antibody screening of the patient is performed to detect circulating antibodies that have specificity for HLA antigens. The presence of antibodies to HLA antigens will restrict the patient's compatibility with potential donors. These tests and their significance to transplantation will be discussed in greater detail (see Immunological evaluation of the potential transplant recipient on page 380).

    I. **The human leukocyte antigen system and the immune response to transplantation**

        A. HLA is a term derived from the discovery, in 1952, of this antigen system on blood leukocytes. These antigens are present on all nucleated cells. HLA antigens are cell-surface heterodimeric glycoprotein molecules that are the products of a group of closely associated genetic loci on chromosome 6 known as the major histocompatibility complex (MHC). The HLA antigens are classified into class I and class II by their different structures. HLA class I antigens have an α chain inserted into and crossing the cell membrane that is noncovalently coupled with β_2-microglobulin at the cell surface. HLA class II antigens have two chains that associate with one another extracellularly and cross the cell membrane. Both of these HLA antigen structures have a similar cleft-like groove distal to the cell membrane created by two juxtaposed alpha helices. It is within these grooves that peptide antigens, derived from both self- and foreign antigens, are bound. Thus, HLA antigens play a key role in the functioning of the immune response by serving as the molecules that display both foreign and self-peptides to T lymphocytes. Moreover, HLA antigens are themselves highly immunogenic molecules that can trigger vigorous immune responses in allogeneic transplantation, transfusion, and pregnancy (see The immune response to transplantation). Consequently, in transplanting an HLA-bearing organ, the closer that the identity of the donor HLA is to that of the recipient, the more acceptable it is immunologically and the smoother the clinical course will be for the patient.

Major histocompatibility complex class I antigens are products of the HLA genes named A, B, and C and are present on all nucleated cells and on platelets. **MHC class II antigens** are products of the HLA-DR, DQ, and DP multigene loci that are expressed on immunologically competent cells such as B lymphocytes, activated T lymphocytes, monocytes, macrophages, and dendritic cells. The most striking feature of the genes of the HLA system is their great polymorphism. More than 100 distinct HLA antigens (alleles) have been identified by serological typing (Table 16.1). By the molecular techniques of gene cloning and DNA sequencing, the number of defined alleles is approaching 1,000 as a result of sequencing both the exons and introns of these genes, making the MHC the most polymorphic genetic system in humans. During the initial development of the HLA system by serological typing, the HLA antigens were named with a letter representing the genetic locus coding for the antigen followed by an accession number (e.g., A3, B45, DR18, DQ4, etc.). Currently, new HLA alleles of these same loci are assigned numbers based on the similarity of their nucleic acid sequences to previously defined alleles rather than on their reactivity with HLA typing sera.

B. **The immune response to transplantation.** The primary functions of the immune system are to recognize any potentially infective nonself material and to respond via multiple effector mechanisms so that the foreign material is rendered inactive. The function of HLA antigens is to display peptide fragments derived from both self- and nonself-protein molecules. The types of cells functioning as antigen-presenting cells (APCs) include dendritic cells, monocytes, macrophages, and B lymphocytes, among others, i.e., those cells involved in immunoregulatory processes. HLA class I molecules most often present peptides derived from intracellular proteins, mainly of self or viral origin, having bound the processed peptides while traversing the golgi–endoplasmic reticulum secretory pathway on their way to the cell surface. HLA class II antigens bind peptides from exogenous foreign antigens that have been taken into the APCs and processed into peptide fragments via the endosomal pathway of degradation. At the surface, the peptide antigen bound within the cleft of the MHC molecule is presented to immune system effector cells (i.e., helper and cytotoxic T lymphocytes). Foreign antigens are recognized only in the context of self-HLA antigens, a process referred to as HLA restriction. Self-peptides can also be bound in the groove and may, under some aberrant immune responses, initiate the processes of autoimmunity.

C. **Immune recognition.** The first step in the immune response is the recognition by T helper cells (CD4⁺ T cells) of the foreign peptide presented by the self-MHC molecule. The T-cell receptor (TCR) must be precisely specific for that antigen–MHC complex for recognition to occur. Upon cell contact, a trimolecular complex is formed consisting of the TCR and the foreign peptide-plus-MHC molecule on the APC. Interaction between T cells and the APC is aided by other lymphocyte and APC cell surface molecules such as CD4, CD8, CD28, and CD11a/CD18 (leukocyte function-associated

Table 16.1. Human leukocyte antigen specificities[a]

A	B	C	DR	DQ	DP
A1	B5	Cw1	DR1	DQ1	DPw1
A2	B7	Cw2	DR103	DQ2	DPw2
A203	B703	Cw3	DR2	DQ3	DPw3
A210	B8	Cw4	DR3	DQ4	DPw4
A3	B12	Cw5	DR4	DQ5(1)	DPw5
A9	B13	Cw6	DR5	DQ6(1)	DPw6
A10	B14	Cw7	DR6	DQ7(3)	
A11	B15	Cw8	DR7	DQ8(3)	
A19	B16	Cw9(w3)	DR8	DQ9(3)	
A23(9)	B17	Cw10(w3)	DR9		
A24(9)	B18		DR10		
A2403	B21		DR11(5)		
A25(10)	B22		DR12(5)		
A26(10)	B27		DR13(6)		
A28	B35		DR14(6)		
A29(19)	B37		DR1403		
A30(19)	B38(16)		DR1404		
A31(19)	B39(16)		DR15(2)		
A32(19)	B3901		DR16(2)		
A33(19)	B3902		DR17(3)		
A34(10)	B40		DR18(3)		
A36	B4005		DR51		
A43	B41		DR52		
A66(10)	B42		DR53		
A68(28)	B44(12)				
A69(28)	B45(12)				
A74(19)	B46				
A80	B47				
	B48				
	B49(21)				
	B50(21)				
	B51(5)				
	B5102				
	B5103				
	B52(5)				
	B53				
	B54(22)				
	B55(22)				
	B56(22)				
	B57(17)				
	B58(17)				
	B59				
	B60(40)				
	B61(40)				
	B62(15)				
	B63(15)				
	B64(14)				
	B65(14)				
	B67				
	B70				
	B71(70)				
	B72(70)				
	B73				
	B75(15)				
	B76(15)				
	B77(15)				
	B7801				
	B8101				
	B8201				
	Bw4				
	Bw6				

[a] HLA antigens as recognized by the World Health Organization. Antigens listed in parentheses are the most common forms of the antigens; those followed in parentheses are the variant forms of the antigens. Antigens of the Dw series are omitted because they are not the products of specific major histocompatibility complex genes.

antigen 1 [LFA-1]) on T cells with APC molecules such as B7, CD40, and intercellular adhesion molecule 1 (ICAM-1). Through the interactions of the receptors and their ligands, T cells become activated via multiple biochemical signaling pathways. Genes that code for cell surface receptors and other immunomodulatory molecules such as cytokines are turned on, transcribed, and translated into active products. In the early stage of activation, the cytokines interleukin 2 (IL-2) and interferon-γ (IFN-γ) are produced, resulting in the clonal expansion of the responding T cells. Macrophages and B cells are also recruited that contribute additional cytokines and chemokines, broadening the response by stimulating B cells to mature to antibody-producing plasma cells. Thus, both the cellular and humoral arms of the immune response are engaged in reaction to the foreign HLA antigens of a transplanted organ.

In the transplant setting, allorecognition and activation of clones of specific **alloreactive** T cells can lead to acute rejection episodes, impairment of graft function, and to chronic rejection, ultimately resulting in graft loss. Two distinct cellular mechanisms, known as the direct and indirect pathways of allorecognition, operate in the immunogenicity of the foreign HLA antigens of the graft. In the direct pathway, recipient T cells with TCRs that have specificity for donor MHC antigens recognize and are activated by direct contact with the HLA antigens of the graft. It is presumed that the foreign HLA antigen mimics the combination of self-MHC plus foreign antigen so that the TCR is engaged successfully. Meanwhile, donor dendritic cells, arriving as "passenger" leukocytes within the graft, migrate from the graft and home to recipient lymph nodes. In the lymph nodes recipient T cells respond to the foreign MHC and peptides presented by the donor APCs and become activated and proliferate. These activated recipient cells then migrate to and infiltrate the graft and initiate rejection processes easily visible upon biopsy of a deteriorating graft. The response via the indirect recognition pathway requires the processing and presentation of donor antigen by recipient APCs. This can occur both in the lymph nodes as passenger leukocytes invade recipient nodes or at the site of the graft where graft antigen is shed, retrieved, and processed by recipient APCs. The direct recognition pathway is predominantly active in the initial responses to the graft, whereas the indirect pathway assumes increasing importance in maintaining the rejection process as time passes and the passenger leukocytes disappear as a stimulus.

D. **The alloantibody response.** Consequent to transplantation, activated T helper cells can interact with B lymphocytes to stimulate the formation of alloantibodies directed to specific donor HLA antigens. The detection of such antibodies posttransplant can signal the presence of an accompanying cellular rejection response. In addition to the stimulus of transplantation, immune responses to HLA antigens are also elicited from exposure to HLA alloantigens through leukocyte-containing blood transfusion and pregnancy. Patients receiving multiple transfusions and some multiparous women may become immunized to HLA antigens and produce antibodies and activated T-cell clones reactive to specific HLA antigens. Patients whose transplant has failed are frequently found to have high levels of antibodies directed against the HLA antigens of the rejected graft.

Sensitization occurs when antibodies to HLA are formed by a potential transplant recipient, and can be a major impediment to finding a compatible organ donor. Transplantation of an organ bearing the particular HLA antigen(s) to which the patient is sensitized can result in **hyperacute rejection**. In this process, complexes formed by recipient antibody with donor antigen immediately trigger coagulation in the graft vessels, resulting in blockage and immediate cessation of blood flow to and within the graft, thereby destroying it rapidly. For sensitized patients awaiting kidney, heart, and pancreas transplants, there is an absolute requirement to choose a donor that does not bear the target antigens of those preformed alloantibodies. In contrast, liver transplant recipients with measurable anti-donor HLA antibodies do not experience hyperacute rejection for reasons that remain unclear.

Because foreign HLA antigens stimulate immune rejection, matching for HLA antigens between recipient and donor is an effective strategy to facilitate transplant success. HLA matching is often a practical necessity for highly sensitized patients for whom only a donor having no mismatched antigens will be compatible.

E. **Human leukocyte antigen matching.** Matching donor and recipient for HLA antigens reduces the strongest stimulus for immune rejection. The ideal organ donor will have an HLA type closely matched or identical to that of the recipient. For practical purposes, HLA matching for solid organ transplantation is based upon the classical, serologically defined, HLA antigens. Assuming a random assortment of the more than 100 different HLA class I and class II antigens, the likelihood of locating a fully matched unrelated donor can be from 1 in 1,000 to 1 in 1,000,000, depending on the frequency of occurrence of the recipient's antigens in the general population. However, the likelihood of a fully matched sibling donor is 1 in 4 because the inheritance of HLA antigens follows classic mendelian genetics (see Inheritance of human leukocyte antigen below).

In contrast to solid organ transplantation, the requirements for HLA matching for stem cell transplantation are far more stringent. Matching is required at the allele level for HLA class II, especially for HLA-DR and possibly -DQ and -DP, to avoid potentially lethal graft versus host disease. Allele-level matching for HLA class I is highly desirable to avoid both recipient rejection of the graft and graft versus host disease. Registries comprised of several million potential stem cell and bone marrow donors are shared internationally to facilitate searches for acceptable donors for these patients.

F. **Inheritance of human leukocyte antigen.** The best prospect for a well matched, compatible organ donor lies within the immediate relatives of the patient. HLA antigens are inherited in a codominant mendelian fashion as a block of genes (the MHC) on chromosome 6 from each of the two parents (Fig. 16.1). The group of genes is referred to as a "haplotype" and is usually passed en bloc from generation to generation, intact. Genetic recombination within the MHC does occur with an approximate frequency of 1%. Each individual therefore inherits two antigens from each locus, one from the maternal and one from the paternal haplotype. Failure to identify two antigens at a given locus can mean that the individual is homozygous, i.e., has inherited an identical antigen from each parent (e.g., both parents were HLA-A2) or that an antigen is present, but the typing test has no defining antiserum. Molecular-level typing is very successful in determining the nature of these serologically "blank" antigens by examining the genomic DNA of the individual. All of the inherited antigens are codominantly expressed on the cell surface and are referred to as the **HLA phenotype**. For example, a representative **HLA phenotype** is:

A1, A24; B35, B44; Cw4, Cw5; DR6, DR7; DQ2

This HLA phenotype does not indicate which A locus antigen was inherited with which of the two B, C, or DR locus antigens. An **HLA genotype** is the assignment of the HLA antigens of the phenotype according to the inheritance of the block of MHC genes on each chromosome 6. For example, the individual phenotype illustrated above may have been inherited as the following haplotypes:

1. A1, B35, Cw4, DR6, DQ1
2. A24, B44, Cw5, DR7, DQ2

Within a family, the four parental haplotypes, designated as paternal a and b and maternal c and d, can be assorted in four combinations, as shown in Fig. 16.2. HLA identity, meaning the inheritance of the same two parental haplotypes, is thus a 1 in 4 chance occurrence, as is complete non-

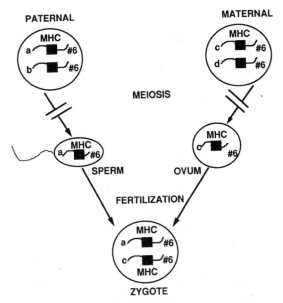

FIG. 16.1. Inheritance of human leukocyte antigen (HLA) haplotypes: A schematic representation of the assortment of parental haplotypes in gametes by the process of meiosis, and the inheritance of one of two possible parental haplotypes, paternal a or b and maternal c or d, by the zygote.

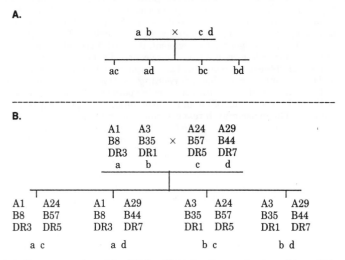

FIG. 16.2. Representation of the **(A)** familial inheritance of paternal (a and b) and maternal (c and d) human leukocyte antigen (HLA) haplotypes. **(B)** Example showing inheritance of HLA antigens on parental haplotypes. The HLA antigens (products of the HLA genes on the chromosomes) are indicated for each haplotype. Note that the HLA antigens of each chromosome are inherited as a unit and are codominantly expressed in the individual. If child ac is the patient, then siblings ad and bc are matched at one haplotype and sibling bd is matched for zero haplotypes.

identity. One-haplotype sibling matches occur with a 1 in 2 frequency and each parent will also be a one-haplotype match with their child.

G. **Human leukocyte antigen matching for transplantation.** For living donor-related transplantation of kidneys, HLA typing is performed to identify the best HLA-matched relative as a potential kidney donor. Parents are one-haplotype matches with their offspring except in the case of genetic recombination in the child. Figure 16.2 illustrates genotyping from parental haplotypes for an individual who is designated as inheriting haplotypes a and c. HLA matching by haplotypes for MHC class I and II antigens in a family implies that all other genetic loci on the haplotype are also identical. HLA identical sibling transplants often require less total immunosuppression to control rejection than unmatched transplants, but do require some treatment to control responses to minor histocompatibility antigens on other (nonidentical) chromosomes.

It is highly advantageous, but extremely difficult, to locate a cadaver donor with the same HLA-A, B, and DR antigens as the patient. Finding such a six-antigen match (or a zero-antigen mismatch) does not signify haplotype identity but rather only that there is identity of the designated HLA antigens (A, B, and DR) between the individuals. True genetic identity of all alleles of the MHC between unrelated donor–recipient pairs is nearly impossible because of the extensive polymorphism of the HLA system. Thus, an HLA-identical sibling transplant is a superior match to a six-antigen-matched organ of identical HLA-A, B, and DR antigens. The projected graft survival half-life ($T_{1/2}$) is dramatically superior in HLA-identical sibling transplants ($T_{1/2}$ of approximately 22 years) compared to unrelated, mismatched cadaver donor grafts ($T_{1/2}$ approximately 5 years). Under current immunosuppression protocols, HLA matching confers minimal graft survival advantage in the short term. However, long-term graft survival is significantly improved by HLA matching, and there is an inverse relationship between the number of mismatched antigens and graft survival.

II. **Immunological evaluation of the potential transplant recipient**
The immune status of potential organ recipients and the suitability of potential donors is determined by three basic tests performed by the histocompatibility laboratory: tissue typing, screening, and cross-matching. **Tissue typing** determines the HLA antigens of the recipient. If the HLA type of the patient and potential donors is known, it allows the selection of a donor whose HLA antigens best match those of the recipient. Tissue typing can be performed by serological and molecular biology methods. **Screening** tests for presence of preformed antibodies to HLA antigens in the serum of the patient. The presence of such antibodies indicates a state of immune sensitization from prior exposure to HLA antigens. **The cross-match test** combines the recipient's serum with prospective donor cells to discover any preformed recipient antibodies that are reactive with donor HLA antigens. Preformed antidonor antibodies have been definitively shown to cause hyperacute rejection of the kidney. **ABO blood group typing** and ABO matching is mandatory for renal transplantation and generally is done for other organs, although exceptions are made for stem cell transplantation and occasionally for emergent liver transplantation.

A. **Tissue typing by serological methods.** The basic serological method for HLA typing is the **lymphocytotoxicity assay**. For HLA class I typing, either peripheral blood lymphocytes (PBLs) or isolated T cells may be used. For HLA class II typing for DR and DQ antigens, B lymphocytes must be isolated from the mixture of mononuclear peripheral blood cells. Aliquots of 2,000 lymphocytes are combined in separate microtest wells with 1 µL of one of a panel of antisera each having a defined HLA specificity. The test is incubated to allow each antibody to bind to its target antigen and form an antigen–antibody complex on the cell surface. Serum complement, usually rabbit serum, is introduced and, after further incubation, a vital dye, such as eosin or acridine orange/ethidium bromide, is added to visualize the live and dead cells. If the antibody has bound to the HLA antigens of the test cell, the cell will be lysed by the activated com-

Table 16.2. Scoring of human leukocyte antigen cytotoxicity test

Percent cells killed	Assigned score	Interpretation
0–10	1	Negative
11–20	2	Doubtful negative
21–50	4	Weak positive
51–80	6	Positive
81–100	8	Strongly positive

From Zachary A, Teresi G, eds. *ASHI laboratory manual*, 2nd ed. Lenexa, KS: American Society for Histocompatibility and Immunogenetics, 1990, with permission.

plement. The presence of dead cells indicates that the cell possesses the HLA antigen corresponding to the specificity of the antibody in the typing serum. The cytotoxicity test is scored as the percentage of dead cells. Tables 16.2 and 16.3 illustrate the test scoring scale and a representative HLA typing test, respectively. The strongly positive scores (8s) indicate the antigens of the subject's HLA phenotype.

B. **Limitations of serological human leukocyte antigen testing.** HLA typing requires a minimum sample of 15 mL of freshly drawn blood for class I typing and at least 30 mL of blood for class II typing to allow for isolation of an adequate number of class II-bearing B cells. The isolated lymphocytes must have a minimum viability of 80%. Biological reagents, such as antisera and serum complement, are subject to variability over time caused by improper storage, contamination, and general deterioration. The main problems inherent in serological typing are the lack of sufficient amount and/or viability of sample and availability of appropriate HLA-typing sera. HLA-typing sera are rare reagents that are discovered by testing many samples of sera from multiparous women on panels of HLA-typed lymphocytes. Antisera for the rare specificities are in short supply and may not be available for use in all laboratories. Consequently, results of HLA typing tests must be interpreted based on the experience of the laboratory with the properties of its antiserum panel. Antisera for HLA class II DR and DQ specificities are especially problematic, and at present, no antisera are available for HLA-DP antigen testing. Serum panels of monoclonal anti-sera have been developed, but these reagents frequently react with multiple HLA antigens (cross-reactivity) and can confuse the interpretation of test results. These limitations are overcome by new methods in molecular tissue typing.

Table 16.3. Scoring of a representative human leukocyte antigen typing test

Serum no.	Antibody specificities	Score[a]
1	A1	8
2	A1, A36	8
3	A1, A3, A11	6
4	A2	1
5	A2, A28	1
6	A3	8
7	A3, A11, B14	8
8	A23, A24	1
9	A24	1

[a] Interpretation: Cell is positive for both A1 and A3.

C. **Molecular methods for human leukocyte antigen typing** utilize isolated DNA from the individual's leukocytes or other tissues rather than the viable blood lymphocytes required by serological testing. The techniques of these molecular methods are based upon the nucleotide sequences of the HLA antigens and focus upon the variations in the sequences. Although HLA antigens have large portions of their sequences in common, these localized differences, termed "epitopes," define the extensive polymorphism of the HLA system. Each HLA antigen is now regarded as being composed of a basic consensus sequence along with a unique selection of these polymorphic epitopes. The sharing of epitopes is the basis for the observation of the serologically defined "cross-reacting groups" (CREGs) (Table 16.4) of antigens. Three methods for DNA typing for HLA are in common use: sequence-specific priming (SSP), sequence-specific oligonucleotide probing (SSOP), and sequence-based typing (SBT). To identify the specific HLA antigens, these methods detect the presence of single or multiple epitopes on a selected template of genomic DNA containing HLA genes. The DNA is amplified to multiple copies through the polymerase chain reaction (PCR).

1. **Polymerase chain reaction** is an automated, DNA polymerase-based method for increasing the number of copies of a known DNA sequence, such as a selected portion of an HLA gene. Microgram quantities of isolated genomic DNA are sufficient for a successful amplification. In this process, two oligonucleotide DNA primers for the polymerase are synthesized that are complementary in sequence to the two flanking sequences of the segment of the HLA gene to be amplified. The primers hybridize to the adjacent regions and initiate the replication of the target sequence by the polymerase. At the end of the first cycle, twice as many copies will have been made as the starting DNA template. In a repetitive process of denaturing the duplex DNA strands, annealing the primers, and repeating the polymerase-driven replication of the sequence, the number of copies of the desired DNA segment exponentially increases to near a million after approximately 25 cycles. In the reaction, the primers can be designed to isolate and amplify sequences that are locus-specific (e.g., all DR antigens), group-specific (e.g., all DR4 antigens), or specific for a particular allele (e.g., DRB1*0404).

2. **In the sequence-specific priming method**, the PCR process itself is used to ascertain the presence or absence of the epitopes that characterize particular HLA antigens. In SSP, the primers are constructed exactly to complement one or more of the unique DNA sequences of each HLA antigen to be identified. For example, primer pairs are designed

Table 16.4. Crossreacting HLA antigen groups (CREGs)

CREG Group	HLA Antigens
1C	A1, 3, 11, 23, 24, 29, 30, 31, 36, 68, 69, 80
2C	A2, 28, 68, 69, 23, 24; B17
10C	A11, 25, 26, 32, 33, 34, 43, 66, 68, 69, 74
5C	B51, 52, 35, 53, 18
7C	B7, 8, 13, 27, 41, 42, 46, 47, 48, 54, 55, 56, 60, 61, 73, 81
8C	B8, 18, 38, 39, 51, 59, 64, 65
12C	B13, 37, 4005, 41, 44, 45, 47, 48, 49, 50, 60, 61
21C	B35, 49, 50, 51, 52, 53, 57, 58, 62, 63, 71, 72, 73, 75, 76, 77, 78
4C	A23, 24, 32; Bw4
6C	Bw6

HLA, human leukocyte antigen.
From Rodey GE. An Approach to High PRA Analysis In: Rodey GE ed. *HLA beyond tears*. Atlanta: DeNovo, 1991.

to hybridize with a specific epitope found on all alleles of DR4. A unique set of primer pairs must be designed to be specific for each epitope of interest and thus the method requires multiple PCR reactions, typically 30 for HLA-DR and -DQ, and 100 to 200 for HLA-A, -B, and -C typing. After the PCR, the products of the amplifications are separated by gel electrophoresis. If the PCR process has resulted in an amplified product, the individual possesses that epitope, whereas the lack of any product shows the absence of that defining epitope. The HLA type is thereby determined by the composite result of multiple amplifications. The method is limited by the ability to design primers that function under standard conditions and that can be adequately specific for the large array of HLA alleles.

3. **Sequence-specific oligonucleotide probing** uses small oligonucleotides (19 to 24 base pairs in length) of single-stranded DNA that are constructed to exactly compliment selected unique sequences of each HLA epitope. PCR-amplified DNA, usually from class I or class II genes, is dotted onto membranes, the probes are exposed to the DNA for hybridization and then the membranes are washed under conditions of high stringency. Hybridization of the probe signifies the presence of the target HLA epitope and antigen(s). The probes can be labeled with radioactive, colorimetric, or chemiluminescent molecules. For some uses, generalized probes can be constructed to recognize sequences shared by subgroups of alleles (group-specific), so that a series of probes can be used in a sequential fashion to define the unknown antigen. An alternate SSOP method, referred to as the "reverse dot blot" method, is available in which the probes are fixed to a solid medium and the isolated DNA, in solution, is allowed to hybridize to them. The SSOP technique requires continual updating of the collection of probes as new HLA alleles are discovered.

In SSOP as in SSP, primers or probes will only identify known alleles and will fail to detect new alleles with unique sequences. The ultimate typing technique that will detect new HLA alleles, as well as all known (i.e., previously sequenced) HLA alleles, is to sequence the DNA of the MHC itself.

4. **Sequence-based typing** is accomplished in two steps of PCR amplification. In the first step, a segment of DNA containing the gene of interest is amplified, followed by a second amplification, the cycle-sequencing process, in which the replication of strands of DNA is terminated upon incorporation of dideoxynucleotide analogs to the normal nucleotide bases. The PCR product will contain DNA chains of varying sizes that have been terminated at each nucleotide base in the sequence. Separation of the chains by size on a gel will reveal the order of the nucleotide bases along the DNA template. Automated sequencing utilizes dye labeling of either the initiating primers or the terminating nucleotides to read the nucleotide sequence. The final sequence can then be compared to a library of all known HLA sequences for identification of the HLA antigen. A sufficient stretch of DNA must be sequenced to detect all possible defining epitopes. Sequencing of the second exon of HLA class II is usually sufficient, whereas class I sequences require the sequencing of exons two and three, as well as some intron regions where further polymorphism has been found.

D. **Cellular methods for histocompatibility testing.** Prior to the development of molecular methods for HLA typing, cellular-based tests, such as the **mixed lymphocyte culture** (MLC) test, were used to select the most compatible donor from among several living candidates. T cells are exquisitely sensitive to the presence of nonself-HLA and foreign peptides as presented by self-HLA. When recipient peripheral blood leukocytes are exposed to donor lymphocytes with mismatched HLA antigens, the recipient T cells proliferate, signaling the presence of HLA nonidentity. A lesser degree of T cell response could indicate a preferable donor among several HLA mismatched donors. The previous advantage of the MLC was that it could reveal HLA class II differences, which may not be serologically detectable because of the lack of appropriate antisera. With the advent of molecular tissue typing and resolution of HLA types at the allele level, the MLC has been abandoned and replaced by routine typing by DNA. Cellular assays do find an application in posttransplant immune monitoring. Investigators report successful use of the MLC to detect posttransplant activation of recipient T cells to donor antigens that, in some instances, can signal incipient rejection.

E. **Testing for presensitization to human leukocyte antigens**
1. **Human leukocyte antigen antibody screening.** Exposure to HLA antigens through transfusion, pregnancy, or transplantation can result in the formation of antibodies specific for HLA antigens (i.e., sensitization). The presence of these antibodies is a contraindication to transplantation if the HLA antigens of the organ donor match the specificity of the patient's antibody (e.g., when the patient has an anti-HLA B8 antibody and the donor is HLA B8-positive). The extent of sensitization can be determined by testing serum from the patient for the presence of HLA antibodies. Test cell panels of 30 to 60 HLA-typed lymphocytes are selected so that the combined HLA phenotypes represent all of the common HLA antigens. The patient's serum is screened for reactivity with these cells using the lymphocytotoxicity assay. An estimate of the extent of sensitization is made by calculating the percent of **panel-reactive antibodies** (PRA): the number of cells that react positively with the serum divided by the number of cells in the test panel, times 100, equals the percent PRA. The percent PRA indicates the likelihood that the patient's antibodies will react with the HLA of a random, (i.e., cadaveric) donor. Patients with PRAs over 80% have difficulty finding a compatible donor and consequently spend many years on the cadaver donor waiting list. Such patients require very well-matched donors to obtain a transplant. Antibodies may fade over time, but such sensitized patients, when transplanted, remain at relatively high risk for rejection of the graft.

Screening for the presence of anti-HLA antibodies (also termed lymphocytotoxic antibodies) is usually performed at the first medical evaluation visit, on additional samples drawn monthly, and subsequent to any immunizing event, such as a transfusion, transplant rejection, pregnancy, or change in immunosuppression therapy.

2. **Antibody specificity.** Determination of the specificity of the anti-HLA antibody is made by examination of the HLA phenotypes of the test cells with which the antibody is reactive. For example, if all of the five cells that reacted positively with the serum have HLA-A1 in their HLA phenotypes, the antibody specificity is considered to be anti-A1. Some antibodies are reactive with epitopes held in common among several HLA antigens. Such antigen groups are known as **CREGs** (Table 16.4) Patients with antibodies to one or two CREGs can have high PRAs. Identification of the antibody specificities of patients awaiting transplant is an important component of the selection of a suitable organ donor. It is accepted practice to avoid transplantation of an organ bearing an HLA antigen to which the patient has been previously sensitized.

Anti-HLA antibodies can have specificity for both HLA class I and class II antigens. Class I antigens (HLA-A, -B, and -C) are present on all lymphocytes used in the standard cytotoxicity assays. Antibodies to HLA class II antigens are frequently found in sera that also contain antibodies to HLA class I. Antibodies to HLA class II antigens react with HLA-DR and -DQ on B lymphocytes and monocytes, and, *in vivo*, have the potential to react with activated (but not resting) T cells, dendritic cells, and graft endothelial cells. To screen for these antibodies by cytotoxicity, the cell panels must be composed of isolated B lymphocytes.

3. **Autoantibodies.** Autoantibodies are defined as antibodies that react with one's own tissues. Autoantibodies are detectable by the cytotoxicity assay, and can produce false-positive reactions in the antibody screening test and also in a cross-match test. Thus, it is critical to screen patients for the presence of autoantibodies by testing their serum with their own cells in the autocross-match test. If the autocross-match is positive, the antibodies are considered to be nonspecific (i.e., not anti-HLA). This conclusion is based upon the assumption that individuals do not make antibodies against their own HLA antigens. Thus, when autoantibodies are detected, they are considered benign to the transplant outcome. Although most autoantibodies are of the immunoglobulin M (IgM) isotype, it is not prudent to dismiss all IgM antibodies as inconsequential to transplantation. Antibodies to HLA antigens can be of the IgG and IgM isotypes. Anti-HLA antibodies of the IgM class can lead to rejection episodes.

Both IgG (of the complement-fixing subtypes) and IgM antibodies are detectable by cytotoxicity.

IgM antibodies can be removed by treating the serum with reducing agents such dithiothreitol (DTT) or by heating the serum to 63°C for several minutes. Alternatively, the serum can be absorbed using the patient's own cells or those of a third party. Care should be taken that the HLA phenotype of the third-party cell has no HLA antigens in common with potential donor(s) so as to avoid absorbing out any HLA antibodies potentially reactive with the donors. The treated serum should then be retested for antibodies reactive with the patient and with any donors. If, upon treatment, the serum activity disappears, the presence of IgM cytotoxic antibodies in the original sample is confirmed. Occasionally, removal of IgM autoantibodies uncovers the presence of an IgG anti-HLA antibody.

4. **Cell-free antibody detection.** The reaction of nonspecific antibodies with molecules on the cell membrane that are not HLA can produce false-positive antibody tests. To overcome this biological problem, methods for the detection of HLA antibodies have been developed that use cell-free preparations of HLA antigens that are fixed to a solid medium. In one method, a pool of HLA molecules is fixed to a plastic plate and a colorimetric enzyme reaction is used in a standard enzyme-linked immunosorbent assay (ELISA) to mark antigen–antibody complexes. This technique allows for efficient automation and high-volume testing. Approximately 40 different sera can be tested in duplicate on a typical ELISA screening plate. A second method binds isolated HLA antigens to microparticles that can be passed through a flow cytometer. Like the ELISA trays, the HLA-coated beads carry a large array of HLA antigens typically found in a standard lymphocyte panel for PRA testing. The beads are exposed to the patient's serum, followed by addition of a fluorescently labeled antihuman IgG antibody to tag any bound antibody. The fluorescent beads are counted by the cytometer and the amount of shift in the fluorescence intensity of the beads compared with the negative control is taken to represent the percent PRA. These two methods are powerful aids in the identification of the specificity of antibodies reactive in the cytotoxicity test, and help to identify those antibodies that are not anti-HLA and that will be benign to transplantation.

D. Cross-matching

1. Selection of a histocompatible donor is ultimately determined by the results of the cross-match test. In the serological cross-match, serum of the recipient is mixed with the cells of the potential donor for the purpose of detecting any preformed antibodies that are reactive with the donor HLA antigens. The cross-match is termed "positive" when antidonor antibodies are found. The presence of such antibodies can

precipitate an immediate, or hyperacute, rejection of the graft. These anti-HLA antibodies will bind to donor antigens on the graft and vascular endothelium, thereby triggering the complement system and activating platelets leading to fibrin clot formation. The vessels occlude and the organ becomes ischemic and necrotic. The goal of cross-matching is to detect antibodies that are potentially harmful and that signal the patient's capacity for future development of antidonor antibodies and cytotoxic T cells.

It is mandatory to select the most current serum of the patient for cross-matching, preferably drawn within 1 month of transplantation. For sensitized patients with current, measurable PRAs or patients having a recent sensitizing event, the serum should be drawn within 24 to 48 hours prior to testing. In addition to the most current serum, a number of previous sera can be selected (commonly, the most reactive serum drawn in the recent past, the "peak"), in order to detect previously formed antibodies that may have disappeared from the current serum. Opinion differs on the relevance of cross-matching sera older than 6 months. For patients with a history of multiple antibodies or with a previous transplantation, two or more previous, stored serum samples should be cross-matched with the selected donor. It should be borne in mind that the formation of memory T and B cells occurs concurrently with the humoral response to HLA. Such specific memory cells may retain the capacity to be reactivated if the original sensitizing antigen is present on the new graft.

2. **Cell targets of the cross-match test.** PBL cross-matching: The simplest cross-match is the PBL cross-match in which isolated donor peripheral blood mononuclear leukocytes are mixed with recipient serum using standard cytotoxicity test methods. PBLs are approximately 60% to 80% T cells and 5% to 20% B cells. HLA class I antigens are expressed on both cell types, whereas HLA class II antigens are restricted to B cells. In a PBL cross-match, weak antibody reactivity could be interpreted as either a weak anti-HLA class I antibody or as indicative of antibodies to HLA class II.

   a. **T-cell cross-matching.** Cross-matching with peripheral blood **T cells** ensures that any HLA antibody detected will be specific to HLA class I antigens. It is universally accepted that a positive IgG antidonor T-cell cross-match is a contraindication to transplantation for all solid organs with the exception of the liver.

   T cells can be isolated from peripheral blood by monoclonal antibodies that negatively select and eliminate non-T cells from PBLs, or by a positive selection technique that uses magnetic microparticles coated with antibodies against T-cell-specific surface molecules, such as CD2, CD4, or CD8. Because of the relative ease of obtaining peripheral T cells and of the proven importance of avoiding of anti-class I antibodies for transplantation, this test is the most widely utilized in the cross-matching of potential donors and recipients.

   b. **B-cell cross-matching.** Because B lymphocytes are normally are present in isolated PBLs at from 5% to 20% of lymphocytes, they must be isolated and purified to more than 80% for the cytotoxicity test to yield strong, definitive results. The same types of monoclonal antibody and microparticle bead selection methods used for T cells are also used for B-cell isolation. B-cell cross-matches are frequently performed using serial dilutions of the serum to determine the strength (titer) of the antibody. High-titered B-cell antibodies are associated with strong graft rejection, whereas low-titer antibodies can be safely ignored for some patients undergoing their first transplant. However, a positive B-cell cross-match indicates a high risk for rejection for the regraft patient. B cells can be used as targets to detect both HLA class I and II antibodies because they have both antigens on their cell surface. B cells are more sensitive targets than T cells for HLA class I antibodies because their surface has a greater density of these antigens. Consequently, a low-titer HLA class I antibody may result in a positive B-cell cross-match, but a negative T-cell cross-match.

The significance of a positive B-cell cross-match to the outcome of first transplants continues to be debated. However, there is general agreement that for regraft patients, a positive B-cell cross-match contraindicates the transplant.

3. **Cross-match techniques**
   a. **Serological.** Several serologically-based methods for cross-matching provide increased sensitivity over the basic method (the National Institutes of Health or "NIH" technique) of simple incubation of cells plus serum followed by complement. Other modifications include extending the incubation times of cells plus serum and of complement, and the addition of one or more wash steps whereby the serum is removed from the cells before the addition of the complement. Further sensitivity is achieved by adding an antibody to human globulin after the wash steps and prior to complement addition. The antihuman globulin (AHG) cross-links the bound antibody and facilitates complement binding and cell lysis.
   b. **Flow cytometry cross-match**. Of all current cross-match methods, the flow cytometry cross-match (FCXM) is the most sensitive. Flow cytometry measures the quantity of patient antibody bound to donor cells by using an indirect antibody assay. After incubation of the donor cells and patient serum, a second antibody (the developing antibody) is added that is directed against the IgG-specific epitope of the patient's anti-HLA antibody. The developing antibody is tagged with a fluorochrome, thereby making the cells fluoresce under laser illumination in the cytometer. The flow cytometer senses and counts the number of fluorescent cells and presents a histogram plotting the number of cells versus fluorescence intensity. The fluorescence intensity is given on the x-axis in units of "channels" or intensity units. The y-axis indicates the number of cells counted in that channel of fluorescence. Figure 16.3 illustrates the differences in the positions of the cell histogram peaks that are seen with negative and positive controls and with a patient serum that has antibodies to donor HLA antigens.

   Specific cell populations can be selectively examined in the flow cytometer by tagging them with labeled monoclonal antibodies directed to a unique surface molecule, such as the CD3 receptor on T cells, or the CD20 molecule on B cells. This population-specific antibody is tagged with a fluorescent molecule emitting light at a different wavelength than that of the developing antihuman Ig antibody (two-color flow cytometry). For example, to look for anti-class I antibodies bound only to T cells, the donor cells and patient serum are first incubated to allow antibody binding, followed by addition of an anti-CD3 monoclonal antibody labeled with phycoerythrin (PE, 580 nm) and the antihuman IgG developing antibody labeled with fluorescein isothiocyanate (FITC, 515 nm). The T cells are selected for examination by setting the flow cytometer to look at only the PE fluorescing cells and then, among those, to measure the number of FITC-labeled cells (cells with antibody) and their fluorescence intensity. The FCXM can be up to 100 times more sensitive than a serological cross-match. However, with this sensitivity, it cannot only detect very low levels of antibody but also other types of antibodies including non-HLA antibodies and antibodies that are noncomplement-fixing (and would be negative

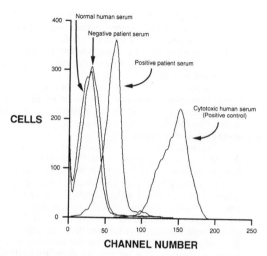

FIG. 16.3. The flow cytometry cross-match histogram. The histogram is produced by counting the number of cells (*y*-axis) of a given fluorescent intensity (*x*-axis, divided into 256 channels). Cells from the potential organ donor are mixed with patient serum to test for the presence of antidonor human leukocyte antigen (HLA) antibody. A second antibody to human IgGF(ab')^2 labeled with a fluorochrome is added to tag any bound antibody. The number of fluorescing cells is counted for each channel of a given intensity. The cell peak containing cells with bound antibody will shift to the right compared with the peak of the same cells exposed to a negative control serum. A shift of greater than 9 to 10 channels indicated a positive test (i.e., the presence of antidonor antibody).

in the cytotoxicity assay). The FCXM has been criticized as being too sensitive and is suspected of depriving some recipients with benign antibodies of a transplant. This circumstance can be countered by ensuring that the true specificity of any donor-reactive antibody is well characterized as an anti-HLA antibody.

c. **Cross-matching with treated serum.** IgG antidonor antibodies are detrimental to transplantation, whereas IgM antibodies are usually benign. IgM antibodies are frequently, but not always, nonspecific autoreactive antibodies. Both immunoglobulin isotypes can fix complement and can result in a positive cross-match. IgM antibodies can be eliminated by breaking the disulfide bonds holding the pentameric IgM molecule together through treatment of the serum with reducing agents, such as DTT, or by heating the serum to 63°C for several minutes. The cross-match is then repeated with treated serum and if the result is negative, transplantation is usually performed. However, some IgM antibodies can be anti-HLA and have the potential of damaging the graft. IgM antibodies with specificity for HLA antigens can be identified by the combination of cytotoxicity tests with the serum treated and untreated to identify the antibody specificity and the immunoglobulin isotype. Unfortunately, screening for IgM anti-HLA antibodies is not a routine procedure in most tissue-typing laboratories.

4. **Cross-matching strategies** for high-risk and low-risk patients. A **high-risk patient** is one who has been sensitized to HLA antigens with a PRA (see Testing for presensitization to human leukocyte antigen on page 384) of 10% or greater, or has been previously trans-

planted regardless of the current PRA status. These patients can have a negative cross-match on a current serum sample but may have anti-donor antibodies in older, stored sera. Cross-matching previously reactive sera can be informative because immune system memory cells may be reactivated to produce these former antibodies against the new graft. In general, more extensive cross-matching is performed for high-risk patients, including T- and B-cell serological testing and flow cytometry cross-matching on multiple sera. Low-risk patients are those candidates for a primary graft with low or no panel-reactive antibodies.

The serum of patients with autoantibodies should always be treated to remove IgM prior to cross-match. If the autoantibody is IgG, the serum can be absorbed prior to testing with the patient's or third-party cells to remove nonspecific antibodies. The third-party cell should not share any antigens with the prospective donor to avoid absorbing out any specific antidonor antibody.

5. **Interpretation of cross-match results.** Cross-matches must always be interpreted in the light of knowledge of the patient's current and past immune profile and the status of the patient as a primary or regraft recipient. Evidence of prior sensitization places the patient at risk for transplant rejection. Table 16.5 summarizes cross-match patterns and generally accepted interpretations of results. Alternate decisions are certainly made by individual programs based on their own experiences and for the special circumstances of an individual patient.

A positive IgG antidonor T-cell cross-match is a contraindication to the transplantation of kidneys, hearts, lungs, and pancreas. A positive B-cell cross-match must be tested further to determine the target antigens of the antibody, either HLA class I or class II or both.

Table 16.5. Crossmatch results and interpretations

| Crossmatch type | | | | Cells | Interpretation of | Transplant |
T[a]	B[a]	FCXM-T	FCXM-B	(D, P)	main antibody type	(yes, no)[b]
−	−	−	−	D	No anti-HLA antibodies, or DTT or heat treated serum	Yes
+	+	+	+	D	IgG anti-class I—high titer	No
−	+/−	+	+	D	IgG anti-class I—low titer	Yes/no[c]
−	+	−	+	D	IgG anti-class II	No
−	−	−	+	D	IgG, possibly weak anti-class II	Yes/no[c]
+	+	−	−	D/P	IgM, autoantibody, nonspecific	Yes
−	−	+	−	D	IgG, probably not anti-HLA	Yes

[a] Crossmatch done by serological methods.
[b] Transplant: These decisions to perform or withhold transplant represent consensus based on knowing that the antibody specificity is anti-HLA. Individual programs may depart from these practices.
[c] Decision is based on primary versus repeat transplant patient and on whether the positive result is found in current or only in historic sera.
FCXM-T, T cell flow cytometry crossmatch; FCXM-B, B cell flow cytometry crossmatch; D, donor; P, patient; HLA, human leukocyte antigen; DTT, dithiothreitol; IgG, immunoglobulin G.

Cross-matches that are negative with donor T cells and positive for donor B cells are interpreted as evidence for an HLA class II antibody. In fact, this result can also occur when a low-titered class I antibody is present.

Rarely, a cross-match will be positive with T cells and negative with B cells. This result is difficult to interpret given the cellular distribution patterns of HLA antigens, and suggests that the antibody is not against HLA. The specificity of the antibody should be further investigated to clarify such a result.

A positive T cell FCXM confirms the presence of anti-HLA class I (A, B, or C) antibodies.

An FCXM that is T cell negative and B cell positive indicates an antibody to HLA class II (DR, DQ, or possibly DP), although as in serology cross-matching, it could also result from a weak anti-class I antibody. It is controversial whether solid organ transplantation in the presence of anti-HLA class II antibodies should take place. Patients at low risk have been successfully transplanted with low-titered anti-class II antibodies, whereas high risk patients, i.e., recipients of second transplants, are generally not transplanted against positive B-cell cross-matches.

If the serological cross-match is negative, and the FCXM with T cells is positive, the risk status of the patient must be considered when interpreting a positive FCXM. A positive FCXM contraindicates transplantation for high-risk patients, although many centers now transplant low-risk patients, particularly those with 0% PRA and no prior transplants, for whom there is no recent sensitizing event. The amount of channel shift is also taken into consideration in deciding which patients to transplant. In a T-cell cross-match, channel shifts of greater than 20 channels (256 channel scale) can indicate increased risk of rejection.

Cross-matches that are positive by serology and negative by flow cytometry indicate that the antibody isotype is IgM. The developing antibody of the flow cytometry cross-match is usually of the anti-IgG specificity.

III. Immunosuppression

Posttransplant immunosuppression therapy is mandatory for all transplant recipients. However, recipients fortunate enough to receive a kidney from an HLA-identical sibling or a zero-HLA antigen-mismatched cadaver donor require significantly less immunosuppression. Foreign HLA antigens trigger a vigorous immune response that must be controlled by immunosuppressive drugs to avoid an acute or accelerated rejection episode that could lead to loss of the graft. Standard immunosuppression regimens use multiple drugs for both pre- and posttransplant management: pretransplant for high-risk patients as a rejection–prophylaxis measure, and posttransplant for maintenance of immunosuppression and for the treatment of rejection episodes. The current drug armamentarium includes corticosteroids, azathioprine, cyclosporine A (CsA), tacrolimus (FK506), sirolimus (SRL, Rapamycin), mycophenolate mofetil (MMF), various monoclonal antibodies such as basiliximab (Simulect) and daclizumab (Zenapax), and polyclonal antibodies such as antithymocyte globulin (ATG), antilymphocyte globulin (ALG), and OKT-3. All of these drugs are associated with significant toxic side effects. These agents act to interrupt one or more of the several processes of immune activation of T lymphocytes or to block effector functions. Thus, appropriate synergistic combinations of these drugs, each used at a decreased dosage, can broaden the immunosuppressive effect and minimize the side effects of an individual drug.

A. Cyclosporine A. CsA is in widespread use in solid organ transplantation for maintenance of immunosuppression. CsA has increased first-year graft survival by 10% to 15% compared to previous regimens that used the combination of prednisone and azathioprine, and has greatly reduced the incidence of acute rejection. The major side effects of CsA are a dose-dependent nephrotoxicity, both acute and chronic, and neurotoxicity. The nephrotoxic effects of CsA are exacerbated by the circumstances responsible for delayed graft function, such as prolonged cold ischemia, organ reperfusion injury, and other non-specific inflammatory insults to the organ. Administration of CsA is often delayed until proper posttransplant function is well established. Blood concentration is continuously monitored, but many recipient factors (such as weight, diet, and metabolic differences) will influence the relationship between drug level and efficacy for individual patients.

Both CsA and tacrolimus (see Tacrolimus below) act by inhibiting calcineurin. Calcineurin is a critical enzyme in the process of intracellular signaling that follows the stimulation of a CD4+ T cell through engagement of its receptor by foreign antigen. The recognition signal is amplified through biochemical pathways leading to the transcription of genes that produce cytokines essential for T-cell activation and proliferation. CsA and tacrolimus bind to cyclophilins (intracellular cis-trans isomerases) and the complex inhibits calcineurin function. By this interaction, CsA and tacrolimus prevent the production of IL-2 and other cytokines essential to the initiation and expansion of inflammatory and allogeneic cellular and humoral immune responses. Blocking the production of IL-2, IFN-γ, and lymphotoxin produced by activated T cells prevents the clonal expansion of cytotoxic T cells that are responsive to donor antigens. Current 1-year graft survival with CsA coverage is between 85% and 95%. However, CsA administration apparently has not altered the long-term processes of chronic rejection.

B. **Tacrolimus** (FK506) is functionally similar to CsA as an immunosuppressive agent in transplantation, although it is quite different in structure. Like CsA, FK506 inhibits calcineurin and thereby inhibits the production of cytokines (IL-2, IFN-γ), resulting in inhibition of the activation and proliferation of helper and cytotoxic T lymphocytes. It is between 10 and 100 times more potent than CsA, but has similar nephrotoxic effects that clearly limit its use for rejection therapy in renal transplantation. It is the drug of choice for liver transplantation. Tacrolimus has had dramatic success as a "rescue therapy" in the reversal of both acute and early chronic rejection in liver transplant recipients. When given as primary immunosuppression, tacrolimus results in improved graft and patient survival rates compared with CsA in some studies. Five-year graft survival in patients treated with tacrolimus was significantly improved compared with CsA (63.8% versus 53.8%). Incidence and severity of acute rejection was also significantly improved with tacrolimus. A 2-year trial of combined tacrolimus and MMF demonstrated fewer corticosteroid-resistant rejections and better renal function than regimens using combinations of CsA, MMF, and steroids, or tacrolimus, azathioprine, and corticosteroids. Tacrolimus has shown to be useful as a corticosteroid-sparing agent. A combination of tacrolimus and MMF can allow withdrawal of corticosteroids by day 7 posttransplant with excellent graft survival and renal function.

C. **Mycophenolate mofetil.** MMF, a purine analog, inhibits *de novo* purine synthesis in activated lymphocytes, thereby inhibiting DNA synthesis and interrupting the transition from G1 to S phase of the cell division cycle. MMF prevents the proliferation of reactive T- and B-cell clones. Inhibiting T-cell clonal proliferation blocks antigen-specific rejection, whereas inhibiting B-cell proliferation suppresses donor-specific antibody formation. MMF is effective at reducing both acute and chronic rejection in renal transplant patients. The most prominent dose-dependent side effects of MMF are gastrointestinal tract irritation and bone marrow suppression associated with increased infection.

D. **Sirolimus.** SRL (Rapamycin) is a macrolide antibiotic that is a structural analog of tacrolimus. SRL has potent immunosuppressive effects that synergize with other immunosuppressants. SRL complexes with FK506 binding protein 12 (FKBP12), as does tacrolimus, but its activity differs from the latter in its further interaction in the cell activation process. SRL preferentially binds with FKBP12 and that complex, in turn, binds with a second protein, the mammalian target of rapamycin (mTOR). The result is cell cycle arrest at the G1–S interface due to inhibition of several kinases and decreased production of messenger RNAs (mRNAs) encoding ribosomal proteins. In addition to inhibiting donor-specific T cell proliferation, SRL also prevents B-cell maturation into antibody-producing plasma cells, thereby depressing the humoral arm of the immune response to foreign antigen. SRL is one of a very few agents that can influence antibody production (intravenous gamma globulin, IVIg, is another).

The major toxicity of SRL is an elevation of both triglycerides and cholesterol, with hyperglycemia, hypokalemia, and thrombocytopenia also observed. However, there is no evidence of the nephrotoxicity and hypertension commonly seen in patients receiving the calcineurin inhibitors CsA and tacrolimus, and patient survival and acute rejection rates are comparable to other drug regimens. SRL is a competitive antagonist of tacrolimus because of its similar structure, but it acts synergistically with CsA. CsA and SRL in combination reduce the rate and severity of acute rejection and improve the duration of graft survival normally seen with usage of either SRL or the calcineurin inhibitors alone. Thus, the combination of SRL and CsA blocks both the early phase of cytokine production (by CsA) and the effects on cellular function (by SRL), exerting a potent synergistic double effect to prevent acute rejection. The addition of SRL into the protocol permits a decreased dosage of CsA, thus decreasing the risk of its nephrotoxic side effects.

E. **Corticosteroids.** Corticosteroids have long been recognized for their potent antiinflammatory local and systemic effects. The proinflammatory cytokines, IL-1 and tumor necrosis factor (TNF), are produced by APCs upon their antigen-specific contact with a T helper cell (CD4+ T cell). These cytokines stimulate the production of IL-2 and IFN-γ by the activated T helper cells, thereby initiating the cascade of events leading to donor-antigen-specific organ rejection. Corticosteroids inhibit the transcription of the IL-1 and TNF genes, and thus deflect the immune-mediated rejection process and ameliorate any systemic inflammatory response. Prednisone is used routinely in posttransplantation immunosuppression regimens. High-dose corticosteroid pulses are administered to reverse acute rejection episodes.

The side effects of corticosteroid therapy are well known, including cushingoid facial and body changes, alterations in mood, hypertension, edema, degenerative changes in the hip and other bones, depression of adrenal function, and delayed effects such as the possibility of cataracts, glaucoma, growth retardation in children, and a host of metabolic changes leading to muscle wasting and bone and connective tissue loss. A variety of clinical trials are in progress that have as their goal the eventual complete withdrawal of corticosteroid use.

F. **Azathioprine.** In combination with prednisone, azathioprine was used for transplant immunosuppression for several decades until the advent of cyclosporine. Azathioprine inhibits DNA synthesis by blocking purine metabolism at the level of inosinic acid synthesis. By inhibiting DNA synthesis, azathioprine suppresses T-helper and T-cytotoxic-cell responses in the transplanted recipient. Unlike MMF, azathioprine is not lymphocyte-specific but rather targets rapidly multiplying cells, and it can induce a profound suppression of hemopoietic cells in the marrow. Depression of the bone marrow proliferation can lead to infections and potentially to cancers consequent to a loss of immune surveillance by immunocompetent cells. Therefore, patients on immunosuppressive regimens including azathioprine require blood cell monitoring to check for marrow function.

G. **Monoclonal antibody therapies** have been developed to target specific antigens or epitopes to suppress specific immune responses to transplanted tissue.

1. **OKT-3** is a murine monoclonal antibody with specificity for the CD3 portion of the T-cell receptor complex found on all T lymphocytes. The OKT-3 binds to the T-cell receptor, resulting in the initial disappearance of the receptor from the cell surface, thus rendering the T cell nonfunctional for antigen recognition and activation. Commonly used as a treatment for corticosteroid-resistant rejection, OKT-3 dramatically reduces overall levels of circulating T cells and thereby counteracts the rejection episode. The CD3 receptor returns to the cell surface, as measured by other monoclonal anti-T-cell receptor antibodies, but is functionally blocked by the binding of OKT-3. OKT-3 is also used prophylactically for patients at high risk for rejection. The drug has potent side effects including pulmonary edema and neurologic complications. Certain patients respond to OKT-3 therapy by producing antibodies to the murine determinants on the OKT-3 immunoglobulin molecule, effectively neutralizing the drug's effectiveness, which can be monitored by measuring levels of CD3-bearing cells in the circulation. Repeat administration of OKT-3 for a second rejection episode is possible, but it is essential to test for the presence of any sensitization to the drug prior to treatment.

2. **Daclizumab** is a chimeric monoclonal antibody with specificity for the a subunit (Tac) of the surface antigen CD25, the IL-2 receptor expressed on activated T lymphocytes. A product of recombinant DNA technology, daclizumab is 90% human and 10% murine in composition and as such, it avoids sensitization of the recipient to nonhuman portion of the antibody molecule, unlike OKT-3. By binding to the CD25 molecule, daclizumab blocks the activation signal to the T cell that arises from the binding of IL-2. In combination with other standard immunosuppressants, daclizumab effectively reduces rejection episodes. Its current use is mainly prophylactic rather than as a treatment for acute rejection.

3. **Basiliximab**, like daclizumab, is an engineered chimeric murine–human monoclonal antibody directed against the IL-2 receptor α-chain (CD25, Tac) on activated T lymphocytes. Basiliximab competitively inhibits the binding of IL-2 to CD25. It abrogates T cell proliferation and activation of antidonor T cells. Like daclizumab, basiliximab is used prophylactically to reduce the incidence of rejection in combination with other immunosuppressive drugs. There are no reported drug interactions, nor are there any toxic effects on end organs or bone marrow, or deleterious effects on cellular effector functions such as cytokine release syndrome.

4. Other monoclonal antibodies exist with potential for application to transplantation. Research in the biochemistry of the immune response has revealed key points which could serve as targets for intervention and disruption of the process. In order to be activated to proliferate, T cells require two signals, one from the engagement of their antigen-specific receptors (TCR–CD3 complex) and a second from the binding of an additional receptor by its corresponding ligand on the APC. Monoclonal antibodies directed toward costimulatory T-cell receptors and their corresponding ligands on the APC (e.g., CD28, CTLA4, B7, CD40L [CD154] and CD40, Fas, and Fas ligand) are under investigation. Other potential targets for intervention are cell surface adhesion molecules that enhance the intercellular contact between the T cell and the APC, including LFA-1 and its APC ligand ICAM-1, and the CD4 and CD8 epitopes that interact with the MHC–antigen complex on the APC.

H. **The polyclonal antilymphocyte drugs**, ALG and ATG, are produced in horses and rabbits (respectively) in response to immunization with human lymphocytes or T cells, and thus are heterologous, polyclonal antibody preparations having multiple specificities. These drugs deplete circulating

T lymphocytes and are highly effective for treating acute rejection and for preventing graft rejection. T-cell depletion and generalized immunosuppression by these agents can last for weeks and even months. ATG and ALG are used in place of calcineurin inhibitors immediately post-renal transplant to avoid drug nephrotoxicity, should the kidney exhibit delayed graft function. As function returns, the calcineurin-inhibiting agents are phased in to replace ALG or ATG. Severe T-cell depletion increases the risk to the recipient for infection and can produce other side effects (e.g., thrombocytopenia) due to the inclusion of other antibodies in the preparations. The strength of these reagents can be variable because of their polyclonality and the antibody heterogeneity within the animal serum pools. These antibodies can, in some patients, suppress normal antibody production.

When these antibodies are present in serum samples from patients undergoing treatment for rejection or prophylaxis, they produce false-positive reactions in the standard lymphocytotoxic antibody test and can mask donor-specific antibodies. Care should be taken to avoid performing cytotoxic cross-matching and screening with serum containing these therapeutic antibodies. With such sera, alternative techniques are available for antibody screening, such as ELISA and HLA-coated microparticles.

IV. Immunologic monitoring

   A. Monitoring for graft rejection. Posttransplant monitoring for graft rejection is an essential part of the care of transplant patients. As yet, there are no reliable laboratory tests for the diagnosis of rejection, and biopsy remains the only unequivocal means of detection of both acute and chronic rejection.

   Two approaches can be used to predict a forthcoming rejection episode: monitoring recipient T cells for increased antidonor activity, and screening the recipient's serum for the *de novo* appearance of antidonor antibodies.

   Cellular monitoring for rejection: A cellular-based rejection episode involves the clonal expansion of T cells that react to mismatched HLA antigens of the donor. By combining lymphocytes from the transplant recipient and from the organ donor in the MLC test, the strength of reaction of recipient cells to donor cells may be assessed and compared with that measured prior to transplant. An increase in recipient responsiveness can signal an impending rejection. This method of monitoring requires that a source of donor cells be readily available posttransplant, which can be difficult or impossible with cadaveric transplants.

   Posttransplant monitoring of antibodies in recipient serum is far easier to accomplish routinely than is cellular monitoring by MLC. For most renal transplants, there will have been no detectable antibody reactivity against the organ donor's HLA antigens prior to transplant. The *de novo* appearance of antibody reactive with donor lymphocytes may be a signal of an impending humoral rejection episode. Some programs have reported a correlation between the appearance of antidonor antibody and early rejection. Neither of these monitoring assays is in common use.

   B. Monitoring the absolute numbers of circulating T lymphocytes is an accurate assay to measure the effectiveness of administration of antirejection agents such as OKT-3, thymoglobulin, and other agents designed to decrease the number of alloreactive T cells. T lymphocytes are tagged by fluorescence-labeled antibodies directed to cell surface molecules that are specific for T cells, typically, the CD3 molecule. The percentage of CD3-positive cells is determined by cell counting by flow cytometry. The decrease and increase of T-cell levels provides information on the effectiveness of dosage and duration of administration.

   C. Monitoring for antibodies to nonhuman determinants on therapeutic monoclonal antibodies. Monoclonal and polyclonal antibodies from animal sources can stimulate the formation of recipient antibodies against the species-specific determinants of the immunoglobulin molecules. Such antibodies form complexes with the therapeutic antibodies and inactivate them. When large doses of therapeutic antibodies are ineffective in reducing circulating T-cell levels, the presence of such antibodies must be considered.

D. Monitoring for hemopoietic stem cell engraftment. Tissue typing for HLA antigens can be used to monitor the progress of engraftment of donor stem cells provided that the donor has HLA antigens that are different than those of the recipient. In hematopoietic stem cell transplantation, HLA antigen disparity between donor and recipient, even at the allele level, is carefully avoided, particularly in unrelated stem cell transplants. HLA mismatching of a single nucleotide base (and amino acid) can trigger rejection and graft versus host disease; HLA disparities in class I antigens promote graft rejection, whereas disparities in class II trigger graft versus host disease. Thus, one or two HLA class I antigen differences (and in some cases of parent to child, one-haplotype differences) are acceptable when the recipient has an impaired immune system, such as for children with severe combined immune deficiency disease or patients with aplastic anemia. When stem cell donor and recipient are perfectly matched for HLA at the allele level, other polymorphic genetic systems can be utilized to test for the presence of engrafted donor cells.

Molecular probes exist for non-HLA polymorphic genes and can be used to determine the presence of genomic tandem repeat sequences of variable number (variable-number tandem repeats [VNTRs]) from 30 to 100 base pairs and for short tandem repeats (STRs) of from 2 to 6 base pairs. Typing the patient and donor alleles for these genes and repeated sequences must be done before transplantation in order to identify the genetic loci having unique donor alleles.

If a sex difference exists between donor and patient, several DNA and flow cytometry methods are available to monitor posttransplant samples for the X and Y chromosomes.

V. Human leukocyte antigen, therapeutics, and tolerance in transplantation

T cells become activated upon interaction with HLA molecules and their peptides on self-APCs. For successful activation, the T cells must also receive a second signal from the engagement of accessory molecules, such as the binding of the B7.1 and B7.2 molecules on the APC with the CD28 receptor on the T cell. In the absence of such second signals, T-cell functions are modulated. T cells that interact only with the MHC complex can undergo apoptosis (DNA fragmentation and cell death) or become anergic (nonresponsiveness). Both of these effects can establish a state of apparent tolerance to the graft. Similarly, MHC molecules that are extracted from cells can be used to modulate T-cell responses. These can be prepared as soluble HLAs (sHLAs) alone or in combination with peptides. sHLA molecules can be found in the body fluids of normal individuals and, when formed into aggregates, are very effective at inducing T-cell apoptosis and cell death. Apoptosis of donor-reactive recipient T cells will abrogate immune responses to the graft. Dimers and tetramers of selected MHC plus peptides have been successfully constructed and can bind strongly to T cells restricted by that particular HLA antigen. These constructs can be used diagnostically to detect antigen-specific $CD8^+$ CTL (cytotoxic T lymphocyte) clones by flow cytometry, by quantifying the number of T cells that bind a specific antigen. In a therapeutic clinical situation, the modulation and functions of such identified T-cell clones can be followed with these MHC reagents. Tetramers could be made of the recipient's MHC molecules containing donor HLA peptides that would potentially target and eliminate any recipient T cells that could be activated by the donor antigens in the transplant.

A major role of soluble HLA antigens is to bind antibodies in solution and this process may serve an immunoregulatory function in normal physiology. In transplantation, sHLAs that are shed from the graft may exert a protective effect by binding to the recipient's anti-HLA antibodies and cytotoxic T cells, thereby deflecting their action against the graft itself. This process also decreases the amount of the shed sHLAs and prevents them from being processed and presented by recipient APCs, thus protecting the graft from both cellular and humoral rejection. The liver, in particular, releases large quantities of soluble HLA antigen, a phenomenon that may explain its relative resistance to rejection despite the presence of preexisting recipient anti-HLA antibodies.

HLA offers the potential for both diagnostic and therapeutic strategies. In the transplant setting, the goal is to induce donor-specific tolerance and avoid generalized immune suppression and its concomitant side effects. Utilization of portions or all of the MHC molecules holds the promise of supplementing current immunosuppression protocols and has the potential to replace these drugs entirely. Other avenues of transplant tolerance are being explored concurrently that include modulation of other surface molecules on immunocompetent cells, and the disruption of T-cell signals and cytokine interactions that lead to activation and proliferation of the immune response.

Suggested Readings

Baxter-Lowe L, Colombe BW. *Histocompatibility testing in medical immunology*, 10th ed. Parslow T, Stites D, Terr A, et al., eds. New York: McGraw-Hill-Lange, 2001.

Bidwell JL, Navarrete C, eds. *Histocompatibility testing*. London: Imperial College Press, 2000.

Buell JF, Kulkarni S, Grewal HP, et al. Early corticosteroid cessation at one week following kidney transplant under tacrolimus and mycophenolate mofetil immunosuppression. *Transplantation* 2000;69:S134(abst 88).

Gonwa TA, Johnson C, Ahsan N, et al. Two year follow-up of a randomized multicenter kidney transplant study comparing tacrolimus + azathioprine vs. cyclosporine + mycophenolate mofetil vs. tacrolimus + MMF. *Transplantation* 2000;69:S113(abst 11).

Hansen JA, ed. *The detection and application of DNA polymorphisms, reviews in immunogenetics*. Copenhagen: Munksgaard, 1999:1(2).

Marsh S, Parham P, Barber L, eds. *The HLA facts book*. San Diego: Academic Press, 2000.

McCluskey J, ed. *Immunobiology of the major histocompatibility complex, reviews in immunogenetics*. Copenhagen: Munksgaard, 1999:1(1).

Petersdoft, EW, Gooley TA. Anasetti C, et al. Optimizing outcome after unrelated marrow transplantation by comprehensive matching of HLA class I and II alleles in the donor and recipient. *Blood* 1998;92;3515.

Pirsch JD. Tacrilomus versus cyclosporine in kidney transplantation. *Transplantation* 2000;69:S113(abst 8).

Thorsby E, ed. *Immunogenetics of allorecognition, reviews in immunogenetics*. Copenhagen: Munksgaard, 1999:1(3).

Tilney NL, Strom TB, Paul LC, eds. *Transplantation biology, cellular and molecular aspects*. Philadelphia: Lippincott-Raven, 1996.

17. PRIMARY IMMUNODEFICIENCY DISEASES

Charlotte Cunningham-Rundles

Resistance to infection is necessary for health. The major barriers to infections are the natural physical barriers, skin and the epithelial surfaces of the respiratory, intestinal, and genital tracts, which tend to exclude invading bacteria. Because the mucosal epithelium is a more permeable mechanical barrier than skin, other mechanisms in this location augment resistance, including ciliary clearance, mucus, lysozyme, and lactoferrin. When infectious agents penetrate these barriers, other nonspecific host factors, such as cytokines, complement, and the phagocytic cells (neutrophils and macrophages) provide a second line of defense.

At both mucosal and systemic levels, a third line of immune defenses includes the specialized immune systems: B lymphocytes that produce antibodies, and T-cell-mediated immunity. Defects in one or more of these systems can produce a spectrum of clinical manifestations, depending on the system(s) affected, the extent of impairment, and the compensatory mechanisms that can be recruited.

Deficiencies of the immune system can be congenital or acquired, can occur in children or adults, and can be primary defects or secondary to an underlying disorder. On the other hand, many patients with recurrent infections are immunocompetent. In children especially, allergic rhinitis and/or asthma is one of the most common diseases leading to repeated upper and lower respiratory tract infections. Other diseases, such as cystic fibrosis or the immotile cilia syndrome, may need to be considered to provide an accurate diagnosis and determine the correct therapy. Determining if an immune defect is likely to be present can be problematic, but some guidelines can aid the practicing clinician.

I. **Classification of primary immunodeficiency**
   The overall incidence of these immunodeficiency diseases is estimated at about 1 in 10,000, excluding selective IgA deficiency; for unknown reasons, more than half of the reported immune defects (still excluding IgA deficiency) involve defects in antibody production. To evaluate a patient for immunodeficiency, a basic understanding of the immune system is useful (see Chapter 1). The International Union of Immunologic Sciences (IUIS) has compiled a catalog of the known defects of the immune system that is periodically updated. An overview of major immunodeficiency syndromes, divided by type, is given in Table 17.1. Although exact categorization can sometimes be difficult for individual patients, primary immunodeficiencies can be classified into eight general categories. Within these major headings, recognized clinical syndromes can be grouped, according to the predominant mechanism(s) that is defective.

   A. **Combined cellular and antibody (T and B cell) deficiencies** comprise 20% to 25% of primary immunodeficiencies. This is a heterogeneous group, characterized by the presence of T- and B-cell dysfunction often associated with decreased numbers of T lymphocytes and immunoglobulin levels, as seen in severe combined immunodeficiency disease (SCID). The associated defects can predominate, as in Wiskott-Aldrich syndrome (thrombocytopenia) and DiGeorge syndrome (cardiac abnormalities and hypocalcemia).

   B. **Cellular deficiency (T cell) disorders** account for at most 5% to 10% of primary immunodeficiencies. Although it is operationally useful to classify these as isolated T-cell disorders, when T-cell function is impaired, antibody formation is also deficient.

   C. **Antibody deficiency (B cell) disorders** comprise 50% to 65% of all primary immunodeficiencies and are the most common defects that are diagnosed. This excludes selective IgA deficiency, which has an incidence of approximately 1 in 500 in the general population, although most of these individuals do not have any symptoms. In patients with antibody deficiency, serum immunoglobulin (Ig) levels (IgG, IgA, and/or IgM) may be markedly

Table 17.1. Types of immunodeficiency syndromes

Condition	Comments
COMBINED T-CELL AND B-CELL DEFICIENCY	
Reticular dysgenesis	Generalized hematopoietic hypoplasia
Severe combined immunodeficiency (SCID)	Includes the following immunodeficiency syndromes:
	X-linked SCID, due to defect of chain of IL-2 receptor
	Autosomal-recessive inheritance of unknown kind
	Adenosine deaminase (ADA) deficiency
	Defective recombinase (RAG1, 2) enzyme
	Omenn syndrome, in many cases due to mutation in RAG enzyme
	Cartilage-hair hypoplasia, short-limbed dwarfism, associated with bony defects
	Bare lymphocyte syndrome with poor expression of histocompatibility HLA class II antigens
	Defects in JAK kinase
	IL-7 receptor defect
	Defect of T-cell signal ZAP-70
Hyper-IgM syndrome	IgM normal to elevated; defect in expression of gp39, a T-cell ligand for CD40, the B-cell receptor responsible for isotype switching; associated with neutropenia, pneumocystis pneumonia, high incidence sclerosing cholangitis
Ataxia–telangiectasia	IgE, IgG-2, and/or IgA deficiency common; high incidence of lympho-reticular malignancy; chromosome repair defect
Thymoma	T-cell defect variable; hypogammaglobu-linemia in some
Wiskott-Aldrich syndrome	Thrombocytopenia (small platelets); no carbohydrate antibody responses; eczema; X-linked inheritance; high incidence of lymphoreticular malignancy; CD43+ cells not detected
PRIMARILY T-CELL DEFICIENCY	
DiGeorge syndrome	Characteristic facies; heart lesions (interrupted aortic arch most typical); hypoparathyroidism; T-cell deficiency may be severe enough for associated antibody deficiency; immune defect usually spontaneously improves; thymus is absent in complete form; failure of normal descent nearly always; chromosome 22 defect in most
Inosine phosphorylase (PNP) deficiency	Often associated with primary red cell aplasia
CD3 nonexpression	T cells present but do not express CD3, necessary for T-cell receptor function

Table 17.1. *Continued*

Condition	Comments
PRIMARILY B-CELL DEFICIENCY	
Congenital X-linked agammaglobuline-mia (Bruton) disease (XLA); other causes, defect of μ chain, surrogate light chain, etc.)	Absence of B-cells; clinically presents in first year of life, males for the X-linked form, and male or female for others
Transient hypogammaglobulinemia of infancy	Occurs at 2–6 months of age; difficult to differentiate from the normal nadir of IgG, which occurs during that time
Selective IgA deficiency	IgA less than 10 mg/dL; normal to increased IgG, 12% with IgG2 deficiency; selective deficiency of IgA; most common deficiency (1/500 of Caucasians); associated with inheritance of histocompatibility antigen
Selective IgM deficiency	Quite rare, associated with *Neisseria* infections
Common variable immuno-deficiency	Antibody defect prominent; B cells present; T-cell deficiency may be present and increase with time
IgG subclass deficiency	Caused by genetic deletion of Ig heavy chain genes, or deficient production of selected IgG isotypes; asymptomatic or associated with infections if antibody production is impaired
COMPLEMENT DEFECTS	
Complement deficiency	May mimic antibody deficiency syndromes; C3 deficiencies clinically similar to pan-hypogammaglobulinemia; deficiencies of complement components, particularly C6–C9, associated with recurrent infec-tions with *Neisseria* species
PHAGOCYTIC DEFECTS	
	Caused by low numbers of phagocytes, lack of chemotaxis, lack of intracellular killing
STRUCTURAL DEFECTS	
Ciliary dysmotility	Mimics antibody deficiency syndromes; recurrent otitis and chronic pulmonary infections with bronchiectasis are characteristic
DEFECTS OF ADHESION	
Cell adhesion molecule deficiency (LFA-1/Mac-1)	Mimics antibody deficiency syndromes somewhat; delayed separation of the um-bilical cord, poor inflammatory response, periodontitis, recurrent septic episodes
DEFECTS OF UNKNOWN ORIGIN	
Hyper-IgE syndrome	Job-Buckley syndrome (hyper-IgE); skin and organ abscesses, bone abnormalities, dental abnormalities
Chronic mucocutaneous candidiasis	Granulomatous skin lesions; often associ-ated with hypoadrenalism, hypopara-thyroidism, or other endocrinopathy; recurrent infection with antibody defi-ciency may appear

IL, interleukin; RAG1, 2, recombination activation gene 1 or 2; HLA, human leukocyte antigen; JAK-3, janus kinase-3; ZAP-70, zeta-associated phosphoprotein-70; IgE, immunoglobulin E; CD43⁺, cluster of differentiation 43⁺; LFA, leukocyte function-associated antigen; PNP, purine nucleoside phosphorylase.

decreased or completely absent. It is important to note that the majority of subjects with significant antibody defects are adult. Very much more rarely, antibody deficiency with normal serum immunoglobulin concentrations may also occur. Antibody deficiency in these cases can be broad (both protein and polysaccharide antigens) or more restricted (e.g., to carbohydrate bacterial capsular antigens).

D. **Complement deficiencies** can result in inadequate coating of bacteria with antibody (opsonization,) reduced or absent phagocytosis, or lysis of microorganisms. These defects lead to infections that are often characterized by sepsis. The most common complement defect, however, is of the C1 inhibitor, which results in recurrent attacks of swelling, but not infections. Complement disorders account for a small percentage of primary immunodeficiencies (less than 2%) and may coexist with autoimmune diseases, such as systemic lupus erythematosus (SLE).

E. **Phagocytic disorders** (granulocytes, monocytes) constitute approximately 10% to 15% of all primary immunodeficiencies. Defects of neutrophil and monocyte maturation and differentiation, chemotaxis, phagocytosis, and intracellular killing have been described. The most common of these are diseases that lead to neutropenia, followed by chronic granulomatous disease (CGD).

F. **Defects of cell surface adhesion** can produce immune dysfunction. A good example are leukocyte adhesion defects, in which leukocytes fail to form normal attachments to endothelial cell surfaces, and cannot migrate into tissues effectively to fight infections.

G. **Structural defects.** Although not a part of the immune system, a defect of ciliary structure can result in poor mucous clearance, and frequent sinopulmonary infections.

H. **Unknown defects.** Some of the established immune deficiency syndromes are not yet understood from a biochemical or molecular point of view, and the primary immune function that is defective has not been identified.

II. **Clinical findings in immunodeficiency disorders**

The most frequent clinical indicator of an immune defect is the occurrence of "too many infections." This is the main manifestation of infants and children with immune deficiency, and presents a significant challenge to the pediatrician because infections are so common in normal childhood. When **frequent and prolonged infections are coupled with failure to thrive, or if unusual infections** appear, an evaluation of the immune system is in order. A confirmed report of an immunodeficiency disease occurring in a sibling or first-degree relative should also prompt careful clinical assessment and laboratory investigation, even without a history of severe or unusual infections. The causes of some of the more common primary immunodeficiency disorders are unknown. The onset of symptom may be in infancy, childhood, or later in adult life. Some common clinical findings of primary immunodeficiencies are listed in Table 17.2.

A. **History**

1. **Sinopulmonary infections.** These are a common symptom of many immunodeficiency diseases. In most cases, sinopulmonary infections are due to common respiratory bacterial pathogens, such as *Streptococcus pneumoniae, Haemophilus influenzae, Moraxella catarrhalis, Staphylococcus aureus,* and *Pseudomonas aeruginosa.* Although frequent (6 to 10 per year) upper respiratory infections are common in normal young children, especially if there is exposure to older siblings or to other children (e.g., daycare centers,) or coexisting respiratory allergies, there are some distinguishing characteristics of infections that may suggest abnormal host resistance (such as the presence of fever, more purulent secretions, lack of clear allergy symptoms, lymphadenopathy, positive family history for immunodeficiency, or need for frequent antibiotics). These infections may become chronic and lead to complications, such as perforated tympanic membranes, otitis media with mastoiditis, restrictive lung disease, or bronchiectasis.

Table 17.2. Clinical features of immunodeficiency

Usually present
  Recurrent upper respiratory infections
  Severe bacterial infections
  Persistent infections with incomplete or no response to therapy
Often present
  Failure to thrive or growth retardation for infants or children
  Weight loss for adults
  Intermittent fever
  Infection with unusual organisms
  Skin lesions, such as rash, seborrhea, pyoderma, necrotic abscesses, alopecia,
    eczema, telangiectasia
  Recalcitrant thrush
  Diarrhea and malabsorption
  Persistent sinusitis or mastoiditis
  Hearing loss due to chronic otitis
  Chronic conjunctivitis
  Arthralgia or arthritis
  Bronchiectasis
  Recurrent bronchitis or pneumonia
  Evidence of autoimmunity, especially autoimmune thrombocytopenia or hemolytic
    anemia
  Hematologic abnormalities: aplastic anemia, hemolytic anemia, neutropenia, and
    thrombocytopenia
Occasionally present
  Paucity of lymph nodes and tonsils
  Lymphadenopathy
  Hepatosplenomegaly
  Severe viral disease (e.g., varicella or *Herpes simplex*)
  Chronic encephalitis
  Recurrent meningitis
  Autoimmune disease such as autoimmune thrombocytopenia, hemolytic anemia,
    rheumatologic disease, alopecia, thyroiditis, pernicious anemia
  Pyoderma gangrenosum
  Adverse reaction to vaccines
  Delayed umbilical cord detachment
  Chronic stomatitis or peritonitis

From Stiehm ER. Immunodeficiency disorders: general considerations. In: Stiehm ER, ed. *Immunologic disorders in infants and children,* 3rd ed. Philadelphia: WB Saunders, 1996, with permission.

2. **Other bacterial infections** (e.g., deep infections such as cellulitis, osteomyelitis, meningitis, or sepsis). Although severe infections can occur in healthy individuals, two severe infections of this kind suggest the possibility of immunodeficiency. Recurrent neisserial infections characterized by sepsis suggest a deficiency of terminal complement component.

3. **Infections with opportunistic organisms**, such as *Pneumocystis carinii, Aspergillus fumigatus, Giardia lamblia,* cryptosporidia, atypical mycobacteria, or *Candida albicans,* suggest cell-mediated dysfunction. Infections with *Aspergillus* or *Candida* are also commonly found in individuals with phagocytic disorders.

4. **Failure to thrive** often occurs in infants in children, but its absence does not exclude an immunodeficiency. Failure to thrive is particularly frequent in cell-mediated immunodeficiency disorders, especially when

diarrhea develops. In adults, weight loss or loss of subcutaneous fat is a more common manifestation.

5. **Gastrointestinal disease.** Chronic or prolonged diarrhea, with or without malabsorption, is frequently present in all types of immunodeficiency disorders. Infectious etiologies, such as *Giardia lamblia*, *Campylobacter*, *Cryptosporidium*, enteropathic *Escherichia coli*, *Helicobacter pylori*, or viruses (e.g., rotavirus and cytomegalovirus) occur. Other causes of diarrhea include intestinal lymphoid nodular hyperplasia, disaccharidase deficiency, sprue-like syndrome, inflammatory conditions resembling Crohn disease, or intestinal lymphoma.

6. **Surgery.** Sinus surgical procedures may have been performed for recurrent infections. Other surgeries may have included incision and drainage, tonsillectomy and adenoidectomy, lymph node biopsies, lobectomies, and intestinal biopsies. A retrospective pathology review of lymphoid tissue (tonsils, adenoids, and intestine) can help to evaluate the absence of germinal centers and plasma cells, or both.

7. **Family history.** Table 17.3 lists the inheritance patterns of selected primary immunodeficiency disorders. As illustrated, some of these disorders are inherited as either X-linked or autosomal-recessive inherited traits. A history of consanguinity should be sought and, if possible, a family genealogic tree constructed. Important clues in other family members include fetal death, autoimmune disorders, and lymphoreticular malignancies.

B. **Physical examination**

The physical examination can reveal pertinent clues to the nature of an immune defect (Table 17.4). The physical examination should include the following:

1. **Height and weight.** Failure to thrive in children is a common feature of cell-mediated immune deficiencies, especially when associated with chronic diarrhea. An active, well-nourished, well-developed child is not as likely to have a serious (T and B cell) immunologic deficiency, although children with B-cell immune deficiencies may grow normally. For children, growth charts can serve as a guide to the effectiveness of therapy (see Appendix IX for growth charts). An apparent appearance of normality can be misleading, because a substantial immune defect can be documented in adults who look perfectly normal.

2. **Lymphoid tissue.** Small or absent peripheral lymph node tissues may be found in both T- and B-cell immunodeficiency syndromes. However, as a result of chronic infectious stimulation with accompanying immune dysregulation, lymphadenopathy may be found. Hepatosplenomegaly is also quite common.

3. **Oral examination.** Periodontitis can be sign of neutrophil disorders. Mucosal ulcerations of the tongue or oral mucosa appear in many immunodeficiency syndromes. Retention of primary teeth is an indicator of the hyper-IgE syndrome.

4. **Mucocutaneous candidiasis.** Although candidiasis involving the oral pharynx is common in young infants, it is not seen after about 1 year of age in a healthy infant. It is the most common presentation in cell-mediated immunodeficiencies (e.g., SCID, DiGeorge syndrome, and Wiskott-Aldrich syndrome). Several features distinguish candidiasis in the immunocompromised host, including lack of predisposing conditions such as concomitant antibiotic or corticosteroid usage and breast-feeding, persistence of candidal involvement in the older infant, resistance to appropriate antifungal therapy, reappearance after appropriate treatment, presence of candidal esophagitis, and persistent cutaneous involvement.

5. **Eczema and/or seborrheic dermatitis.** Skin lesions are commonly found in patients with T-cell abnormalities. Weeping scalp seborrheic dermatitis is also common in (especially young) patients with hyper-

Table 17.3. Inheritance pattern of primary immunodeficiency diseases

Designation	Inheritance
Combined immunodeficiencies	
Severe combined immunodeficiencies (SCID)	
Reticular dysgenesis	AR
Defect in common γ chain of cytokine receptors	XL
RAG1/RAG2 mutation	AR
Adenosine deaminase deficiency (ADA)	AR
Nucleoside phosphorylase deficiency	AR
MHC class II deficiency	AR
JAK-3 kinase	AR
CD3 (T cell) deficiency	AR
ZAP-70 deficiency	AR
IL-7 receptor defect	AR
Wiskott-Aldrich syndrome	XL
DiGeorge syndrome	AD? Variable penetrance
Ataxia telangiectasia	AR
X-linked lymphoproliferative disorder	XL
Antibody immunodeficiencies	
X-linked (Bruton) agammaglobulinemia	XL
Ig deficiency with increased IgM (hyper-IgM immunodeficiency syndrome)	XL, AR
Common variable immunodeficiency	Unknown
IgA deficiency	Unknown
IgG subclass deficiency	Unknown
Transient hypogammaglobulinemia of infancy	Unknown
Phagocytic immunodeficiencies	
Chronic granulomatous disease	
Cytochrome b558 absent	XL
Cytosol factors absent	AR
Hyperimmunoglobulin E syndrome (hyper-IgE syndrome)	Unknown
Chédiak-Higashi syndrome	AR
Other Defects	
Tap1/Tap2 defect	AR
Leukocyte adhesion defect	AR
Mucocutaneous candidiasis with or without endocrine disease	AR; unknown

AR, autosomal recessive; AD, autosomal dominant; XL, X-linked; RAG1 2, recombination activation gene 1 or 2; MHC, major histocompatibility complex; CD, cluster of differentiation; JAK-3, janus kinase-3; ZAP-70, zeta-associated phosphoprotein-70; Ig, immunoglobulin; Tap1, transporter-associated protein.

IgE syndrome. Severe diaper rash is common in infants with combined T- and B-cell defects, or T-cell defects.

6. **Clubbing of the fingers** or chest examination demonstrating increased **anterior to posterior diameter**. Persistent crackles suggest the complications of chronic pulmonary disease (e.g., bronchiectasis) commonly seen in primary immunodeficiency syndromes.

7. **Fungal nail infections.** Nail infections are common in mucocutaneous candidiasis, hyper-IgE syndrome, combined T- and B-cell defects, and in T-cell defects.

8. **Otitis and sinusitis.** Purulent discharge from the ear, with or without tympanic membrane perforations and scarring, are frequent findings. Sinus tenderness, with or without purulent rhinitis are common.

Table 17.4. Special clinical features associated with immunodeficiency disorders

Clinical features	Disorders	Associated findings
Dermatologic		
Eczema	T- or B-cell immune deficiency	Recurrent infections, diarrhea
	Wiskott-Aldrich syndrome	Thrombocytopenia
Sparse, hypo-pigmented hair	Cartilage hair hypoplasia	Short-limb dwarfism, severe varicella infections
Telangiectasia	Ataxia-telangiectasia	Ataxia, malignancies
Oculocutaneous albinism	Chédiak-Higashi syndrome	
Seborrheic dermatitis	T-cell defects	Severe diarrhea
	SCID with acute GVHD	Hepatosplenomegaly, diarrhea, adenopathy, alopecia
Scleroderma	SCID with chronic GVHD	Hepatosplenomegaly, diarrhea, adenopathy, alopecia
Recurrent abscesses	Hyper-IgE syndrome	Coarse facies, thrush, eczema
	Chronic granulomatous disease	Granulomata of stomach (vomiting) and colon (colitis)
	Leukocyte adhesion defect	Delayed umbilical cord separation, perio-dontitis, stomatitis
Oral ulcers	Severe T-cell immune defects	Thrush, diarrhea, FTT
	Hyper-IgM syndrome	Neutropenia, spleno-megaly, immune thrombocytopenia
Peridontitis, stomatitis	Neutrophil defects	Recurrent abscesses
Candidiasis	T-cell immune defects; combined defects; muco-cutaneous candidiasis	Recurrent infections/ autoimmune disease
Vitiligo	B-cell defects	Recurrent infections
Alopecia	B-cell defects	Recurrent infections
Chronic conjunctivitis	B-cell defects	Recurrent infections
Extremities		
Clubbing of the nails	Chronic lung disease due to antibody defect	Rales, wheeze, purulent sputum Recurrent infections
Fungal nail infection	T-cell defect, combined defects; mucocutaneous candidiasis	
Arthritis	Antibody defects; Wiskott-Aldrich, hyper-IgM	Recurrent infections
Endocrinologic		
Hypoparathyroidism	DiGeorge syndrome	Unusual facies, cardiac defects
Endocrinopathies (autoimmune)	Mucocutaneous candidiasis	Thrush, nail dystrophy, pernicious anemia

Table 17.4. *Continued*

Clinical features	Disorders	Associated findings
Growth hormone deficiency	X-linked agamma-globulinemia	
Gonadal dysgenesis	Mucocutaneous candidiasis	
Hematologic		
Hemolytic anemia	B- and T-cell immune defects	Splenomegaly
Thrombocytopenia	Wiskott-Aldrich syndrome	Purpura, echymosis
Immune thrombo-cytopenia	B-cell immune defects	Splenomegaly
Skeletal		
Short-limb dwarfism	Short-limb dwarfism with T- and/or B-cell immune defects	
Bony dysplasia	ADA-deficiency associated SCID	

SCID, severe combined immunodeficiency; GVHD, graft-versus-host disease; FTT, failure to thrive; IgM, immunoglobulin M; ADA, adenosine deaminase.

9. **Cutaneous abscesses** can occur, especially in neutrophil disorders. This includes rectal abscesses and the presence of previously healed abscesses or fistulae.
10. **Arthritis** is a frequently associated manifestation in patients with antibody-deficiency disorders, but it may appear in combined immune defects such as Wiskott-Aldrich syndrome and in hyper-IgM syndrome.
11. **Chronic conjunctivitis** due to nontypable *H. influenzae* and other polysaccharide-encapsulated bacteria is often present, especially in the antibody deficiency syndromes.
12. **Delayed umbilical cord detachment** is observed in leukocyte adhesion defects secondary to CD11/CD18 integrin deficiency, which produces poor phagocytic inflammatory responses.

III. **Test for the evaluation of the immune system**

When an immune defect is suspected, the next questions are what part of the immune system should be investigated, what tests are needed, and how far one should carry these investigations. **The selection of immunologic tests must be guided by clinical suspicion based on the clinical history and physical examination.** The evaluation of the immune system is best approached in stages, performing the basic screening tests first, and turning to more complex testing as indicated. An overview of this staged approach is given in Table 17.5.

A. **Initial screening investigations**

1. **Previous medical records and a complete blood count and differential.** Aside from the initial history taking and physical examination, including measuring the height and weight, the first immune test is the complete blood count. A white blood count and differential will provide information on the number of each cell type. Part of the first visit should also include obtaining all the previous medical records, including pathology reports or slides, and results of previous cultures and radiologic studies.
2. **Serum immunoglobulins.** Because antibody deficiency diseases are more common that other immune defects, the first emphasis should be placed on the investigation of immunoglobulins and antibody production. The relevant test is quantitative immunoglobulins, which gives the serum levels of IgG, IgA, and IgM. Because immunoglobulin values increase with age, comparison to age-matched controls is necessary for correct interpretation (see Appendix V).

Table 17.5. Laboratory tests for immunodeficiency

	Initial	Second level	Advanced
B cell	Quantitative immunoglobulins: IgG, IgA, and IgM Preexisting antibodies to prior immunizations: tetanus, diphtheria, rubella, *Haemophilus influenzae,* and polio Isohemagglutinins IgG subclass levels	IgE level, B-cell enumeration Antibody responses to pneumococcal polysaccharide vaccination, and protein antigens tetanus diptheria	Molecular studies Genetic studies Antibody responses to bacteriophage ΦX 174 (primary and secondary) antibody responses, IgM/IgG isotype switching
T cell	Total lymphocyte count Delayed-type hypersensitivity skin tests	T-cell and subpopulation enumeration Proliferative responses to mitogens, antigens, allogeneic cells Acquisition of activation molecules; *in situ* hybridization for chromosome 22 defect	Cytokine synthesis Cytotoxicity assays ADA and PNP levels in RBC Genetic studies
Phagocytic	WBC count and morphology IgE level	Nitroblue tetrazolium reduction; oxidative burst by flow cytometer	Phagocytic assay Chemotaxis assay Chemiluminescence Genetic studies
Complement	CH$_{50}$ C3 and C4 levels	Individual complement levels	Serum opsonic and chemotactic assays; Alt50

Alt50, 50% activity, alternative pathway; IgG, immunoglobulin G; ADA, adenosin deaminase; PNP, purine nucleoside phosphorylase; RBC, red blood cell; CH$_{50}$, 50% hemolyzing dose of complement.

3. **Pulmonary function.** Immune deficiency, especially if it has persisted for some time, will often affect lung function. Complete lung function with volumes, flows, and diffusion capacity should be tested, even if the chest x-ray is normal. Patients with both T- and B-cell defects are subject to pulmonary infections, resulting in bronchospasm, restrictive or obstructive disease, or combinations of these abnormalities.

4. **Delayed-type hypersensitivity.** Commonly used to assess T-cell function, delayed-type hypersensitivity skin tests have been widely used in general screening. Although these tests are not always easy to interpret, perhaps due to use of nonstandardized reagents, they may yield some information. A positive test with recall antigens can rule out a more severe T-cell defect, but such tests are not useful for infants younger than the age of 2 years, because appropriate exposure has not yet occurred. In adults, about 85% will have one or more positive re-

actions. The usual reagents used are *Candida* extract (1:100 dilution), tetanus (1:100 dilution), and mumps antigen (undiluted).

5. **Sweat chloride** determinations should be done as a screening test if cystic fibrosis is suspected clinically, especially in a patient with a history of repeated respiratory infections, a history suggestive of malabsorption, and failure to thrive. Values greater than 60 mEq per L are abnormal. In questionable cases, request DNA evaluations to determine possible genetic defects that occur in approximately 70% to 75% of patients with cystic fibrosis.

B. **Second-level measurements**

1. **Antibody production.** To resolve the clinical significance of somewhat reduced serum immunoglobulin IgG levels, one measures specific antibody responses to previously administered or naturally occurring antigens. When a possible B-cell immunodeficiency is suspected, measurements of antibody responses to both protein and polysaccharide antigens are essential in order to assess B-cell function. This is particularly important if treatment with immunoglobulin is being considered. It is important to try to complete the evaluation prior to administering immunoglobulin, otherwise it will be difficult to verify the need for immunoglobulin therapy without stopping and reassessing antibody production after 5 or more months have elapsed.

   a. **Antibody responses to protein antigens.** Determining antibody titers to diphtheria and tetanus toxoids pre- and postimmunization (2 to 4 weeks) of diphtheria, tetanus toxoids, pertussis (DPT), diphtheria, tetanus (DT), immunization (in adolescents and adults) is helpful to assess IgG antibody responses to protein antigens. Typically, patients have already received their primary DPT immunizations, thus this is a measure of amnestic antibody responses. Antibody responses following immunization to killed poliomyelitis and hepatitis B vaccines can also be used. **Immunization with live viral vaccines is contraindicated in patients with suspected immune disorders; these include measles, mumps, rubella, all attenuated polio, bacilli bilié de Calmette-Guérin (BCG), and chicken pox vaccines.** If the child or adult has received the usual immunizations in the past, antibody titers for these vaccine antigens can be quantified. If the child has not been immunized, or for adults in whom more time has elapsed since vaccination, a measurement of the response after booster vaccine administration should be performed. There is no consensus on how to interpret each response; in general, an increase of 2- to 3-fold or more over baseline, and/or the establishment of protective levels of antibody, signify an adequate response to these vaccines.

   b. **Antibody responses to polysaccharide antigens.** To measure antibody responses to polysaccharide antigens, the pneumococcal vaccine, free of carrier proteins, is used. Antibody titers are determined before and 3 to 4 weeks postimmunization. Antibody responses to carbohydrate antigens are typically poor in children younger than 2 years old and may be depressed up to 5 years of age. Thus, polysaccharide vaccines are not useful in infants.

   c. **Isohemagglutinins** (anti-A or anti-B blood group substance) can be used as a test of antibody production, for subjects who are blood group A (who have anti-B antibody), or for those who are blood group B (who have anti-A), or for blood group O subjects (who have both.) These antibodies develop in subjects older than the age of 2 years, and are usually found in a titer of 1:16 or greater.

   d. **Immunoglobulin G subclasses.** IgG consists of four subclasses, IgG1 through IgG4, distinguished by both structural and biological differences. Although individual roles for each IgG subclasses, as distinct from each other, have not been established, antibodies to many bacterial cell wall antigens are concentrated in the IgG2 subclass. Measurement of IgG subclasses may be indicated in patients with repeated bacterial sinopulmonary infections who have normal or mildly subnormal IgG levels or selective IgA deficiency. Deficiency of IgG2, which comprises approximately 20% of the total serum IgG, can occur alone or in association with selective IgA deficiency and/or IgG4 deficiency. However, determinations of functional antibody responses to polysaccharide antigens, such as *S. pneumoniae*, are essential and more clinically relevant. Absence of an IgG2 response could result in a failure to develop protective immunity against bacterial infection. Despite these indicators, the biological significance of IgG1 or IgG2 subclass deficiency is not always clear; the case for IgG3 and IgG4 deficiency is much more tenuous. To determine the biological significance of IgG subclass deficiency, testing of specific antibody production, usually by administering vaccines such as tetanus, diphtheria, *Haemophilus*, and a pneumococcal vaccine, is mandatory. Antibody deficiency to polysaccharide antigens with normal IgG2 levels has been frequently observed. Also, IgG2 deficiency (due to G2 heavy-chain deletion) has also been found in rare normal healthy individuals.

   e. IgE level can help to distinguish between allergic and immunodeficiency disease. Very high levels of IgE with eosinophilia may indicate severe allergy, allergic aspergillosis, or hyper-IgE syndrome.

2. Quantification of T, B, and natural killer cells. (See Chapter 19.) Analysis of lymphocyte phenotypes using monoclonal antibodies and flow cytometry has identified a great number of cell surface proteins, some of which are unique to certain lymphocyte populations; specific antibodies identify T- and B-cells, subpopulations of T-cells, natural killer (NK) cells, and monocytes/macrophages. Immunodeficiency diseases may result in defective generation of T cells (CD3+ cells), or low numbers of CD4+ and/or CD8+ T cells. If an immune defect is suspected, this panel of T-cell markers is examined and the absolute number of cells in each set determined, in comparison to the laboratory-established normal controls of similar age. Sixty-five percent to 70% of peripheral lymphocytes are T cells; about 60% are CD4+ cells and the remainder are CD8+ T cells. About 10% to 20% of peripheral blood lymphocytes are B cells (CD20+) in older children and adults, but there are somewhat higher numbers in young infants. Monocytes (CD16+) and NK cells (CD56+) are also identified by specific markers, and form the remaining cell types.

3. T-cell functional assessment. (See Chapter 19.) Delayed hypersensitivity skin tests are commonly used as measures of T-cell function, because they measure the ability to recognize and present the antigen, mobilize the T cells, and generate a specific inflammatory response. However, there are major shortcomings in using skin tests; the results are often difficult to interpret, and infants have not had sufficient exposure to respond to antigens. More definitive insight into the functional capability of T cells can be obtained by testing *in vitro* proliferative responses to specific stimuli, mitogens, and antigens. In these analyses T lymphocytes are exposed to mitogens, antigens, or allogeneic cells; the cells are transformed into large, blast-like cells with synthesis of DNA and eventual cell division (blastogenesis). Lymphocyte activation is usually measured by the uptake of a radiolabeled nucleotide, ^{3}H- or ^{14}C-labeled thymidine, into DNA for 6 to 18 hours, followed by precipitation of the radiolabeled DNA and subsequent liquid scintillation counting. Mitogens are plant extracts that stimulating both CD4- and CD8-positive T lymphocytes to divide the specific antigens. Tetanus, diphtheria, and *Candida* are commonly used to study specific T cell responses. Sufficient exposure to the antigen is required for a positive response; proliferation to antigenic stimuli is uncommon in infant during the first year of life.

4. **Complement deficiency assessment.** (See Chapter 19.) Although deficiencies of complement proteins are uncommonly found, they can lead to recurrent bacterial infection, or in some cases, to autoimmune disease. Screening tests include total hemolytic complement (called CH_{50}) C3, C4, and a functional test of the entire classical complement cascade. It is important that the serum or plasma obtained for these analyses reach the laboratory in optimum condition for testing, which may mean simply frozen.

5. **Polymorphonuclear leukocyte analyses.** (See Chapter 19.) Aside from neutropenia, a major polymorphonuclear leukocyte disorder is CGD. In the presence of a suggestive history, this diagnosis should be considered on the first clinic visit. A test called the nitroblue tetrazolium test (NBT) is the classic laboratory method for screening for CGD, but has been replaced in many laboratories by a flow cytometer equivalent, the neutrophil oxidative index (NOI), that is better suited to the study of clinical samples. The hyper-IgE syndrome is phenotypically somewhat similar to CGD; however, defective polymorphonuclear leukocyte (PMN) function is not a clear feature of this disease. The diagnosis is suggested by the demonstration of IgE levels higher than 2,000 IU/mL (but as high as 20,000 to 60,000 IU/mL) with the appropriate clinical manifestations.

C. Advanced testing

1. **Enzyme measurements.** Deficiencies of two enzymes related to purine metabolism are associated with severe immune deficiency. SCID is caused by a deficiency of the enzyme adenosine deaminase (ADA) in approximately 25% of infants. ADA and the enzyme purine nucleoside phosphorylase (PNP, which is an even rarer cause of SCID), are usually measured in erythrocyte lysates. If blood transfusions have been given within the prior 3 months, the assay for these enzymes may be unreliable, and skin fibroblasts, grown from a skin biopsy, must be tested instead.

2. **Lymph node biopsy** is generally not necessary to establish the diagnosis of an immunodeficiency, but it can be helpful in equivocal cases and to exclude reticuloendothelial malignancy in immunodeficient patients with lymphadenopathy. Optimally, the biopsy should be performed 5 to 7 days after local antigen stimulation (e.g., tetanus immunization). Specimens from patients with antibody deficiency show few plasma cells, an increased number of primary lymphoid follicles, cellular disorganization, a thin cortex, and absence of germinal centers. An increased number of histiocytes and other reticuloendothelial elements can be present.

3. **Rectal and intestinal biopsies.** Small intestinal biopsies are indicated for evaluation of chronic diarrhea and malabsorption to exclude villous atrophy or cryptosporidial and *Giardia lamblia* infections.

4. **Analysis of additional surface markers on leukocytes.** Additional cell membrane proteins can be assessed by flow cytometry to characterize the level of maturation, differentiation, and activation of lymphocytes; these developmentally regulated cell-surface markers are termed the cluster of differentiation (CD) antigens. These CD antigens possess biological activity and may be useful in the evaluation of certain immunologic diseases such as the T and B cell immunodeficiencies (Table 17.1). Interpretation of lymphocyte phenotype markers must be carefully based on normal age-related values and the quality control for each laboratory, because small variations in technique can alter the final results.

5. **Advanced laboratory evaluation for complement and opsonic deficiencies.** If the complement screening tests results are abnormal

or the clinical history suggests a complement deficiency, other more detailed studies can be done in selected research laboratories. These studies include measurement of individual complement components (immunochemical and functional assessment), assays of the alternative complement pathway, and assays of the patient's serum to determine its ability to generate chemotactic factors as well as to provide opsonic activity. An opsonic deficiency is demonstrated by the inability of the test serum to enhance phagocytosis of yeast particles or bacteria by normal leukocytes.

6. **Additional polymorphonuclear leukocyte analyses.** Aside from chronic granulomatous disease, other defects of neutrophils include myeloperoxidase deficiency, and disorders of cell adhesion, and of cell movement. Myeloperoxidase deficiency, inherited as an autosomal-recessive defect, is of unknown clinical significance, having been described both in asymptomatic as well as infection-prone individuals. Abnormalities of neutrophil, monocyte, and macrophage cell adhesion appear if there are defects of the integrin CD18, the common β-chain of LFA-1, Mac-1, and p150,95 molecules. The presence of the CD18 molecule can be sought using flow cytometry.

   Congenital defects of neutrophil movement occur in the above adhesion defect diseases, as well as in additional quite rare neutrophil diseases, Shwachman syndrome, Chédiak-Higashi syndrome, and specific granule deficiency. The first two may be accompanied by anemia, thrombocytopenia, pancreatic insufficiency; oculocutaneous albinism is a feature of Chédiak-Higashi syndrome. Morphologic examination of stained neutrophils shows the characteristic abnormalities in specific granule deficiency.

7. Assessment of **neutrophil chemotaxis** is a technically difficult laboratory test, and erratic results can simply be a laboratory artifact. Full evaluation of movement disorders requires close correlation with the overall clinical picture and extensive clinical experience. Leukocyte mobility may be evaluated by directed migration through membrane filters or under agarose. Further tests to assess neutrophil mobility involve injections of epinephrine and steroids, which cause neutrophils to demarginate and leave the marrow reserves. The Rebuck skin window technique (in which the skin is abraded gently with a scalpel) shows the timing and cell characteristics of skin migration, and was used in the past to describe the inflammatory response, but has not had much clinical application.

8. **Molecular genetics and prenatal diagnosis.** Molecular techniques are useful for the diagnosis of immune deficiency and in determining carrier status in X-linked diseases and in a few other conditions where the gene defect has been identified. The most prevalent test is *in situ* hybridization for the chromosome 22 abnormality present in DiGeorge syndrome; many larger hospitals and also commercial laboratories can perform this test, which analyzes if the region often deleted in this syndrome is present.

   Genes for a number of immune deficiency diseases have been identified, and can be clinically tested and used in confirming diagnoses for suspected disorders. In addition, genes are used for prenatal diagnosis using chorionic villous sampling or amniocentesis material. Female carriers of some X-linked immunodeficiency disorders do not inactivate the X-chromosome in a random manner in cells which are affected by the disease; thus, assessment of nonrandom X inactivation can be also used in these cases to predicted carrier status.

IV. **Treatment of immunodeficiency disorders**
   A. **Antibiotics in acute illness.** Antibiotics should be started immediately for fevers and other manifestations of infection after blood and other appropri-

ate cultures have been obtained. These cultures are important to direct further therapy if the infection does not respond to the initial antibiotic chosen. The choice and dose of antibiotic for a specific infection are usually identical to those used in immunocompetent patients. If the infection does not respond to antibiotics, the possibility of viral, fungal, mycobacterial, or protozoan infection or mycoplasma infections should be considered.

B. Management of specific infections. Chronic **otitis media** should be treated aggressively in both infants and adults, with antibiotics and with myringotomy tube placement, when indicated. Special attention should be directed to hearing loss, incorporating routine audiologic evaluations into the treatment plan. **Sinusitis** requires aggressive antibiotic therapy and topical decongestant therapy during acute episodes. If symptoms continue, daily lavage procedures using nasal irrigators with adaptors and saline solutions are useful. If these fail, consider conservative surgical treatment (such as lavage or endoscopic sinus surgery) to treat as well as to identify the infecting organism(s). Aggressive sinus operations should be avoided unless absolutely needed. Patients with **chronic pulmonary disease** should be followed with yearly pulmonary function testing (or more frequently if evidence of deteriorating pulmonary function is seen) and chest radiographs or chest computed tomography (CT) scans as required. The importance of a home treatment program of postural drainage and inhalation therapy should be emphasized in patients with respiratory damage such as bronchiectasis.

C. Prophylactic antibiotics can be of benefit in immunodeficiency syndromes, especially for subjects with chronic lung disease. One useful regimen employs several antibiotics in alternating cycles at 1- to 2-month intervals. This regimen allows suppression of infection while minimizing emergence of resistant organisms. A satisfactory combination of antibiotics includes amoxicillin–clavulanate, erythromycin, trimethoprim and sulfamethoxazole, or a cephalosporin. In adults, amoxicillin–clavulanate, trimethoprim and sulfamethoxazole, tetracyclines, or a cephalosporin are useful. The newer quinolones, with fewer daily doses can also be used, but are best saved to treat acute infections.

D. Immune globulin replacement therapy is the primary treatment of antibody-deficiency disorders. Commercially available intravenous immunoglobulin (IVIg) preparations contain predominantly IgG antibodies (with trace amounts of IgA and IgM) in concentrations sufficient to protect against sepsis and to reduce recurrent or chronic pulmonary infections. Products available commercially are listed in Table 17.6. IVIg is indicated in humoral immunodeficiency diseases, such as X-linked agammaglobulinemia, common variable immunodeficiency disease, hyper-IgM syndrome, and combined immunodeficiency disorders, such as SCID and Wiskott-Aldrich syndrome. Most children who are diagnosed with the disorder known as "transient hypogammaglobulinemia" do not require IVIg. Some patients with IgA deficiency require immunoglobulin treatment because of significantly reduced antibody production; in these cases (and in some with common variable immunodeficiency) IVIg products with very low levels of IgA frequently are required if anti-IgA antibodies are present.

1. **Dosage.** There are a number of commercially available IVIg preparations (Table 17.6). These preparations, containing intact IgG antibodies, are generally well tolerated and effective in restoring IgG antibody to patients with antibody immunodeficiency disorders. The usual starting dose of IVIg is approximately 300 to 400 mg/kg/month, given every 3 or 4 weeks. Trough serum IgG levels 4 weeks after treatment should be maintained at greater than 500 mg per dL (approximately low normal levels). Some studies have found that dosages up to 600 mg/kg/month better control chronic pulmonary infections and improved pulmonary functions when compared with lower dosages. Individualization of the dosage and dosing frequency is based on clinical response and

Table 17.6. Current intravenous immunoglobulins

Category	Venoglobulin-S	Gammar-PIV	Gammagard S/D	Polygam S/D	Gamimune N	Iveegam	Sandoglobulin
Manufacturer*	Alpha Therapeutic Corp.	Aventis Behring	Baxter Healthcare Corp.	Distributed by American Red Cross (ARC)	Bayer	Baxter Healthcare Corp.	Norvartis
Contra-indication	Antibodies to IgA	IgA deficiency with antibodies to IgA	None (caution with IgA deficiency)	None (caution with IgA deficiency)	IgA deficiency with antibodies to IgA	IgA deficiency with antibodies to IgA	IgA deficiency with antibodies to IgA
IgA content	15.1 µg/mL	25 µg/mL	<3.7 µg/mL	<3.7 µg/mL	270 µg/mL	15–20 µg/mL	720 µg/mL
pH (after reconstitution)	5.2–5.8	7.0	6.8	6.8	3.25	7.0	6.6
Plasma source	Plasmapheresis >10,000 donors	Plasmapheresis >8,000 donors	Plasmapheresis >10,000 donors	>10,000 volunteer donors via the ARC	>2,000 donors	Plasmapheresis >6,000 donors	>16,000 volunteer donors
Half-life, days	33.5 ± 7	21	24	24	21	23–29	21
Solvent detergent treatment	Yes	No	Yes	Yes	No	No	No
Pasteurization	No	Yes	No	No	No	No	No
IgG subclass, %	65.7–67.2	69	67	67	60.0	64.1	60.5
IgG1	65.7–67.2	69	67	67	60.0	64.1	60.5
IgG2	23.7–25.3	23	25	25	29.4	30.3	30.2
IgG3	5.7–5.9	6	5	5	6.6	0	6.6
IgG4	3.0–3.4	2	3	3	4.1	1.5	2.8

S/D, solvent/detergent; IgA, immunoglobulin A.

determination of trough serum IgG levels. Serial immunoglobulin assays are generally not necessary to gauge the effectiveness of treatment, although many immunologists test serum IgG levels at 4- to 6-month intervals to ensure maintenance of adequate trough levels. During acute infections, gamma globulin metabolism increases, and extra infusions may be required.

2. **Adverse effects.** Fever, chills, nausea, vomiting, and back pain may occur with IVIg, especially during or after the first several infusions. These are often related to the rate of infusion or concomitant host infection. More severe reactions, such as anaphylactic reactions (hypotension, flushing, or bronchospasm) are very unusual, but may occur. They may be due to aggregated IgG or more rarely, anti-IgA antibodies. Some individuals have reactions when IVIg products are switched from one brand to another. Severe systemic reactions require immediate treatment (see Chapter 10). For subsequent IVIg administration in patients with severe reactions, the following measures should be taken:

   a. **Reassess the need for intravenous immunoglobulin G.** Is the patient truly IgG-deficient and will he or she benefit from IVIg administration?

   b. **Determine if the brand of intravenous immunoglobulin G has been changed**, and return to a better-tolerated product.

   c. **Test for anti-immunoglobulin G antibodies to IgA** (at commercial laboratories or the American Red Cross). Although IgE anti-IgA antibodies may be a cause of anaphylactic reactions, subjects who have IgE anti-IgA also have IgG anti-IgA, so these individuals at risk can be identified. If the reaction is due to anti-IgA antibodies, IVIg products depleted of IgA (Gammagard S/D or Polygam S/D) can be used. The first infusions in such a circumstance should be done in a controlled setting, using only a small dose.

   d. **Consider pretreatment.** Some practitioners pretreat with diphenhydramine (Benadryl) and/or corticosteroids before infusions. Although effective in preventing severe reactions in some patients, pretreatment can also mask early systemic manifestations.

   e. **Substitution of slow subcutaneous administration of intravenous immunoglobulin G** over 24 hours by an infusion pump through a 23-gauge butterfly needle or via a needle adapted for subcutaneous infusions is another very useful method of eliminating infusion reactions. It is also very successfully employed if venous access is poor. This method is preferred over the insertion of an indwelling port.

E. **Specific treatment for cellular deficiency.** Specific treatment for T-cell immune deficiencies is complicated because these disorders often involve heterogeneous defects; some are very severe, and others are more mild. This heterogeneity makes it difficult to determine the exact requirements for complete immunologic reconstitution. As a result, a number of treatment approaches are currently employed. Because of the complexity of diagnosis and treatment, such patients are usually cared for by referral centers with an investigative capacity and interest in the specific immunodeficiency diseases.

   1. **Bone marrow/stem cell transplantation.** Bone marrow, mobilized stem cells, and placental blood contain postthymic T cells and pluripotent stem cells that can differentiate into the hematopoietic, lymphoid, phagocytic, and megakaryocytic cell series. Bone marrow, peripheral blood, and placental stem cell transplants, providing precursors for a variety of cell systems, have been used successfully to treat severe combined immunodeficiency, Wiskott-Aldrich syndrome, and other T-cell deficiencies, as well as CGD (X-linked form) and congenital neutropenia. Extensive medical support is required to care for the severely immunosuppressed patient before and after transplantation. Transplantation should be done in medical centers equipped to provide adequate clinical and research services.

a. **For bone marrow transplantation**, multiple small aspirates are made from the iliac crest of the donor under general anesthesia. This preparation is then given to the patient intravenously. Although this procedure is relatively simple, successful bone marrow transplantation requires detailed tissue typing and matching to avoid fatal graft versus host disease (GVHD). Ideally, the donor is a sibling, or other genotypically HLA-matched relative. Phenotypically matched but unrelated HLA-matched donors can also be used, although GVHD is then a greater problem (see Chapter 15).

b. **Haploidentical T-cell-purged bone marrow transplantation** (usually from a parent) has also been widely used to successfully reconstitute immunodeficiencies. This procedure requires large volumes of bone marrow from the donor and stem cells concentrated by purification procedures. This technique has been successful in reconstituting T-cell immunity in SCID, but has been less successful in establishing permanent B-cell antibody function.

c. **Mobilized peripheral blood stem cells** can also be used to reconstitute immunity in primary immunodeficiency. Cytokine therapy with granulocyte colony-stimulating factor (G-CSF) or granulocyte macrophage colony-stimulating factor (GM-CSF) is given to the donor and the emerging stem cells are obtained by leukophoresis; peripheral blood may contain a larger quantity of more mature progenitors, which may be the reason for a more rapid return of granulocytes and platelets in the recipient.

d. **Placental/umbilical cord blood** has been used for allogeneic bone marrow replacement since 1988. For this procedure, placental blood can be collected, tested, frozen, and then used for related or unrelated patients in need of hematopoietic stem cell replacement. This resource has been applied most often to younger patients who have no HLA match.

F. Other replacement therapies

1. **Enzyme replacement.** The autosomal-recessive form of SCID can occur due to ADA deficiency. Enzyme replacement therapy using bovine ADA, modified by conjugation with polyethylene glycol (PEG-ADA) can be used. This preparation allows for markedly increased amounts of plasma ADA, resulting in significant clinical improvement accompanied by varying degrees of immunologic improvement.

2. **Gene therapy.** Investigators at the National Institutes of Health first performed historic studies by transfecting peripheral blood T lymphocytes of two patients with ADA-deficient SCID, who did not have HLA-compatible bone marrow donors. This approach is considered experimental, and the results have remained equivocal. More recently, using a different vector in X-linked SCID, much more promising results have been obtained in this disease.

3. **Thymic hormones.** A variety of peptide hormones of thymic origin or that are thymus-dependent have been purified, including thymosin and thymopoietin. Thymosin, a 28 amino acid peptide extracted from bovine thymus, exerts *in vitro* and *in vivo* effects that appear to require the presence of a precursor cell responsive to thymosin. Results with thymosin therapy in DiGeorge syndrome have been difficult to assess.

4. **Cytokines.** In theory, as a number of cytokines have been studied and in some cases made available for clinical studies, one might presume that these biological agents could provide a useful adjunct therapy in the primary immunodeficiency diseases. In practice, only a few instances of benefit are clear.

   a. Interferon IFN-γ is useful in chronic granulomatous disease.

   b. In SCID and in common variable immunodeficiency, some patients demonstrate enhanced T-cell function when treated with low doses of interleukin 2 (IL-2).

    c. Interferon alfa (IFN-alfa) has been demonstrated to have some success in Epstein-Barr virus (EBV)-induced B-cell lymphomas.

    d. Other cytokines, such as G-CSF and GM-CSF, have been used to stimulate neutrophil and/or monocyte bone marrow maturation in congenital neutropenias and as adjunctive treatment following immunosuppression.

    e. IL-12 has been used in subjects with IL-12 receptor defects to overcome an abnormal binding affinity.

  5. Trace elements. A rare inborn error of metabolism that prevents the normal absorption of zinc from the gastrointestinal tract results in a form of severe combined immunodeficiency associated with acrodermatitis enteropathica. The clinical manifestations of this disease include severe skin lesions, gastrointestinal malfunction with malabsorption and diarrhea, and bizarre, irritable behavior. Treatment with zinc in sufficient amounts by parental or oral routes corrects all manifestations of the disease, which is often fatal if untreated. In other cases of congenital immunodeficiency, if chronic diarrhea persists, zinc deficiency can add to the existing immune deficiency, particularly affecting the T-cell system.

  6. Cultured thymic epithelium and fetal thymus transplantation. Thymic epithelial or tissue transplant has been performed in the DiGeorge syndrome, in some cases resulting in reconstitution of T-cell immunity. The fetal thymus tissue (obtained from a fetus of less than 14 weeks gestation in order to minimize the possibility of GVHD) has been given as an organ implant into a muscle in the anterior abdominal wall, as a cell suspension by either the intravenous or intraperitoneal route, or as thymic fragments by the intraperitoneal route.

G. Specific treatment of phagocytic disorders. Specific cellular or enzyme replacement for phagocytic disorders, such as CGD, myeloperoxidase deficiency, and Chédiak-Higashi syndrome, is even less well defined than that for T-cell disorders.

  1. Interferon gamma (Actimmune, manufactured by InterMune Pharmaceuticals, Inc.) is a standard treatment of CGD, although the mechanism of immune enhancement is not well understood.

  2. Antibiotic therapy. Most subjects with neutrophil defects such as CGD or hyper-IgE syndrome are maintained on chronic antibiotic treatment, a common regimen being trimethoprim sulfa every day. If fungal infections have been present in the past, the addition of itraconazole is a common measure, although its usefulness on an ongoing basis has not been proven. Antibiotic therapy for **acute illness** should be given early and by the intravenous route during an active infection, after appropriate cultures are taken. Patients with phagocytic disorders are at a significant risk of fulminant, overwhelming sepsis and should be treated aggressively during acute illnesses.

  3. Granulocyte transfusions, together with antibiotics, may be beneficial for severe infections. This therapy has been used in CGD and in hyper-IgE syndrome, in cases of aggressive bacterial or fungal infections where antibiotic and or surgical therapy was not sufficient to control the infection.

H. Specific treatment for complement deficiency

  1. Fresh-frozen plasma from normal donors can replace specific complement components in patients with isolated complement component defects and increased susceptibility to a wide range of microorganisms. Patients with deficiency or dysfunction of C5 protein and patients with C3 or C3b inactivator deficiency have shown clinical and laboratory improvement following such infusions. Plasma infusion is also useful for surgical or dental prophylaxis in subjects with C1 inhibitor deficiency (hereditary angioedema, see Chapter 9).

  2. Investigational concentrates of C1 inhibitor have shown benefit in patients with C1-inhibitor deficiency during acute attacks.

3. **Anabolic steroids** such as danazol and stanozolol can induce production of C1-esterase inhibitor and can prevent dangerous attacks of angioedema. It is not useful for treatment of an attack, because it has a slow on set of action (see Chapter 9).

V. General considerations

A. **Diet.** No special dietary limitations are necessary except in patients with malabsorption and diarrhea. In these patients, professional dietary consultation is helpful to ensure that the diet is adequate in calories, protein, trace elements, and vitamins for normal growth and development. Chronic malnutrition can further depress a variety of immune functions.

B. **Avoidance of pathogens.** Patients with immunodeficiencies, especially if T-cell functions are impaired, should be protected from unnecessary exposure to infection. "Germ-free" care of individuals with significant T-cell immune defects, although effective in reducing or eliminating contact with microorganisms, is technically demanding and expensive. Less vigorous isolation is of some benefit and includes limiting exposure to other young family members, sleeping in a separate location, and isolation from persons with respiratory or other infections, especially *Herpes simplex* and varicella-zoster. Patients with antibody deficiency can have a normal life span with gamma globulin therapy, and should not be overprotected. An affected child should be encouraged to go outdoors, to play with other children in small groups, and to attend nursery school and regular school. Special avoidance measures are necessary for patients of any age who have CGD; marked susceptibility to certain fungi, such as *Aspergillus*, found in moldy vegetation (hay, grass clippings, raked leaves), makes avoidance of exposure quite important.

C. **Avoid whole blood transfusions** in patients who have or are suspected of having a cellular immunodeficiency, because infused donor lymphocytes can cause a fatal graft versus host reaction. If transfusion is necessary, the blood should be irradiated (3,000 cGy) before administration. In addition, cytomegalovirus-free and hepatitis-virus-free blood products should be used.

D. **Avoid the administration of live virus vaccines** (e.g., poliovirus, measles, mumps, and rubella) and BCG in all immunodeficient patients, but especially those with a cellular immunodeficiency. These vaccines carry the risk of vaccine-induced infection. In the past, parents, siblings, and other household members were not given smallpox vaccine (when widely used) because of the high risk of spreading the infection to the patient. Similarly, oral live attenuated poliovirus vaccine should be withheld from household members to prevent spread; the inactivated-virus preparation can be substituted (see Tables 20.1 and 20.2, Chapter 20). Vaccines using inactivated organisms have generally been safe, and their use for stimulating a measurable antibody response is of diagnostic value. However, less-purified inactivated vaccines such as typhoid and paratyphoid have produced shock in patients with Wiskott-Aldrich syndrome, probably from endotoxin activation of complement by the alternative pathway in patients whose titers of "natural" antibodies are too low to prevent this reaction. Consequently, such vaccines should be used with caution in immunodeficient patients.

E. **Tonsillectomy** and **adenoidectomy** should be performed rarely and then only with strict indications. Similarly, **splenectomy** is contraindicated except in the most severe and unusual circumstances, such as to control bleeding secondary to thrombocytopenia in Wiskott-Aldrich syndrome, extreme hypersplenism, or uncontrollable autoimmune cytopenias in common variable immunodeficiency or other immune defect. The addition of the phagocytic defect (absence of the spleen) to an already existing immunologic defect can significantly increase the risk of sudden, overwhelming sepsis.

F. **Strict indications for the use of corticosteroids and other immunosuppressive** agents should be observed in immunodeficient patients.

G. **Psychosocial support.** Because of the severe psychological and financial demands placed on severely affected patients and their families, attention must be paid to these areas. The school should be made aware of the problems and provide tutors to help make up for school absences. Financial counselors can give the patient or the family information about agencies that can provide partial or complete financial support for medical care. Agencies for crippled children in many states can provide help for immunodeficient patients.

The Immune Deficiency Foundation (40 W. Chesapeake Avenue, Suite 308, Towson, MD, 21204; phone: 410-321-6647 and 800-296-4433; fax: 410-321-9165; www.primaryimmune.org) provides educational information to patients and parents and helps sponsor patient support groups through its regional affiliates. The Jeffrey Modell Foundation (phone: 800-JEFF-844; 212-919-0200; fax: 212-764-4180; http://wwwjmfworld.com) provides information, supports scientific meetings, and offers additional support services. The International Patient Organization is an international group with an interactive web site giving information about news and publications in primary immunodeficiency diseases, bulletin boards, and a chat room (www.ipopi.org). The National Organization of Rare Diseases (NORD Inc., 100 Route 37, P.O. Box 8923, New Fairfield, CT 06812-1783; phone: 203-746-6518; www.raredisease.org) is another organization that has been an additional resource for support.

Selected Readings

Buckley RH. Advances in immunology: primary immunodeficiency diseases due to defects in lymphocytes. *N Engl J Med* 2000;343:1313–1324.

Buckley RH, Schiff RI, Schiff SE, et al. Human severe combined immunodeficiency: genetic, phenotypic, and functional diversity in one hundred eight infants. *J Pediatr* 1997;130:378–387.

Chapel HM, Spickett GP, Ericson D, et al. The comparison of the efficacy and safety of intravenous versus subcutaneous immunoglobulin replacement therapy. *J Clin Immunol* 2000;20:94–100.

Cunningham-Rundles C, Bodian C. Common variable immunodeficiency: clinical and immunological features of 248 patients. *Clin Immunol* 1999;92:34–48.

Fischer A. Gene therapy of lymphoid primary immunodeficiencies. *Curr Opin Pediatr* 2000;12:557–562.

Grimbacher B, Holland SM, Gallin JI, et al. Hyper-IgE syndrome with recurrent infections—an autosomal dominant multisystem disorder. *N Engl J Med* 1999;340:692–702.

Hammarstrom L, Vorechovsky I, Webster D. Selective IgA deficiency (SIgAD) and common variable immunodeficiency (CVID). *Clin Exp Immunol* 2000;120:225–231.

Lee ML, Gale RP, Yap PL. Use of intravenous immunoglobulin to prevent or treat infections in persons with immune deficiency. *Ann Rev Med* 1997;48:93–102.

Lekstrom-Himes JA, Gallin JI. Advances in immunology: immunodeficiency diseases caused by defects in phagocytes. *New Engl J Med* 2000;343:1703–1714.

Patel DD, Gooding ME, Parrott RE, et al. Thymic function after hematopoietic stem-cell transplantation for the treatment of severe combined immunodeficiency. *N Engl J Med* 2000;342:1325–1332.

Minegishi Y, Rohrer J, Conley ME. Recent progress in the diagnosis and treatment of patients with defects in early B-cell development. *Curr Opin Pediatr* 1999;11:528–532.

Primary immunodeficiency diseases. Report of a WHO scientific group. *Clin Exp Immunol* 1997;109:1–28.

Smart BA, Ochs HD. The molecular basis and treatment of primary immunodeficiency disorders. *Curr Opin Pediatr* 1997;9:570–576.

Stiehm ER. Human intravenous immunoglobulin in primary and secondary antibody deficiencies. *Pediatr Infect Dis J Rev* 1997;16:696–707.

Stiehm ER. Immunodeficiency disorders: general considerations. In Stiehm ER, ed. *Immunologic disorders in infants and children*, 3rd ed. Philadelphia: WB Saunders, 1996:157–195.

18. HUMAN IMMUNODEFICIENCY VIRUS DISEASE AND RELATED OPPORTUNISTIC INFECTIONS

John M. Boggs

Human immunodeficiency virus (HIV) produces a spectrum of illness, from asymptomatic carriage to the full-blown **acquired immunodeficiency syndrome** (AIDS). The status of disease is defined by the measurement of **immunologic** (cluster of differentiation 4 [CD4] cell count) and **virologic** (HIV viral burden, HIV RNA) parameters, and by the occurrence of **opportunistic infections** or **neoplasms** resulting from **immunosuppression**. AIDS was first described in 1981, when increasing cases of *Pneumocystis carinii* pneumonia (PCP) and Kaposi sarcoma (KS) were appearing in young, otherwise healthy homosexual men in Los Angeles, New York, and San Francisco. Additional cases among blood transfusion recipients, injection drug users, and heterosexual partners of affected patients fueled the search for a transmissible agent, which was discovered as HIV in 1984. By the following year, serologic testing became available to screen blood donors and identify infected individuals. This greatly facilitated research and development of potential drug candidates. With the expansion of antiretroviral therapy to several classes of agents used in combination (known collectively as **highly active antiretroviral therapy** [HAART]), significant strides have finally been made in restoring some immune function, delaying the development of opportunistic infections, and prolonging and improving the quality of life for HIV-infected patients. As these therapies remain largely unaffordable and unavailable to the vast majority of infected individuals in the developing countries where the epidemic is progressing most rapidly, prospects for global control still rest with effort at changing high-risk behaviors and development of effective vaccines.

The fast-moving nature of this field renders it almost impossible to capture the most current recommendations in a published book format. Several helpful websites are therefore included at the end of this chapter (see Suggested Readings).

I. Human immunodeficiency virus disease
A. Epidemiology and transmission

HIV probably originated in Africa, as suggested by serologic data as well as virologic studies of similar simian lentivirus strains. Through sexual transmission and parenteral spread by infected needles, the pandemic now extends throughout the world, contributing significantly to morbidity and mortality, especially among young and middle-aged adults. As of December 1997, more than 500,000 cases of AIDS had been reported in the United States. Although the number of cases among gay men appears to have reached a plateau, steady increases continue among injection drug users and among heterosexual partners in developing countries of Africa and Southeast Asia. Through 1997, more than 60% of those previously diagnosed with AIDS had died. Since the advent of combination antiretroviral therapy, including protease inhibitors in 1995, AIDS-associated mortality has begun to decrease, as has the occurrence of opportunistic infections.

HIV is transmitted predominantly by sexual contact, by parenteral exposure to contaminated blood or blood products, or perinatally. The virus has been detected in a variety of body fluids, including saliva, cerebrospinal fluid, blood, semen, amniotic fluid, and breast milk.

Sexual transmission represents the predominant spread of HIV worldwide. In the United States and Europe, homosexual men account for approximately two-thirds of all AIDS cases. In Sub-Saharan Africa and Southeast Asia, however, heterosexual transmission is the major route of disease spread. Risk factors for transmission in gay men include a history of receptive anal intercourse and multiple sexual partners. Vaginal intercourse is the major route of male to female transmission of HIV.

Sexually transmitted diseases, particularly those that produce ulcerative genital lesions, are important cofactors in increasing the transmission of HIV during sexual contact. Gonorrhea, syphilis, human papillomavirus infection, and chancroid all cause cervical ulcerations, which can increase the risk of HIV transmission during intercourse.

Injection drug use has been associated with HIV transmission by needles contaminated with blood. Injection drug users constitute the largest population of HIV-positive heterosexuals in the United States and Europe. Aside from parenteral exposure, use of drugs such as heroin and cocaine often accompanies promiscuous sexual behavior, increasing the probability of HIV transmission.

Perinatal transmission is seen in approximately 30% of women who are HIV infected. Recent data suggest that the majority of perinatal infections occur during passage of the fetus through the infected birth canal, although breastfeeding also increases the risk of perinatal transmission. Additional risk factors for perinatal transmission include high viral burden in the mother and degree of CD4 cell depression at the time of pregnancy. The role of neutralizing antibodies in preventing perinatal infection is controversial, but recent experience shows that peripartum antiretroviral drug treatment can decrease perinatal transmission.

Blood products can also transmit HIV. Before the testing of all blood products in 1985 with commercial HIV kits, 80% of hemophiliacs in the United States became infected after receiving HIV-contaminated factor VIII. Transplantation of HIV-infected organs has also resulted in HIV infection. Following transplantation of an infected organ, such as a cornea, heart, liver, or kidney, the risk of seroconversion in a recipient is essentially 100%.

B. Pathogenesis

Improvements in treatment and monitoring of HIV disease have occurred together with better understanding of the virology and immunology of HIV pathogenesis. Studies of viral dynamics show high rates of continuous HIV replication, especially in lymphoid tissues, in equilibrium with rates of clearance by the immune system. Even in individuals with "undetectable" plasma viral RNA, viral replication persists at lower levels, in "reservoirs" of latently infected CD4+ cells.

HIV enters cells following binding of viral glycoprotein GP120 to the CD4 molecule and to one of several recently identified chemokine coreceptors (CXCR4 for T-cell-tropic strains, CCR5 for macrophage-tropic strains, and possibly others). Mechanisms of CD4 cell depletion induced by HIV infection include:

1. Autoimmune destruction of CD4 cells
2. Direct viral cytopathic effects on host CD4 cells
3. Syncytium formation (fusion between infected and uninfected cells to form multinucleate giant cells)
4. Toxicity of viral proteins and cytokines, leading to bone marrow toxicity and inhibition of lymphopoiesis
5. Apoptosis (programmed cell death)

The degree of CD4 cell depletion has served as an important clinical barometer of immune status in human immunodeficiency virus-infected individuals. Data from several large cohorts confirm a direct correlation between the CD4 cell count and risk of AIDS-defining opportunistic infections. Prophylaxis for opportunistic infections such as PCP is started when CD4 cell counts reach the 200 to 250 cells per mm^3 range. Similarly, patients with HIV infection with CD4 cells < 50/mm^3 have a significantly increased risk of developing cytomegalovirus (CMV) retinitis or *Mycobacterium avium* complex (MAC) infection. While HAART produces significant increases in peripheral blood CD4 cell counts in many patients, this repletion probably reflects expansion of certain resting memory cell populations, but incomplete reconstitution of the native repertoire of CD4 cells from which certain clonal types have been deleted.

Cells other than CD4 are also factors in the pathogenesis of HIV infection. Monocytes and macrophages infected with HIV can deliver virus to sites in the central nervous system (CNS). Follicular dendritic cells can be infected with HIV and may also play a role in pathogenesis. Studies of lymph nodes from HIV-infected individuals show that large amounts of virus are sequestered around infected dendritic cells in germinal centers. Despite the absence of virus in peripheral blood, lymph nodes are centers for massive viral replication during "silent stages" or asymptomatic stages of HIV infection. Furthermore, infected mononuclear cells show decreased functional responses such as reduced chemotaxis and reduced killing of organisms. Release of cytokines, such as tumor necrosis factor (TNF), from HIV-infected monocytes may contribute to marked wasting and cachexia in patients with advanced disease. B-lymphocyte hyperactivation and dysregulation manifests as polyclonal hypergammaglobulinemia, as an overall increase in immunoglobulin E (IgE) levels, and possibly by increased susceptibility to Epstein-Barr virus (EBV)-induced lymphomas. Natural killer cells (NK) may play a role in inhibiting HIV replication by cell-mediated killing and by secretion of inhibitory chemokines. Thus, though HIV infection leads to immunodeficiency, this occurs gradually in the setting of general hyperactivation of the immune system as the virus subverts host machinery to its own advantage.

C. Natural history and clinical manifestations

HIV infection usually begins with an acute, self-limited, febrile viral syndrome, followed by a long, clinically latent period with signs and symptoms suggestive of chronic, slowly progressive immunosuppression (Fig. 18.1). The time course for progression of disease is quite variable. The majority of individuals remain asymptomatic for 5 to 10 years following infection, even in the absence of antiretroviral therapy. Several studies suggest that development of potent CD8+ cytotoxic T lymphocyte (CTL) responses may be associated with long-term survival and slower progression.

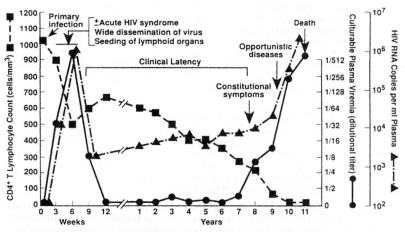

FIG. 18.1. Typical course of human immunodeficiency virus (HIV) infection. The complex, multifactorial multiphasic, and overlapping factors of the immunopathogenic mechanisms of human immunodeficiency virus (HIV) disease are shown. Throughout the course of HIV infection, virus replicates and immunodeficiency progresses steadily, despite the absence of observed disease during the so-called clinical latency period. Immune activation and cytokine secretion vary among HIV-infected persons, sometimes increasing dramatically as disease progresses. Immune activation and cytokine secretion play a major role in pathogenesis. From Pantaleo G, et al. New concepts in the immunopathogenesis of human immunodeficiency virus infection. *N Engl J Med* 1993;328:327–335, with permission.

There are two widely used classification schemes for HIV infection. In 1993, the Centers for Disease Control and Prevention (CDC) changed criteria to include a diagnosis of AIDS on the basis of a CD4 cell count less than 200 per mm^3 (Table 18.1). Many opportunistic viral, fungal, and protozoan infections are recognized as AIDS-defining diagnoses, as are recurrent bacterial pneumonias and invasive cervical cancer (in the presence of HIV infection). In addition, malignancies such as KS or B-cell lymphomas are considered diagnostic for AIDS.

Following acute infection, most patients enter a prolonged asymptomatic phase. Decline in CD4 cells is estimated at 50 to 100 per mm^3 cells per year, with accelerated rates of decline following opportunistic infections. Progression rates in various risk groups, including intravenous (i.v.) drug users and recipients of blood transfusions, are similar. Following acute retroviral infection, high levels of infectious virus may be isolated from plasma. Infectious virus disappears from the blood after several weeks, coincident with the appearance of CD8-positive CTL in the peripheral circulation. Clearance of the virus is not associated with neutralizing antibody, although these antibodies are seen following disappearance of the virus from peripheral blood. Despite clearance from the bloodstream, the virus then localizes in lymphatic tissues such as nodes, liver, and spleen. After a prolonged period of latent disease, containment of the virus in the lymphoreticular system breaks down and the viral infection rapidly spreads. Markers of immune activation and viral replication increase as the disease progresses, and are measured to "stage" patients, as well as monitor response to therapy. The most commonly used laboratory tests for staging disease include the absolute CD4 cell count and the quantitative measurement of plasma HIV RNA (viral load, or viral burden). Symptoms such as fevers, sweats, and weight loss also represent independent predictors of immunologic decline.

D. Laboratory diagnosis of human immunodeficiency virus infection
The standard serologic method for the diagnosis of HIV infection detects virus-specific antibodies by enzyme immunoassay (EIA, or enzyme-linked immunosorbent assay [ELISA]) or Western blot (WB) (see Chapter 19). For practical purposes, most current tests are directed at finding infection due to human immunodeficiency virus type 1 (HIV-1). HIV-2 can cause a syndrome of immunodeficiency similar to HIV-1, but is found primarily in West Africa and is thought to be exceptionally rare in other areas at the present time. Alternative methods for identifying HIV infection include direct detection of viral antigens or nucleic acids or direct isolation by culture of HIV from peripheral blood.

Table 18.1. 1993 revised classification system for human immunodeficiency virus infection and expanded acquired immunodeficiency syndrome surveillance case definition for adolescents and adults[a]

CD4 + T-cell categories	Clinical categories		
	(A)[b] Asymptomatic, acute (primary) HIV, or PGL	(B) Symptomatic, not (A) or (C) conditions	(C) AIDS-indicator conditions
(1) ≥500/mm^3	A1	B1	C1
(2) 200–499/mm^3	A2	B2	C2
(3) <200/mm^3 (AIDS-indicator T-cell count)	A3	B3	C3

[a] Including the expanded AIDS surveillance case definition. Persons with AIDS-indicator conditions (category C), as well as those with CD4$^+$ counts <200/mm^3 (categories A3 or B3) are reportable as AIDS cases in the United States and Territories, effective January 1, 1993.
[b] Clinical category A includes acute (primary) HIV infection.

1. Enzyme-linked immunosorbent assay and Western blot

a. EIA confirmed by WB is the most widely accepted method for screening of individuals with suspected HIV infection. The sensitivity and specificity of the commercially available HIV antibody kits are both greater than 99%. False-positive reactions do occur, especially in populations with a low prevalence of HIV infection, and following immunizations such as influenza vaccine. The WB test, a very sensitive and highly specific assay to detect antibodies to HIV, is not used for screening because it is a more expensive and time-consuming procedure. Positive WB tests are defined as those that contain at least one antibody to proteins of env, gag, and pol genes. The presence of one or two bands is considered indeterminate and requires further testing. Most laboratories regard a combination of p24, p31, gp41, and gp120/gp160 as positive for HIV infection.

2. Additional methods for human immunodeficiency virus detection

a. Nucleic acid detection assays

Polymerase chain reaction (PCR) and other **nucleic acid detection assays** are relatively new technologies that depend on amplification of genomic DNA or RNA from HIV. Use of these assays to measure viral load (or viral burden) has revolutionized the monitoring and assessment of treatment efficacy in patients on highly active antiretroviral therapy. The major advantage of PCR or other diagnostic procedures is the extreme sensitivity of the methods in detecting minute quantities of HIV RNA or DNA. The major problem with widespread use of PCR is carry-over contamination. **Branched DNA** (bDNA) techniques utilize synthetic DNA for binding and detection of viral sequences in plasma and cells. Though not quite as sensitive as PCR, these assays depend on chemiluminescent reactions that are easily quantified by luminometry, and may also be used in assessing viral load. It is recommended that the same type of assay, and preferably the same laboratory, be used when following serial viral load measurements in a given individual.

b. Human immunodeficiency virus (p24) antigen tests screen for the presence of viral antigen. This sensitive assay can detect picogram quantities of p24. Complexing of p24 with anti-p24 antibody can occur, which decreases the sensitivity of the assay. Newer p24 assays incorporate an acid-dissociation step, which breaks down immune complexes of HIV for detection of p24 antigen. Though now largely supplanted by assays for HIV RNA, p24 antigen testing may be useful in screening patients for acute HIV-seroconversion syndrome when antibodies are not detectable.

3. Viral culture

remains a very sensitive and specific means of detecting HIV infection, but is now mainly a research tool because of the expense and lack of standardized technique. Virus can be cultured from plasma both qualitatively and quantitatively, or quantitatively by peripheral blood mononuclear cell micro-coculture.

E. Antiretroviral therapy and management of human immunodeficiency virus disease

The availability of a variety of active antiretroviral agents over the past 5 years and their use in combination have had profound effects on the clinical course of HIV infection. Although the actual choices of agents for initial therapy vary with the individual, consensus guidelines have been developed to help codify the overall approach. Nevertheless, several studies suggest improved outcomes for patients cared for by more experienced HIV care providers, reflecting the complexities of current treatment and monitoring approaches.

1. Approach to therapy

Agents currently available are shown in Table 18.2. The three classes of currently approved antiretroviral agents are

Table 18.2. Antiretroviral agents

Drug (trade name)	Dose (adult)	Common side effects	Comments
NUCLEOSIDE RTI			
Zidovudine, AZT (Retrovir)	300 mg b.i.d.	Nausea, headache, neutropenia, anemia, rarely myopathy	
Didanosine, ddI (Videx)	200 mg b.i.d., 400 mg q.d.	Peripheral neuropathy, pancreatitis	
Stavudine, d4T (Zerit)	40 mg b.i.d.	Peripheral neuropathy, less commonly hepatitis, pancreatitis	
Lamivudine, 3TC (Epivir)	150 mg b.i.d.	Rash	
Zalcitabine, ddC (Hivid)	0.75 mg t.i.d.	Peripheral neuropathy, aphthous ulcers, pancreatitis	Less commonly used now
Zidovudine, lamivudine (Combivir)	300 mg/150 mg b.i.d.	As per individual drugs	
Abacavir (Ziagen)	300 mg b.i.d.	Hypersensitivity, with fever, nausea, vomiting, rash, potentially severe (2%–5%)	Rechallenge after drug interrupted or discontinued is contraindicated
Zidovudine, lamivudine, abacavir (Trizivir)	300 mg/150 mg/ 300 mg b.i.d.	As per individual drugs	
NONNUCLEOSIDE RTI			
Efavirenz (Sustiva)	600 mg q.h.s.	Rash, CNS disturbances (vivid dreams, dizziness, headache)	
Nevirapine (Viramune)	200 mg q.d. × 14 d, then 200 mg b.i.d.	Rash	
Delavirdine (Rescriptor)	400 mg t.i.d.	Rash	
PROTEASE INHIBITORS			
Saquinavir (softgel, Fortovase)	1200 mg t.i.d.	Nausea, vomiting, diarrhea, headache	Preferred over hardgel; much better bioavailability
Saquinavir (hardgel, Invirase)	800 mg t.i.d.	Nausea, vomiting, diarrhea, headache	Now used mainly in combination with ritonavir
Indinavir (Crixivan)	800 mg t.i.d.	Kidney stones, hyperbilirubinemia (indirect)	

(continued)

Table 18.2. *Continued*

Drug (trade name)	Dose (adult)	Common side effects	Comments
Nelfinavir (Viracept)	750 mg t.i.d., or 1250 b.i.d.	Diarrhea	
Ritonavir (Norvir)	600 mg b.i.d.	Nausea, vomiting, diarrhea, abdominal pain, paresthesias	Potent inhibitor of cytochrome P450 system, useful in boosting levels of other PI
Amprenavir (Agenerase)	1200 mg b.i.d.	Nausea, vomiting, diarrhea, rash, paresthesias	
Lopinavir, ritonavir (Kaletra)	400 mg/100 mg b.i.d.	Nausea, vomiting, diarrhea	Higher dose of 530 mg/130 mg b.i.d. recommended in combinations containing efavirenz

RTI, reverse transcriptase inhibitor; CNS, central nervous system; PI, protease inhibitor.

a. **Nucleoside reverse transcriptase inhibitors** (nRTI), which inhibit viral replication by acting as nucleoside analogues and interfering with DNA chain formation by viral reverse transcriptase
b. **Nonnucleoside reverse transcriptase inhibitors** (nnRTI), which allosterically inhibit reverse transcriptase function by binding to sites distinct from nucleoside binding
c. **Protease inhibitors** (PI), which interfere with processing and cleavage of polyproteins by viral protease, resulting in production of defective viral particles

    Both the Department of Health and Human Services (DHHS) and the International AIDS Society-USA (IAS-USA) have advocated similar approaches to timing and choices of treatment (Tables 18.3, 18.4).

    Though much is still controversial in approaching antiretroviral therapy, several general principles have emerged:

(1) The patient must be ready to embark on therapy with intent of complete adherence, in order to achieve greatest benefit, minimize side effects, and to avoid encouragement of resistant viral strains. This choice involves considerations of pill burden per day, frequency and conditions of administration, and potential interactions with other medications.
(2) Because backup regimens are generally less successful once initial therapy fails (as evidenced by decreasing CD4 counts, increasing viral load, or signs and symptoms of opportunistic infections), the initial regimen should be chosen to be maximally effective, with the goal of suppression of viral replication below the level of detection in plasma.
(3) The initial regimen should utilize combinations of at least three drugs shown to be effective, without antagonism or overlapping side effect profiles.

Table 18.3. Indications for initiation of antiretroviral therapy

Clinical Category	CD4+ T-cell count and HIV RNA	Recommendation
DHHS GUIDELINES		
Acute HIV syndrome or < 6 months after seroconversion	All	Treat
Symptomatic (AIDS, thrush, unexplained fever)	All	Treat
Asymptomatic	CD4+ T cells < 500/mm³ or HIV RNA > 10,000 (bDNA) or > 20,000 (RT-PCR)	Treatment should be offered. Strength of recommendation is based on prognosis for disease-free survival and willingness of patient to accept therapy
Asymptomatic	CD4+ T cells > 500/mm³ and HIV RNA < 10,000 (bDNA) or 20,000 (RT-PCR)	Many experts would delay therapy and observe; however, some would treat

CD4 Count/mm³	VL < 5000	VL 5,000–30,000	VL > 30,000
IAS-USA RECOMMENDATIONS			
< 350	Treat	Treat	Treat
350–500	Consider	Treat	Treat
> 500	Defer	Consider	Treat

DHHS, Department of Health and Human Services; HIV, human immunodeficiency virus; AIDS, acquired immunodeficiency syndrome; bDNA, branched DNA; RT-PCR, reverse transcriptase-polymerase chain reaction; IAS-USA, International AIDS Society-USA; VL, viral load, as measured by HIV RNA copies/mm³ plasma. CD4, cluster of differentiation 4; PGL, persistent generalized lymphadenopathy.

(4) In changing a regimen, at least two agents should be changed simultaneously, and preferably be new for the patient, or of different classes compared with agents previously used, to avoid cross-resistance with previous, failing regimens. Testing for resistance using genotypic or phenotypic assays can help with this decision-making, and appears to add benefit compared with regimens chosen on the basis of medication history alone.

2. **Monitoring**

Laboratory testing can aid in assessing efficacy of treatment as well as toxicity. The most useful measures of efficacy are

a. CD4 cell count, which is a marker of immune function status and informs decision-making regarding prophylaxis for opportunistic infections, and

b. HIV RNA, or viral load, as obtained by either PCR or bDNA assays. These two measurements are usually checked every 2 to 3 months if a regimen is stable, or more frequently as treatment is initiated or changed. Effective regimens can produce significant increases in CD4 count, which results in improved immune function and decreased risk of opportunistic infections, such that in some cases prophylaxis may be safely discontinued. The goal of treatment is suppression of viral load to "undetectable" levels (less than 50 copies

Table 18.4. Recommended initial antiretroviral regimens

	Column A	Column B
DHHS GUIDELINES (ONE FROM COLUMN A AND ONE FROM COLUMN B IN PREFERRED CATEGORY)		
Preferred	Efavirenz	D4T/3TC
	Indinavir	AZT/ddI
	Nelfinavir	AZT/3TC
	Ritonavir/Saquinavir	D4T/ddI
Alternative	Abacavir	DdI/3TC
	Amprenavir	AZT/ddC
	Delavirdine	
	Nevirapine	
	Ritonavir	
	Saquinavir (Fortovase)	
	Nelfinavir/Fortovase	
No recommendation (insufficient data)	Hydroxyurea	
	Ritonavir/Indinavir	
	Ritonavir/Nelfinavir	
Not recommended	Saquinavir (Invirase)	DdC/ddI
		DdC/d4T
		DdC/3TC
		AZT/d4T

IAS-USA RECOMMENDATIONS

Preferred
  2 nRTI and a PI
  2 nRTI and an nnRTI

Under evaluation
  3 nRTI
  Consider in patients with CD4 count < 50/mm^3 or VL > 100,000 copies/mL
    2 nRTI + 2 PI
    2 nRTI + PI + nnRTI

nRTI, nucleoside reverse transcriptase inhibitor; nnRTI, nonnucleoside reverse transcriptase inhibitor; PI, protease inhibitor; VL, viral load; CD4, cluster of differentiation 4.

per mm^3 by current assays), or to as low a level as possible; a decrease of greater than 1 log in HIV RNA is considered a significant beneficial effect. Progressive increases in viral load, conversely, herald failure of a regimen, and often reflect the presence of drug resistance mutations in the host's strains of HIV.

Monitoring for toxicity depends on the agents used. Practically, complete blood count, chemistry panels, and liver function tests are obtained routinely to watch for the more common side effects of myelo- or hepatotoxicity, and for metabolic abnormalities, as discussed below.

F. **Side effects and long-term complications of antiretroviral therapy** With the significant gains in quality of life associated with newer combination regimens has come the recognition of a variety of longer-term complications and delayed side effects. Metabolic abnormalities are common, and include lipid disorders, most notably hypertriglyceridemia, as well as increases in total and low-density lipoprotein (LDL) cholesterol; insulin resistance, with an increased propensity to develop diabetes mellitus; and changes in body fat composition (prominent abdominal or visceral obesity, cervicodorsal fat pad, female breast enlargement, and peripheral fat wasting). This group of abnormalities is sometimes collectively referred to as lipodystrophy. Debate continues as to whether these result from use of protease inhibitors or reflect metabolic changes associated with viral suppression and immune reconstitution.

A more recently recognized syndrome with considerable morbidity is characterized by lactic acidosis and hepatomegaly with steatosis. Vague complaints of nausea, vomiting, fatigue, and abdominal pain often occur with elevated creatine kinase, alanine aminotransferase (ALT), and lactate dehydrogenase (LDH). Computed tomography (CT) scans of the abdomen may reveal hepatic steatosis. The exact cause remains undefined, but a greater statistical association with certain nRTI agents has raised the question of drug-related mitochondrial toxicity.

Avascular necrosis of the femoral head can occur as a late complication of antiretroviral therapy. Whether this represents another metabolic aberration remains unclear, but it seems to arise more commonly in patients previously treated with corticosteroids, and those with a history of hyperlipidemia or alcohol abuse.

G. **Drug–drug interactions**

Because of the importance of reliable absorption and maintenance of drug levels to maximize antiretroviral efficacy and minimize toxicity, coadministration of other drugs must be undertaken with caution. Some interactions may be predicted based on known binding to serum proteins or effects on the cytochrome P450 system, but up-to-date resources should always be consulted.

II. **Opportunistic infections**

Directly and indirectly, opportunistic infections (OI) still account for the majority of deaths in HIV-infected patients. Although antiretroviral therapy clearly prolongs survival, the management and prophylaxis of opportunistic disease can be equally critical.

The most common opportunistic pathogens observed in HIV-infected patients include *P. carinii*, MAC, *Mycobacterium tuberculosis*, *Cryptococcus neoformans*, *Candida* spp., *Toxoplasma gondii*, *Histoplasma capsulatum*, herpesviruses (e.g., CMV, EBV, varicella-zoster virus [VZV], and *Herpes simplex* virus [HSV]), hepatitis C, and a variety of other bacterial, fungal, and protozoal pathogens.

A. ***Pneumocystis carinii*** pneumonia remains the most common opportunistic pulmonary disorder in patients with advanced HIV disease. Studies using ribosomal RNA homology show this organism is more closely related to fungi than to protozoa. However, on the basis of response to chemotherapeutic agents, *P. carinii* behaves more like a protozoan than a fungus. **PCP is rarely observed in patients with CD4 cell counts less than 200 per mm³**. Reactivation of latent disease usually acquired in childhood is the presumed pathogenesis of the disease in most cases.

1. **The most common clinical findings** include fever, shortness of breath, nonproductive cough, and hypoxemia. Most patients have bilateral interstitial infiltrates on chest x-rays, although radiographic patterns can be normal or atypical, especially if the patient has been taking prophylactic aerosolized pentamidine. Pleural effusions are rare with PCP and should suggest other diseases such as pulmonary KS, tuberculosis (TB), or bacterial pneumonia. Apical disease, cavitary lesions, or spontaneous pneumothoraces are also seen more often in patients receiving aerosolized pentamidine prophylaxis.

2. **Diagnosis** of PCP is based on identification of organisms in the sputum or from bronchoalveolar lavage (BAL) samples by means of silver or other staining techniques. Transbronchial biopsy is rarely indicated because the diagnostic yield from BAL is approximately 90% to 95%. Sputum induction is a very useful diagnostic technique in the setting of HIV infection, but a negative test does not rule out PCP.

3. **Treatment** for PCP includes oral or intravenous **trimethoprim–sulfamethoxazole** (TMP-SMX) (15 to 20 mg per kg p.o. or i.v. daily, divided every 6 to 8 hours) or i.v. **pentamidine** (3 to 4 mg/kg/day i.v.); either are typically administered for 21 days. Adjunctive corticosteroids are indicated for patients with moderate to severe disease as defined by a Po_2 less than 70 mm Hg. Prednisone (40 mg p.o. every 12 hours) or the equivalent intravenous corticosteroid dose is given for 5 to 7 days and then gradually tapered over 3 weeks.

Alternative therapies for sulfa-intolerant adult patients include **dapsone** (100 mg p.o. q.d.) combined with **trimethoprim** (15 mg per kg p.o. q.d.) or **primaquine** (30 mg base p.o. q.d.) combined with **clindamycin** (600 mg i.v. p.o. every 8 hours). The recently approved antimalarial, **atovaquone** (Mepron), is an alternative therapy for sulfa-intolerant adult patients (750 mg p.o. b.i.d.). Atovaquone is less effective than TMP-SMX for treatment of acute PCP, but is also less toxic. Variability in absorption may account in part for its lack of equivalence with TMP-SMX. Administration of atovaquone with fatty meals may improve absorption. **Trimetrexate** (45 mg per m^2 i.v. daily) **with folinic acid** (20 mg per m^2 i.v./p.o. q.d.) presents another alternative therapy possibly useful following TMP-SMX failure.

Adverse reactions to TMP-SMX and pentamidine are seen in 25% to 80% of patients and include fever, rash, leukopenia, hepatitis, and azotemia. Oral desensitization procedures can be used successfully in sulfa-intolerant patients when necessary for refractory disease or intolerance to alternatives. Pentamidine is associated with hypo- and hyperglycemia, as well as pancreatitis in approximately 2% to 5% of patients. Dapsone and primaquine can induce hemolysis in glucose-6-phosphate dehydrogenase (G6PD)-deficient individuals.

4. **Prophylaxis.** Preventive, or long-term suppressive therapy is recommended as secondary prophylaxis for all patients with a history of PCP, or as primary prophylaxis for patients with no prior diagnosis of PCP but with CD4 cell counts less than 200 per mm^3 (or less than 20% of total lymphocyte count). Without PCP prophylaxis, relapse rates of up to 25% to 60% are observed within 1 year of the initial episode. Patients with fever and/or oral thrush with CD4 cell counts of 300 to 350 per mm^3 should also receive PCP prophylaxis. TMP-SMX (1 DS tab, 160 mg trimethoprim/800 mg sulfamethoxazole, q.d. or t.i.w.) is the drug of choice. Dapsone (50 to 100 mg p.o. q.d.), atovaquone (1500 mg p.o. q.d.), or aerosolized pentamidine (300 mg every month) are alternatives for sulfa-intolerant patients. Regimens that provide additional prophylaxis for PCP and toxoplasmosis include TMP-SMX, dapsone plus pyrimethamine (50 mg p.o. every week) with folinic acid (25 mg p.o. every week), and atovaquone. Problems associated with aerosolized pentamidine include higher relapse rates (20% per year versus 4% to 5% for TMP-SMX), bronchospasm, apical disease, extrapulmonary disease, and subpleural infection resulting in spontaneous pneumothorax.

B. *Mycobacterium avium* **complex disease.** Prior to the use of HAART, disseminated infection with MAC was a frequent complication of advanced HIV infection, limiting both survival and quality of life. Case-controlled studies suggest that survival decreases in patients with disseminated infection compared with noninfected controls and that antimycobacterial treatment, although imperfect, results in symptomatic relief and can increase survival.

The risk of MAC disease is greatest when CD4 cell counts are markedly depressed. Observational cohort studies suggest that risk of developing MAC disease is approximately 8% per year with CD4 counts less than 100 per mm^3. It is relatively rare for patients to develop disseminated infection with CD4 counts greater than 100 per mm^3. Because these organisms are commonly found in soil and water, the most likely source of exposure in immunocompromised patients is contaminated water.

1. **Diagnosis** and treatment of MAC infection focuses on patients who are symptomatic with disseminated, or bacteremic infection, as manifested by positive blood cultures. The mere detection of organisms in stool or bronchial washings is not an absolute indication for therapy, because this may indicate colonization rather than true infection. Repeated isolation from the same site (e.g., lung or stool), however, probably represents true infection. Only patients with fever, weight loss, and other constitutional symptoms should be treated in the absence of positive blood cultures.

2. **Treatment** usually includes clarithromycin or azithromycin plus ethambutol (Table 18.5). Additional drugs such as rifabutin, amikacin, or a fluoroquinolone (e.g., ciprofloxacin) may be added if disease is severe or extensive, or has developed during prophylaxis. Most patients show improvement in fever and quantitative bacteremia within 2 to 4 weeks of initiating treatment. Clofazamine is no longer used because it is associated with no significant benefit and with excess mortality. Optimal duration of therapy is unclear, but most experienced clinicians treat for at least 1 year.

   Prophylaxis for MAC should be considered in patients at risk for MAC disease (i.e., less than 50 CD4 cells per mm^3). Clarithromycin, azithromycin, and rifabutin are all effective; choice is often based on consideration of interactions with the patient's other medications (e.g., HAART). Risk of disease also decreases markedly with increasing CD4 count in response to antiretroviral therapy, such that current guidelines support discontinuing prophylaxis if a significant, durable CD4 increase occurs.

C. *Mycobacterium tuberculosis* **infection.** The dramatic worldwide increase in TB has been linked to the HIV pandemic. Large numbers of HIV-infected individuals appear to be coinfected with *M. tuberculosis*, particularly intravenous drug users living in urban areas.

1. **Clinical presentation.** Extrapulmonary disease is more common in patients with HIV infection. Subjects with higher CD4 cell counts

Table 18.5. Antimycobacterial agents for *Mycobacterium avium* complex

Agent	Dose	Side effects	Comments
Clarithromycin	500 mg p.o. b.i.d.	GI intolerance	
Azithromycin	500–600 mg p.o. q.d.	GI intolerance	
Ethambutol	15–25 mg/kg p.o. q.d.	Rash, optic neuritis	Patient should note any change in vision
Rifabutin	300–600 mg p.o. q.d.	Uveitis, hepatitis, GI intolerance	Uveitis more common if used with clarithromycin or fluconazole
Amikacin	10–15 mg/kg i.v. q.d.	Auditory, vestibular, renal toxicity	
Ciprofloxacin	750 mg p.o. b.i.d.	GI intolerance	

GI, gastrointestinal.

usually present with pulmonary TB, which is similar to presentation in non-HIV-infected individuals. With lower CD4 cell counts, atypical presentations such as **tuberculous lymphadenitis** or disseminated disease are more common.

2. **Diagnosis** of *M. tuberculosis* depends on recovery of the organism from appropriate specimens. Samples of sputum, blood, urine, and bone marrow may all be used to make the diagnosis. Tuberculin skin testing with purified protein derivative (of tuberculin) (PPD) is problematic in HIV-infected individuals because of anergy associated with CD4 cell decline.

3. **Treatment and prophylaxis.** The usual initial regimen consists of isoniazid, rifampin (or rifabutin), and pyrazinamide, with ethambutol added if drug resistance is suspected (as in most urban areas) (Table 18.6).

Addition of pyridoxine 50 mg daily is recommended to prevent peripheral neuropathy in HIV-infected patients if isoniazid acid hydrazide (INH) is used. Patients should be treated for at least 6 months with appropriate combination therapy based on *in vitro* drug susceptibilities. As with the treatment of MAC disease, choice of treatment should take into account drug–drug interactions with antiretroviral agents. HIV-infected adults and children with PPD reactions of greater than 5 mm of induration should receive a 9-month course of INH of 300 mg per day (for most adults) and 5 mg/kg/day for children (up to 300 mg). A shorter, 2-month course of rifampin and pyrazinamide has recently been shown to be similarly effective and well tolerated. Individuals with HIV infection who are anergic and are considered at risk for TB infection (institutionalized individuals, immigrants from endemic areas, or individuals with recent contact with an active case) should also receive INH prophylaxis.

Increasing incidence of multidrug-resistant TB in several urban centers throughout the United States has resulted in numerous fatalities. Regimens containing five or more drugs may be needed for an HIV-infected individual suspected of having multidrug-resistant TB;

Table 18.6. First-line antituberculous agents

Isoniazid	5 mg/kg (maximum 300 mg) p.o. q.d.	Elevated transaminases, hepatitis, peripheral neuropathy, fever, hypersensitivity	Pyridoxine 50 mg/d suggested in pregnancy, diabetes mellitus, and HIV infection
Rifampin	10 mg/kg (maximum 600 mg) p.o. q.d.	Orange discoloration of tears, urine and secretions; hepatitis, GI intolerance	
Ethambutol	15–25 mg/kg p.o. q.d.	Rash, optic neuritis	Patient should note any change in vision
Pyrazinamide	15–30 mg/kg p.o. q.d.	Rash, hepatitis, hyperuricemia, arthralgia	
Rifabutin	150–450 mg p.o. q.d.	Hepatitis, orange discoloration of secretions, rash, GI intolerance	Uveitis more common if used with clarithromycin or fluconazole

HIV, human immunodeficiency virus; GI, gastrointestinal.

prior consultation with experts from local public health departments is advised.

D. Protozoal infections

1. **Toxoplasmosis** usually occurs in HIV-infected patients as a consequence of reactivation of latent infection. Focal, space-occupying cerebral lesions are the most common presentation of *T. gondii* infection in AIDS patients. Among the most frequent clinical manifestations are fever, altered mental status, headache, seizures, and focal neurologic deficits.

   a. **Diagnosis.** CNS imaging with either CT or magnetic resonance imaging (MRI) usually reveals multiple ring-enhancing toxoplasmic brain abscesses. Cerebrospinal fluid findings are nonspecific and helpful only in excluding other opportunistic CNS infections such as cryptococcal meningitis. Extraneural infections can occur, such as toxoplasmic chorioretinitis, peritonitis, pneumonitis, and lymphadenitis.

   Definitive diagnosis of toxoplasmosis depends on visualization of tachyzoites in tissue biopsy specimens. Serologic testing for anti-toxoplasma IgG antibodies may be helpful in assessing risk, but is complicated in AIDS patients because approximately 15% of patients with HIV infection and acute toxoplasmosis do not have detectable IgG antibodies.

   b. **Treatment and prophylaxis.** The treatment of choice for toxoplasmosis is sulfadiazine (1 to 2 g p.o. q6h) in combination with pyrimethamine (100 to 200 mg p.o. loading dose, followed by 50 to 100 mg p.o. q.d.); folinic acid (leucovorin, 10 mg p.o. q.d.) is added to reduce the risk of marrow suppression. High-dose clindamycin (900 mg q6h i.v. or 600 mg q6h p.o. in adults; 16 to 20 mg/kg/day in four divided doses for children) is an alternative to sulfadiazine for sulfa-intolerant patients. Other alternative regimens include the new macrolide antibiotics, azithromycin (1200 mg p.o. q.d.) or clarithromycin (1 g p.o. b.i.d.). Atovaquone (750 mg p.o. t.i.d.) has also been shown to be active against *T. gondii*. Because definitive diagnosis requires brain biopsy, and response to treatment of toxoplasmosis is usually prompt (within 1 to 2 weeks), empiric therapy for toxoplasmosis is often started in the absence of a specific tissue diagnosis if the clinical presentation is suggestive. Acute therapy is continued for at least 6 weeks and suppressive therapy at lower doses is continued indefinitely.

   The optimum regimen for **prophylaxis** is unknown, but trimethoprim–sulfamethoxazole (1 DS tab q.d. or t.i.w.) or pyrimethamine (50 mg p.o. every week)/folinic acid (25 mg every week) plus dapsone (50 to 100 mg p.o. q.d.) are effective, and also cross-protect against PCP. Prophylaxis is recommended for all HIV-seropositive patients with positive IgG for toxoplasmosis and CD4 count less than 100 per mm^3.

2. **Cryptosporidiosis** is caused by *Cryptosporidium parvum*, a ubiquitous animal pathogen that causes a self-limited diarrheal disease in immunocompetent hosts. Patients with AIDS, however, often have watery diarrhea associated with severe abdominal cramping, malabsorption, and dehydration.

   a. **Diagnosis** is by demonstration of organisms in stool samples or in small-bowel biopsies.

   b. **There is no known effective therapy for cryptosporidiosis.** Accumulating evidence, however, suggests that diarrhea and nutritional status may improve dramatically in those who respond well to HAART. Multiple antibiotics have been tried without demonstrated success. Somatostatin analogues (Sandostatin) may decrease fluid loss from the bowel by decreasing secretion, and together with anti-motility agents such as Lomotil, may improve diarrheal symptoms in some patients. Cryptosporidial infection in AIDS can be associated with a sclerosing cholangitis-like illness.

3. **Isosporiasis** occurs more commonly in patients from the Caribbean, but accounts for disease in less than 1% of patients with HIV infection in the United States. *Isospora belli* infection presents **clinically** as a syndrome of watery diarrhea and abdominal cramping similar to cryptosporidiosis.

   a. **Diagnosis** is made by stool examination, but this may be difficult due to the paucity of organisms.

   b. **Trimethoprim–sulfamethoxazole** is the treatment of choice for patients with this bowel pathogen, usually producing symptomatic improvement within 7 to 10 days. Relapse is frequent if TMP-SMX is not continued suppressively, but in those responding to HAART, this can be discontinued successfully after 3 to 4 weeks.

4. **Cyclosporiasis**, caused by *Cyclospora cayetanensis*, consists of a diarrheal syndrome quite similar to those above.

   a. **Diagnosis** is by stool examination for oocysts.

   b. Good response to TMS is usually seen, and as with *Isospora*, maintenance therapy may be required.

5. **Microsporidiosis.** *Enterocytozoon bieneusi* and *Encephalitozoon* (formerly *Septata*) *intestinalis* are most commonly associated with diarrhea in AIDS patients, although *E. intestinalis* can cause disseminated disease.

   a. **Diagnosis.** Although the organisms are small, they can be found in stool or duodenal biopsies.

   b. **Treatment.** *E. intestinalis* often responds to albendazole 400 mg p.o. b.i.d. Response is less reliable after treatment of *E. bieneusi*, but experimental fumagillin has been helpful anecdotally.

E. **Herpesvirus infections**

1. **Epstein-Barr virus. Oral hairy leukoplakia** is an orolingual lesion associated with latent infection with EBV. Oral lesions may simulate candidiasis in appearing white and plaque-like. These lesions usually occur along with grooves on the lateral surface of the tongue and buccal mucosa.

   a. **Diagnosis** of oral hairy leukoplakia is based on the appearance of the lesions. Further conformation is obtained by the presence of EBV, as demonstrated by immunohistochemical staining of biopsy specimens.

   b. Regression of oral hairy leukoplakia can occur spontaneously or following use of antiviral drugs such as acyclovir or ganciclovir.

   Patients with HIV infection are at increased risk for non-Hodgkin lymphoma, which has been associated with EBV infection. The tumors are believed to be related to malignant transformation of lymphoid tissue infected with EBV. Lymphomas associated with EBV infection are treated with systemic chemotherapy and radiation therapy.

2. **Herpes simplex virus.** Prolonged and severe mucocutaneous HSV infection was one of the original clinical findings observed in AIDS patients. Serologic studies have shown an extremely high prevalence of HSV infection in HIV-infected men.

   a. **Diagnosis** of HSV infection associated with HIV is similar to that in other settings, usually by viral culture of a specimen obtained by swabbing the base of a lesion.

   b. **Treatment** of recurrent HSV infection is with **acyclovir** (200 mg p.o. 5 times daily, or 400 mg t.i.d.), **valaciclovir** (500 mg b.i.d.), or **famciclovir** (125 to 250 mg b.i.d.) at standard doses used in non-immunocompromised patients. Clinical responses may be slower, however, often mandating longer duration of treatment, and even increased doses in the settings of acyclovir resistance or primary (initial) infection. Patients with acyclovir-resistant HSV often have diminished activity of viral-specific thymidine kinase, which phosphorylates acyclovir and allows it to act as a DNA-polymerase inhibitor. Foscarnet and cidofovir are active against acyclovir-resistant HSV, but side effects are more frequent and may be significant.

3. **Varicella-zoster virus** reactivation (shingles) is often an early clinical finding in HIV disease. Recurrent episodes of localized VZV as well as multidermatomal VZV can occur. Unusual manifestations of VZV infection include acute retinal necrosis syndrome and zoster-associated esophagitis. Disseminated varicella, particularly in children with HIV infection, can result in multiorgan failure, including pneumonia and death.

    a. **Diagnosis** of VZV is based on clinical manifestations and culture of the virus. Giant intranuclear inclusion bodies may also be noted on histopathology.

    b. **Treatment** of VZV is initiated with high-dose oral acyclovir (800 mg p.o. 5 times daily), valaciclovir (1000 mg p.o. t.i.d.), or famciclovir (500 mg p.o. t.i.d.). As with HSV, acyclovir-resistant VZV can emerge, and can be treated with foscarnet or cidofovir. Indications for parenteral acyclovir therapy include ocular involvement, severe esophagitis, and occasionally multidermatomal infection.

    Patients with facial zoster should be monitored carefully for ocular involvement. Any patient with potential ocular involvement should be hospitalized with close ophthalmologic evaluation. Adjunctive topical therapy with trifluridine may be indicated.

4. **Cytomegalovirus.** CMV infection is common in the general population. Seroprevalence rates range from 40% to 100%, depending on the geographic and associated economic population studied. Among HIV-infected individuals, the most common clinical manifestation of CMV is retinitis, occurring primarily in patients with advanced HIV disease (CD4 cell counts less than or equal to 100 per mm^3). Retinitis can be bilateral and is often sight threatening. Presenting symptoms include a change in vision, visual field defects, or asymptomatic flame hemorrhages seen on funduscopy. Following hematogenous dissemination, CMV localizes in retinal vascular arcades and causes hemorrhage and necrosis. Lesions that are initially small can enlarge and destroy increasing areas of the retina, resulting in progressive visual loss or retinal detachment.

    CMV can also cause extraocular disease in patients with HIV infection. At autopsy, 90% of AIDS patients have CMV infection documented in the GI tract, lungs, liver, or CNS. CMV can cause acute inflammation in the GI tract of patients with HIV infection, presenting as severe esophagitis or colitis. Other manifestations of CMV include neuropathy, ventriculitis, global CNS dysfunction, and rarely, pneumonitis. CMV is implicated in a form of polyradiculopathy associated with neutrophilic CSF pleocytosis sometimes suggestive of acute bacterial meningitis. These patients usually present with bowel and bladder dysfunction and ascending paralysis.

    a. **Diagnosis** of CMV retinitis is made on the clinical appearance of the lesions noted by funduscopy and the exclusion of other OIs that can affect the retina such as ocular pneumocystosis, toxoplasmic chorioretinitis, and syphilitic retinitis.

    b. **Treatment** of CMV disease is with either ganciclovir or foscarnet, initially, both of which inhibit viral polymerase. A more recent, highly effective alternative is the surgically implanted intraocular ganciclovir release device (Vitrasert). This acts locally and thus does not prevent extraocular disease, but may be given together with the oral form for slightly better systemic coverage. Because relapse is common without maintenance therapy, all patients who are treated for CMV should continue indefinitely on suppressive maintenance regimens. Both drugs appear to be effective, although foscarnet may confer some survival benefit because concurrent therapy with nucleoside analogues such as zidovudine is better tolerated. Combined therapy with zidovudine and ganciclovir increases the risk of synergistic myelosuppression.

Upon diagnosis, a 2- to 3-week course of intravenous "induction therapy" is begun. Ganciclovir is administered at a dose of 10 mg/kg/day during induction, then is reduced to a dose of 5 to mg/kg/day given 5 to 7 days per week as chronic suppressive therapy. Therapy is usually administered through a central catheter because of the need for long-term intravenous therapy. The main side effect of ganciclovir is myelosuppression, particularly neutropenia, which can limit the use of the drug or interrupt its use periodically to allow the neutrophil count to recover. The use of colony-stimulating factor drugs such as granulocyte macrophage colony-stimulating factor (GM-CSF) or granulocyte colony-stimulating factor (G-CSF) may allow for the continuation of ganciclovir when neutropenia occurs.

Foscarnet is used both as primary therapy for CMV retinitis, as well as for those patients who do not tolerate ganciclovir or have refractory disease. Foscarnet is administered at a dose of 60 mg/kg/day q8h during the induction phase and then a lower dose (90 to 120 mg/kg/day) is administered daily as suppressive therapy. The drug must be given as a controlled infusion and has significant side effects including nephrotoxicity, anemia, and electrolyte abnormalities, particularly of calcium and phosphorus. Neurotoxicity associated with symptomatic hypocalcemia during the infusion can occur in the induction phase, probably due to the phosphate-like activity of foscarnet. Renal function must be monitored carefully during foscarnet therapy, and dose adjustments must be made if alterations in glomerular filtration rate are noted.

Cidofovir is a nucleotide analogue with potent activity against CMV. Initial dosing is 5 mg per kg i.v. given weekly for 2 weeks, then every 2 weeks. Prehydration and careful monitoring are mandatory to prevent dose-limiting renal toxicity.

Although it is less effective than intravenous therapy, oral ganciclovir can be used especially in patients with non-sight-threatening lesions, obviating the need for intravenous access and thus improving the quality of life for some patients. The recently approved prodrug of ganciclovir, valganciclovir, demonstrates efficacy similar to intravenous ganciclovir and will probably replace oral ganciclovir as the oral alternative of choice.

As increasingly recognized with other OIs, maintenance therapy can be discontinued safely in patients whose CD4 cell counts increase to greater than 100 per m^3 following HAART.

Treatment for **extraocular CMV disease** is similar to that used for retinitis.

F. Hepatitis C virus

Coinfection with HIV and hepatitis C virus (HCV) is estimated to occur in approximately 30% of those infected with HIV. The prevalence of coinfection varies considerably, however, with the setting and risk group: 50% to 90% of those acquiring HIV from injection drugs are HCV-infected, whereas coinfection is less common (2% to 10%) among HIV-infected men having sex with men. Because the natural history of liver disease appears aggravated in those infected with HIV, hepatitis C was designated an OI in HIV-infected persons by the U.S. Public Health Service in 1999. In some U.S. urban centers, end-stage liver disease caused by hepatitis C has become a major cause of hospital admissions and death among those coinfected with HIV.

The impact of HCV on the natural history of HIV infection is less clear. Some groups have found a less robust increase in CD4 count following antiretroviral treatment, or a more rapid deterioration in immune function in coinfected patients. Furthermore, liver enzyme abnormalities and hepatotoxicity can complicate treatment of either infection.

1. **Diagnosis.** All HIV-infected persons should be screened for HCV infection with an enzyme immunoassay for HCV antibody in blood. Those seropositive should then undergo confirmatory testing by either recombinant immunoblot assay (RIBA) or qualitative testing for HCV RNA.

2. **Treatment.** The treatment of individuals coinfected with HIV and HCV requires a considerable degree of monitoring and frequent follow-up, usually warranting referral to those with particular experience or expertise. In general, the current recommendations for medical treatment of HCV infection in HIV-infected persons do not differ fundamentally from that of non-HIV-infected persons, although the threshold for treatment might be lower due to the accelerated natural history of HCV disease. Indications for treatment include persistent elevation of ALT, detectable HCV RNA, histologic evidence of portal or bridging fibrosis, or moderate degrees of inflammation or necrosis. Liver biopsy is often, but not always, obtained to assess stage of disease and appropriateness of treatment. Best results to date in HIV-uninfected patients have occurred with the use of interferon (IFN)-alfa combined with oral ribavirin, but the efficacy of this combination in coinfected patients is still under study.

   Contraindications to treatment with IFN include several conditions that occur frequently in coinfected patients, such as major depressive illness or psychoses, active illicit drug or alcohol use, and baseline abnormalities in cell counts. Coinfected patients should be immunized for both hepatitis A and B, if found susceptible on serologic testing, to prevent any additional superimposed liver injury.

G. Fungal infections

Severe fungal infections are frequent and severe complications of advanced HIV disease. Individuals residing in endemic areas are at increased risk for histoplasmosis, coccidioidomycosis, and blastomycosis. *C. neoformans* affects HIV-infected patients worldwide because of the ubiquitous presence of fungal spores in soil and bird droppings. Patients with fungal infections usually respond initially to amphotericin B, but the majority relapse following primary treatment unless chronic suppressive therapy is maintained.

1. **Candidiasis**

   a. **Oral mucosal candidiasis** is seen in virtually all HIV-infected patients. Among HIV-infected women, candidal vaginitis is common and is often difficult to treat. The clinical manifestations of mucosal candidiasis are easily recognized. Less common forms of oral candidiasis include atrophic disease and angular cheilitis, which present as cracking at the edge of the lips. *C. albicans* can also affect the esophagus, presenting with odynophagia and difficulty swallowing. The absence of oral thrush does not exclude candidal infection of the esophagus.

   b. **Diagnosis** of candidiasis requires the visualization of yeast forms on wet preparations of material scraped from mucosal surfaces, and treated with KOH to dissolve cellular debris. Diagnosis of esophagitis is often made presumptively by the characteristic clinical presentation. Endoscopy can more definitively show ulcerations and white or yellow plaques compatible with the diagnosis, or can be used to obtain specimens for histopathologic evidence of *Candida*.

   c. **Treatment** of oral candidiasis may be topical or systemic. A variety of agents including nystatin suspension, clotrimazole troches, and other azole drugs are used to treat candidiasis. Those who do not respond to local treatment are often switched to oral ketoconazole, fluconazole, or itraconazole. Ketoconazole is used less often now because of its poor absorption in the absence of gastric acid and its side effect of adrenal suppression. Patients with HIV infection often have gastropathy associated with decreased acid production, which may be exacerbated by concomitant use of antacids or H_2 blockers. Fluconazole does not depend on gastric acid for absorption and is therefore preferred for treatment of candidal infections of the mouth and esophagus. For patients with refractory esophagitis, short courses (7 to 10 days) of low-dose i.v. amphotericin B (0.3 mg/kg/day) may be effective.

2. **Cryptococcosis**. *C. neoformans* is a ubiquitous encapsulated yeast, and the second most common fungal infection in patients with AIDS.

   a. **Meningitis** is the most common form of cryptococcal disease in patients with HIV infection. Patients with cryptococcal meningitis present with headache, fever, altered mental status, and less commonly, seizures and coma. Poor prognostic factors at presentation include altered mental status, very high titers of cerebrospinal fluid (CSF) cryptococcal antigen, depressed CSF white blood cell count (less than 20 per mm³), age less than 35 years, positive blood cultures for *Cryptococcus*, and focal neurologic deficits. Other sites of infection include the lung (producing bilateral patchy infiltrates), retina, skin, bone, prostate, and other organs.

   b. **Diagnosis** of cryptococcal meningitis requires detection of the organism in CSF. Isolation of the fungus from blood, bone marrow, and other tissues can also reveal extraneural infection. The use of cryptococcal antigen testing has greatly facilitated diagnosis of cryptococcal infection in patients with HIV disease. Approximately 90% of patients with cryptococcal meningitis have a positive CSF cryptococcal antigen test. Patients with cryptococcal meningitis can have a relatively low-grade CSF pleocytosis despite extremely high antigen titers.

   c. **Amphotericin B** is the drug of choice for patients with severe cryptococcal infection, with or without 5-flucytosine (5FC; doses should be less than or equal to 150 mg/kg/day p.o. to reduce bone marrow suppression, which is more common in AIDS patients). Amphotericin is given parenterally, and the dose is gradually increased to 0.6 to 0.8 mg/kg/day. An alternative choice is **fluconazole**, 400 mg per day, which can be appropriate for patients with mild disease or who lack poor prognostic factors. Following a 2- to 6-week course of amphotericin, patients can be switched to oral fluconazole for continuation of acute therapy for an additional 6 to 10 weeks. Repeated lumbar punctures may be necessary in patients developing symptoms or signs of hydrocephalus (recurrent headache or altered mental status).

   All patients with documented cryptococcal disease must be maintained on effective maintenance therapy in order to prevent relapse. Randomized clinical trials have clearly shown that fluconazole is superior to amphotericin in terms of relapse rate and tolerability. Oral doses of 200 to 400 mg per day help prevent recurrent disease following primary therapy.

3. **Histoplasmosis.** Disseminated disease caused by *H. capsulatum* in patients with HIV infection is especially common in geographically specific areas where the fungus is endemic. In the United States, these areas include the central and midwestern states. Histoplasmosis in AIDS patients, however, is occasionally observed in individuals who have only minimal contact in or brief travel through endemic areas.

   a. **Clinical presentation** is generally nonspecific, but can be life threatening, with multisystem disease including headache, cough, fever, weight loss, lymphadenopathy, and organomegaly.

   b. Diagnosis is made by culture of appropriate specimens, including
   lymph node tissue, blood, and bone marrow. Measurement of urinary *Histoplasma* antigen is quite useful in detecting histoplasmosis and in monitoring therapy once the diagnosis has been
   established.

   c. Amphotericin B is the treatment of choice for patients with disseminated histoplasmosis. Doses in excess of 2 g per day are usually required for induction therapy before maintenance therapy
   begins. Although considerably more expensive, liposomal forms of
   amphotericin B appeared to be as effective as amphotericin B de-
   oxycholate and generally better tolerated. Itraconazole is effective
   in treatment of patients with mild to moderate histoplasmosis.

4. Coccidioidomycosis occurs in patients with HIV infection residing
   in the southwestern United States. The disease often presents with
   pulmonary disease or meningitis, which responds to parenteral amphotericin or fluconazole. Maintenance therapy with fluconazole or itraconazole is required.

5. Aspergillosis usually presents as invasive pulmonary disease, with
   cough, shortness of breath, fever, and cavitary lung disease, often with
   diffuse infiltrates. Amphotericin B and/or itraconazole are marginally
   effective, but prognosis is poor in the absence of immune reconstitution in response to HAART.

6. *Penicillium marneffei* infection occurs most often in patients from
   endemic areas of southeast Asia, characteristically presenting as fever,
   pneumonitis, or as disseminated disease involving lymph nodes, skin,
   and mucosa in a syndrome similar to histoplasmosis. Fungus can be
   isolated from involved sites including blood, sputum, or bone marrow.
   Amphotericin B is preferred for severe disease, but mild to moderate
   cases can respond to itraconazole 400 mg p.o. q.d. Maintenance therapy with itraconazole is recommended after initial response.

H. Bacterial infections
   Recurrent bacterial infections appear with increased frequency in HIV-
   infected persons. Pyogenic organisms, including *Streptococcus pneumoniae*, *Haemophilus influenzae*, *Staphylococci*, and Gram-negative rods such
   as *Pseudomonas* commonly infect patients with HIV. These bacterial infections are associated with frequent relapses after treatment, a higher incidence of bacteremia, and multiorgan involvement. Other pathogens often
   seen are *Nocardia*, *Listeria*, *Shigella*, and *Salmonella* sp, and *Bartonella
   henselae* (cat scratch bacillus).

   Patients with HIV infection are at increased risk for community-acquired
   pneumonia associated with *S. pneumoniae* and *H. influenzae*. The source of
   these organisms may be the sinuses because these patients often have **recurrent episodes of bacterial sinusitis**. *Salmonella* and *Campylobacter*
   infections usually present with GI disease, but can also present with persistent or relapsing bacteremia and metastatic foci of infection.

   Infections with *B. henselae* or *B. quintana* often cause skin lesions (bacillary angiomatosis). Originally described as epithelial angiomatosis, these
   lesions are often confused with KS of the skin and respond to treatment with
   erythromycin, other macrolides, or tetracyclines. Fever, bacteremia, and
   metastatic lesions to bone, liver, lung, and the CNS can also occur.

   The increase in incidence of **syphilis** in the United States can largely be
   ascribed to cases diagnosed in HIV-infected individuals. Clinical manifestations of syphilis are generally similar to those seen in non-HIV-infected
   individuals, but atypical presentations are more frequent. In particular,
   negative or equivocal serologic tests can be seen in HIV-infected patients
   with documented secondary syphilis. The decision to sample CSF in subjects
   with positive syphilis serologies is controversial. Relapse following standard
   therapy, particularly with oral antibiotics, is more commonly observed in
   patients with HIV infection. Clinical trials of a variety of therapeutic

agents are now being conducted to determine the optimum treatment for the syphilis-infected patient with HIV disease. To date, no reliably effective alternative to penicillin has been found. In patients with history of penicillin allergy, penicillin skin testing and desensitization are recommended.

III. **Neoplastic complications of human immunodeficiency virus infection**

A. **Kaposi sarcoma** is the most common malignancy seen in patients with HIV infection. Recent evidence strongly suggests the causative agent to be human herpesvirus type 8 (HHV-8). About 15% to 20% of gay men with HIV infection develop KS during the progression of their disease, but KS is uncommon in women and children. The incidence of KS is declining in cohorts of gay men studied since the beginning of the epidemic in the early 1980s.

1. **Clinically**, KS can present with localized cutaneous lesions or disseminated visceral disease. Cutaneous KS is characterized by nodular skin lesions that are usually purplish in color. Painless lesions can be found in the oropharynx, including the gingival and buccal mucosal surfaces. Sites of visceral involvement include the lung, lymph nodes, liver, and GI tract. GI KS lesions can produce chronic blood loss and acute hemorrhage. Pulmonary involvement can mimic OIs such as PCP. KS in the lung often presents with nodular coarse infiltrates bilaterally, often associated with pleural effusions. These infiltrates can be difficult to distinguish from pneumonitis caused by opportunistic pathogens.

2. **Diagnosis** of KS is based on the clinical appearance of the lesions, as well as characteristic histopathologic features on biopsy. Lesions of the mucosal surfaces that mimic KS include cutaneous fungal infections (*Cryptococcus*) and bacillary angiomatosis associated with *Bartonella* sp. Diagnosis of visceral disease is often established by endoscopic visualization of the lesions in the respiratory or GI tracts. Biopsy of these lesions is rarely done because of their propensity to bleed.

3. **Treatment** of KS depends on the extent of the disease. Isolated cutaneous lesions can regress on their own or following HAART. Intralesional injection of Vinca alkaloids often suffices for cutaneous lesions. Cryotherapy and other topical remedies have also been successful. Radiation therapy can provide significant palliation from local mechanical discomfort due to bulky lesions in the oral cavity or airway, or when regional lymph node disease causes venous obstruction.

    More extensive KS can be treated with intravenous Vinca alkaloids on an intermittent basis. Treatment with IFN-γ has also been shown to be effective in patients with CD4 cell counts greater than 400 per mm^3; however, it is often associated with a flu-like syndrome and with myelosuppression.

    Patients with extensive visceral involvement can warrant treatment with multiple chemotherapeutic agents. The immunosuppressive effects of chemotherapy can preclude its use in effective doses, particularly with concurrent use of certain antiretroviral agents. Treatment regimens including bleomycin, Adriamycin, and Vinca alkaloids are partially successful in treating disseminated KS. The role of any antiviral therapy directed at HHV-8 is unclear.

B. **Non-Hodgkin and Hodgkin lymphomas.** Patients with HIV infection are at increased risk of developing lymphomas, particularly non-Hodgkin lymphoma, which historically respond poorly to standard chemotherapeutic regimens. Survival appears to be improving in the era of HAART. Lymphomas are opportunistic malignancies in immunosuppressed patients, such as transplant recipients and those receiving immunosuppressive drugs for autoimmune diseases. Patients with HIV infection and non-Hodgkin lymphomas are particularly vulnerable to the side effects of chemotherapeutic regimens, especially drugs that cause bone marrow suppression. Because HIV infection itself, as well as concomitant antiretroviral therapy and OIs, affects the bone marrow, tolerance to multichemotherapeutic regimens is generally poor.

1. **Primary central nervous system lymphoma** is the most common CNS opportunistic malignancy in patients with HIV infection. CNS lymphomas are extremely aggressive and are very difficult to treat. Patients with mass lesions on CNS imaging must be evaluated for CNS lymphoma or other OIs such as toxoplasmosis.
2. **Diagnostically**, a single mass lesion appearing on CT or MRI scan is very suggestive of a lymphoma. Definitive diagnosis requires biopsy, but PCR on CSF for EBV may be positive in up to 90% of CNS lymphomas, thus supporting a presumptive diagnosis noninvasively.
3. **Radiation therapy** can reduce tumor size but is not curative. Because chemotherapy is only palliative in these patients, it is often deferred because of the advanced state of HIV disease usually present when CNS lymphoma is detected.

   Recent data suggest that the addition of G-CSF or GM-CSF to chemotherapeutic regimens using agents such as bleomycin, methotrexate, doxorubicin, cytoxan, vincristine, and dexamethasone can limit myelosuppression, but the effect of colony-stimulating factors on ultimate outcome in these malignancies is unclear.

   An increased incidence of Hodgkin disease has also been noted in HIV-infected cohorts. Response to therapy is less favorable than that seen in patients with Hodgkin disease without HIV infection.

C. **Other neoplastic disorders.** Other malignancies reported in association with HIV infection include **carcinoma of the genital tract**, including the anus, rectum, and cervix, as well as **EBV-associated Burkitt lymphoma**. Squamous cell carcinomas of the anus and cervix probably arise from concomitant infection with subtypes of human papillomavirus (HPV), which are known to be associated with malignant transformation. Recent studies suggest that increasing numbers of men and women with HIV infection have HPV-associated carcinomas. Therapy for these malignancies can be ablative, surgical, or require systemic chemotherapy.

Selected Readings

American Thoracic Society/Centers for Disease Control and Prevention Statement Committee on Latent Tuberculosis Infection. Targeted tuberculin testing and treatment of latent tuberculosis infection. *MMWR Morb Mortal Wkly Rep* 2000;49(RR-06):1–54.

Bartlett JG. *Medical management of HIV infection.* Baltimore: Johns Hopkins University, 2000.

Carpenter CCJ, Cooper DA, Fischl MA, et al. Antiretroviral therapy in adults: Updated recommendations of the International AIDS Society-USA Panel. *JAMA* 2000;283: 381–390.

Centers for Disease Control and Prevention. 1999 USPHS/IDSA guidelines for the prevention of opportunistic infections in persons infected with human immunodeficiency virus. US Public Health Service (USPHS) and Infectious Diseases Society of America (IDSA). *MMWR Morb Mortal Wkly Rep* 1999;48:1–59,61–66.

Cohen O, Cicala C, Vaccarezza M, et al. The immunology of human immunodeficiency infection. In: Mandell GL, Bennett JE, Dolin R, eds. *Principles and practice of infectious diseases*, 5th ed. Philadelphia: Churchill Livingstone, 2000:1374–1397.

El-Sadr WM, Burman WT, Grant LB, et al. Discontinuation of prophylaxis for Mycobacterium avium complex disease is HIV-infected patients who have a response to antiretroviral therapy. *N Engl J Med* 2000;342:1085–1092.

Fauci AS. Immunopathogenic mechanisms of HIV infection. *Ann Intern Med* 1996; 124:654–663.

Furrer H, Egger M, Opravil M, et al. Discontinuation of primary prophylaxis against Pneumocystis carinii pneumonia in HIV-1 infected adults treated with combination antiretroviral therapy. *N Engl J Med* 1999;340:1301–1306.

Hirsch MS, Brun-Vezinet F, D'Aquila RT, et al. Antiretroviral drug resistance testing in adult HIV-1 infection: Recommendations of an International AIDS Society-USA Panel. *JAMA* 2000;283:2417–2426.

Jacobson MA. Treatment of cytomegalovirus retinitis in the acquired immunodeficiency syndrome. *N Engl J Med* 1997;337:105–112.

Kahn JO, Walker BD. Acute human immunodeficiency virus type 1 infection. *N Engl J Med* 1998;339:33–39.

Ledergerber B, Mocroft A, Erard V, et al. AIDS-related opportunistic illnesses occurring after initiation of potent antiretroviral therapy. *JAMA* 1999;282:2220–2226.

Loutit JS. Bartonella infections. In Remington JS, Swartz MN, eds. *Current clinical topics in infectious diseases*. Boston: Blackwell Science, 1997;17:269–290.

Martin DF, Kupperman BD, Wolitz RA, et al. Oral ganciclovir for patients with cytomegalovirus retinitis treated with a ganciclovir implant. *N Engl J Med* 1999;340: 1063–1070.

Mellors JW, Munoz A, Giorgi JV, et al. Plasma viral load and CD4+ lymphocytes as prognostic markers of HIV-1 infection. *Ann Intern Med* 1997;126:946–954.

Palella FJ Jr, Delaney KM, Moorman AC, et al. The HIV outpatient study investigators. Declining morbidity and mortality among patients with advanced human immunodeficiency virus infection. *N Engl J Med* 1998;338:853–860.

Pantaleo G, et al. New concepts in the immunopathogenesis of human immunodeficiency virus infection. *N Engl J Med* 1993;328:327–335.

Saag MS, Holodniy M, Kuritzkes DR, et al. HIV viral load markers in clinical practice. *Nat Med* 1996;2:625–629.

Weiss LM, Keohane EM. The uncommon gastrointestinal protozoa: Microsporidia, Blastocystis, Isospora, Dientamoeba, and Balantidium. In: Remington JS, Swartz MN, eds. *Current clinical topics in infectious diseases*. Boston: Blackwell Science, 1997;17:147–187.

Zaitseva M, Blauvelt A, Lee S, et al. Expression and function of CCR5 and CXCR4 on human Langerhans cells and macrophages: Implications for HIV primary infection. *Nat Med* 1997;3:1369–1377.

Useful Internet Websites

The Johns Hopkins University AIDS Service (www.hopkins-aids.edu)

UCSF AIDS Program (www.hivinsite.ucsf.edu)

HIV/AIDS Treatment Information Service (www.hivatis.org)

International AIDS Society-USA (www.iasusa.org)

19. DIAGNOSTIC IMMUNOLOGY

Thomas A. Fleisher and Jack J. H. Bleesing

Techniques for evaluation of immunologic function have expanded dramatically in recent years as our understanding of the immune system has increased. The application of these studies is useful for the evaluation of immune deficiency diseases and evaluating a patient for autoimmune, allergic, or malignant diseases. This chapter is directed at general concepts and appropriate applications of methods used to characterize and quantify immunoglobulins and specific antibodies, evaluate lymphocyte phenotype and function, study neutrophil function, assay complement, and assess allergic disease.

I. **Characterization and quantitation of immunoglobulins and specific antibodies.** Immunoglobulins are glycoproteins that are secreted by differentiated B lymphocytes (plasma cells). Specific immunoglobulins (antibodies) are normally produced following antigenic stimulation, yielding a variety of antibody molecules, all of which react with varying strengths to the specific antigen. This type of response is referred to as polyclonal, because it involves multiple B cell clones. The basic molecular structure of each of these classes consists of two identical heavy chains (α, δ, ϵ, γ, or μ) and two identical light chains (κ or λ) that together form a Y-shaped monomer (see Chapter 1). There are five different classes or isotypes of immunoglobulin that are determined by the heavy chain used in the molecule (e.g., immunoglobulin G [IgG] contains two identical γ heavy chains). The arms of the Y, referred to as the Fab portion, form the antigen-combining sites, and the stem, referred to as the Fc portion, contains the other sites of biologic function, such as complement component binding. IgG, the most prevalent immunoglobulin in serum, is found as a monomer, and constitutes the major antibody class produced in secondary antibody responses. Both IgE, the antibody of allergic response, and IgD, a principal B-cell surface immunoglobulin, are also present in serum as monomers and are found in low concentrations. IgA is found in serum and secretions as a dimer, together with a J chain and secretory component. The secretory component is synthesized by mucosal epithelial cells and joined to the dimeric IgA molecule as it passes through the epithelium. IgM, normally present in serum as a pentamer, is the immunoglobulin class produced early during a primary antibody response to an antigen. Evaluation of immunoglobulins consists of qualitative and quantitative tests that can be directed at evaluating immunoglobulin classes and their subclasses and/or antigen-specific antibody. There is an age-dependent change in the levels of immunoglobulins that must be taken into account when interpreting results (see Appendices IV and V). Alterations in the level of a serum protein, such as an immunoglobulin, can result from impaired synthesis, altered utilization, and/or increased loss.

A. **Electrophoresis**

1. **Zone electrophoresis.** This technique allows for the separation of proteins based on electrical charge. The sample (solution) to be tested is placed on a buffer-saturated support medium (e.g., paper, agarose) and subjected to an electropotential gradient. **Serum electrophoresis** normally yields five bands consisting of albumin, alpha-1, alpha-2, beta, and gamma globulin fractions (Fig. 19.1). The bands can be assessed with a densitometer that generates a tracing from which the relative percentage of each fraction is determined. Immunoglobulins normally fall in the gamma globulin band, although they also migrate into the beta and alpha-2 globulin bands. Zone electrophoresis can also be performed on other body fluids, including cerebrospinal fluid (CSF) and urine. This semiquantitative technique is useful for assessing total protein status and can be used to screen for monoclonal

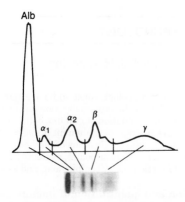

FIG. 19.1. Zone electrophoresis. The electrophoretic pattern and densitometric tracing demonstrate the five major bands (albumin plus alpha-1, alpha-2, beta, and gamma globulins) from a normal serum sample.

immunoglobulins, although this technique may miss low-level monoclonal antibodies seen in early myelomas.

2. **Immunoelectrophoresis** is a two-step method in which proteins are electrophoretically separated in a gel and then antiserum is directed against one immunoglobulin heavy chain (α, δ, ε, γ, or μ) protein, or one light chain (κ or λ) protein is loaded into a trough in the gel and is allowed to diffuse into the gel containing these separated proteins. The antibody combines with the appropriate protein (immunoglobulin), resulting in the formation of a precipitin arc(s) of the antibody–antigen complex (in the area of the gel where antigen and antibody concentrations are at equivalence) (Fig. 19.2). This is not a quantitative test, and it requires considerable experience for proper interpretation. It is used primarily for the characterization of monoclonal immunoglobulins.

3. **Immunofixation electrophoresis** uses zone electrophoresis followed by overlaying of the electrophoretically separated proteins with antibodies directed against specific immunoglobulin heavy or light chains. This results in immunoprecipitation of the antibody–antigen complex (at equivalence), which can then be stained (e.g., imido black) and visualized (Fig. 19.3). Polyclonal immunoglobulins give a diffuse band, and

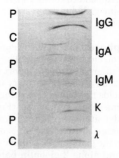

FIG. 19.2. Immunoelectrophoresis. This gel demonstrates a normal pattern with the control (C) serum and μ heavy chain and κ light chain spurs with the patient (P) sample compatible with IgM-κ monoclonal gammopathy.

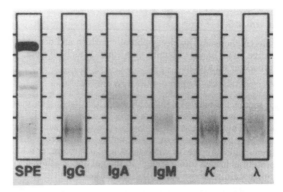

FIG. 19.3. Immunofixation electrophoresis. Demonstrates a normal pattern with antibodies to the major heavy-chain and light-chain proteins. A clonal immunoglobulin would result in a darker staining band in a heavy-chain and light-chain zone.

a monoclonal immunoglobulin produces an intense narrow band often within the diffuse band in the background. This technique is easier to interpret and more sensitive than immunoelectrophoresis, but also is not quantitative. The test currently is used by many laboratories instead of immunoelectrophoresis for the identification of monoclonal or oligoclonal immunoglobulins.

B. Double gel diffusion is another semiquantitative test that evaluates the relationship between specific antibodies or antigens in solutions. Comparison between a reference material and unknown serum allows a comparative assessment for identity, partial identity, or nonidentity. This method currently is used by some laboratories in evaluating autoimmune disorders for the presence or absence of autoantibodies to extractable nuclear antigens (ENA), including (anti-Sm), anti-nuclear ribonuclear protein (anti-RNP), anti-Sjögren syndrome A (anti-SS-A), anti-Sjögren syndrome B (anti-SS-B), anti-Scl-70, and anti-Jo-1 (see Chapter 14). Although it lacks the detection sensitivity of many quantitative methods, the test is technically easy, can be performed with antigen preparations that are only partially purified, is highly specific, and serves as a useful screening test for the presence of an antibody or antigen.

C. Single radial immunodiffusion allows quantification of a protein (antigen) by adding serum (or other fluid) to wells cut into agarose that contains specific antiserum. An immunoprecipitin ring of immune complexes is formed as the relevant serum protein (antigen) diffuses into the antibody containing agarose and precipitates at the region of antibody–antigen equivalence. Thus, the diameter of this ring is proportional to the concentration of the protein (antigen) being evaluated because the concentration of the antiserum is constant throughout the gel. The concentration of the unknown is then determined by plotting the ring diameter on a concentration curve produced from a series of standards with know protein (antigen) concentration. **Radial immunodiffusion (RID)** is a simple and reliable method to quantify immunoglobulins (including IgG subclasses), complement components (e.g., C3, C4, and factor B), and other proteins. Low-level RID kits are available that extend the detection level to as low as 0.03 mg per L. At least three situations may result in erroneous results using conventional RID kits: (i) **low molecular weight or monomeric IgM** (e.g., Waldenström macroglobulinemia and ataxia telangiectasia) will be reported incorrectly high, because the low molecular weight IgM diffuses more rapidly than the heavier pentameric IgM standard; (ii) **high concentrations of IgG**

rheumatoid factor can produce complexes of IgG that diffuse more slowly than the IgG standard, resulting in an underestimation of the IgG level; (iii) **the presence of antibovida (e.g., goat) species antibodies**, which may be seen in IgA-deficient patients, that can bind the antiserum (in the support medium) if it is from a bovidae source. This generates a precipitin ring that might be interpreted as signifying the presence of IgA, although it is actually absent. Using an alternate source of anti-IgA (e.g., rabbit) in the support medium can remedy this problem.

D. **Nephelometry**, a method to quantify proteins in a solution, is based on the scattering of light from soluble immune complexes generated by the addition of specific antibody to the sample to be tested. In contrast to precipitin reactions, nephelometry is performed in the antibody excess region of the precipitin curve (rather than equivalence) and this procedure is readily amenable to automated instrumentation. There are two general approaches, rate and fixed-time nephelometry, both of which enable accurate measurement of IgG and IgG subclasses, IgA, IgM, C3, C4, factor B, C-reactive protein (CRP), and a number of other serum proteins. This method is adaptable for the determination of low-level proteins, including those in the CSF. At least one system is capable of measuring IgE levels (normally present in nanogram per milliliter quantities). Nephelometry is the standard method for quantifying immunoglobulin in most clinical laboratories because of the high-volume capabilities of modern nephelometers.

E. **Immunoassays**

1. **The radioimmunoassay** (RIA) was initially described more than 30 years ago and originally was developed to measure insulin in serum, which was undetectable by other methods available at the time. The original RIA was based on a competitive binding assay in which a constant amount of antigen-specific antibody is placed together with a small amount of the antigen that has been radiolabeled. Next, the sample, which contains an unknown concentration of the antigen, is added. Antibody binding antigen from the sample displaces the labeled antigen, and this decrease in radioactivity (in the immune antibody–antigen complexes) correlates with the concentration of the antigen in the sample (Fig. 19.4).

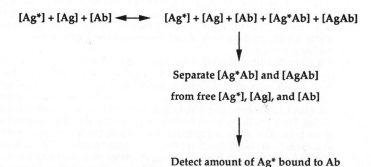

$$[Ag^*] + [Ag] + [Ab] \longleftrightarrow [Ag^*] + [Ag] + [Ab] + [Ag^*Ab] + [AgAb]$$

Separate [Ag*Ab] and [AgAb]

from free [Ag*], [Ag], and [Ab]

Detect amount of Ag* bound to Ab

FIG. 19.4. Competitive binding radioimmunoassay (RIA). This approach involves incubating a fixed amount of a radionuclide-labeled antigen with specific antibody and either a standard or an unknown sample containing the antigen (unlabeled). The resulting immune complexes are precipitated, and the amount of labeled antigen in the complexes is determined. There is a decrease in the amount of labeled antigen-bound (radioactivity) as the concentration of the free (unlabeled) antigen increases. This method can also be adapted to the use of enzyme-labeled or fluorescent-labeled antigen. Ag*, labeled antigen (radionuclide-, enzyme-, or fluorescent-labeled); Ag, antigen in unknown sample or standard; Ab, test antibody.

The competitive binding test can also be reversed by using a fixed concentration of purified antigen together with labeled antibody to evaluate for specific antibody concentration in an unknown sample. A further modification of this method uses a **solid phase** to immobilize one of the reactants (antigen or antibody) and can be performed as an indirect or sandwich assay (see Enzyme-linked immunosorbent assay below). RIA remains a very sensitive method for quantification of specific antigens or antibodies. However, it has the disadvantage of requiring expensive equipment and relatively expensive radioactive reagents, which have defined shelf life that may be rather limited and require special means for disposal.

2. **Enzyme-linked immunosorbent assay** (ELISA) is an immunoassay method that uses polystyrene plates, tubes, or beads as the solid phase to provide a binding site for the specific antigen under study. Serum (or other fluid) is added to the antigen-coated plate (tube, beads), which enables antibody to bind to the specific antigen immobilized on the solid phase. The presence of bound immunoglobulin from the sample following a wash step is then detected using a second antibody (reactive with the bound immunoglobulin), which is enzyme labeled. Following another wash step, the appropriate chromogenic substrate is added, resulting in enzyme-dependent generation of color (Fig. 19.5). The intensity of this reaction can be measured and is proportional to the antibody concentration present in the sample. The method can be altered using a "sandwich" technique to detect antigen with a test system that has antigen-specific antibody immobilized on the solid phase. This "capture" antibody is used to bind antigen in an unknown sample. This is followed by a second antigen-specific antibody that is enzyme labeled (Fig. 19.5). Addition of the appropriate chromogenic substrate will yield color that is proportional to the antigen concentration.

The sensitivity of an ELISA can be made comparable to that of an RIA. This method can be used for quantifying a number of specific anti-

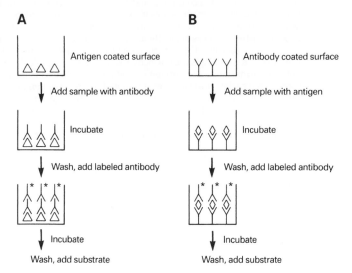

FIG. 19.5. Solid-phase enzyme-linked immunosorbent assay (ELISA): **(A)** indirect assay; **(B)** "sandwich" assay. The label (*) on the antibody can be an enzyme plus substrate (as shown), a radionuclide (solid-phase radioimmunoassay), or a fluorochrome (solid-phase fluorescence immunoassay).

bodies or antigens and has the advantages of being simple to perform, requiring no radioactive isotopes, and having excellent reproducibility. It is currently the standard assay in many laboratories for antiviral antibody testing, including initial human immunodeficiency virus (HIV) antibody testing, and also testing for a number of other immunologic proteins (including IgG subclasses and IgE). Alternatives to the enzyme-based test system include immunoassays that employ either a fluorescent or a chemiluminescent detection system. The latter approach has the advantage of providing amplification to the signal, extending the detection range of the immunoassay.

F. **Immunoblot (Western blot)** is primarily a qualitative method to identify specific antibodies. In this technique antigens of interest are separated using polyacrylamide gel electrophoresis. The separated proteins are then transferred to a nitrocellulose membrane. This is followed by overlaying the membrane with the antibody (e.g., serum) sample of interest and evaluating for the presence of bound immunoglobulin (specific antibodies) using a second labeled antibody (radioactive or enzyme) to human immunoglobulin. Although this method is not quantitative, it does allow for the detection of antibodies reactive with electrophoretically distinct protein antigens. The availability of commercial test kits has simplified the performance of these assays, and has allowed the widespread use of the Western blot as a confirmatory test in assessing HIV serologic status and by many laboratories in characterizing the antibody response to *Borrelia burgdorferi* (Lyme disease). Other clinical laboratory applications of this technology are relatively limited at this time.

G. **Other methods for detecting specific antibodies**

1. **Indirect immunofluorescence assays** usually use a tissue section or cell line on a microscope slide as a source of the antigen(s) of interest. The substrate is overlaid with the unknown sample, allowing any specific antibody to bind to the antigen(s). The presence of bound antibody is determined with a fluorochrome-labeled antibody reactive with bound antibody, followed by visual examination using fluorescence microscopy. This method is commonly used to test for antinuclear antibody (ANA) and a variety of virus-specific antibodies. The technique is fairly sensitive, relatively quantitative, and technically simple to perform.

2. **Agglutination assays** typically are performed using either red blood cells or latex particles that are coated with the antigen of interest. The presence of antigen-specific antibody results in macroscopically detectable agglutination of the antigen-coated particles. These tests are currently used to detect antithyroglobulin and antimicrosomal antibodies (by hemagglutination), rheumatoid factor (by latex agglutination), and various other antibodies. These assays are technically easy to perform and relatively quantitative, but are less sensitive than immunoassays. Interpretation of negative results in certain tests (e.g., antithyroglobulin antibody) must take into account the prozone effect, which renders a false-negative result in samples with significant antibody excess; this can be ruled out by testing a wider range of dilutions for unknown samples.

II. **Leukocyte phenotyping** identifies cells based on the presence of specific cell surface antigens (receptors), and provides clinically important data for disease status in HIV infection and the characterization of leukemia and lymphoma. This technique also is used as an adjunct in the evaluation of immune deficiencies, immune-mediated diseases, and in the monitoring of transplant and immune-based therapy patients. The present approach to lymphocyte phenotyping utilizes fluorochrome-labeled monoclonal antibodies specific for lymphocyte surface antigens and employs flow cytometry to quantitate the cell populations.

A. **Monoclonal antibodies** are produced by fusing an immortal murine myeloma cell line with normal murine plasma cells to yield hybridoma cells that effectively are immortal and can be selected for appropriate antibody specificity before cell expansion. This approach leads to virtually an un-limited supply of antigen-specific antibodies. There is an ever-increasing number of monoclonal antibodies to lymphocyte cell surface antigens, which are categorized according to a **cluster of differentiation (CD) numerical convention** (Table 19.1). These reagents allow for significant progress in the understanding of lymphocyte differentiation and maturation. In addition, other monoclonal antibodies have been produced, yielding information about mechanisms of cell adhesion and activation. In the area of lymphocyte phenotyping, monoclonal antibodies enable more complete evaluation of cell lineage, differentiation, activation, and functional capacity. These reagents provide important pieces of information regarding the presence of particular cells and their potential function, but they do not evaluate the actual function of the cell. More recently, intracellular staining for specific proteins including cytokines has become a standard approach that supplements immunophenotyping.

Table 19.1. Selected lymphocyte surface antigens

T-CELL SURFACE ANTIGENS

CD1	Found on cortical thymocytes
CD2	Alternative pathway for T-cell activation; SRBC receptor also referred to as LFA-2, found on all circulating T cells
CD3	Multichain receptor associated with the T cell antigen receptor (TCR); found on all circulating T cells
CD4	Cytoadhesion molecule for MHC (HLA) class II molecules; found on approximately two-thirds of the circulating T cells
CD5	Single-chain molecule found on most circulating T cells; also found on some B cells
CD7	Present on T-cell precursor and throughout T-cell differentiation
CD8	Cytoadhesion molecule for MHC (HLA) class I molecules; found on approximately one-third of the circulating T cells
CD25 (Tac, IL-2R, p55)	Alpha chain of the interleukin-2 (IL-2) receptor; found on activated T cells and B cells
CD28 (9.3)	Mediates a comitogenic signal for T cell proliferation, found on most CD4$^+$ T cells and a subset of CD8$^+$ T cells
CD38	Found on thymocytes, activated T cells, pre-B cells, activated B cells, and plasma cells
CD45RA	Isoform of the CD45 molecule found on "naïve" CD4 T cells
CD45RO (UCHL1)	Isoform of CD45 found on "memory" CD4 T cells
CD95 (Fas)	Receptor that is a member of the tumor necrosis receptor super family that is expressed by activated T (and B) cells and induces lymphocyte apoptosis
CD154 (CD40 ligand)	Expressed by T cells following activation and interacts with CD 40 on B cells to facilitate isotype switch and CD40 on monocytes in response to selected opportunistic organisms

continued

Table 19.1. *Continued*

B-CELL SURFACE ANTIGENS

Surface immunoglobulin	IgM found on immature B cells; IgM and IgD is found on mature B cells; the appearance of IgG, IgA, or IgE develops later after isotype switching
HLA-DR	MHC class II molecule found on all B cells; also present on monocytes and activated T cells
CD5	Present in low density on a B cell subpopulation (presence of which is inversely related to age) and on the majority of B cell CLL cells (also found at high density on most T cells)
CD10 (CALLA)	Found only on pre-B cells and on common acute leukemia cells
CD19	Expressed on pre-B cells and present throughout B cell differentiation; augments B cell proliferation
CD20	Present throughout B cell differentiation but is expressed after CD19 appears on the pre-B cell
CD21	Complement receptor for C3d (CR2), also is the EBV receptor, found on the majority of circulating B cells
CD22	Found on the majority of circulating B cells, also found in high density on hairy cell leukemia cells
CD23	Low-affinity IgE Fc receptor (FcεRII)
CD32	IgG Fc receptor (FcγRII)
CD40	Interacts with CD40 ligand (CD154) on T cells; activation enables B cells to undergo isotype switching; also present on monocytes
CD72	Expressed on very early B cells and lost during differentiation; CD5 ligand

NK-CELL SURFACE ANTIGENS

CD2	Found on 40%–70% of NK cells
CD8	Low level expression found on 30%–50% of NK cells
CD16	Low-affinity IgG Fc receptor (FcγRIII)
CD56 (NKH-1)	Found on the majority of NK cells, also found on a small subset of T cells that function as non-MHC-restricted cytotoxic cells
CD57 (HNK-1)	Found on approximately 50% of NK cells; also found on T-cell subpopulations

CD1; cluster of differentiation 1; SRBC, sheep red blood cell; LFA-2, leukocyte function associated antigen 2; MHC, major histocompatibility complex; HLA, human leukocyte antigen; IgM, immunoglobulin M; CLL, chronic lymphocytic leukemia; EBV, Epstein-Barr virus; NK, natural killer.

B. Fluorochromes are compounds that absorb light of a defined wavelength and convert this energy into light of a longer defined wavelength (lower energy). There are currently two fluorochromes routinely used in clinical phenotyping: **fluorescein isothiocyanate (FITC)** and **phycoerythrin (PE)**. Both of these compounds are excited by blue light (488 nm), with FITC generating green light and PE emitting orange light. A new fluorochrome, peridinin chlorophyll protein (PerCP) and certain double (tandem) fluorochromes, which rely on energy transfer from one component to the other, are also excited by blue light and produce a red signal. The combination of these fluorochromes directly conjugated to different monoclonal antibodies allows for three-color studies with one excitation (blue) light source, and this approach has become common in the clinical laboratory. Other fluorochromes, including Texas red, rhodamine, and allophycocyanin, are used primarily in research settings because they require a second excitation wavelength.

C. The **flow cytometer** is an instrument that allows for the rapid evaluation of multiple fluorescent and nonfluorescent measurements on a large number of cells in a solution. This enables assessment of multiple cell surface characteristics (parameters) for each cell, which can provide population and subpopulation information. The combination of multiple parameter assessment on each individual cell, together with a rapid analysis, provides significant advantages over conventional fluorescence microscopy for determining lymphocyte phenotypes. In addition, this type of instrumentation can be used to evaluate total cellular DNA as part of cell cycle analysis and other intracellular parameters using a variety of newer fluorescent probes.

D. **Lymphocyte phenotyping** utilizes fluorochrome-conjugated monoclonal antibodies directed at specific cell surface antigens and flow cytometry to differentiate lymphocyte subpopulations. Most clinical laboratories add two or more fluorochrome-conjugated monoclonal antibodies to small volumes of whole blood. After sufficient time to allow the antibody to react with the appropriate cell surface antigen, the red blood cells are lysed, the sample is washed, and the cells are evaluated by the flow cytometer. The proper characterization of lymphocytes requires differentiating these cells from the other leukocytes (i.e., monocytes and granulocytes). This process is referred to as **lymphocyte gating** and, if done incorrectly, will invalidate the results of the study.

The data generated from lymphocyte phenotyping should be expressed both as the percentage and absolute number of each cell subpopulation evaluated. In addition, data must be interpreted in the context of appropriate controls, because normal phenotypes vary with age, race, and sex. A simple approach to validate results depends on the axiom "the whole is the sum of its parts" (T cells + B cells + natural killer [NK] cells = 100%). This simple check can be applied to any phenotyping study that reports all three major lymphocyte groups. In normal adults approximately three-fourths of the circulating lymphocytes are T cells with the **ratio of CD4 cells to CD8 cells normally 1.5–2.0 : 1**, the remaining non-T lymphocytes are generally equally divided between B and NK cells.

The most commonly requested flow cytometric test is a CD4 count, used to obtain prognostic data regarding HIV infection and to make decisions regarding therapy. The evaluation of clonal excess, cell lineage, and state of differentiation by flow cytometry is becoming a standard approach in the assessment of leukemia and lymphoma. Additional applications of this methodology include evaluation for absence of cell subpopulations in specific immune deficiencies or increased levels of cell activation in a variety of immunologically mediated diseases. Flow cytometry generally does not provide diagnostic data, but rather supportive information, and in many settings it is used for investigative types of studies.

III. **Functional evaluation of lymphocytes**

A. **B cells**

1. *In vivo* **studies of B cell function**

a. **Quantitative immunoglobulin** levels represent the first-line screening in evaluating B cell function. The most common methods used to evaluate immunoglobulin levels are automated **nephelometry and radial immunodiffusion**. Results must be interpreted with age-matched controls, because there are significant changes with age (see Appendices IV and V) as well as minor differences based on sex and race. It is important to remember that most reference ranges have a 95% confidence interval, meaning that 5% of controls fall outside of these results (i.e., 2.5% are above and 2.5% are below the range).

b. Immunoglobulin G subclass levels are performed to detect more subtle abnormalities in B-cell function. This is clinically important in certain patients with recurrent infections who have normal or modestly decreased total IgG levels but have selective depression of one or more IgG subclasses. IgG subclass testing is moderately expensive and should be reserved for investigating cases with a history of recurrent bacterial infections that are suggestive of an immune disorder in conjunction with a normal or low normal total IgG level. Because the majority of individuals with IgG subclass deficiency are clinically well, identifying a decrease in IgG subclasses still requires **demonstration of functional antibody abnormality** to make the diagnosis of immune deficiency.

c. Functional antibody production evaluates B-cell immunity by determining the *in vivo* antibody response to specific antigens. This approach consists of measuring pre- and postimmunization titers to protein antigen (e.g., tetanus toxoid, diphtheria toxoid) and polysaccharide antigen (e.g., pneumococcal polysaccharide [Pneumovax]). Quantification of antibodies to these antigens is available through selected commercial laboratories and may be available through state health laboratories. These studies help provide definitive evidence for an abnormality in B-cell function and, in the absence of panhypogammaglobulinemia, give critical information before initiating intravenous immunoglobulin therapy. Differentiating normal from abnormal responses to polysaccharide antigens in young children (especially under 2 years of age) remains unclear and should be considered in the context of the clinical circumstance.

2. *In vitro* studies of B-cell function consist of testing B cells for the capacity to undergo proliferation, terminal differentiation, and immunoglobulin secretion following nonspecific (mitogen) or specific (antigen) stimuli in a culture system. These studies, generally performed in investigational laboratories, are reserved for research applications.

B. T cells

1. *In vivo* studies of T-cell function

a. The absolute lymphocyte count gives information in evaluating T-cell function because T cells comprise approximately 75% of the circulating peripheral lymphocytes. A significant decrease in T cells is far more likely to affect the overall lymphocyte count compared with a decrease in the smaller population of B cells or NK cells. It is important to consider the absolute lymphocyte count in the context of an age appropriate reference range.

b. Delayed hypersensitivity skin testing assesses the capacity of T cells to initiate an inflammatory response upon intradermal introduction of a recall antigen that induces a mononuclear cell response to cytokines released by memory T cells. Measurement of erythema and induration at the injection site is done at 48 or 72 hours. Failure to respond can be the result of immune dysfunction or lack of previous exposure to the test antigen. To minimize the latter possibility, a panel of antigens should be used that can include *Candida* antigen, tetanus toxoid, diphtheria toxoid, dermatophyton (*Trichophyton*) antigen, mumps antigen, and purified protein derivative (PPD) (see Chapter 17). Absence of reactivity to a group of recall antigens is compatible with anergy and, in the presence of opportunistic infections, suggests a deficiency in T-cell function.

A recent history of poison ivy or other contact sensitivity (e.g., nickel contained in clothing or jewelry) is additional evidence for functional T cells.

2. *In vitro* studies of T-cell function

a. **Proliferative assays** represent an *in vitro* correlate to delayed-type hypersensitivity testing. T-cell proliferation is essential for a variety of immune functions and is evaluated by assessing DNA synthesis in lymphocytes in culture following one or more stimuli. These stimuli include polyclonal activators (mitogens including phytohemagglutinin [PHA] and concanavalin A [conA]) and antigens (alloantigens or exogenous recall antigens such as tetanus toxoid). At the end of the response period, proliferation is evaluated by quantifying the incorporation of a radioactive-labeled nucleoside (e.g., tritiated thymidine) into newly synthesized DNA. The results are usually expressed as counts per minute (cpm) or disintegrations per minute (dpm) or as a stimulation index (cpm of stimulated cells/cpm of unstimulated cells). Mitogen stimulation activates a significant proportion of normal T cells and can be assessed after 3 days of culture, whereas antigen stimulation is limited to T cells with the specific antigen receptor and is evaluated at 6 or 7 days. As with delayed-type hypersensitivity skin testing, a panel of antigens should be used to ensure prior exposure to the test antigen. When whole blood assays are used for testing lymphocyte proliferation rather than separated mononuclear cells, it is important to consider the absolute lymphocyte count because this can significantly affect the results. Alternative detection methods include flow cytometric measurements of activation antigens, cell cycle, or bromodeoxyuridine (BrDu) incorporation.

Studies of patients with HIV infection have demonstrated that unresponsiveness to recall antigens can be present early when there is a relatively subtle T-cell disorder. Progression of the T-cell defect is associated with loss of T-cell response to alloantigens followed by loss of the response to PHA. The extent of T-cell deficiency may be reflected by the degree of the proliferative defect, with PHA unresponsiveness indicative of a very profound T-cell abnormality.

b. **Cytotoxicity** testing evaluates the capacity of T cells to kill target cells in either major histocompatibility complex (human leukocyte antigen [HLA])-restricted or in non-MHC-restricted assays (see Chapter 16). The assay most commonly is used to test MHC-restricted, α/β + T-cell receptor (TCR), CD8+ T cells that recognize endogenously processed antigens (i.e., viral antigen or alloantigen) in the context of class I MHC molecules (HLA-A, B, or C molecules). CD4+ cytotoxic T cells recognize antigens in the context of class II MHC molecules, whereas γ/δ + TCR T cells typically mediate non-MHC-restricted cytotoxicity.

In standard assays the target cells are labeled with a radioactive probe (^{51}Cr). T-cell lysis of the target cell is assayed by measuring radioactivity released into the cell-free supernatant. In MHC (HLA)-restricted systems, the T cells must have prior exposure to the antigen in order to generate active cytotoxic cells. This type of T-cell response is particularly important for host defense against viruses and other intracellular pathogens. Non-MHC-restricted T-cell cytotoxicity is mediated by a small percentage of the circulating T cells and is very similar to NK cell cytotoxicity, because it does not require prior sensitization (see Natural immunity/natural killer cells on page 452). The *in vitro* cytotoxicity assay system used to test all of these various forms of cytotoxicity utilizes a similar technique. Labeled target cells are mixed with the effector cells at varying effector to target ratios, and the degree of lysis is quantified in comparison to known normal cells. These assays are used primarily in characterizing immune defects.

      c. Soluble products are produced by activated lymphoid cells and can be assessed in the cell-free supernatant following cell stimulation and culture. Assay methods for quantitating these proteins (e.g., cytokines) include commercially available immunoassays and functional assays, which are technically more complicated. The evaluation of cytokine levels *in vivo* is complicated because of the short half-life of most cytokines and the high affinity binding of these proteins to their cell receptors. An alternative method evaluates the presence of cytokines in the cytoplasm of lymphocytes following a short-term *in vitro* activation with mitogen (phorbol myristate acetate and ionomycin) or antigen that is followed by intracellular fluorochrome-labeled antibody staining for specific cytokines and detection by flow cytometry.

C. Natural immunity/natural killer cells

1. **Natural killer cell** cytotoxicity does not require prior sensitization of the effector cells. Susceptible target cells consist of a number of different cell lines, and the assay system is essentially identical to the approach described in Cytotoxicity (see page 451). The NK cell is one of a number of different cell types that mediates a cytotoxic function referred to as **antibody-dependent cellular cytotoxicity** (ADCC). In this process, the cytotoxic effector cells are bound via their IgG Fc receptors to the IgG antibody-coated target cells. This increases the range of susceptible target cells and can be tested in a standard cytotoxicity assay system using antibody-coated targets. The NK cell appears to be important in responding to viral infections, graft rejection, and tumor rejection. Absence of NK cell activity is very rare, although diminished function can be seen in a number of clinical situations, including patients with cancer.

2. **Cytokine-enhanced cytotoxicity** uses the NK cell assay but introduces a preincubation step with specific cytokines, including interferons and interleukin-2. Addition of interferon enhances *in vitro* NK cell cytotoxicity within hours. Preincubation with interleukin-2 for 24 hours or longer increases not only the level of cytotoxicity, but also the range of susceptible target cells to include targets that are not killed in standard NK cell assays (autologous tumor cells). These stimulated cells are referred to as **lymphokine-activated killer (LAK)** cells.

IV. Functional evaluation of phagocytic cells

A. Monocyte/macrophage function

can be evaluated for a number of specific functions, including antigen presentation for T-cell proliferation, ADCC, tumor cell cytotoxicity, chemotaxis, and microbial killing. In addition, cytokine production can be evaluated following monocyte activation. These tests evaluate the monocyte role in antigen processing and presentation, tumor cell cytotoxicity, microbial phagocytosis, cytokine receptor expression, and elaboration of cytokines. The clinical indications for testing monocyte function include deficiency of T-cell function and unusual or atypical infections with opportunistic, intracellular microorganisms.

B. Neutrophil function

can be separated into specific aspects of cell function including chemotaxis, phagocytosis, generation of the oxidative burst, microbial killing, and presence of surface adhesion molecules.

1. **Neutrophil chemotaxis** can be studied by isolating peripheral blood neutrophils and using an apparatus called a **Boyden chamber**. This device is designed with a filter that separates the cells from the chemoattractant (e.g., C5a) or control material. After a predetermined period of time, the filters are removed and examined for the presence of neutrophil migration in response to the chemoattractant. An alternative approach involves evaluating chemotaxis in a soft agar system in response to standard chemoattractants. *In vivo* chemotaxis can be studied with the **Rebuck skin window method**. With this test, the skin is abraded with a scalpel, and a laboratory cover slip is placed over the abraded

areas for 24 hours. The cover slip is then stained and analyzed microscopically. An immune deficiency may be present if there is an abnormality of neutrophils or monocytes displayed either by their absence or their inability to migrate to intracellular sites of antigen within 12 hours. Abnormalities of chemotaxis have been found in the **Chédiak-Higashi syndrome**, the **Pelger-Huët anomaly**, and some patients with the **hyper-IgE syndrome**. Demonstration of a significant decrease in neutrophil response to chemoattractants *in vitro* is usually associated with a diminished inflammatory response *in vivo*.

2. **The oxidative burst** is the process that follows neutrophil activation and phagocytosis and results in increased hexose monophosphate shunt activity, oxygen consumption, hydrogen peroxide production, and superoxide radical formation. Functional testing of this process can be performed using the **nitroblue tetrazolium (NBT) test**, the **dihydrorhodamine 123 (DHR) assay** or the **chemiluminescence assay**. In the NBT test, activation of the neutrophils induces phagocytosis of NBT dye. The oxidative burst, associated with activation and phagocytosis, reduces the NBT dye within the cell and generates blue insoluble crystals of formazan, which can easily be detected by microscopic examination. **Absence of NBT dye reduction is a classic finding in patients with chronic granulomatous disease (CGD)**. A more quantitative test involves the use of an intracellular fluorochrome, DHR, which upon contact with intracellular hydrogen peroxide is oxidized and emits a fluorescent signal that can be detected using a standard flow cytometer. The dye-loaded granulocytes are activated with PMA and evaluated for increased fluorescence within 15 minutes of exposure to the stimulus. The **DHR assay has proven to be extremely accurate in diagnosing patients with CGD and X-linked carriers of CGD**. An alternative test involves evaluation of chemiluminescence, the oxidative burst-dependent generation of light (energy) by activated neutrophils. Addition of ingestible particles (such as zymosan) activates neutrophils and induces phagocytosis, which results in the release of light (energy). The chemiluminescence obtained with patient cells is measured and compared with the response obtained from normal cells. The results from this method usually parallel the findings of the NBT test and the DHR assay.

3. **Microbial killing assays** mix neutrophils with opsonins and bacteria *in vitro* to evaluate actual killing of specific microorganisms. Different types of microorganisms can be used in the evaluation of killing. Cells from patients with CGD demonstrate markedly diminished killing of *Staphylococcus aureus* in this assay. The accuracy of this test depends on well-defined controls and an experienced laboratory.

4. **Adhesion molecule assessment** is directed at identification of three specific cell surface receptors on neutrophils: leukocyte function-associated antigen 1 (LFA-1), Mac-1, and p150,95. These can be identified by flow cytometry using monoclonal antibodies to the individual α chains (CD11a, CD11b, CD11c) and to the common β chain (CD18) that form the three heterodimeric adhesion molecules. Patients with leukocyte adhesion defects (LAD) have a defect in CD18 that manifests as decreased or absent expression of these surface antigens in both resting and activated neutrophils. Additional features in this disorder include the presence of peripheral neutrophilia and reduction of cell adherence, chemotaxis, and phagocytosis. Because the neutrophils of patients with LAD fail to move to the site of inflammation and are functionally deficient, the clinical features include recurrent infections, delayed wound healing, and absence of pus at infection sites.

V. **The complement system** is comprised of circulating glycoproteins that are activated in a cascade-like fashion. There are three different mechanisms of complement activation: the classical, the alternative, and the lectin pathway.

The complement system is a part of the host defense through its lytic, chemotactic, and opsonic activity, its effects on catabolism of circulating immune complexes, and its role in immunoregulation.

A. **Complement activity** of the classical pathway can be evaluated with the total hemolytic complement (CH_{50}) assay. In this test, various dilutions of patient or control sera are added to sheep red blood cells that are bound (sensitized) by anti-red cell antibody (hemolysin). The serum provides a source of complement, and the degree of red cell lysis is plotted on a standard curve. CH_{50} results are reported as the inverse of the serum dilution that produces 50% red cell lysis. Currently, there are modifications of the traditional CH_{50} tube test that employ microtiter plates or immunoassays that detect unique components derived during complement activation to simplify the procedure. The biological activity of complement components is labile, and **improper handling or storage of a serum sample can result in diminished complement activity**.

The CH_{50} is a very effective means of screening for the absence of a complement component and is particularly useful in diagnosing terminal component defects associated with recurrent neisserial infections. It is also frequently used to evaluate for complement activation, although it is less sensitive in this capacity. This approach has been clinically useful in following patients with SLE and nephritis. Assaying for the presence of complement cleavage proteins is theoretically the optimal approach to test for complement activation, and studies are currently underway to explore this possibility.

Assessment of the **alternative complement pathway** and the lectin pathway are usually not performed in clinical laboratories because there are few clinical situations where these data are required.

B. **Complement component testing** is usually included in the laboratory evaluation of immune-mediated inflammatory diseases and when there is a suspected genetic deficiency of one of the complement components.

   1. **Immunoassays** for complement components are technically the simplest means of assessing their concentration, and usually involve radial immunodiffusion, immunoassay, or nephelometric testing. Most clinical laboratories use these methods to assess complement components. This approach is fully satisfactory except in conditions that have a functionally deficient complement component that is antigenically indistinguishable from a normal complement component in the immunoassay. For example, in approximately 15% of patients with **hereditary angioedema**, the immunoassay for C1-esterase inhibitor yields normal levels of this protein because the abnormal protein is antigenically indistinguishable from the normal protein, yet the functional assay shows decreased or absent activity. In these uncommon patients, the functional assay (but not the immunoassay) correlates with the clinical findings.

   2. **Functional assays** evaluate the actual activity of a complement component in an unknown sample. The indicator system is a CH_{50} assay that is constructed to contain all but one complement component. The unknown sample is the putative source of this component, and the degree of hemolysis is compared with that from a known normal. These assays are difficult and are generally performed only in specialized laboratories. The main use of this testing is to identify the actual component defect in an individual with clinical disease and a depressed CH_{50}. Additional functional testing can be directed toward the various complement regulatory proteins, including the C1-esterase inhibitor.

C. **Immune complex assays** consist of a number of different techniques for determining the concentration of nonspecific antigen–antibody immune complexes in serum. Certain methods detect (bind) activated C3 and its cleavage products that are fixed to the antigen–antibody complex. In the

Raji cell assay, immune complexes are immobilized with a cell line that has receptors for C3bi and C3d. In the **anti-C3 assay**, antibodies directed toward immune complexes fix C3, and in the **bovine conglutinin assay**, a bovine protein (conglutinin) binds immune complex-fixed C3. The next step involves addition of a labeled antibody to human immunoglobulin as the detection step for the immune complexes. An alternative approach is the **C1q binding assay** that uses the complement component, C1q, which is radio-labeled or immobilized on a solid phase to bind the immune complexes and allow for their detection. Recently, a solid-phase immunoassay system has been developed that uses an antibody to C3 cleavage products to capture immune complexes that have the derivatives of C3. Detection of the complexes is dependent on labeled antiimmunoglobulin antibodies. More than one method is recommended for reliable detection of circulating immune complexes, although the clinical significance and utility of the results have not been clearly identified.

VI. *In vitro* allergy testing

A. **Immunoglobulin E quantification** has been a challenge because of the low levels of this immunoglobulin isotype compared with IgG, IgA, and IgM (see Appendix IV and V). There is an **age-dependent variation in the normal levels of IgE** (see Appendix IV). Currently, the most common method for IgE detection involves a solid-phase immobilized antibody that binds IgE contained in a test sample. This step is followed by the addition of a labeled second antibody to IgE, allowing for the quantitation of IgE in the sample (see Immunoassays on page 444). The World Health Organization standard for IgE was developed in an attempt to standardize the various assays being used to quantify levels.

The measurement of total IgE is not a useful screen for allergy because there is significant overlap between allergic and nonallergic subjects. It does appear that infants with elevated IgE levels have increased risk for allergies, and adults with very low IgE levels (less than 50 ng per mL) are unlikely to have allergies. **Serial IgE levels are useful in assessing response to therapy in allergic bronchopulmonary aspergillosis.** Marked elevation in IgE levels is seen in patients with the Wiskott-Aldrich syndrome and hyper-IgE syndrome as well as in some patients with parasitic infections and atopic dermatitis.

B. **Allergen-specific immunoglobulin E** assessment is usually performed with epicutaneous and (if necessary) intradermal skin tests. *In vitro* **testing for allergen-specific IgE** is usually reserved for situations that include extraordinary sensitivity to allergen, abnormal skin conditions, and required medication that interferes with skin test results. This approach may also prove to be useful in the assessment of possible food allergies. The standard *in vitro* test uses specific allergen attached to a solid-phase support (allergosorbent) as the substrate. Test serum is added to this substrate, which allows specific antibody to bind. Unbound antibody is removed, labeled anti-IgE antibody is added, and the amount of bound label is measured as a reflection of the allergen-specific IgE concentration. This test is called a **radioallergosorbent test (RAST)** when the anti-IgE antibody is labeled with a radionuclide. Alternatively, an enzyme or fluorochrome can be used to label the anti-IgE antibody in an allergosorbent test for allergen-specific IgE, and this is the most common approach in the clinical laboratory. The application of *in vitro* testing for allergen specific IgE is useful in certain clinical situations, with recent data suggesting particular utility in children with food allergies as well as in research applications.

Basophil histamine release assay is another approach to assess allergen-specific IgE. This test measures IgE-mediated histamine release *in vitro*, and theoretically is more representative of an allergic reaction. The indicator system consists of allergen-sensitized whole blood or separated leukocytes which contain basophils. Test serum is added to the cell source, and specific IgE cross-links the allergen bound to the basophil, inducing mediator release. Histamine is measured in the supernatant and is compared with the total basophil histamine content. This test can be used to examine the effect of drugs and other substances on the allergic response. This test is difficult to perform, and its clinical utility has not been established.

Selected Readings

Buckley RH. Primary immunodeficiency diseases due to defects in lymphocytes. *N Engl J Med* 2000;343:1313–1324.

Fleisher TA, Tomar R H. Introduction to diagnostic immunology. *JAMA* 1997;278: 1823–1834.

Frank MM. Complement deficiencies. *Pediatr Clin North Am* 2000;47:1339–1354.

Hamilton RG. Assessment of human allergic disease. In Rich RR, Fleisher TA, Schwartz BD, et al., eds. *Clinical immunology: principles and practice,* 2nd Edition. London: Mosby, 2001; 124.1–124.14.

Houston D. Diagnostic laboratory immunology. *Immunol Allergy Clin North Am* 1994;14:199–481.

Lekstrom-Himes JA, Gallin JI. Immunodeficiency diseases caused by defects in phago-cytes. *N Engl J Med* 2000;343:1703–1714.

Ownby DR. Allergy testing, in vivo versus in vitro. *Pediatr Clin North Am* 1988;55: 995–1009.

Rose NR, et al., eds. *Manual of clinical laboratory immunology*, 5th ed. Washington DC: American Society for Microbiology, 1996.

Shearer WT, Buckley RH, et al. Practice parameters for the diagnosis and management of immunodeficiency. *Ann Allergy Asthma Immunol* 1996;76:280–294.

Woroniecka M, Ballow M. Office evaluation of children with recurrent infection. *Pediatr Clinic North Am* 2000;47:1211–1224.

20. IMMUNIZATION AND IMMUNOPROPHYLAXIS

Edina Moylett and William T. Shearer

The practice of immunization has greatly impacted childhood health in the 20th century. Immunoprophylaxis can be defined as the development of protection against an infectious agent by increasing the body's immune response. This may be accomplished via active immunization, in which an antigen is administered to mimic natural infection, or passively, via the administration of preformed antibody.

I. **Active immunization**
   A. **Vaccines.** A number of vaccines are currently licensed for use in the United States (Table 20.1). The principal distinction between vaccines is that some are live, whereas others are inactivated. Each type has specific advantages and disadvantages (Table 20.2).
      1. An **attenuated live vaccine** consists of an entire or partial organism (virus or bacteria) which is subjected to a process of attenuation. Attenuation reduces the viability of the organism as an infectious agent, but still allows it to generate an effective immune response, and often results in lifelong immunity. Attenuated live vaccines are believed to induce an immunologic response more similar to that resulting from natural infection than do killed vaccines.
      2. **Killed vaccines** (bacteria, viruses, or *Rickettsia*) are composed of killed microorganisms (e.g., cholera and pertussis), which result in an initial large antigen load followed by a plateau. Because the immune response is inferior to that stimulated by live vaccines, these agents usually require repeat administration.
      3. **Subunit vaccines** are comprised of a constituent of the whole organism, such as a bacterial capsular component (e.g., *Streptococcus pneumoniae*) or a viral protein (e.g., hepatitis B surface antigen). The advantage of subunit vaccines is their safe administration to young children, in whom live vaccines may be either too virulent or over-attenuated, resulting in diminished immunogenicity.
      4. **Toxoid vaccines** are rendered nontoxic but retain the ability to stimulate production of antibody.
      5. **Conjugate vaccines.** Pure polysaccharide vaccines are poorly immunogenic in children less than 2 years of age. Covalent linkage of the polysaccharide to a carrier protein enhances the immune response.
   B. **Novel approaches to immunization**
      1. **Recombinant vaccines.** Recombinant vector vaccines are produced when one or more genes encoding for critical determinants of immunity from pathogenic microorganisms are inserted into a vector. Candidate vectors include both viruses (e.g., poxviruses vaccinia, canarypox, adenovirus) and bacteria (e.g., *Salmonella* or bacillus Calmette-Guérin [BCG]). Potential human immunodeficiency virus (HIV) recombinant vaccine is an example of a recombinant vaccine under development. Other novel approaches include microencapsulation of critical antigens in polymers, which results in sustained or intermittent release of the antigens. This approach mimics the effects of multiple injections of an antigen over a several-month period.
      2. **DNA vaccines** utilize nucleic acids that encode for critical antigens, thereby eliminating the risks associated with live viral vaccine. Safety issues applicable to DNA or nucleic acid vaccines include the formation of anti-DNA antibodies, unexpected consequences of the persistent expression of foreign material, and the potential for a transformation

(text continues on page 467)

Table 20.1. Currently licensed vaccines in the United States

Vaccine	Type	Indication	Efficacy[a]	Dosing	Route	Major adverse effects
Adenovirus Anthrax	Live virus Inactivated bacteria	Available only to U.S. armed forces U.S. military active and reserve personnel; any person in contact with contaminated materials or environment	90% cutaneous infection	0.5 mL at 0, 2, and 4 weeks and again at 6, 12, 18 mo followed by annual booster	p.o. s.c.	
BCG	Live bacteria	To be considered for infants with prolonged exposure to TB, especially if MDR, in addition HCW, where MDR TB is a problem	80% CNS/ miliary TB 50% pulmonary TB	Single dose	i.d. or s.c.	Regional adenitis, disseminated BCG infection, osteitis due to the BCG organism
Cholera	Inactivated bacteria	50% efficacy, only administered to satisfy travel requirements for certain countries	50%	Two doses 1 week, apart, 6 monthly boosters to maintain immunity	s.c., i.m. or i.d.	
Diphtheria–tetanus (dT, DT)	Toxoids	DT (where pertussis-containing vaccine is contraindicated) is indicated for infants and young children as part of the primary series; dT is indicated for children > 7 yr and adults	90%	DT, beginning at 8 weeks, 4–8 week intervals for three doses; a fourth dose 6–12 mo after the third dose, a fifth dose at 4–6 yr, dT booster at 11–12 yr and 10-yearly thereafter	i.m.	

Vaccine	Type	Indications	Efficacy	Schedule	Route	Adverse effects
DTP DTaP	Toxoid and inactivated bacterial component	Primary immunization series of infants and children	90%	6 weeks to 7 yr of age, 4–8 week intervals for three doses; a fourth dose 6–12 months after the third dose, a fifth dose at 4–6 yr; 7 yr or older, dT at 4–8 week intervals with a third dose at 6–12 mo	i.m.	Bacterial or sterile abscesses at the injection site, seizures, hypotonic–hyporesponsive states, fever > 104.8°F, prolonged crying, anaphylaxis; all of the above are less frequent following DTaP than DTP
Hepatitis A	Inactivated viral antigen	Any person 2 yr or older at increased risk of hepatitis A infection, residents of or travelers to endemic areas, IVDUs, male homosexuals, primate handlers, daycare staff, sewer workers, regular recipients of blood or blood products; patients with chronic underlying liver disease	94%–100%	Single dose followed by 6–12 monthly booster for prolonged immunization; recommended 2 weeks prior to travel	i.m.	
Hepatitis B Energix-B Recombivax HB	Inactivated viral antigen	Primary immunization series; adolescents not previously vaccinated; adults	95% infants and children 75%–90% adults	Infants, Energix-B, (10 µg) at 0, 1, 2, and 12 mo or Recombivax HB	i.m.	Anaphylaxis rarely, (1 in 600,000 patients)

continued

Table 20.1. *Continued*

Vaccine	Type	Indication	Efficacy[a]	Dosing	Route	Major adverse effects
		at increased risk of infection, residents and staff of institutions for developmentally disabled, immigrants from areas of high HBV endemnicity, hemodialysis patients, IVDUs, homosexual males, household contacts of HBV carriers, blood product recipients, Alaskan natives and Pacific Islanders, male prisoners, HCWs with frequent blood contact		(5 μg) at 2, 4, and 12–15 mo; adolescents (11–19 yr), two doses separated by 4 weeks, a third dose 4–6 mo later or two 10 μg doses of Recombivax HB separated by 4–6 mo; adults (> 20 yr), 10μg Recombivax HB or 20 μg Energix-B, two doses separated by 4 weeks, a third dose 4–6 mo later		
Haemophilus influenzae type b PRP-D (Prohibit) HbOC (HibTITER) PRP-T (ActHIB or OmniHIB) PRP-OMP (PedvaxHIB)	Polysaccharide–protein conjugate	Primary immunization series (see Table 1). PRP-D (Prohibit) is not recommended <18 mo of age; the remaining three licensed conjugate vaccines are all interchangeable	93%–100%	See Table 3	i.m.	

Vaccine	Type	Efficacy	Indications	Schedule	Route	Adverse effects
Influenza	Whole virus, disrupted, or split virus	60%–80% 20%–30% in nursing home setting	All persons 50 yr of age and older; other at risk individuals, residents of long-term care facilities, pregnant women, patients 6 mo to 18 yr on chronic aspirin therapy, persons with chronic illness, e.g., cardiopulmonary, renal, metabolic, hemoglobinopathies, immunosuppression	Annually, beginning in September in temperate regions; 6–35 mo (0.2 mL) one or two* doses; 3–8 yr (0.5 mL) one or two* doses; 9–12 yr (0.5 mL) one dose*; >12 yr (0.5 mL) one dose *one dose only if the child received vaccine during a prior season	i.m.	Lower febrile potential associated with split-product vaccines; anaphylaxis to egg protein
Japanese encephalitis	Inactivated virus	91%	Expatriates living in Asia, travelers to endemic areas for >30 d especially if activity is in rural areas; not indicated for routine visitors to Asia	Primary series is three doses, 1 mL each, on days 0, 7, and 30 (the third dose may be administered at 14 days); for children 1–3 yr 0.5 mL, no data on children <12 mo	s.c.	Vaccine-associated hypersensitivity, 0.3% (urticaria, angioedema)
Lyme disease	Inactivated protein	58%–86%	Individuals of 15–70 yr of age, who reside, work, or recreate in geographic areas of high or moderate risk; those who visit areas of high risk during peak Lyme disease transmission	Primary series is three doses, 0, 1, and 12 mo	i.m.	

continued

Table 20.1. *Continued*

Vaccine	Type	Indication	Efficacy[a]	Dosing	Route	Major adverse effects
Measles	Live virus (Edmonston-Enders strain)	Primary immunization series (as MMR); all persons born after 1957 should have documentation of at least one dose of MMR or evidence of measles immunity; adults at increased risk of infection, college students, HCWs, international travelers	95%	First dose on or after 12 mo, second dose at 4–6 yr old; 11–12 yr health visit if no documentation of previous two doses	s.c.	
Meningococcal (serotypes A, C, Y, and W-135)	Polysaccharide	Individuals >2 yr old with functional or anatomic asplenia, C5–C8 or properdin deficiency; travelers to areas with endemic vaccine-preventable disease, and college students; all U.S. military recruits receive the vaccine	90%	Single 0.5 mL dose	s.c.	

MMR	Live virus	As for measles	98%	As for measles	s.c.	Thrombocytopenia, (One case per 30,000 to 40,000 vaccines)
Mumps	Live virus	As for measles	90%–97%	As for measles	s.c.	
Plaque	Inactivated bacteria	Persons whose occupation places them at increased risk of infection, travelers to endemic areas		Primary series is three doses, the second and third doses are given 1–3 and 5–6 mo respectively, after the first; three boosters at 6-monthly intervals for ongoing exposure; additional boosters at 1–2 yearly intervals	i.m.	
Pneumococcal (23-valent) Pneumovax	Polysaccharide	Individuals > 2 yr old with sickle cell disease, functional or anatomic asplenia, nephrotic syndrome or chronic renal failure, immunosuppression, HIV infection, CSF leaks, chronic cardiorespiratory disease, diabetes mellitus, chronic liver disease; Alaskan natives, certain Native Americans; persons >65 yr	60%–70% invasive disease	Single 0.5 mL dose; routine reimmunization of immunocompetent persons is not recommended; reimmunization of persons at highest risk of severe disease 5 yr or more after the first dose	i.m.	

continued

Table 20.1. *Continued*

Vaccine	Type	Indication	Efficacy[a]	Dosing	Route	Major adverse effects
Pneumococcal (serotypes 4, 6B, 9V, 14, 19F and 23F) Prevnar	Polysaccharide–protein conjugate	Primary immunization series for all children < 24 mo; children 24–59 mo at high risk for invasive pneumococcal infection as outlined for polysaccharide vaccine; adult patients or older children at risk for invasive pneumococcal disease	88% bacteremia, 82% meningitis, 71% otitis media	See Table 20.5	i.m.	
Poliovirus	Inactivated virus (IPV) Live virus (trivalent OPV)	Primary immunization series with IPV exclusively (since 2000 in U.S.); OPV to be considered for unvaccinated children traveling to polio-endemic area in <4 weeks; consider vaccination of some adults, travelers to endemic areas, select lab workers and HCWs	IPV 99% OPV 95%	IPV at 2, 4, and 6–18 mo, fourth dose at school entry if third dose before fourth birthday; an all IPV schedule is preferable, IPV may follow prior OPV immunization	IPV s.c. OPV p.o.	VAPP following OPV, increased risk following the first dose, in persons >18 yr of age, and immunodeficient patients, especially humoral immunodeficiency

Vaccine	Type	Indications	Efficacy	Dosage	Route	Adverse reactions
Rabies (human diploid cell, vaccine, HDCV rabies vaccine adsorbed, purified chick embryo cell)	Inactivated virus	Postexposure prophylaxis; preexposure prophylaxis with high-risk rabies exposure such as veterinarians, certain lab workers, visitors to countries with high incidence of dog rabies	100%	Postexposure: 1 mL on day 1 postexposure and days 3, 7, 14, and 28; preexposure: 1 mL on days 0, 7, and 21 or 28	i.m. i.d. as alternative for HDCV	Immune-complex-like reactions in persons receiving booster doses of HDCV
Rubella	Live virus	Primary immunization >12 mo; susceptible adolescents and adults without documented evidence of rubella immunity; nonpregnant women of child-bearing age	95%	Two doses as combination MMR at least 4 weeks apart; all older children and susceptible adults should receive one dose	s.c.	Rubella vaccine, arthropathy, acute joint symptoms in 25% of adult women, frank arthritis in 10%
Tetanus	Toxoid	Primary immunization of all children; indicated for all persons residing in the U.S.; usually given in combination with diphtheria; indicated for tetanus-prone wounds if immunization status unknown or > 10 yr since last booster	95%	<12 mo, DTaP/DTP/ DT 2, 4, and 6 mo, 12–15 mo and at school entry; all other persons DT/dT two doses 4–8 weeks apart, third dose 6–12 mo later; 10-yearly dT boosters	i.m.	Arthus-like reaction with multiple doses of toxoid, rarely brachial plexus neuropathy, rarely GBS
Typhoid	Inactivated bacteria	Travelers to endemic areas, prolonged exposure to carriers, certain lab workers	50%–80%	Two doses ≥4 weeks apart, boosters every 3 yr as per risk	s.c.	

continued

Table 20.1. *Continued*

Vaccine	Type	Indication	Efficacy[a]	Dosing	Route	Major adverse effects
	Capsular polysaccharide (ViCPS)	Ty21a not recommended <6 yr; ViCPS not recommended <2 yr, phenol-inactivated bacteria >6 mo		Single dose, boosters every 2 yr as per risk	s.c. i.d./boosters	
	Live bacteria (Ty21a)			Four doses on alternate days, repeat course every 5 yr as per risk	p.o.	
Varicella	Live virus	Primary immunization of all children; susceptible adults such as workers in institutions where transmission increased, schools, prisons and daycare, international travelers, nonpregnant females of child-bearing age	86% (any varicella) 100% (severe disease)	Single dose at 12–18 mo; >13 yr old, two doses 4–8 weeks apart	s.c.	
Yellow fever	Live virus	Travelers to yellow-fever endemic areas, not recommended <4 mo of age	High	Single dose, 10-yearly boosters	s.c.	Rarely, encephalitis encephalopathy

[a] Percentage expressed applies to a completed series.

p.o., oral; s.c., subcutaneous; i.d., intradermal; i.m., intramuscular; TB, tuberculosis; MDR, multidrug-resistant; HCW, healthcare worker; IVDU, intravenous drug user; CSF, cerebrospinal fluid; BCG, bacilli-Calmette-Guérin; CNS, central nervous system; HBV, hepatitis B virus; MMR, measles, mumps, rubella; HDCV, human diploid cell rabies vaccine; VAPP, viral associated paralytic polio; GBS, Guillain Barré syndrome.

Table 20.2. Advantages and disadvantages of live versus inactivated vaccines

Live: advantages
Prolonged protection following single vaccine
Stimulates multiple components of the immune system including T-cell response
and mucosal-mediated IgA
Usually involves herd immunity (i.e., spread to nonvaccinees)

Live: disadvantages
May cause illness in undiagnosed immunocompromised individuals
May revert to virulence by mutation or interserotypic recombination
Cannot vaccinate in early infancy owing to interference by maternal antibody
Requires storage and transportation at low temperature (4°C) to retain potency

Inactivated: advantages
Safe to administer without risk of reversion to virulence
Easy to produce and store
May be administered in early infancy without interference by preexisting antibody

Inactivated: disadvantages
Requires repeat administration to maintain protection
Poor induction of cellular and mucosal immunity
May occasionally potentiate disease due to imbalanced immune response induction

IgA, immunoglobulin A.

event. Examples of microorganisms for which DNA vaccines are under
research include influenza virus, HIV, and *Herpes simplex* virus.

C. **Constituents of immunizing agents**

1. **Adjuvants.** An adjuvant is a substance that, when combined with inactivated microorganisms or their products (e.g., toxoids), aids in boosting the immune response. Adjuvants function to boost immunity in
several ways: (i) by producing an antigen depot that is slowly released
over time; (ii) by recruitment of cells involved in antigen presentation;
and (iii) by stimulating the production of cytokines or costimulatory
molecules important for the immune response. The only licensed adjuvant in the United States at this time is the weak adjuvant aluminum
hydroxide.

2. **Suspending fluid.** Sterile water or normal saline serve as suspending
fluids for vaccines. However, during the attenuation process this fluid
may contain small amounts of protein derived from the medium or biologic system in which the immunizing agent is produced (e.g., serum
proteins, egg antigens, cell-culture derived antigens).

3. **Preservatives, antibiotics, and stabilizers.** These components
serve to ensure that vaccines remain stable and sterile prior to use.
Thimerosal (mercurial) is the most frequently used preservative that
inhibits bacterial growth in virus vaccines. Because of concerns regarding pediatric mercury exposure, thimerosal-free vaccines are now in
production. Allergic reactions may occur if the recipient is sensitive to
any of these additives.

D. **Vaccine administration**

1. **Combination vaccines.** To improve upon vaccine uptake, combination vaccines are available that have been demonstrated to be at least
as immunogenic with similar reactogenicity to the individual vaccine
components. A number of vaccine combinations have been proven to be
efficacious and safe, including diphtheria, tetanus, and acellular pertussis (DTaP); diphtheria, tetanus, and whole cell pertussis (DTwP);
DTwP and *Haemophilus influenzae* type b (Hib) vaccine (DTwP-Hib);
Hib and hepatitis B (Hep B) vaccine (Hib-Hep B); measles, mumps, and
rubella (MMR); and trivalent inactivated vaccine (IPV). Three different

Hib vaccines are currently licensed for primary immunization use in the United States, which consist of the Hib capsular polysaccharide (polyribosylribotol phosphate [PRP]) conjugated to a carrier protein. Because the immune response may differ depending on the vaccine employed, each Hib vaccine has its own primary vaccination schedule (Table 20.3). In addition, because the immune response to the Hib component of DTaP-Hib or diphtheria, tetanus, and pertussis (DTP)-Hib combination is lower in infants, Hib alone should be administered for the primary immunization series at 2, 4, and 6 months.

2. **Interchangeability.** Vaccines produced by different companies may differ in their components and immune response. Vaccines that can be used interchangeably according to their licensed indication during a vaccine series include diphtheria and tetanus toxoids, live and inactivated polio vaccines, hepatitis A vaccines, hepatitis B vaccines, and rabies vaccines. Any of the licensed Hib conjugate vaccines may be used interchangeably for primary as well as booster immunization series. No data exist for the interchangeability of the different DTaP products; therefore, it is preferable to use the same product during the primary vaccination series. In cases for which the history is unknown or the previously administered vaccine is unavailable, it is deemed safe to administer any of the available DTaP products.

3. **Simultaneous vaccine administration.** The majority of vaccines available for primary childhood immunization can safely be administered together (DTaP, IPV, MMR, varicella, hepatitis B, and Hib). Oral polio vaccine (OPV) (which is no longer administered as part of the primary schedule in the United States) should not be coadministered with cholera or yellow fever vaccines. Similarly, cholera and yellow fever vaccine administration should be separated by at least 3 weeks.

4. **Active immunization with immune globulin administration.** Coadministration of immunoglobulin (Ig) preparations with inactivated vaccines or toxoids does not impair the immune response to the vaccine and is indicated for hepatitis B, tetanus, and rabies postexposure prophylaxis. In contrast, Ig administration does impair the immune response to certain live viral vaccines. It is recommended that if Ig must be administered within 14 days of receipt of measles, mumps, or varicella vaccine, the patient should be tested for seroconversion or revaccinated. No contraindications exist concerning Ig administration and yellow fever or cholera vaccines.

5. **Routes of administration**
   a. **Intramuscular** (i.m.) vaccines should be administered into the anterolateral thigh area of children less than 1 year; in older children the deltoid muscle is usually large enough. The upper, outer aspect of the thigh should not be used for active immunization because of uncertain extent of absorption. A 22- to 25-gauge needle is appropriate for most i.m. vaccines.
   b. **Subcutaneous** (s.c.) vaccines can be administered in the anterolateral aspect of the thigh or upper arm by inserting the needle into a fold of skin. A 23- or 25-gauge needle, $\frac{5}{8}$- to $\frac{3}{4}$-inch long is recommended.
   c. **Intradermal** vaccines should be administered on the volar aspect of the forearm. Owing to the limited amount of antigenic material administered, it is essential that the correct technique be maintained, with elevation of a wheal following immunization.

E. **Immunization recommendations**
   1. **Children.** Recommendations for childhood immunization schedules are proposed and updated annually by the American Academy of Pediatrics (AAP), Committee on Infectious Diseases (Table 20.4). If an immunization has been missed during a primary series, the patient should

(*text continues on page 472*)

Table 20.3. Recommended regimens for routine *Haemophilus influenzae* type b immunization[a,b]

Age at immunization	Vaccine product	Carrier protein	Total no. of doses	Recommended regimen
2–6 mo	HbOC	CRM$_{197}$ (a nontoxic mutant diphtheria toxin)	Four	Three doses at 2-mo intervals initially, fourth dose at 12–15 mo of age
2–6 mo	PRP-T PRP-OMP	Tetanus toxoid OMP (an outer membrane protein of *Neisseria meningitidis*)	Three	Two doses at 2-mo interval initially, same vaccine recommended for dose one and two, third dose 12–15 mo of age

[a] PRP-D is not recommended for use in children <12 mo.
[b] In Native American and Alaskan Native children, because of their increased risk for disease in early infancy, PRP-OMP is recommended for the first dose in a series because of the substantial antibody response after one dose.
From recommendations of the American Academy of Pediatrics (AAP) and Advisory Committee on Immunization Practices (ACIP), with permission. (See *Morb Mortal Wkly Rep* 1994; 43:1–38.)

Table 20.4. Recommended childhood immunization schedule, United States, January–December 2001[a,b]

Vaccine ▼	Birth	1 mo	2 mo	4 mo	6 mo	12 mo	15 mo	18 mo	24 mo	4–6 yr	11–12 yr	14–18 yrs
Hepatitis B[c]		Hep B #1										
			Hep B #2			Hep B #3					Hep B[c]	
Diphtheria, tetanus, pertussis[d]			DTaP	DTaP	DTaP		DTaP[d]			DTaP	Td	
Haemophilus influenzae type b[e]			Hib	Hib	Hib	Hib						
Inactivated polio[f]			IPV	IPV	IPV[f]					IPV[f]		
Pneumococcal conjugate[g]			PCV	PCV	PCV	PCV						
Measles, mumps, rubella[h]						MMR				MMR[h]	MMR[h]	
Varicella[i]							Var				Var[i]	
Hepatitis A[j]									Hep A-in selected areas[j]			

[a] Vaccines are listed under routinely recommended ages. Bars indicate range of recommended ages. Any dose not given at the recommended age should be given as a "catch-up" immunization at any subsequent visit when indicated and feasible. Ovals indicate vaccines to be given if previously recommended doses were missed or given earlier than the recommended minimum age.

[b] This schedule indicates the recommended ages for routine administration of currently licensed childhood vaccines, as of 11/1/00, for children through 18 yr of age. Additional vaccines may be licensed and recommended during the year. Licensed combination vaccines may be used whenever any components of the combination are indicated and its other components are not contraindicated. Providers should consult the manufacturers' package inserts for detailed recommendations.

[c] Infants born to HBsAg-negative mothers should receive the first dose of hepatitis B (Hep B) vaccine by age 2 mo. The second dose should be at least 1 mo after the first dose. The third dose should be administered at least 4 mo after the first dose and at least 2 mo after the second dose, but not before 6 mo of age for infants. Infants born to HBsAg-positive mothers should receive hepatitis B vaccine and 0.5 mL hepatitis B immune globulin (HBIG) within 12 h of birth at separate sites. The second dose is recommended at 1–2 mo of age and the third dose at 6 mo of age.

Infants born to mothers whose HBsAg status is unknown should receive hepatitis B vaccine within 12 h of birth. Maternal blood should be drawn at the time of delivery to determine the mother's HBsAg status; if the HBsAg test is positive, the infant should receive HBIG as soon as possible (no later than 1 week of age).

All children and adolescents who have not been immunized against hepatitis B should begin the series during any visit. Special efforts should be made to immunize children who were born in or whose parents were born in areas of the world with moderate or high endemicity of hepatitis B virus infection.

[d] The fourth dose of DTaP (diphtheria and tetanus toxoids and acellular pertussis vaccine) may be administered as early as 12 mo of age, provided 6 mo have elapsed since the third dose and the child is unlikely to return at age 15–18 mo. Td (tetanus and diphtheria toxoids) is recommended at 11–12 yr of age if at least 5 yr have elapsed since the last dose of DTP, DTaP, or DT. Subsequent routine Td boosters are recommended every 10 yr.

[e] Three Haemophilus influenzae type b (Hib) conjugate vaccines are licensed for infant use. If PRP-OMP (PedvaxHIB or ComVax [Merck]) is administered at 2 and 4 mo of age, a dose at 6 mo is not required. Because clinical studies in infants have demonstrated that using some combination products may induce a lower immune response to the Hib vaccine component, DTaP/Hib combination products should not be used for primary immunization in infants at 2, 4, or 6 mo of age, unless FDA-approved for these ages.

[f] An all-IPV schedule is recommended for routine childhood polio vaccination in the United States. All children should receive four doses of IPV at 2 mo, 4 mo, 6–18 mo, and 4–6 yr of age. Oral polio vaccine (OPV) should be used only in selected circumstances. [See Morb Mortal Wkly Rep 2000;49:1–22.]

[g] The heptavalent conjugate pneumococcal vaccine (PCV) is recommended for all children 2–23 mo of age. It also is recommended for certain children 24–59 mo of age. [See Morb Mortal Wkly Rep 2000;49:1–35.]

[h] The second dose of measles, mumps, and rubella (MMR) vaccine is recommended routinely at 4–6 yr of age but may be administered during any visit, provided at least 4 weeks have elapsed since receipt of the first dose and that both doses are administered beginning at or after 12 mo of age. Those who have not previously received the second dose should complete the schedule by the 11–12 yr old visit.

[i] Varicella (Var) vaccine is recommended at any visit on or after the first birthday for susceptible children, i.e., those who lack a reliable history of chickenpox (as judged by a health care provider) and who have not been immunized. Susceptible persons 13 yr of age or older should receive two doses, given at least 4 weeks apart.

[j] Hepatitis A (Hep A) is recommended for use in selected states and/or regions, and for certain high risk groups; consult your local public health authority. [See Morb Mortal Wkly Rep 1999;48:1–37.]

Approved by the Advisory Committee on Immunization Practices (ACIP), the American Academy of Pediatrics (AAP), and the American Academy of Family Physicians (AAFP), with permission.

Hep, hepatitis; DTaP, diphtheria, tetanus, pertussis vaccine; Td, tetanus, diphtheria toxoid; Hib, Haemophilus influenzae type B vaccine; IPV, inactivated poliomyelitis vaccine; PCV, pneumococcal conjugate vaccine; MMR, measles, mumps, rubella vaccine; Var, varicella; HBsAG, hepatitis B surface antigen; DTP, diphtheria, tetanus, pertussis vaccine; FDA, U.S. Food and Drug Administration.

receive the missed dose as soon as possible and complete the recommended number of doses in the series according to schedule. Children without immunization records should be immunized as though disease-susceptible, because there is no evidence suggesting that administering MMR, Hib, varicella, Hep B, or poliovirus vaccine to a previously immunized patient is harmful. If the patient is older than 7 years, D tetanus immunization should consist of adult-type diphtheria and tetanus toxoids, dT (less diphtheria toxoid than contained in dT as used for infants and younger children).

2. **Adolescents.** The 11- to 18-year-old well child care visit is an opportunity to vaccinate with (i) tetanus, diphtheria toxoid, adult type (dT) booster for children who received their primary series and the last tetanus, diphtheria toxoid vaccine was given at age 5 years, (ii) second MMR if not received, (iii) varicella vaccine to susceptible patients, (iv) three-dose Hep B series if not received, and (v) influenza virus vaccine, pneumococcal vaccine, meningococcal vaccine (college students living in dormitories), and hepatitis A, if indicated.

3. **Adults.** All adults should be vaccinated against tetanus and diphtheria and, if never immunized, should receive a primary series followed by boosters every 10 years thereafter. The MMR vaccine should be given to patients not previously immunized against measles, mumps, or rubella. A history of clinical illness is inadequate unless supported by a physician's examination. All women of childbearing age should be immunized against rubella. Adults over 65 years of age as well as adults with chronic disease should receive annual influenza immunization. The pneumococcal vaccine is indicated for all adults older than 65 years.

4. **Healthcare workers.** Although no standard vaccination program exists for all healthcare workers, the Advisory Committee on Immunization Practices (ACIP) and the Hospital Infection Control Practices Advisory Committee (HICPAC) has made recommendations for healthcare workers. Diseases for which immunization is strongly recommended, owing to ease of nosocomial spread, include influenza, hepatitis B, measles, mumps, rubella, and varicella. ACIP does not recommend routine immunization of healthcare workers against hepatitis A, pertussis, meningococcal disease, typhoid fever, or vaccinia. However, immunoprophylaxis for these diseases in special circumstances may be indicated.

5. **Travel.** The Centers for Disease Control (CDC) and the World Health Organization (WHO) publish standard references for travel immunization recommendations. Yellow fever vaccine is the only vaccine currently required by the WHO. The yellow fever vaccine is a live attenuated viral vaccine derived from chick embryo cultures and a single dose confers immunity for 10 years. The vaccine should not be administered to patients who have known allergy to eggs, infants less than 9 months old, pregnant or lactating women, or immunocompromised patients. Vaccines that are recommended prior to travel (depending on destination and exposure risk) include hepatitis A immune globulin, typhoid fever, cholera, meningococcal quadrivalent vaccine, and rabies virus vaccine. Japanese encephalitis is a mosquito-transmitted viral infection endemic in Asia, and Japanese encephalitis vaccine is recommended for individuals traveling to endemic (especially rural) areas. Lyme disease vaccine received U.S. Food and Drug Administration (FDA) approval in 1999. The majority of cases of Lyme disease in the United States have been reported in the northeast, upper midwest, and Pacific coastal areas. The vaccine is recommended for individuals aged 15 to 70 years who anticipate travel to endemic areas, particularly if they plan to engage in camping or prolonged outdoor activity.

6. **Pregnancy.** The most important factor relating to maternal immunization is safety for both mother and the developing fetus. The goal of immunizing expectant mothers is to provide the newborn with adequate

organism-specific antibodies to combat infection during the susceptible neonatal period. Vaccines currently recommended for pregnant women include dT toxoid and inactivated influenza virus vaccine. Vaccines recommended in special circumstances (high risk owing to underlying conditions, probable exposure during epidemics, or travel to an endemic area) include poliovirus vaccine, pneumococcal polysaccharide, meningococcal polysaccharide, hepatitis A and B, and yellow fever.

7. **Immunocompromised patients.** Guidelines for immunizations depend on the type of immunodeficiency, severity of immune compromise, and the expected duration of compromised immune status.

   a. **Primary immunodeficiency.** Patients with **T-cell immunodeficiencies** should not receive live vaccines. Similarly, patients with **humoral immunodeficiency** should not receive live vaccines; however, no contraindications exist regarding inactivated vaccines. Patients with IgA deficiency, however, may receive live vaccines with the exception of OPV. Patients with humoral immunodeficiency who are receiving IG replacement therapy do not require active immunizations. Patients with **early or late complement deficiencies** may receive both live and inactivated vaccines. In addition, because complement-deficient patients are at risk for infections with encapsulated bacteria, they should be vaccinated against pneumococcus and meningococcus. Patients with **phagocyte function defects** should not be administered live bacterial vaccines (BCG, Ty21a *Salmonella typhi*), but can be safely given all other vaccines.

   b. **Secondary immunodeficiency.** Owing to the potential severity of viral infections in **HIV-infected patients**, MMR and varicella vaccines are recommended for patients with asymptomatic HIV infection who show no evidence of severe immunosuppression. MMR vaccination of symptomatic HIV-infected persons should be considered if they lack evidence of measles immunity and have no evidence of severe immunosuppression. Although live viral vaccines are not administered to severely immunocompromised HIV-infected patients, immunization with inactivated vaccines should be commenced as soon as possible. Following **cancer chemotherapy**, viral vaccines are usually withheld for a period of 3 months or until immune reconstitution occurs. Patients receiving **high-dose systemic corticosteroids** (greater than 2 mg per kg body weight) for 2 weeks or longer should have live virus vaccines deferred until they have been off of steroids for at least 1 month. Patients with **asplenia** are at greater risk for infection with encapsulated organisms such as meningococcus and pneumococcus and should therefore receive pneumococcal and meningococcal vaccines.

8. **Children undergoing transplantation.** Owing to limited clinical data, there are no standard immunization schedules for transplant recipients. In general, patients older than 12 months of age who are scheduled to receive solid organ transplant should have serum antibody titers checked against measles, mumps, rubella, and varicella; if susceptible, immunization should be planned at least 1 month prior to transplantation. Response to diphtheria and tetanus antigens may be maintained following bone marrow transplant (BMT) by administering a booster to the donor pretransplant and to the recipient immediately following transplant. A similar response may be anticipated for Hib vaccine. Alternatively, diphtheria and tetanus toxoids may be administered as determined by posttransplant titers or following transplant at 12, 14, and 24-month intervals. Patients less than 7 years of age should receive DTaP. Pneumococcal polysaccharide vaccine should be administered 12 and 24 months posttransplant. MMR may be given to BMT recipients 24 months following transplant if they are considered immunocompetent. Patients with graft versus host disease should not be given MMR. Varicella vaccine is generally contraindicated following BMT.

IPV may be administered 12, 14, and 24 months following BMT; household contacts should not be given OPV and all should be immunized against hepatitis A, influenza, MMR, and varicella.

F. Contraindications and precautions

1. Absolute contraindications. Anaphylaxis to a component contained within a vaccine or following a previous dose of a vaccine is an absolute contraindication to further administration of that vaccine. For pertussis vaccine, encephalopathy without obvious cause within 7 days of immunization is an absolute contraindication to further dosing. DT should be used to complete the series unless true anaphylaxis to DTP/DTaP occurred.

2. Temporary contraindications. Women should avoid becoming pregnant within 3 months of receiving MMR or rubella vaccine and within 1 month of mumps or varicella vaccination. Accidental immunization with a live virus vaccine is not an indication for termination because no data exist to link live virus immunization with fetal anomalies. Breastfeeding mothers may receive live virus vaccines. Patients with a primary or secondary immunodeficiency should not be administered live vaccines. Caveats include MMR vaccine for pediatric HIV-infected patients with mild or moderate immunosuppression, and varicella vaccine for immune competent/asymptomatic HIV-infected patients. OPV should not be given to household contacts of an immunosuppressed individual. Immunogenicity of certain live virus vaccines is diminished following receipt of IG preparations or whole blood products. The same effect is not observed for inactivated vaccines and in certain circumstances, such as postexposure tetanus prophylaxis, is recommended. Guidelines concerning measles immunization are available from the CDC; similar guidelines are recommended for varicella and rubella immunization. IG preparations or blood products do not appear to impact the immune response to OPV or yellow fever vaccines. Severe acute illness usually warrants deferral of immunization until resolution of the acute phase.

3. Precautions. When DTaP/DTP is administered, each case should be evaluated on an individual basis. If the risk of adverse events following immunization exceeds those of infection, immunization should be not be offered. Conversely, during an epidemic situation, immunization should be strongly considered. Precautions that warrant careful consideration include:
   - Temperature of 40.5°C within 48 hours of prior immunization with DTP/DTaP
   - Collapse or shock-like state within 48 hours of prior immunization with DTP/DTaP
   - Seizures within 3 days of prior immunization with DTP/DTaP
   - Persistent inconsolable crying lasting 3 hours or more within 48 hours of prior immunization with DTP/DTaP
   - Guillain-Barré syndrome within 6 weeks of immunization with DTP/DTaP
   - Thrombocytopenia temporally related to receipt of MMR

4. Allergic reactions to egg-related antigens is thoroughly discussed in Chapter 13.

G. Adverse events

1. Local. Local reactions, which are inflammatory in nature, consist of localized pain and swelling at the injection site. Symptoms usually resolve within 48 hours and are more frequently associated with intradermal vaccinations.

2. Systemic. As a general rule, systemic adverse events are also inflammatory in nature and usually associated with a local reaction. Systemic symptoms following a vaccination may include fever, malaise, myalgia, and headache. Symptoms usually resolve within 48 hours. Very rarely, patients may manifest an immunoglobulin E (IgE)-mediated allergic reaction following an immunization; this may occur in response to any type of vaccination. These reactions may include the symptoms urticaria, angioedema, or anaphylaxis immediately following the injection. Immune complex-mediated reactions (serum sickness) have also been rarely reported following immunizations.

3. **Rare adverse events.** Certain vaccines are associated with more specific adverse events; these events are generally extremely rare. OPV has been associated with paralytic poliomyelitis in healthy recipients as well as in previously undiagnosed immunodeficient patients. MMR vaccine can, in rare circumstances, cause clinically apparent thrombocytopenia within 2 months of vaccination. Incidence ranges from 1 case per 30,000 vaccinated children in Finland (with temporal clustering of cases) to 1 per million in the United States (with passive reporting). DTP vaccine can cause acute encephalopathy with an estimated risk of 0 to 10.5 episodes per million vaccinations. An association between immunization and the following adverse event remains scientifically unfounded at this time:
  - MMR and childhood autism or other behavioral disorders
  - MMR and inflammatory bowel disease
  - Hepatitis B and multiple sclerosis
  - DTP and sudden infant death syndrome

H. **Adverse event reporting**

Adverse events following immunization may be reported by passive surveillance or actively as mandated by the National Childhood Vaccine Injury Act of 1986. The Vaccine Adverse Event Reporting System (VAERS) was created in 1990 by the CDC and the FDA. Because VAERS is an open reporting system, all persons, including patients, their parents, and health professionals can report adverse events. Information relating to vaccine safety can be obtained at the following web sites: www.cdc.gov/nip/vacsafe; www.healthfinder.gov; and www.immunofacts.com.

I. **Vaccine storage**

To maintain optimal immunogenicity and efficacy, vaccines need to be stored in the correct manner at the recommended temperature.
  - Oral polio and varicella vaccines should be stored at –18°C or 5°F or lower.
  - MMR, DTaP/DTP, DT, Td, Hib, Hep A, Hep B, influenza, IPV, and pneumococcal vaccines should be stored at 2 to 8°C or 35 to 46°F.
  - Vaccines should be refrigerated immediately upon receipt; vaccines should not be stored in the door of the refrigerator.
  - Protect MMR vaccine from light.
  - Maintain correct temperatures in the refrigerator, (2 to 8°C or 35 to 46°F) and the freezer compartment (–14°C or 7°F or lower).
  - Vaccines should only be removed from the refrigerator when ready for use.

J. **Newly licensed vaccines**

A **Lyme disease vaccine** was licensed by the FDA in 1998 for persons 15 to 70 years of age. Use of this vaccine is targeted for individuals residing in or anticipating travel to tick endemic areas but should not replace established personal protection practices. The FDA approved the **rhesus rotavirus tetravalent vaccine (Rotashield)** in 1998. Owing to the subsequent association of this vaccine use with intussusception, the vaccine was withdrawn from the market in October 1999. A vaccine to prevent rotavirus infection is not currently available. The FDA approved the use of a **protein conjugate heptavalent pneumococcal vaccine (Prevnar)** in April 2000 for children less than 24 months of age. Prevnar should be routinely administered to all individuals less than 24 months at 2, 4, 6, and 12 to 15 months. Details concerning catch-up immunization as well as immunization of high-risk individuals greater than 24 months is available from the American Academy of Pediatrics Committee on Infectious Diseases (Table 20.5).

Table 20.5. Recommended immunization schedule
for pneumococcal conjugate vaccine

Age at first dose	Primary series (0.5 mL per dose)	Booster
2–6 mo	Three doses, 6–8 weeks apart	One dose 12–15 mo old
7–11 mo	Two doses, 6–8 weeks apart	One dose 12–15 mo old
12–23 mo	Two doses, 6–8 weeks apart	
>24 mo	One dose	

From the recommendations of the American Academy of Pediatrics (AAP) and Advisory Committee on Immunization Practices (ACIP), with permission. (See Morb Mortal Wkly Rep 2000;49:1–38.)

II. Passive immunization

A. Immune serum globulin.
Administration of fractionated immune globulin by the intravenous or intramuscular routes provides immediate transfer of passive immunity. IG is prepared by alcohol fractionation, is sterile, and is not known to transmit hepatropic viruses, HIV, or any other infectious disease agent. IG primarily contains IgG with only trace amounts of IgA and IgM.

1. **Intravenous immunoglobulin.** Prior to 1997, IVIg was widely used for patients with primary immunodeficiencies as well as many other indications. However, since 1997 there has been a national shortage (withdrawal of product due to possible contamination with Creutzfeldt-Jakob disease agent, waste, excessive use, and export) in the United States, which necessitated the implementation of strict restrictions on IVIg use, per the FDA and National Institutes of Health (NIH).

   a. **Indications for use**
   - Primary immunodeficiencies
   - Kawasaki disease
   - Pediatric HIV infection (scheduled use)
   - Chronic B-cell lymphocytic leukemia
   - Recent bone marrow transplantation in adults
   - Immune-mediated thrombocytopenia
   - Chronic inflammatory demyelinating polyneuropathy

   b. **Adverse effects**
   Five percent of patients receiving IVIg experience adverse events. Most of these events are mild and self-limited in nature, and include:
   - Pyrogenic reactions—fever and chills
   - "Flu-like" symptoms—headache, nausea, malaise
   - Vasomotor changes with tachycardia, flushing, and changes in blood pressure
   - Aseptic meningitis
   - Hypersensitivity reactions
   - Acute renal failure

   c. **Precautions**
   - Patients with hypogammaglobulinemia may be sensitized to the small amount of IgA present in IVIg and develop an anaphylactic reaction. The latter is of particular importance for IgA-deficient patients with an IgG subclass deficiency.
   - Caution should be exercised when administering large volumes of fluid to seriously ill patients or patients with compromised cardiac function.

   d. **Practice guidelines**
   - Slowing infusion rates may minimize mild reactions; patients may be premedicated with an antipyretic and/or antihistamine for febrile reactions.

- More severe and persistent infusion-related reactions may be pretreated with intravenous hydrocortisone (1 to 2 mg per kg 1 hour preinfusion).
- Emergency resuscitative measures should be available, especially for patients with a history of adverse reactions to IVIg.

2. **Immune globulin** is a preparation of pooled human immunoglobulins intended for **intramuscular administration**. Although IG was once used routinely for replacement therapy in humoral immunodeficiency, it is now primarily used as postexposure prophylaxis for hepatitis A and measles. **Hyperimmune globulin** contains high titers of a desired antibody and preparations are available for clinical use against hepatitis B, rabies, tetanus, varicella, cytomegalovirus, and respiratory syncytial virus (Table 20.6).

   a. **Adverse effects**
      - Pain at the injection site
      - Chest pain, dyspnea, anaphylaxis (rare)
      - IgA-deficient patients may be sensitized to the small quantity of IgA present in IG

   b. **Practice guidelines**
      - IG is recommended for intramuscular administration only. To limit pain at the injection site, IG should be administered deep into a large muscle mass.
      - The amount of discomfort experienced is limited if the product is at room temperature.
      - A maximum of 5 mL (adult) and 1 to 3 mL (child) should be administered at any one time.
      - Although allergic reactions are rare, immediate resuscitative measures should be available.

B. **Human plasma**

   Few indications exist for the use of fresh frozen plasma (FFP) as a form of immunoprophylaxis.

C. **Animal antisera and antitoxins**

   Because of the possibility of serious adverse events, products of animal origin should only be administered to humans when there are no alternative treatment options available (Table 20.7). Prior to initiating therapy with animal antisera (antitoxins), a thorough medical history highlighting the following should be obtained: asthma, allergic rhinitis, urticaria, prior injections of animal sera, and horse sensitivity. Patients who have received antisera previously are at an increased risk of developing allergic reactions and serum sickness on reexposure. All patients who are to receive animal sera should have skin testing performed prior to administration. A prick test should be performed with a 1:10 dilution of the antiserum, with a test deemed positive if the wheal is at least 3 mm greater in diameter than the saline control. If the prick test is negative, intradermal testing should begin with 0.02 mL of a 1:1000 dilution of the antiserum. If this test is negative, the test should be repeated with a 1:100 dilution. Positive skin tests indicate hypersensitivity and should be followed by desensitization, if treatment is indicated. Although intravenous, subcutaneous, intradermal, or intramuscular routes have all been used, intravenous desensitization is preferable because it is probably safest. A suggested protocol for intravenous desensitization is outlined in Table 20.8.

   The following adverse effects may follow antisera administration:
   - Acute febrile reactions are usually mild and can be treated with antipyretics or tepid sponging.
   - Acute IgE-mediated reactions, including urticaria, angioedema, or anaphylaxis can occur. Skin testing performed prior to administration should help avoid the occurrence of these reactions.
   - Serum sickness, which may occur 7 to 10 days after receiving animal serum, is manifested by fever, urticaria, maculopapular rash, arthritis

(*text continues on page 481*)

Table 20.6. Hyperimmunoglobulin preparations and indications

Product (trade name)	Indication	Dose	Additional therapy
Hepatitis B Ig (H-BIG) (Hyperhep) (Hep-B-Gammagee)	**Postexposure** prophylaxis Sexual contact Blood contact **Perinatal**[a] Infant of HBsAg-positive mother	0.06 mL/kg i.m. 0.5 mL i.m.	HBV series if nonimmune Initiate HBV series within 12 h of birth
Rabies IG (Imogam Rabies-HT) (BayRab)	**Postexposure** prophylaxis following contact with rabid animal	20 IU/kg infiltrated around the wound, excess administered i.m.	In conjunction with rabies vaccine
Respiratory syncitial virus IG (Respigam)	**Prevention**[b] of RSV disease in infants/children <24 mo with chronic lung disease or history of premature birth (<35 weeks gestation)	15 mL/kg i.v., monthly, just prior to the RSV season and throughout	Palivizumab, (monoclonal antibody directed against the F-glycoprotein of RSV), may be used **alternatively** to Respigam, 15 mg/kg i.m. monthly during RSV season
Tetanus IG (Hyper-Tet Tetanus Immune Globulin)	Management of tetanus-prone wounds Treatment of tetanus infection	250–500 IU i.m.	To be used in conjunction with tetanus-diphtheria toxoids.[c] To be administered at separate site to toxoid

			To be administered within 96 h of exposure
Varicella zoster IG (VZIG)	Postexposure prophylaxis Immunocompromised Infants born to mothers who develop varicella 5 d pre- to 3 d postdelivery pregnant patients	3000–6000 IU[d] ≤10 kg 125 IU i.m. 10. 1–20 kg 250 IU 20. 1–30 kg 375 IU 30. 1–40 kg 500 IU >40 625 IU	
Cytomegalovirus IG (CytoGam)	Prevention of cytomegalovirus infection in solid organ transplant recipients	i.v. administration, <72 h post transplant 150 mg/kg; weeks 2, 4, 6, 8, 100 mg/kg weeks 12, 16, 50 mg/kg	

[a] For preterm infants <2 kg whose mother's HBsAg status cannot be determined within the first 12 h, H-BIG should be administered in addition to the HBV series.

[b] Respigam and Palivizumab are not licensed for use in children with congenital heart disease, or as treatment for RSV infection. Palivizumab or RSV IG may be considered for patients with severe immunodeficiencies. Given the large number of children born at 32–35 weeks gestation, use of RSV IG or Palivizumab should be guided by additional risk factors.

[c] For children less than 7 yr, DTaP or DTP (DT if pertussis vaccine is contraindicated) is preferred to tetanus toxoid alone. For persons 7 yr and older, dT is preferred to tetanus toxoid alone.

[d] Optimal dose unknown, doses as low as 500 IU effective for tetanus neonatorum.

Ig, immunoglobulin; i.m., intramuscular; HBV, hepatitis B vaccine; RSV, respiratory syncytial virus; HBsAg, hepatitis B surface antigen; DTaP, diphtheria, tetanus, pertussis vaccine; Td, tetanus, diphtheria toxoid; DTP, diphtheria, tetanus, pertussis vaccine.

Table 20.7. Indications for administration of animal antisera

Product (Trade name)	Indication	Dose[a]	Additional therapy
Botulinum antitoxin, trivalent A, B, E (Botox)	Botulism	One vial i.v., and one vial i.m.; dose may be repeated in 4 h for severe or progressive cases	Human botulinum IG not routinely available outside infant botulism trials; (contact the Infant Botulism Prevention Program, California State Department of Health Services, 510-540-2646)
Diphtheria antitoxin[b]	Diphtheria	20,000–40,000 IU pharyngeal or laryngeal disease of 48 h duration; 40,000 to 60,000 IU nasopharyngeal lesions; 80,000 to 120,000 IU extensive disease of 3 or more days duration and for anyone with brawny swelling of the neck	Administration by i.v. route over 60 min for severe infection, i.m. administration for moderate infection
Tetanus antitoxin[c]	Tetanus	50,000–100,000 IU, 20,000 IU administered by i.v. route, remainder i.m.	Tetanus Ig plus tetanus toxoid at alternative sites
Latrodectus antivenin	Black widow spider bite	One vial, by slow i.v. infusion, usually curative; may cause anaphylaxis	
Crotalidae antivenin	Rattlesnake bite	Five vials minimum dose, by infusion in normal saline, at increasing rate dependent on patient tolerance; may cause anaphylaxis	

[a] Skin testing with antiserum is mandated prior to use regardless of the severity of clinical illness.
[b] Diphtheria antitoxin is no longer licensed in the United States, but a European-licensed product is available from the National Immunization Program of the Centers for Disease Control and Prevention by calling 404-639-8200.
[c] Not available in the United States.
i.v., intravenous; i.m., intramuscular; Ig, immunoglobulin.

Table 20.8. Desensitization to animal serum via intravenous route

Dose number	Dilution of serum in isotonic sodium chloride	Amount of i.v. injection (mL)
1	1:1000	0.1
2	1:1000	0.3
3	1:1000	0.6
4	1:100	0.1
5	1:100	0.3
6	1:100	0.6
7	1:10	0.1
8	1:10	0.3
9	1:10	0.6
10	Undiluted	0.1
11	Undiluted	0.3
12	Undiluted	0.6
13	Undiluted	1.0

i.v., intravenous.

or arthralgia, and lymphadenopathy. Less frequent events include angioedema, Guillain-Barré syndrome, pyelonephritis, peripheral neuritis, and myocarditis. The onset of symptoms is earlier and more frequent for patients who have previously received animal products. Treatment includes antihistamines and antipyretics for milder symptoms and steroid therapy (1 to 2 mg per kg prednisone for 1 to 2 weeks) for more severe manifestations.

Selected Readings

American Academy of Pediatrics: Report of the Committee on Infectious Diseases. Elk Grove Village, IL: American Academy of Pediatrics, 2000.

Atkinson W, Wolfe C, Humiston S, et al., eds. *Epidemiology and prevention of vaccine-preventable diseases*, 6th ed. Atlanta: Centers for Disease Control and Prevention, 2000.

Feigin RD, Cherry JD, eds. *Textbook of pediatric infectious diseases*, 4th ed. Philadelphia: WB Saunders, 2000.

Mandell GL, Bennett JE, Dolin R, eds. *Principles and practice of infectious diseases*, 5th ed. St. Louis, MO: Churchill Livingstone, 2000.

Pneumococcus vaccination: recommendations for the prevention of pneumococcal infections, including the use of pneumococcal conjugate vaccine (Prevnar), pneumococcal polysaccharide vaccine, and antibiotic prophylaxis. *Pediatrics* 2000;106:362–366.

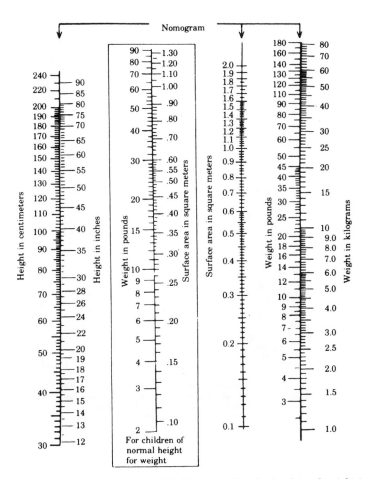

Surface area is indicated where a straight line connecting the height and weight intersects the surface area column, or, in a person of normal proportions, from weight alone (boxed column). From West CD. Electrolyte imbalance and parenteral fluid therapy. Procedures in use at Children's Hospital Medical Center, Cincinnati, OH, with permission.

B. NOMOGRAM FOR PREDICTING THE OPTIMUM TIDAL VOLUME FROM THE BREATHING FREQUENCY, BODY WEIGHT, AND SEX OF THE PATIENT*

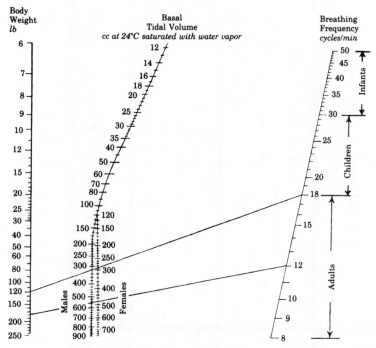

* Corrections to be applied to tidal volume as required: Daily activity, add 10%; fever, add 5% for each degree F above 99° (rectal); altitude, add 5% for each 2,000 feet above sea level; tracheotomy and endotracheal intubation, subtract a volume equal to half the body weight. From Radford EP, et al. Clinical use of a nomogram to estimate proper ventilation during artificial respiration. *N Engl J Med* 1984;251:877, with permission.

Alvin M. Sanico, Bruce S. Bochner, and Sarbjit S. Saini

I. **Percutaneous (also known as epicutaneous, prick, or puncture) skin testing**
Percutaneous skin testing can be done using one of several different devices and methods.

A. **"Drop and puncture" procedure.** Clean the skin area to be tested with alcohol and allow it to dry. Mark and label the test sites on the volar aspect of the forearm or on the upper back at least 2 to 3 cm apart, to avoid any overlapping of positive skin reactions. Place a drop of predetermined allergen solution (e.g., at a dilution of 1:10 or 1:20 w/v) at each mark. Similarly apply positive and negative control solutions (histamine phosphate 0.1% and diluent such as phosphate-buffered saline with 0.4% phenol, respectively). Superficially puncture the skin through each drop of test material, using one of the commercially available devices manufactured for this purpose. These include metal bifurcated needles (ALO Laboratories, Columbus, OH) or plastic devices such as the Duotip-Test (Lincoln Diagnostics, Decatur, IL), Greer-Pick (Greer Laboratories, Lenoir, NC), Morrow Brown needle (Alkaline Corporation, Oakhurst, NJ), or Sharp-Test applicator (Panatrex, Placentia, CA). The skin should not be punctured so deep as to cause bleeding. It has been a common practice to use a single metal bifurcated needle to test multiple allergens on the same patient. In this method, the needle tip is wiped clean with alcohol, typically using both hands, between punctures. In accordance with Occupational Safety and Health Administration recommendations, this technique should be avoided to prevent potential exposure of the tester to blood-borne pathogens. Cleaning the needle using a one-handed technique with a holding apparatus can reduce the chance of accidental direct contact with the contaminated tip. Another safer alternative is to use one of the aforementioned plastic devices that is discarded after a single puncture.

B. **"Dip and puncture" procedure.** This method is similar to the above, except that no drop of test material is placed on the skin before the latter is punctured. Instead, the tip of the puncture device is first dipped into a small well containing the allergen or control solution, and then is introduced into the skin. This particular method can also be employed to apply several different test materials in one operation, using a device with multiple tips attached to a rigid frame. The tips are first dipped into their corresponding wells in a tray, and then are simultaneously pressed onto the skin. These disposable plastic devices include the Multi-Test (Lincoln Diagnostics), Quanti Test System (Panatrex), and Quintest (Hollister-Stier, Spokane, WA). Of note, studies comparing the various skin test devices have demonstrated significant differences among them in terms of the size of wheal and erythema that they produce, using either saline or histamine. It is, therefore, imperative to consistently adhere to the criteria for negative and positive reactions when interpreting results with any of these products. In choosing a skin test device, the practitioner can consider several factors including reliability, safety, cost, convenience, and patient comfort.

II. **Intracutaneous (also known as intradermal) skin testing**
Intracutaneous skin testing could be considered only after a negative percutaneous test result is obtained despite a history strongly suggestive of allergen sensitivity and of relevant exposure. **This method, however, should not be done in the evaluation of possible food sensitivity to avoid either false-positive results or systemic reactions in nonallergic or highly allergic individuals, respectively.** The allergen concentration used in this method is

typically 1/1000 to 1/100 of that used for percutaneous skin testing. The negative and positive controls consist of the diluent solution and histamine phosphate 0.01%, respectively. Clean and mark the skin test area as previously described. Draw approximately 0.1 mL of test material into a sterile tuberculin syringe, and expel any air bubble if present. Stretch the skin taut and introduce the needle into the skin at a 45° angle with the bevel facing downward. Advance the needle until its bevel is completely under the skin. Inject approximately 0.02 mL of the solution, creating a 1- to 3-mm bleb in the process. If no such bleb is formed, due to a delivery that is either too deep or too superficial as to cause leakage, repeat the procedure at another site.

III. Measurement and interpretation of results

Fifteen to 20 minutes after administering the skin test, **measure the longest and orthogonal diameters of any resultant wheal, and record the average of the two.** Do the same procedure for any resultant erythema. Marking the boundaries of these skin changes with a pen can facilitate their evaluation. Note any **pseudopod** formation because this denotes a significantly positive reaction. An average wheal diameter greater than or equal to 3 mm larger than that of the diluent control is considered positive. A grading system can be applied to describe the degree of skin test reactivity. For example, the allergic reaction can be designated 4+ if the wheal size is greater than, 3+ if it is the same as, 2+ if it is two thirds, and 1+ if it is one third that of the histamine control. In interpreting the clinical relevance of the skin test results, the patient's history and other pertinent findings should be considered. Also note that percutaneous skin testing is generally less sensitive, but more specific, than the intracutaneous method. Skin testing with mixtures of allergens (e.g., several different tree pollen extracts in one solution) can be useful for screening purposes, but may potentially be associated with false-negative results. As such, further testing with individual specific allergens could be considered if warranted by a strong clinical history and if allergen immunotherapy is intended.

Selected Readings

Nelson HS, Lahr J, Buchmeier A, et al. Evaluation of devices for skin prick testing. *J Allergy Clin Immunol* 1998;101:153–156.

Corder WT, Hogan MB, Wilson NW. Comparison of two disposable plastic skin test devices with the bifurcated needle for epicutaneous allergy testing. *Ann Allergy Asthma Immunol* 1996;77:222–226.

   I. Collection of specimen. Instruct the patient to blow his or her nose into a piece of wax paper (6 × 6 in.). Place a glass microscope slide on top of the mucus, or apply and spread the mucus from the paper to the slide with a cotton-tipped applicator. Alternatively, place a cotton-tipped applicator into the anterior nasal cavity and leave in place for 2 to 3 minutes. Then remove the applicator and smear the adherent mucus on a glass microscope slide.

  II. Staining of the nasal smear. Conjunctival mucus and sputum can be similarly stained.

    A. Allow the smear to air-dry.

    B. Hansel stain (preferred for demonstration of eosinophils).

      1. Cover the slide with methyl alcohol and allow it to dry.

      2. Flood the slide with Hansel stain* (methanol 95%, eosin, methylene blue, glycerin 5%) and allow the stain to incubate for 30 seconds.

      3. Add a small volume of distilled water (five drops) for 30 seconds (may be mixed by blowing gently to dilute the stain, where a sheen of "oil" appears on the surface).

      4. Pour off the stain and wash with distilled water.

      5. Flood with methyl alcohol to decolor (until specimen appears to have a pale green color).

      6. Air-dry.

    C. Wright stain (used alternatively).

      1. Flood the slide with Wright stain (eosin and sodium bicarbonate diluted in methyl alcohol and added to methylene blue) and incubate for 2 to 3 minutes.

      2. Layer on phosphate buffer (pH 6.4) and blow gently to mix. Allow to stand for 2 to 3 minutes.

      3. Wash with distilled water.

      4. Air-dry.

 III. Examination of the smear. Examine with a microscope under low power (100 ×) first to determine the adequacy of the specimen and the areas of interest. Then examine under a high-power lens and oil immersion (1,000×). Count the number of eosinophils (pink cytoplasmic granules with blue, bilobed nuclei) and the total number of polymorphonuclear leukocytes (PMN) (which have pale-pink cytoplasm and blue, multilobed nuclei) in five separate fields. Express as the ratio of eosinophils to PMNs. Nasal epithelial cells have unlobulated, blue nuclei and abundant pale-blue cytoplasm.

 IV. Interpretation

    A. If there are 10% or more eosinophils, allergic rhinitis is suggested.

    B. A predominance of PMNs suggests infection (eosinophils can be present in moderate amounts).

    C. Acellular specimens without predominance of eosinophils or PMNs suggest vasomotor rhinitis.

---

* Lide Laboratories, 515 Timberwyck, St. Louis, MO 63131.

B. EXAMINATION OF NASAL OR CONJUNCTIVAL EPITHELIUM SPECIMENS

Alfredo A. Jalowayski and Robert S. Zeiger

I. **Collection of specimens.** Instruct the patient to clear the nose of excess secretions. In infants, a rubber bulb may be used to aspirate excess mucus. Using a disposable plastic curette (e.g., Rhino-probe[a]) or a similar device, and under direct illumination and visualization of the nasal cavity, sample the medial or inferior portion of the inferior turbinate posteriorly, avoiding the anterior bulb area. Gently press the cupped tip of the probe on the mucosal surface and move outward 2 to 3 mm. Repeat the motion twice and withdraw the probe without touching the nasal vestibule to prevent contamination. To obtain conjunctival specimens, invert the inferior lid, have the patient look up, and gently scrape the palpebral conjunctiva 1 to 2 mm with the same type of probe used to obtain mucosal epithelial cells. A topical ophthalmic anesthetic (e.g., Ophthetic[b]) can be used for the sensitive patient. The specimen is gently spread over a small area of a microscope slide and fixed quickly in a jar containing 95% ethyl alcohol for 1 minute or until stained.

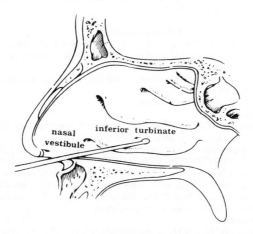

II. **Staining of the epithelial specimens.** Staining may be achieved with the Wright-Giemsa dip method as described below. Hansel stain can be used if eosinophils are the only cells of interest. Wright stain may be used for eosinophils and metachromatic cells with variable results. See Appendix III.A.
   A. Remove the slide(s) from the jar and drain excess alcohol, but do not allow the cells to air-dry.
   B. Dip the slide(s) in Wright-Giemsa (e.g., Volu-Sol[a]) stain for 10 to 15 seconds.
   C. Drain the excess stain, then dip the slide(s) in Volu-Sol buffer for 15 to 30 seconds.
   D. Drain the excess rinse and air-dry the specimens.
III. **Examination of nasal and conjunctival cytograms.** Examine with a microscope under low power (100 ×) first to determine the adequacy of the specimens and the areas of interest. Grade the cytogram under a high-power lens and oil immersion (1,000 ×) quantitatively as the mean number of cells/10 high-power

[a] Apotex Scientific, Inc., Springville, UT 84663.
[b] Allergan Pharmaceuticals, Inc., Irvine, CA 92715.

fields examined, or grade qualitatively, on a scale of 0 to 4+, as suggested in Grading of nasal cytograms below. Normal epithelium consists of numerous epithelial cells (ciliated columnar, nonciliated columnar, goblet, and basal cells) stained light blue, and contains no eosinophils or metachromatic cells (basophils or mast cells); however, a few neutrophils and bacteria can usually be seen.

IV. Grading of nasal cytograms

Quantitative Analysis[a]

Grade[b]	Eosinophils, neutrophils	Metachromatic cells (basophils/mast cells)	Goblet cells[c]
0	0–1.0	0–0.3	0
1+	1.1–5.0	0.4–1.0	1–24
2+	6.0–15.0	1.1–3.0	25–49
3+	16.0–20.0	3.1–6.0	50–74
4+	>20.0	>6.0	75–100

Qualitative Analysis[d]

Grade	Eosinophils, neutrophils, metachromatic cells (basophils/mast cells)
0	No cells seen
1+	Few cells seen
2+	Moderate number of cells seen
3+	Many cells seen
4+	Large number of cells seen

V. Interpreting nasal cytograms

Cellular type	Suggested disorder
Increased eosinophils[e]	Allergic rhinitis, eosinophilic nonallergic rhinitis (ENR) or nonallergic rhinitis with eosinophils (NARES), rhinitis associated with non-IgE-mediated asthma, aspirin sensitivity, Churg-Strauss syndrome, nasal polyps
Increased metachromatic cells (basophils/mast cells)	Conditions listed for increased eosinophils, nonallergic basophilic rhinitis, or primary nasal mastocytosis
Increased neutrophils[f] with:	
1. Intracellular bacteria	Infectious nasopharyngitis or sinusitis
2. Ciliocytophoria[g]	Viral upper respiratory tract infection (URI)
3. No bacteria	Viral URI, irritant rhinitis, or chemically induced rhinitis or sinusitis (or both), may be associated with eosinophils in allergic rhinitis
Increased goblet cells[h]	Allergic rhinitis, infectious rhinitis, or possibly vasomotor rhinitis

[a] Mean number of cells/10 high-power fields (1,000 ×).
[b] Comparative reference for qualitative analysis.
[c] Ratio of goblet cells to epithelial cells, expressed as a percent. The presence of over 50% goblet cells on the nasal cytogram is considered increased.
[d] See relative numbers of cells in quantitative analysis above.
[e] 1+ or greater quantitatively or qualitatively.
[f] Mean number of cells/10 high-power fields (1,000 ×).
[g] Epithelial cells with clumping of chromatin material.
[h] Greater than 50%.

VI. Interpreting conjunctival cytograms

The presence of inflammatory cells within the conjunctival mucosa (superficial epithelial scraping) suggests certain disorders depending on the specific cell types present.

Cellular type	Suggested disorder
Eosinophils, metachromatic cells, (basophils/mast cells)	Allergic, vernal, or giant papillary conjunctivitis or keratoconjunctivitis
Neutrophils	Infectious (bacterial) or irritant conjunctivitis, may be associated with eosinophils in allergic conjunctivitis
Lymphocytes	Viral conjunctivitis

Appendix IV. NORMATIVE TOTAL SERUM IMMUNOGLOBULIN E LEVELS AS DETERMINED BY A NONCOMPETITIVE SOLID-PHASE IMMUNOASSAY

Reference and study group	Sex	Age	Total no.	Total serum IgE (IU/mL)[a] Geometric mean	Upper 95% confidence limit
Barbee et al.:	M	6–14 yr	72	42.7	527
White adults	F		73	4.3	344
in United	M	15–24 yr	109	33.6[c]	447
States[b]	F		121	18.6	262
	M	25–34 yr	108	16.8	275
	F		89	16.6	216
	M	35–44 yr	62	21.7	242
	F		67	19.3	206
	M	45–54 yr	88	19.2	254
	F		97	13.3	177
	M	55–64 yr	105	21.3[c]	354
	F		172	11.7	148
	M	65–74 yr	145	21.2[c]	248
	F		199	11.5	122
	M	75+ yr	69	18.4[c]	219
	F		87	9.2	124
	All M	6–75 yr	758	22.9[c]	317
	All F		905	14.7	189

[a] All total serum IgE levels reported were measured with a noncompetitive paper disk RIST marketed by Pharmacia Diagnostics.

[b] Anglo White subjects living in Tucson, AZ, who had negative skin prick test to house dust, Dematiacease mold mix, Bermuda grass, tree mix, and weed mix. Similar normative values were obtained by using the paper disk RIST for 425 nonallergic subjects in a tristate area (Florida, Georgia, and Alabama).

[c] Mean serum IgE for males significantly greater than mean levels for females.

M, male; F, female; IgE, immunoglobulin E; SPRIA, solid-phase immunoassay; RIST, radioimmunosorbent test.

Appendix V. LEVELS OF IMMUNOGLOBULINS IN SERA OF NORMAL SUBJECTS BY AGE

Age	IgG		IgM		IgA		Total immunoglobulin	
	mg/dL	Percent of adult level	mg/dL	Percent of adult level	mg/dL	Percent of adult level	mg/dL	Percent of adult level
Newborn	1031 ± 200[a]	89 ± 17	11 ± 5	11 ± 5	2 ± 3	1 ± 2	1044 ± 201	67 ± 13
1–3 mo	430 ± 119	37 ± 10	30 ± 11	30 ± 11	21 ± 13	11 ± 7	481 ± 127	31 ± 9
4–6 mo	427 ± 186	37 ± 16	43 ± 17	43 ± 17	28 ± 18	14 ± 9	498 ± 204	32 ± 13
7–12 mo	661 ± 219	58 ± 19	54 ± 23	55 ± 23	37 ± 18	19 ± 9	752 ± 242	48 ± 15
13–24 mo	762 ± 209	66 ± 18	58 ± 23	59 ± 23	50 ± 24	25 ± 12	870 ± 258	56 ± 16
25–36 mo	892 ± 183	77 ± 16	61 ± 19	62 ± 19	71 ± 37	36 ± 19	1024 ± 205	65 ± 14
3–5 yr	929 ± 228	80 ± 20	56 ± 18	57 ± 18	93 ± 27	47 ± 14	1078 ± 245	69 ± 17
6–8 yr	923 ± 256	80 ± 22	65 ± 25	66 ± 25	124 ± 45	62 ± 23	1112 ± 293	71 ± 20
9–11 yr	1124 ± 235	97 ± 20	79 ± 33	80 ± 33	131 ± 60	66 ± 30	1334 ± 254	85 ± 17
12–16 yr	946 ± 124	82 ± 11	59 ± 20	60 ± 20	148 ± 63	74 ± 32	1153 ± 169	74 ± 12
Adults	1158 ± 305	100 ± 26	99 ± 27	100 ± 27	200 ± 61	100 ± 31	1457 ± 353	100 ± 24

[a] One standard deviation.
IgG, immunoglobulin G.
From Stiehm ER, Fudenberg HH. Serum levels of immune globulins in health and disease: a survey. *Pediatrics* 1966;37:715, with permission.

Joseph L. McGerity

A. Principal Pollens, by Region*

Region I (North Atlantic)

Connecticut, Maine, Massachusetts, New Hampshire, New Jersey, New York, Pennsylvania, Rhode Island, Vermont

Trees (pollinating season: late winter through spring)

Box elder/maple (*Acer* sp)

Birch (*Betula* sp)

Oak (*Quercus* sp)

Hickory (*Carya ovata*)

Ash (*Fraxinus americana*)

Pine (*Pinus strobus*)

Sycamore (*Platanus occidentalis*)

Cottonwood/poplar (*Populus deltoides*)

Elm (*Ulmus americana*)

Mulberry (*Morus* sp)

Walnut (*Juglans* sp)

Liquid amber (*Liquidambar*)

Cypress (*Cupressus* sp)

Grasses (pollinating season: spring through summer)

Redtop (*Agrostis alba*)

Orchard (*Dactylis glomerata*)

Fescue (*Festuca elatior*)

Timothy (*Phleum pratense*)

Bluegrass/June grass (*Poa* sp)

Weeds (pollinating season: summer through early fall)

Lamb's-quarters (*Chenopodium album*)

Ragweed, giant and short (*Ambrosia* sp)

Cocklebur (*Xanthium strumarium*)

Plantain (*Plantago lanceolata*)

Dock/sorrel (*Rumex* sp)

Sagebrush (*Artemisia* sp)

Pigweed/careless weed (*Amaranthus* sp)

Region II (Mid-Atlantic)

Delaware, District of Columbia, Maryland, North Carolina, Virginia

Trees (pollinating season: late winter through spring)

Box elder/maple (*Acer* sp)

Birch (*Betula nigra*)

Cedar/juniper (*Juniperus virginiana*)

Oak (*Quercus* sp)

Hickory/pecan (*Carya* sp)

Walnut (*Juglans nigra*)

Mulberry (*Morus* sp)

---

* Figure VI.1 presents maps which divide the United States into 17 regional floristic zones and Canada into 4 regional floristic zones. These zones are established on similarity of climatic and geographical features. The resulting floral growth pattern in a given zone tends to be similar, although with localized fluctuations in climate, elevation, and soil, differences do exist within each zone. Each floristic zone is listed with the allergenic pollinating plants and their seasons of pollination most common to that zone. Alaska and Hawaii are listed, but they are not represented on the floristic map. See Chapter 3 for a more complete description of factors affecting pollen distribution.

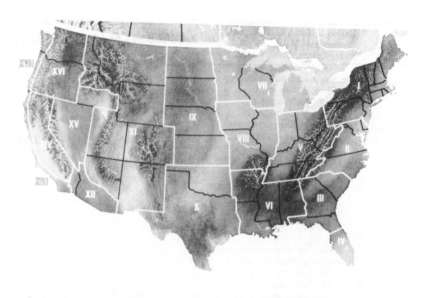

FIG. VI.1. Floristic regional zones in the United States (top) and Canada (bottom). From *Pollen guide for allergy*. Spokane, WA: Hollister-Stier Laboratories, 1978, with permission.

Ash (*Fraxinus americana*)
Cottonwood/poplar (*Populus deltoides*)
Hackberry (*Celtis occidentalis*)
Elm (*Ulmus americana*)
Pine (*Pinus* sp)
Alder (*Alnus incana*)
Sycamore (*Platanus* sp)
Grasses (pollinating season: spring through early summer)
Redtop (*Agrostic alba*)
Vernal grass (*Anthoxanthum* sp)
Bermuda grass (*Cynodon dactylon*)
Orchard grass (*Dactylis glomerata*)

Ryegrass (*Elymus* and *Lolium* sp)
Timothy (*Phleum pratense*)
Bluegrass/June grass (*Poa* sp)
Johnson grass (*Sorghum halepense*)
Weeds (pollinating season: summer through early fall)
    Pigweed (*Amaranthus retroflexus*)
    Lamb's-quarters (*Chenopodium album*)
    Mexican firebush (*Kochia scoparia*)
    Ragweed, giant and short (*Ambrosia* sp)
    Cocklebur (*Xanthium strumarium*)
    Plantain (*Plantago lanceolata*)
    Dock/sorrel (*Rumex* sp)
Region III (South Atlantic)
  Florida (north, above Orlando), Georgia, South Carolina
    Trees (pollinating season: late winter through spring)
      Box elder/maple (*Acer* sp)
      Birch (*Betula nigra*)
      Cedar/juniper (*Juniperus virginiana*)
      Oak (*Quercus* sp)
      Hickory/pecan (*Carya* sp)
      Walnut (*Juglans nigra*)
      Mesquite (*Prosopis juliflora*)
      Mulberry (*Morus* sp)
      Ash (*Fraxinus americana*)
      Cottonwood/poplar (*Populus deltoides*)
      Hackberry (*Celtis occidentalis*)
      Elm (*Ulmus americana*)
    Grasses (pollinating season: spring through early summer)
      Redtop (*Agrostis alba*)
      Sweet vernal grass (*Anthoxanthum* sp)
      Bermuda grass (*Cynodon dactylon*)
      Orchard grass (*Dactylis glomerata*)
      Ryegrass (*Elymus* and *Lolium* sp)
      Fescue (*Festuca elatior*)
      Timothy (*Phleum pratense*)
      Bluegrass/June grass (*Poa* sp)
      Johnson grass (*Sorghum halepense*)
    Weeds (pollinating season: summer through early fall)
      Lamb's-quarters (*Chenopodium album*)
      Ragweed, giant and short (*Ambrosia* sp)
      Sagebrush (*Artemisia* sp)
      Cocklebur (*Xanthium strumarium*)
      Plantain (*Plantago lanceolata*)
      Dock/sorrel (*Rumex* sp)
Region IV (Subtropic Florida)
  Southern Florida (below Orlando)
    Trees (pollinating season: winter through spring)
      Box elder (*Acer negundo*)
      Cedar/juniper (*Juniperus virginiana*)
      Oak (*Quercus* sp)
      Pecan (*Carya pecan*)
      Privet (*Ligustrum lucidium*)
      Palm (*Cocos plumosa*)
      Australian pine (beefwood) (*Casuarina equisetifolia*)
      Sycamore (*Platanus occidentalis*)
      Cottonwood/poplar (*Populus deltoides*)
      Elm (*Ulmus americana*)
      Brazilian peppertree (Florida holly) (*Schinus terebinthifolius*)
      Bayberry (wax myrtle) (*Myrica* sp)

Melaleuca (*Melaleuca* sp)
Cypress (*Cupressus* sp)
Pine (*Pinus* sp)
Grasses (pollinating season: spring through early summer)
Redtop (*Agrostis alba*)
Bermuda grass (*Cynodon dactylon*)
Salt grass (*Distichlis* sp)
Bahia grass (*Paspalum notatum*)
Canary grass (*Phalaris minor*)
Bluegrass/June grass (*Poa* sp)
Johnson grass (*Sorghum halepense*)
Weeds (pollinating season: summer through early fall)
Pigweed (*Amaranthus spinosus*)
Lamb's-quarters (*Chenopodium album*)
Ragweed, giant and short (*Ambrosia* sp)
Sagebrush (*Artemisia* sp)
Marsh elder/poverty weed (*Iva* sp)
Dock/sorrel (*Rumex* sp)
Plantain (*Plantago lanceolata*)
Nettle (*Urtica* sp)
Region V (Greater Ohio Valley)
Indiana, Kentucky, Ohio, Tennessee, West Virginia
Trees (pollinating season: late winter through spring)
Box elder/maple (*Acer* sp)
Birch (*Betula nigra*)
Oak (*Quercus rubra*)
Hickory (*Carya ovata*)
Walnut (*Juglans nigra*)
Ash (*Fraxinus americana*)
Sycamore (*Platanus occidentalis*)
Cottonwood/poplar (*Populus deltoides*)
Elm (*Ulmus americana*)
Mulberry (*Morus* sp)
Pine (*Pinus* sp)
Cypress (*Cupressus* sp)
Liquid amber (*Liquidambar*)
Grasses (pollinating season: spring through early summer)
Redtop (*Agrostis alba*)
Bermuda grass (*Cynodon dactylon*)
Orchard grass (*Dactylis glomerata*)
Fescue (*Festuca elatior*)
Ryegrass (*Lolium* sp)
Timothy (*Phleum pratense*)
Bluegrass/June grass (*Poa* sp)
Johnson grass (*Sorghum halepense*)
Weeds (pollinating season: summer through early fall)
Waterhemp (*Acnida tamariscina*)
Pigweed (*Amaranthus retroflexus*)
Lamb's-quarters (*Chenopodium album*)
Ragweed, giant and short (*Ambrosia* sp)
Sagebrush (*Artemisia* sp)
Cocklebur (*Xanthium strumarium*)
Dock/sorrel (*Rumex* sp)
Plantain (*Plantago lanceolata*)
Nettle (*Urtica* sp)
Region VI (South Central)
Alabama, Arkansas, Louisiana, Mississippi
Trees (pollinating season: late winter through early spring)
Box elder/maple (*Acer* sp)
Cedar/juniper (*Juniperus virginiana*)

Oak (*Quercus* sp)
Hickory/pecan (*Carya* sp)
Walnut (*Juglans nigra*)
Ash (*Fraxinus americana*)
Sycamore (*Platanus occidentalis*)
Cottonwood/poplar (*Populus deltoides*)
Elm (*Ulmus americana*)
Grasses (pollinating season: spring through early summer)
Redtop (*Agrostis alba*)
Bermuda grass (*Cynodon dactylon*)
Orchard grass (*Dactylis glomerata*)
Ryegrass (*Lolium* sp)
Timothy (*Phleum pratense*)
Bluegrass/June grass (*Poa* sp)
Johnson grass (*Sorghum halepense*)
Weeds (pollinating season: summer through early fall)
Pigweed (*Amaranthus retroflexus*)
Lamb's-quarters (*Chenopodium album*)
Ragweed, giant and short (*Ambrosia* sp)
Sagebrush (*Artemisia* sp)
Cocklebur (*Xanthium strumarium*)
Dock/sorrel (*Rumex* sp)
Plantain (*Plantago lanceolata*)
Region VII (Northern Midwest)
Michigan, Minnesota, Wisconsin
Trees (pollinating season: late winter through spring)
Box elder/maple (*Acer* sp)
Alder (*Alnus incana*)
Birch (*Betula* sp)
Oak (*Quercus rubra*)
Hickory (*Carya ovata*)
Walnut (*Juglans nigra*)
Ash (*Fraxinus americana*)
Sycamore (*Platanus occidentalis*)
Cottonwood/poplar (*Populus deltoides*)
Elm (*Ulmus americana*)
Cypress (*Cupressus* sp)
Mulberry (*Morus* sp)
Pine (*Pinus* sp)
Willow (*Salix* sp)
Grasses (pollinating season: spring through early summer)
Redtop (*Agrostis alba*)
Brome (*Bromus inermis*)
Orchard grass (*Dactylis glomerata*)
Fescue (*Festuca elatior*)
Ryegrass (*Lolium* sp)
Canary grass (*Phalaris arundinacea*)
Timothy (*Phleum pratense*)
Bluegrass/June grass (*Poa* sp)
Weeds (pollinating season: summer through early fall)
Waterhemp (*Acnida tamariscina*)
Lamb's-quarters (*Chenopodium album*)
Russian thistle (*Salsoal kali*)
Ragweed, giant and short (*Ambrosia* sp)
Marsh elder/poverty weed (*Iva* sp)
Cocklebur (*Xanthium strumarium*)
Dock/sorrel (*Rumex* sp)
Pigweed (*Amaranthus retroflexus*)
Plantain (*Plantago lanceolata*)

Sagebrush (*Artemisia* sp)
Nettle (*Urtica* sp)

Region VIII (Central Midwest)

Illinois, Iowa, Missouri

Trees (pollinating season: late winter through spring)
Box elder/maple (*Acer* sp)
Birch (*Betula nigra*)
Oak (*Quercus* sp)
Hickory (*Carya ovata*)
Walnut (*Juglans nigra*)
Mulberry (*Morus* sp)
Ash (*Fraxinus americana*)
Sycamore (*Platanus occidentalis*)
Cottonwood/poplar (*Populus deltoides*)
Elm (*Ulmus americana*)
Liquid amber (*Liquidambar*)
Cypress (*Cupressus* sp)
Willow (*Salix* sp)
Pine (*Pinus* sp)

Grasses (pollinating season: spring through early summer)
Redtop (*Agrostis alba*)
Bermuda grass (*Cynodon dactylon*)
Orchard grass (*Dactylis glomerata*)
Ryegrass (*Lolium* sp)
Timothy (*Phleum pratense*)
Bluegrass/June grass (*Poa* sp)
Johnson grass (*Sorghum halepense*)
Corn (*Zea mays*)

Weeds (pollinating season: summer through early fall)
Pigweed (*Amaranthus retroflexus*)
Lamb's-quarters (*Chenopodium album*)
Mexican firebush (*Kochia scoparia*)
Russian thistle (*Salsoa kali*)
Ragweed, giant, short, and western (*Ambrosia* sp)
Marsh elder-poverty weed (*Iva* sp)
Plantain (*Plantago lanceolata*)
Dock/sorrel (*Rumex* sp)
Water hemp (*Acnida tamariscina*)
Nettle (*Urtica* sp)

Region IX (Great Plains)

Kansas, Nebraska, North Dakota, South Dakota

Trees (pollinating season: later winter through spring)
Box elder/maple (*Acer* sp)
Alder (*Alnus incana*)
Birch (*Betula* sp)
Hazlenut (*Corylus americana*)
Oak (*Quercus macrocarpa*)
Hickory (*Carya ovata*)
Walnut (*Juglans nigra*)
Ash (*Fraxinus americana*)
Cottonwood/poplar (*Populus deltoides*)
Elm (*Ulmus americana*)
Cypress (*Cupressus* sp)

Grasses (pollinating season: spring through early summer)
Quack grass/wheatgrass (*Agropyron* sp)
Redtop (*Agrostis alba*)
Brome (*Bromus inermis*)
Orchard grass (*Dactylis glomerata*)

Ryegrass (*Elymus* and *Lolium* sp)
Fescue (*Festuca elatior*)
Timothy (*Phleum pratense*)
Bluegrass/June grass (*Poa* sp)
Weeds (pollinating season: summer through early fall)
Water hemp (*Acnida tamariscina*)
Pigweed (*Amaranthus retroflexus*)
Lamb's-quarters (*Chenopodium album*)
Mexican firebush (*Kochia scoparia*)
Russian thistle (*Salsola kali*)
Ragweed, false, giant, short, and western (*Ambrosia* sp)
Sagebrush (*Artemisia* sp)
Marsh elder/poverty weed (*Iva* sp)
Cocklebur (*Xanthium strumarium*)
Plantain (*Plantago lanceolata*)
Dock/sorrel (*Rumex* sp)
Nettle (*Urtica* sp)
Region X (Southwestern Grasslands)
Oklahoma, Texas
Trees (pollinating season: late winter through spring)
Box elder (*Acer negundo*)
Cedar/juniper (*Juniperus virginiana*)
Oak (*Quercus virginiana*)
Mesquite (*Prosopis juliflora*)
Mulberry (*Morus* sp)
Ash (*Fraxinus americana*)
Cottonwood/poplar (*Populus deltoides*)
Elm (*Ulmus americana*)
Birch (*Betula* sp)
Pine (*Pinus* sp)
Cypress (*Cupressus* sp)
Liquid amber (*Liquidambar*)
Hickory (*Carya* sp)
Sycamore (*Platanus* sp)
Grasses (pollinating season: spring through early summer)
Quack grass/wheatgrass (*Agropyron* sp)
Redtop (*Agrostis alba*)
Bermuda grass (*Cynodon dactylon*)
Orchard grass (*Dactylis glomerata*)
Fescue (*Festuca elatior*)
Ryegrass (*Lolium* sp)
Timothy (*Phleum pratense*)
Bluegrass/June grass (*Poa* sp)
Johnson grass (*Sorghum halepense*)
Weeds (pollinating season: summer through early fall)
Water hemp (*Acnida tamariscina*)
Careless weed/pigweed (*Amaranthus* sp)
Saltbush/scale (*Atriplex* sp)
Lamb's-quarters (*Chenopodium album*)
Mexican firebush (*Kochia scoparia*)
Russian thistle (*Salsola kali*)
Ragweed, false, giant, short, and western (*Ambrosia* sp)
Sagebrush (*Artemisia* sp)
Marsh elder/poverty weed (*Iva* sp)
Cocklebur (*Xanthium strumarium*)
Dock/sorrel (*Rumex* sp)
Plantain (*Plantago lanceolata*)
Nettle (*Urtica* sp)

Region XI (Rocky Mountain Empire)
  Arizona (mountainous), Colorado, Idaho (mountainous), Montana, New Mexico, Utah, Wyoming
    Trees (pollinating season: late winter through spring)
      Box elder (*Acer negundo*)
      Alder (*Alnus incana*)
      Birch (*Betula fontinalis*)
      Cedar/juniper (*Juniperus scopulorum*)
      Oak (*Quercus gambelii*)
      Ash (*Fraxinus americana*)
      Pine (*Pinus* sp)
      Cottonwood/poplar (*Populus deltoides, P. sargentii*)
      Elm (*Ulmus* sp)
      Mulberry (*Morus* sp)
      Cypress (*Cupressus* sp)
      Willow (*Salix* sp)
    Grasses (pollinating season: spring through early summer)
      Quack grass/wheatgrass (*Agropyron* sp)
      Redtop (*Agrostis alba*)
      Brome (*Bromus inermis*)
      Bermuda grass (*Cynodon dactylon*)
      Orchard grass (*Dactylis glomerata*)
      Ryegrass (*Elymus* and *Lolium* sp)
      Fescue (*Festuca elatior*)
      Timothy (*Phleum pratense*)
      Bluegrass/June grass (*Poa* sp)
    Weeds (pollinating season: summer through early fall)
      Water hemp (*Acnida tamariscina*)
      Pigweed (*Amaranthus retroflexus*)
      Saltbush/scale (*Atriplex* sp)
      Sugarbeet (*Beta vulgaris*)
      Lamb's-quarters (*Chenopodium album*)
      Mexican firebush (*Kochia scoparia*)
      Russian thistle (*Salsola kali*)
      Ragweed, false, giant, short, and western (*Ambrosia* sp)
      Sagebrush (*Artemisia* sp)
      Marsh elder/poverty weed (*Iva* sp)
      Cocklebur (*Xanthium strumarium*)
      Plantain (*Plantago lanceolata*)
      Dock/sorrel (*Rumex* sp)
Region XII (Arid Southwest)
  Arizona, Southern California (southeastern desert)
    Trees (pollinating season: winter through spring)
      Cypress (*Cupressus arizonica*)
      Cedar/juniper (*Juniperus californica*)
      Mesquite (*Prosopis juliflora*)
      Ash (*Fraxinus velutina*)
      Olive (*Olea europaea*)
      Cottonwood/poplar (*Populus fremontii*)
      Elm (*Ulmus parvifolia*)
    Grasses (pollinating season: spring through early summer)
      Brome (*Bromus* sp)
      Bermuda grass (*Cynodon dactylon*)
      Salt grass (*Distichlis* sp)
      Ryegrass (*Elymus* and *Lolium* sp)
      Canary grass (*Phalaris minor*)
      Bluegrass/June grass (*Poa* sp)
    Weeds (pollinating season: summer through early fall)
      Careless weed (*Amaranthus palmeri*)
      Iodine bush (*Allenrolfea occidentalis*)

Saltbush/scale (*Atriplex* sp)
Lamb's-quarters (*Chenopodium album*)
Russian thistle (*Salsola kali*)
Alkali blite (*Suaeda* sp)
Ragweed, false, slender, and western (*Ambrosia* sp)
Sagebrush (*Artemisia* sp)
Silver ragweed (*Dicoria canescens*)
Burro brush (*Hymenoclea salsola*)

Region XIII (Southern Coastal California)
  Trees (pollinating season: late winter through spring)
    Box elder (*Acer negundo*)
    Cypress (*Cupressus arizonica*)
    Oak (*Quercus agrifolia*)
    Walnut (*Juglans* sp)
    Acacia (*Acacia* sp)
    Mulberry (*Morus* sp)
    Eucalyptus (*Eucalyptus* sp)
    Ash (*Fraxinus velutina*)
    Olive (*Olea europaea*)
    Sycamore (*Platanus racemosa*)
    Cottonwood/poplar (*Populus trichocarpa*)
    Elm (*Ulmus* sp)
    Pine (*Pinus* sp)
    Alder (*Alnus* sp)
  Grasses (pollinating season: spring through early summer)
    Oats (*Avena* sp)
    Brome (*Bromus* sp)
    Bermuda grass (*Cynodon dactylon*)
    Orchard grass (*Dactylis glomerata*)
    Salt grass (*Distichlis* sp)
    Ryegrass (*Elymus* and *Lolium* sp)
    Fescue (*Festuca elatior*)
    Bluegrass/June grass (*Poa* sp)
    Johnson grass (*Sorghum halepense*)
  Weeds (pollinating season: summer through early fall)
    Careless weed/pigweed (*Amaranthus* sp)
    Saltbush/scale (*Atriplex* sp)
    Lamb's-quarters (*Chenopodium album*)
    Russian thistle (*Salsola kali*)
    Ragweed, false, slender, and western (*Ambrosia* sp)
    Sagebrush (*Artemisia* sp)
    Cocklebur (*Xanthium strumarium*)
    Plantain (*Plantago lanceolata*)
    Dock/sorrel (*Rumex* sp)

Region XIV (Central California Valley)
  Sacramento Valley, San Joaquin Valley
    Trees (pollinating season: late winter though spring)
      Box elder (*Acer negundo*)
      Alder (*Alnus rhombifolia*)
      Birch (*Betula fontinalis*)
      Cypress (*Cupressus arizonica*)
      Oak (*Quercus lobata*)
      Pecan (*Carya pecan*)
      Walnut (*Juglans* sp)
      Ash (*Fraxinus velutina*)
      Olive (*Olea europaea*)
      Sycamore (*Platanus acerifolia*)
      Cottonwood/poplar (*Populus fremontii*)
      Elm (*Ulmus* sp)
      Mulberry (*Morus* sp)

Pine (*Pinus* sp)
Hickory (*Carya* sp)
Liquid amber (*Liquidambar*)
Grasses (pollinating season: spring through early summer)
Redtop (*Agrostis alba*)
Oats (*Avena* sp)
Brome (*Bromus* sp)
Bermuda grass (*Cynodon dactylon*)
Orchard grass (*Dactylis glomerata*)
Salt grass (*Distichlis* sp)
Ryegrass (*Elymus* and *Lolium* sp)
Fescue (*Festuca elatior*)
Canary grass (*Phalaris minor*)
Timothy (*Phleum pratense*)
Bluegrass/June grass (*Poa* sp)
Johnson grass (*Sorghum halepense*)
Weeds (pollinating season: summer through early fall)
Pigweed (*Amaranthus retroflexus*)
Saltbush/scale (*Atriplex* sp)
Sugarbeet (*Beta vulgaris*)
Lamb's-quarters (*Chenopodium album*)
Russian thistle (*Salsola kali*)
Ragweed, false, slender, and western (*Ambrosia* sp)
Sagebrush (*Artemisia* sp)
Cocklebur (*Xanthium strumarium*)
Plantain (*Plantago lanceolata*)
Dock/sorrel (*Rumex* sp)
Sedge (*Cyperacus* sp)
Nettle (*Urtica* sp)
Region XV (Intermountain West)
Idaho (southern), Nevada
Trees (pollinating season: late winter through spring)
Box elder (*Acer negundo*)
Alder (*Alnus incana*)
Birch (*Betula fortinalis*)
Cedar/juniper (*Juniperus utahensis*)
Ash (*Fraxinus americana*)
Sycamore (*Platanus occidentalis*)
Cottonwood/poplar (*Populus trichocarpa*)
Elm (*Ulmus* sp)
Mulberry (*Morus* sp)
Oak (*Quercus* sp)
Pine (*Pinus* sp)
Cypress (*Cupressus* sp)
Grasses (pollinating season: spring through early summer)
Quack grass/wheatgrass (*Agropyron* sp)
Redtop (*Agrostis alba*)
Brome (*Bromus inermis*)
Bermuda grass (*Cynodon dactylon*)
Orchard grass (*Dactylis glomerata*)
Salt grass (*Distichlis* sp)
Ryegrass (*Elymus* and *Lolium* sp)
Fescue (*Festuca elatior*)
Timothy (*Phleum pratense*)
Bluegrass/June grass (*Poa* sp)
Weeds (pollinating season: summer through early fall)
Pigweed (*Amaranthus retroflexus*)
Iodine bush (*Allenrolfea occidentalis*)
Saltbush/scale (*Atriplex* sp)
Lamb's-quarters (*Chenopodium album*)

Mexican firebush (*Kochia scoparia*)
Russian thistle (*Salsola kali*)
Ragweed, false, slender, and western (*Ambrosia* sp)
Sagebrush (*Artemisia* sp)
Marsh elder/poverty weed (*Iva* sp)
Cocklebur (*Xanthium strumarium*)
Plantain (*Plantago lanceolata*)
Dock/sorrel (*Rumex* sp)

Region XVI (Inland Empire)
  Oregon (central and eastern), Washington (central and eastern)
    Tree (pollinating season: late winter through spring)
      Box elder (*Acer negundo*)
      Alder (*Alnus incana*)
      Birch (*Betula fontinalis*)
      Oak (*Quercus garryana*)
      Walnut (*Juglans nigra*)
      Pine (*Pinus* sp)
      Cottonwood/poplar (*Populus trichocarpa*)
      Willow (*Salix lasiandra*)
    Grasses (pollinating season: spring through early summer)
      Quack grass/wheatgrass (*Agropyron* sp)
      Redtop (*Agrostis alba*)
      Vernal grass (*Anthoxanthum* sp)
      Brome (*Bromus inermis*)
      Orchard grass (*Dactylis glomerata*)
      Ryegrass (*Elymus* and *Lolium* sp)
      Velvet grass (*Holcus lanatus*)
      Timothy (*Phleum pratense*)
      Bluegrass/June grass (*Poa* sp)
    Weeds (pollinating season: summer through early fall)
      Pigweed (*Amaranthus retroflexus*)
      Saltbush/scale (*Atriplex* sp)
      Lamb's-quarters (*Chenopodium album*)
      Mexican firebush (*Kochia scoparia*)
      Russian thistle (*Salsola kali*)
      Ragweed, false, giant, short, and western (*Ambrosia* sp)
      Sagebrush (*Artemisia* sp)
      Marsh elder/poverty weed (*Iva* sp)
      Plantain (*Plantago lanceolata*)
      Dock/sorrel (*Rumex* sp)

Region XVII (Cascade Pacific Northwest)
  California (northwestern), Oregon (western), Washington (western)
    Trees (pollinating season: late winter through spring)
      Box elder (*Acer negundo*)
      Alder (*Alnus rhombifolia*)
      Birch (*Betula fontanalis*)
      Hazelnut (*Corylus cornuta*)
      Oak (*Quercus garryana*)
      Walnut (*Juglans regia*)
      Ash (*Fraxinus oregona*)
      Cottonwood (*Populus trichocarpa*)
      Willow (*Salix lasiandra*)
      Elm (*Ulmus pumila*)
      Cypress (*Cupressus* sp)
      Sycamore (*Platanus* sp)
      Pine (*Pinus* sp)
    Grasses (pollinating season: spring through early summer)
      Bent grass (*Agrostis maritima*)
      Sweet vernal grass (*Anthoxanthum* sp)
      Oats (*Avena* sp)

Brome (*Bromus inermis*)
Bermuda grass (*Cynodon dactylon*)
Orchard grass (*Dactylis glomerata*)
Salt grass (*Distichlis* sp)
Ryegrass (*Elymus* and *Lolium* sp)
Fescue (*Festuca elatior*)
Velvet grass (*Holcus lanatus*)
Canary grass (*Phalaris arundinacea*)
Timothy (*Phleum pratense*)
Bluegrass/June grass (*Poa* sp)
Weeds (pollinating season: summer through early fall)
Pigweed (*Amaranthus retroflexus*)
Saltbush/scale (*Atriplex* sp)
Lamb's-quarters (*Chenopodium album*)
Russian thistle (*Salsola kali*)
Ragweed, false, giant, short, and western (*Ambrosia* sp)
Sagebrush (*Artemisia* sp)
Cocklebur (*Xanthium strumarium*)
Plantain (*Plantago lanceolata*)
Dock/sorrel (*Rumex* sp)
Nettle (*Urtica* sp)
Region C-I (Atlantic Provinces and Quebec)
New Brunswick, Newfoundland, Nova Scotia, Prince Edward Island, Quebec
Trees (pollinating season: late winter through spring)
Box elder (*Acer negundo*)
Hard maple (sugar) (*Acer saccharum*)
Tag alder (speckled) (*Alnus incana*)
Paper birch (white) (*Betula papyrifera*)
Beech (*Fagus grandifolia*)
White ash (*Fraxinus americana*)
Green ash (*Fraxinus pennsylvanica*)
Butternut (*Juglans cinerea*)
Sycamore (*Planatus occidentalis*)
Balsam poplar (*Populus balsamifera*)
Trembling aspen (*Populus tremuloides*)
Bur oak (*Quercus macrocarpa*)
Black willow (*Salix nigra*)
American elm (*Ulmus americana*)
Grasses (pollinating season: spring through early summer)
Quack grass (*Agropyron repens*)
Redtop (*Agrostis alba*)
Brome (*Bromus* sp)
Orchard grass (*Dactylis glomerata*)
Ryegrass (*Elymus* and *Lolium* sp)
Timothy (*Phleum pratense*)
Bluegrass (*Poa* sp)
Weeds (pollinating season: summer through early fall)
Pigweed (*Amaranthus retroflexus*)
Ragweed (*Ambrosia* sp)
Lamb's-quarters (*Chenopodium album*)
Plantain (*Plantago lanceolata*)
Dock/sorrel (*Rumex* sp)
Russian thistle (*Salsola kali*)
Region C-II (Ontario)
Trees (pollinating season: late winter through spring)
Box elder (*Acer negundo*)
Hard maple (sugar) (*Acer saccharum*)
Tag alder (speckled) (*Alnus incana*)
Paper birch (white) (*Betula papyrifera*)
Beech (*Fagus grandifolia*)

White ash (*Fraxinus americana*)
Green ash (*Fraxinus pennsylvanica*)
Butternut (*Juglans cinerea*)
Sycamore (*Platanus occidentalis*)
Balsam poplar (*Populus balsamifera*)
Aspen (*Populus tremuloides*)
Bur oak (*Quercus macrocarpa*)
Black willow (*Salix nigra*)
American elm (white) (*Ulmus americana*)
Chinese elm (Siberian) (*Ulmus pumila*)

Grasses (pollinating season: spring through early summer)
Quack grass (*Agropyron repens*)
Redtop (*Agrostis alba*)
Brome (*Bromus* sp)
Orchard grass (*Dactylis glomerata*)
Ryegrass (*Elymus* and *Lolium* sp)
Timothy (*Phleum pratense*)
Bluegrass (*Poa* sp)

Weeds (pollinating season: summer through early fall)
Pigweed (*Amaranthus retroflexus*)
Ragweed (*Ambrosia* sp)
Lamb's-quarters (*Chenopodium album*)
English plantain (*Plantago lanceolata*)
Dock/sorrel (*Rumex* sp)
Russian thistle (*Salsola kali*)

Region C-III (Prairie Provinces and Eastern British Columbia)
Alberta, British Columbia (eastern), Manitoba, Saskatchewan

Trees (pollinating season: late winter through spring)
Box elder (*Acer negundo*)
Tag alder (speckled or mountain) (*Alnus incana*)
Paper birch (white) (*Betula papyrifera*)
Green ash (*Fraxinus pennsylvanica*)
Balsam poplar (*Populus balsamifera*)
Trembling aspen (*Populus tremuloides*)
Bur oak (*Quercus macrocarpa*)
Willow (yellow) (*Salix* sp)
Chinese elm (Siberian) (*Ulmus pumila*)

Grasses (pollinating season: spring through early summer)
Quack grass/wheatgrass (*Agropyron* sp)
Redtop (*Agrostis alba*)
Common wild oats (*Avena fatua*)
Brome (*Bromus* sp)
Orchard grass (*Dactylis glomerata*)
Ryegrass (*Elymus* and *Lolium* sp)
Timothy (*Phleum pratense*)
Bluegrass (*Poa* sp)

Weeds (pollinating season: summer through early fall)
Pigweed (*Amaranthus retroflexus*)
Ragweed (*Ambrosia* sp)
Lamb's-quarters (*Chenopodium album*)
Sagebrush (*Artemisia* sp)
Marshelder/poverty weed (*Iva* sp)
English plantain (*Plantago lanceolata*)
Dock/sorrel (*Rumex* sp)
Russian thistle (*Salsola kali*)

Region C-IV (Western British Columbia and Vancouver Island)
Trees (pollinating season: late winter through spring)
Box elder (*Acer negundo*)
Red alder (*Alnus rubra*)
Sitka alder (*Alnus sinuata*)

Paper birch (white) (*Betula papyrifera*)
Sycamore (*Platanus occidentalis*)
Black cottonwood (*Populus trichocarpa*)
Trembling aspen (*Populus tremuloides*)
Douglas fir (*Pseudotsuga menziesii*)
Garry's oak (*Quercus garryana*)
Yellow willow (Pacific) (*Salix lasiandra*)
Chinese elm (Siberian) (*Ulmus pumila*)
Grasses (pollinating season: spring through early summer)
Quack grass (*Agropyron repens*)
Redtop (*Agrostis alba*)
Tall oats grass (*Arrhenatherum elatius*)
Common wild oats (*Avena fatua*)
Brome (*Bromus* sp)
Orchard grass (*Dactylis glomerata*)
Ryegrass (*Elymus* and *Lolium* sp)
Timothy (*Phleum pratense*)
Bluegrass (*Poa* sp)
Weeds (pollinating season: summer through early fall)
Pigweed (*Amaranthus retroflexus*)
Ragweed (*Ambrosia* sp)
Lamb's-quarters (*Chenopodium album*)
Marshelder/poverty weed (*Iva* sp)
English plantain (*Plantago lanceolata*)
Dock/sorrel (*Rumex* sp)
Russian thistle (*Salsola kali*)
Alaska
Trees (pollinating season: spring)
Alder (*Alnus incana*)
Aspen (*Populus tremuloides*)
Birch (*Betula papyrifera*)
Cedar (*Thuja plicata*)
Hemlock (*Tsuga hetrophylla*)
Pine (*Pinus contorta*)
Balsam poplar (*Populus balsamifera*)
Spruce (*Picea sitchensis*)
Willow (*Salix* sp)
Grasses (pollinating season: late spring and summer)
Bluegrass/June grass (*Poa* sp)
Brome (*Bromus inermis*)
Canary grass (*Phalaris arundinacea*)
Fescue (*Festuca rubra*)
Orchard grass (*Dactylis glomerata*)
Quack grass/wheatgrass (*Agropyron* sp)
Redtop (*Agrostis alba*)
Ryegrass (*Lolium perenne*)
Timothy (*Phleum pratense*)
Weeds (pollinating season: summer)
Bulrush (*Scirpus* sp)
Dock/sorrel (*Rumex* sp)
Lamb's-quarters (*Chenopodium album*)
Nettle (*Urtica dioica*)
Plantain (*Plantago lanceolata*)
Sagebrush/wormwood (*Artemisia* sp)
Sedge (*Carex* sp)
Spearscale (*Atriplex patula*)
Hawaii (all islands) (pollinating season: less defined than for continental regions)
Trees
Acacia (*Acacia* sp)
Australian pine (beefwood) (*Casuarina equisetifolia*)

Cedar/juniper (*Juniperus* sp)
Monterey cypress (*Cupressus macrocarpa*)
Date palm (*Phoenix dactylifera*)
Eucalyptus (gum) (*Eucalyptus globulus*)
Mesquite (*Prosopis juliflora*)
Paper mulberry (*Broussonetia papyrifera*)
Olive (*Olea europaea*)
Privet (*Ligustrum* sp)
Grasses
Bermuda grass (*Cynodon dactylon*)
Corn (*Zea mays*)
Finger grass (*Chloris* sp)
Johnson grass (*Sorghum halepense*)
Love grass (*Eragrostis* sp)
Bluegrass/June grass (*Poa* sp)
Redtop (*Agrostis alba*)
Sorghum (*Sorghum vulgare*)
Weeds
Cocklebur (*Xanthium strumarium*)
Plantain (*Plantago lanceolata*)
Kochia (*Kochia scoparia*)
Pigweed (*Amaranthus* sp)
Ragweed, slender (*Ambrosia* sp)
Sagebrush (*Artemisia* sp)
Scale (saltbush) (*Atriplex* sp)

B. Incidence of Individual Molds in the United States[a]

Type of mold	Northeast[b] Indoor (%)	Outdoor (%)	Southeast[c] Indoor (%)	Outdoor (%)	Central[d] Indoor (%)	Outdoor (%)
Cladmosporium (Hormodendrum)	56.7	66.8	66.8	96.5	63.3	81.8
Penicillium	37.0	25.1	31.5	22.8	30.1	27.3
Alternaria	23.4	48.2	18.0	54.3	39.1	72.3
Aspergillus	20.0	7.3	14.7	7.9	16.0	6.3
Pullularia	9.5	19.6	5.4	10.5	4.1	9.1
Geotrichum	11.5	5.5	19.4	8.8	6.1	3.4
Fomes	7.1	16.3	5.8	8.8	5.0	18.2
Epicoccum	6.1	12.6	7.0	20.2	4.1	6.8
Fusarium	5.7	15.1	7.0	21.9	6.4	17.6
Sterile Mycelia	5.4	12.3	10.3	12.3	8.1	8.5
Phoma	2.8	12.3	1.4	8.8	3.1	9.7
Rhodotorula	5.3	3.3	4.0		1.7	2.3
Cephalosporium	4.6	9.8	7.2	11.4	3.7	7.4
Stemphylium	4.0	2.5	2.1	3.5	4.0	
Streptomyces	2.4	7.8		8.8	1.2	13.6
Botrytis	3.9	5.0		6.1		
Mucor		7.5	2.8	9.6	1.2	6.3
Poria	3.8	2.8	1.9		2.7	1.7
Trichoderma	2.1	5.0		7.0	2.3	4.0
Helminthosporium	3.6	3.5	5.8	10.5	1.8	4.0
Tetracoccosporium		2.3				
Sporobolomyces	3.1	1.5	1.2		2.0	1.7
Rhodosporium				1.8		
Polyporaceae	1.5					1.7
Curvularia			4.9	6.1		
Nigrospora				1.8		
Rhizopus				1.8	2.3	1.7
Spondylocladium						
Verticillium						
Fusidium						
Chaetomium						
Acremonium						
Monosporium						
Unidentified yeast						
Polyporus						
Pleospora						

[a] Expressed as the percentage of total exposures when a given fungal genus was recovered.
[b] Delaware, Maryland, Connecticut, Massachusetts, New Jersey, Pennsylvania, New York, Maine, New Hampshire, Rhode Island, and Vermont.
[c] Florida, Georgia, South Carolina, North Carolina, West Virginia, Virginia, Kentucky, Alabama, Arkansas, Louisiana, and Tennessee.
[d] Ohio, Michigan, Wisconsin, Minnesota, Illinois, Missouri, Iowa, and Indiana.
From *The Role of Molds in Allergy*. Spokane, WA: Hollister-Stier Laboratories, 1977.

South Central[e]		Northwest[f]		Southwest[g]		West[h]	
Indoor (%)	Outdoor (%)	Indoor (%)	Outdoor (%)	Indoor (%)	Outdoor (%)	Indoor (%)	Outdoor (%)
78.6	92.9	62.5	69.6	63.8	93.0	74.5	68.4
25.2	32.1	41.4	40.6	31.9	35.7	35.1	35.9
41.7	85.7	21.1	27.5	42.6	64.3	39.7	47.0
21.3	17.9	15.1	8.7	4.3	7.1	10.1	11.1
1.9		8.0	11.6	6.4	7.1	6.3	12.8
13.6	3.6	6.8	2.9	6.4		2.9	
		2.0	1.4			1.7	5.1
11.7	10.7	2.0	4.3		7.1	16.6	17.1
5.8	46.6	1.2	10.1	4.3	21.4	4.0	11.1
23.3	25.0	4.0	15.9	4.3		7.7	3.4
	7.1	4.8	10.1	6.4	28.6	2.9	8.5
		2.8	7.2	2.1	7.1	2.2	
5.8	21.4	5.2	5.8	4.3	7.1	7.2	4.3
6.8		5.6	11.6	19.1	21.4	10.1	10.3
1.9	17.9	6.8	17.4		35.7	2.9	13.7
		2.4		2.1		4.3	9.4
		3.2	8.7	2.1		3.4	9.4
		1.2	2.9				
		5.2	13.0	2.1			1.7
28.2	25.0	3.6		6.4	14.3	6.3	8.5
		1.2		6.4		1.4	
	32.1	1.6					1.7
4.9	10.7			2.1			
1.9		2.4		6.4	7.1	3.1	5.1
1.9							
	3.6						2.6
	3.6						
			1.4				
				2.1			
				2.1			
					14.3		
						1.2	1.2
							5.1

[e] Oklahoma and Texas.
[f] Nevada, New Mexico, Idaho, Colorado, Montana, and Utah.
[g] California.
[h] Oregon and Washington.

A. Normal Pulmonary Function in Men

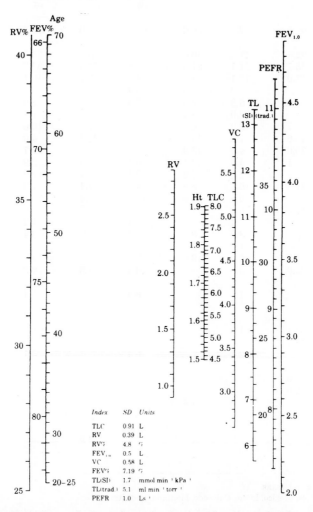

FIG. VII.A. Nomogram relating indices of pulmonary function to height and age for healthy adult men. Ht, height in meters; TLC, total lung capacity; RV, residual volume; RV%, percentage residual volume (RV/TLC × 100); FEV$_{1.0}$, forced expiratory volume in 1 second; VC, vital capacity; FEV%, percentage expired (FEV$_{1.0}$/FVC × 100); TL(SI), transfer factor of gas exchange (international system of measurement); TL (trad.), transfer factor of gas exchange (traditional system of measurement); PEF, peak expiratory flow; SD, standard deviation. The RV% and the FEV% are related only to age, and the TLC only to height. From Cotes JE. Lung function at different stages in Life. In: *Lung function.* London: Blackwell, 1975, with permission.

B. Normal Pulmonary Function in Women

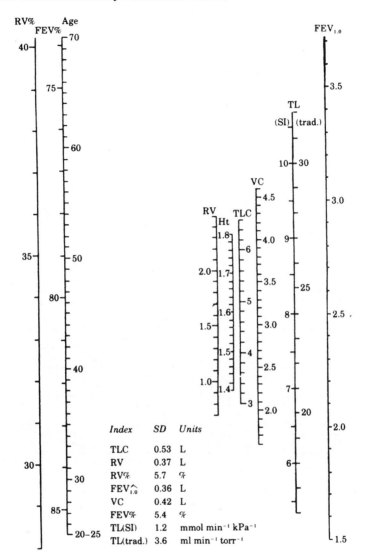

FIG. VII.B. Nomogram relating indices of lung function to height and age for healthy adult women. Ht, height in meters; TLC, total lung capacity; RV, residual volume; RV%, percentage residual volume (RV/TLC × 100); $FEV_{1.0}$, forced expiratory volume in 1 second; VC, vital capacity; FEV%, percentage expired ($FEV_{1.0}$/FVC × 100); TL(SI), transfer factor of gas exchange (international system of measurement); TL (trad.), transfer factor of gas exchange (traditional system of measurement); PEF, peak expiratory flow; SD, standard deviation. The RV% and the FEV% are related only to age, and the TLC only to height. From Cotes JE. Lung function at different stages in Life. In: *Lung function.* London: Blackwell, 1975, with permission.

C. Normal Lung Volumes for Male Children
(function of height in centimeters)

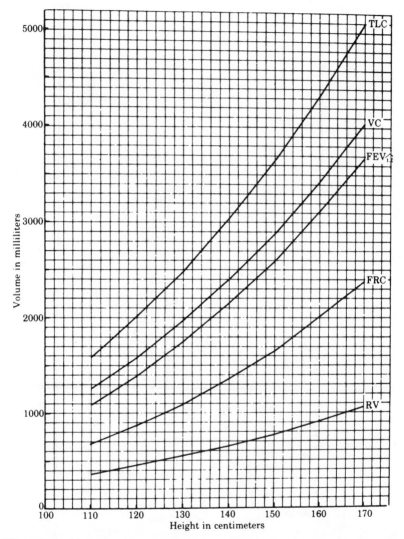

FIG. VII.C. TLC, total lung capacity; VC, vital capacity; FEV$_{1.0}$, forced expiratory volume in 1 second; FRC, functional residual capacity; RV, residual volume. From Polgar G, Promadhat V. Standard values. In: *Pulmonary function testing in children: techniques and standards.* Philadelphia: WB Saunders, 1971, with permission.

D. Normal Lung Volumes for Female Children
(function of height in centimeters)

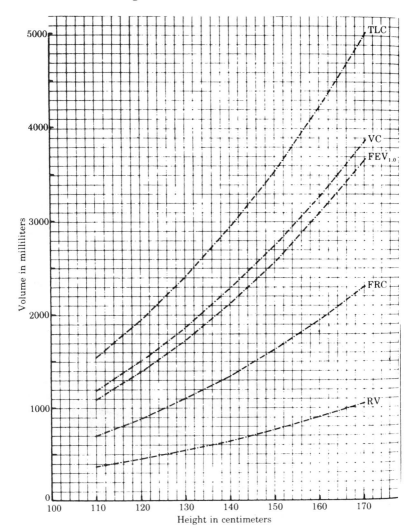

FIG. VII.D.   TLC, total lung capacity; VC, vital capacity; $FEV_{1.0}$, forced expiratory volume in 1 second; FRC, functional residual capacity; RV, residual volume. From Polgar G, Promadhat V. Standard values. In: *Pulmonary function testing in children: techniques and standards.* Philadelphia: WB Saunders, 1971, with permission.

E. Normal Pulmonary Flow Rates for Male and Female Children (function of height in centimeters)

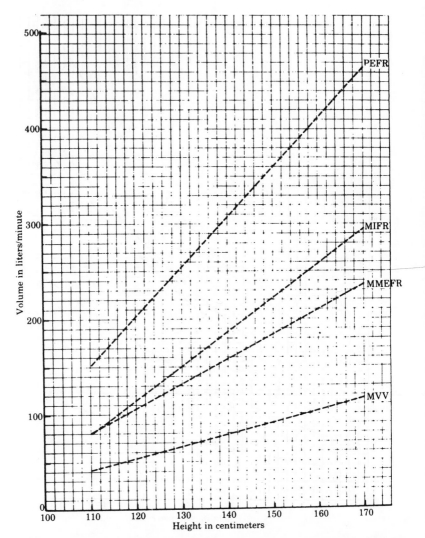

FIG. VII.E. PEF, peak expiratory flow; MIFR, maximal inspiratory flow rate; MMEFR, maximal midexpiratory flow rate; MVV, maximal voluntary ventilation. From Polgar G, Promadhat V. Standard values. In: *Pulmonary function testing in children: techniques and standards.* Philadelphia: WB Saunders, 1971, with permission.

A. Prediction Equation for Arterial Po$_2$ (P$_a$O$_2$)*

$P_aO_2 = 100 - 0.43 \times$ age (years) ± 4.1 standard deviation (SD)

B. Normal Oxygen Dissociation Curves in Humans (pH-dependent at 37°C)

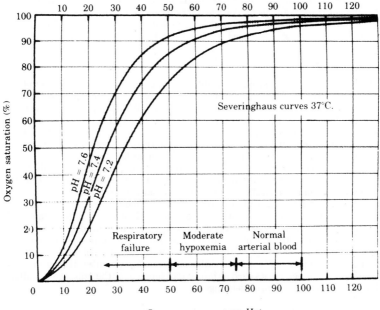

FIG. VIII.1. From Filley GF. Oxygenation and the arterial Po$_2$. In: *Acid-base and blood gas regulation.* Philadelphia: Lea & Febiger, 1971, with permission.

* At sea level; assumes PaCo$_2$ = 38 to 42 mm Hg.

Appendix IX. GROWTH CHARTS

The National Center for Health Statistics (NCHS) has prepared percentiles for assessing physical growth of children in the United States. The NCHS percentiles are based on accurate measurements made on large, nationally representative samples of children. Several groups of experts in physical growth, pediatrics, and clinical nutrition identified the need for new reference data and agreed on the appropriateness of the data used to generate the NCHS percentiles. Seven NCHS percentiles (5th, 10th, 25th, 50th, 75th, 90th, and 95th) are available for two age intervals: birth to 36 months and 2 to 18 years. For the younger age interval, percentiles are presented for body weight for age, length for age, weight for length, and head circumference for age (**A–D**). Data used in generating these percentiles are from the Fels Research Institute, Yellow Springs, Ohio. For the 2- to 18-years age interval, body weight for age and stature for age percentiles are presented (**E** and **F**).

The NCHS percentiles provide reliable reference data for assessment of physical growth. Comparison of the measurements for an individual child against NCHS percentiles indicates where the child ranks relative to all contemporary children in the United States of the same age and sex. Measurements outside the extreme percentiles may be indicative of health or nutritional problems sufficiently severe to affect growth. However, measurements within the central or intermediate percentiles are indicative that growth is within normal limits by current standards.

Use of the NCHS percentiles results in accurate anthropomorphic classification of a child only if the measurement technique is the same as that used to obtain the reference data. Key points regarding the birth to 36 months interval are that body weight should be measured with the infant nude, and length should be measured in the recumbent position. For the 2- to 18-years interval, the child may wear light garments during measurement of body weight, and upright stature is measured in stocking feet. It is necessary to know the age of the child for proper interpretation of measurements. However, weight for stature percentiles are assumed to be independent of age before pubescence and are applicable to most children before, but not after, the appearance of secondary sex characteristics such as breast development or the presence of axillary or pubic hair, regardless of chronologic age.

A. National Center for Health Statistics Percentiles for Length and Weight for Age, Boys, Birth to 36 Months

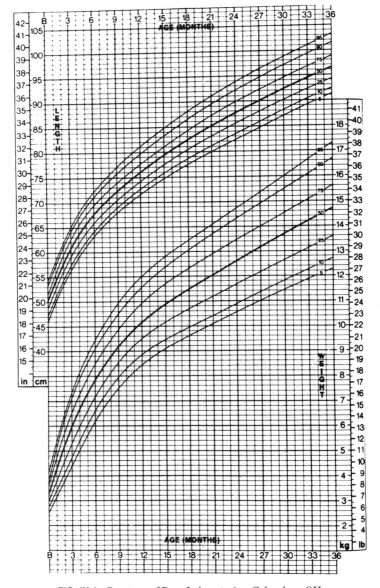

FIG. IX.1. Courtesy of Ross Laboratories, Columbus, OH.

B. National Center for Health Statistics Percentiles for Weight for Length, Boys, Less Than 4 Years, and for Head Circumference, Boys, Birth to 36 Months

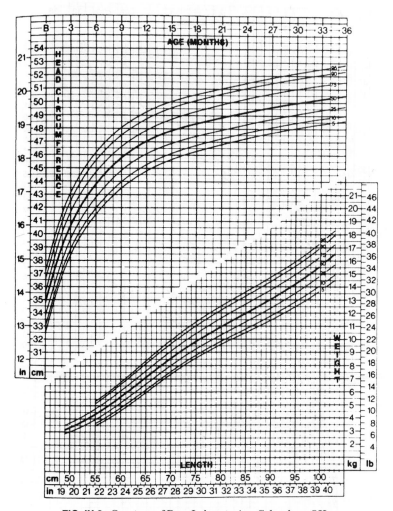

FIG. IX.2. Courtesy of Ross Laboratories, Columbus, OH.

C. National Center for Health Statistics Percentiles for Length and Weight for Age, Girls, Birth to 36 Months

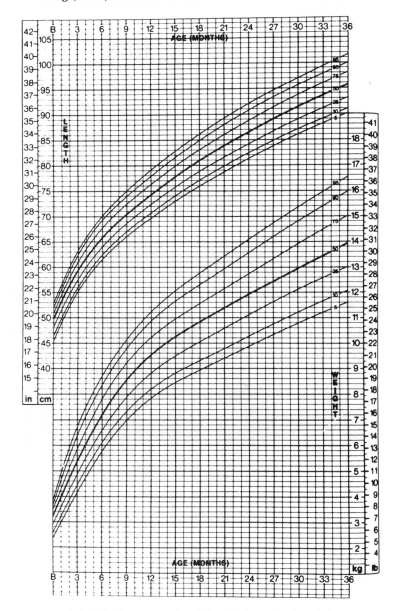

FIG. IX.3. Courtesy of Ross Laboratories, Columbus, OH.

D. National Center for Health Statistics Percentiles for Weight for Length, Girls, Less Than 4 Years, and for Head Circumference, Girls, Birth to 36 Months

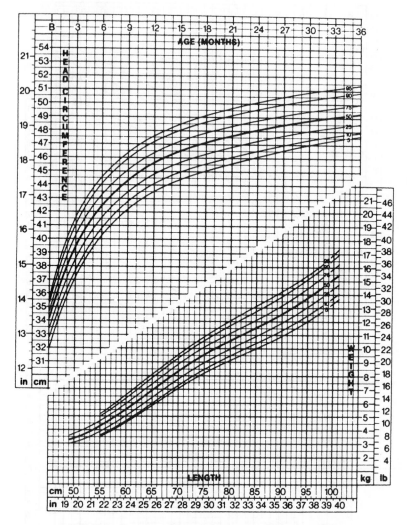

FIG. IX.4. Courtesy of Ross Laboratories, Columbus, OH.

E. National Center for Health Statistics Percentiles for Stature and Weight for Age, Boys, 2 to 18 Years

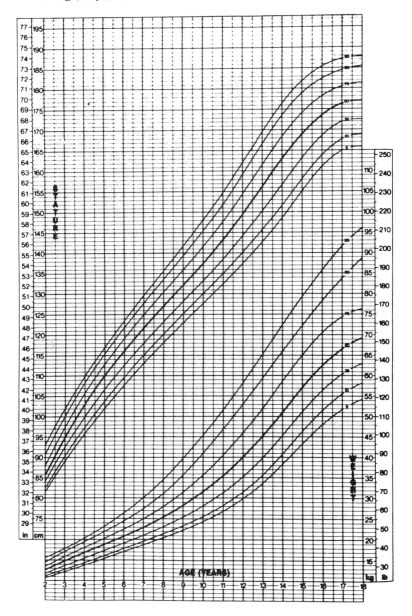

FIG. IX.5. Courtesy of Ross Laboratories, Columbus, OH.

F. National Center for Health Statistics Percentiles for Stature and Weight for Age, Girls, 2 to 18 Years

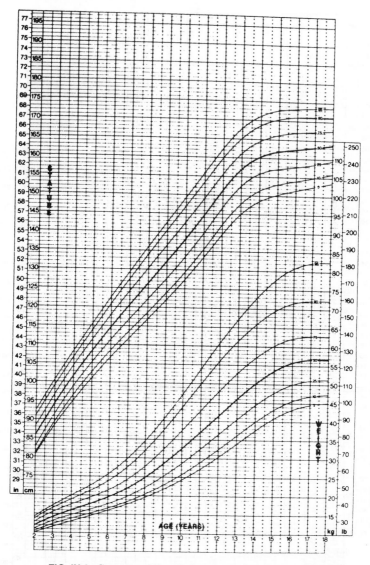

FIG. IX.6. Courtesy of Ross Laboratories, Columbus, OH.

Appendix X. **GLUTEN-FREE DIET**

This diet excludes all products containing gluten. Gluten is in wheat, rye, oats, and barley. These grains and products containing these grains must be omitted from the diet. Gluten may also be present as an incidental ingredient. **It is important to read all labels.** Omit any food or seasoning that lists the following as ingredients: hydrolyzed vegetable protein; flour or cereal products; vegetable protein; malt and malt flavorings; and starch, unless specified as corn or other allowed starch. Flavorings, vegetable gum, emulsifiers, and stabilizers may be derived from or contain wheat, rye, oats, or barley. Foods of unknown composition should be omitted or the manufacturer contacted for complete ingredient information. When dining out, choose foods prepared simply, such as broiled or roasted meats, plain vegetables, and plain salads. Because flour and cereal products are often used in the preparation of foods, it is important to be aware of the methods of preparation as well as the foods themselves. For this reason, all breaded, creamed, or escalloped foods, meatloaf, and gravies are omitted. If these foods are prepared at home using the allowed grains and flours, however, they may be consumed.

Types and amounts of food	Include	Omit
Soups As desired	Homemade broth and un-thickened vegetable soups Cream soups prepared with cream, cornstarch, rice, potato, or soybean flour	Noodle soup, canned soups,[a] bouillon, dehydrated soup mixes
Meat and meat substitutes Three or more servings	Fresh meat, poultry, seafood, plain un-breaded frozen meats, fish, poultry Fish, canned in oil or brine Swiss cheese, cream cheese, cheddar cheese, Parmesan cheese, pure peanut butter, plain dried beans or peas Eggs	Prepared meats that contain wheat, rye, oats, or barley, such as sausage,[a] wieners,[a] bologna,[a] luncheon meats,[a] chili,[a] meatloaf,[a] hamburger with cereal filler,[a] sandwich spreads,[a] pasteurized cheese spreads[a] Canned baked beans[a] Soufflés unless prepared with allowed flours Cottage cheese[a]
Potato and potato substitutes One or more servings	White potato, sweet potato, yams, rice, hominy	Creamed or escalloped potatoes unless pre-pared with allowed flours Macaroni, noodles, spaghetti, lasagna, vermicelli Commercial potato salad,[a] packaged rice mixes[a]
Vegetables One or more servings	All plain, fresh, canned (Include a dark-green or deep-yellow vegetable daily for a source of vitamin A)	Breaded, creamed, or escalloped vegetables unless prepared with allowed flours Commercially prepared vegetables or salads[a]
Breads Three or more servings	Bread or muffins made from: rice flour, corn-starch, tapioca flour, potato flour, soybean flour, and/or arrowroot flour Rice wafers or sticks (usually available at Oriental specialty stores) Pure corn meal tortillas, gluten-free bread mix	All bread and bread prod-ucts containing wheat, rye, barley, oats, bran, or graham, wheat germ, malt, millet, kasha, or bulgar All crackers, Ry-Krisp, rusks, zwieback, pretzels Bread or cracker crumbs Wheat starch

Types and amounts of food	Include	Omit
Cereals 　One or more 　　servings	Only puffed rice, pure corn meal, rice, hominy grits or hominy, cream of rice, Kellog's Puffed Rice, Post's Rice Krinkles, Nabisco Rice Honeys	Snack cereal foods, bran cereals, cream of wheat, farina, Grapenuts, oatmeal, shredded wheat, Ralston, wheatena, pablum, wheat germ, buckwheat, Rice Krispies, corn flakes[a] Cereals with malt added
Fats 　As desired	Butter, cream, margarine, vegetable oil, vegetable shortening, animal fat, pure mayonnaise, home-made salad dressings and gravies prepared with allowed ingredients Bacon	Commercially prepared salad dressings and gravies containing gluten stabilizers or thickened with gluten-containing flours[a] Nondairy creamers
Fruits 　Two or more 　　servings	Fresh, frozen, canned or dried fruits and fruit juices (Include one serving citrus fruit or juice daily for a source of Vitamin C)	Fruits prepared with wheat, rye, oats, or barley
Desserts 　As desired	Homemade cakes, cookies, pastries, pies, puddings (cornstarch, rice, tapioca) prepared with allowed ingredients Gelatin desserts, meringues, custard, fruit ices, whips	Commercial cakes, cookies, pies, doughnuts, pastries, puddings, pie crust, ice cream cones, prepared mixes containing wheat, rye, oats, or barley Icing mixes, ice cream and sherbet containing gluten stabilizers[a]
Milk 　Two or more cups	Fresh, dry, evaporated, or condensed milk, sweet or sour cream	Malted milk, some commercial chocolate drinks, yogurt[a] Ovaltine
Beverages 　As desired	Sanka, instant coffee, coffee, tea, carbonated beverages, fruit juices (fresh or frozen), pure cocoa powder, frozen lemonade concentrate	Fruit punch powders, cocoa powders, ale, beer, gin, whiskey, root beer, Postum, instant coffee[a]

continued

Types and amounts of food	Include	Omit
Miscellaneous As desired	Salt (iodized), sugar, honey, jelly, jam, molasses, pure cocoa, coconut, olives, pure fruit syrup, herbs, extracts, food coloring, cloves, ginger, nutmeg, cinnamon, cornstarch, yeast, sodium bicarbonate, cream of tartar, nuts, dry mustard, monosodium glutamate, cider vinegar, wine vinegar, pure chili pepper	Chili seasoning mix, gravy extracts, starch,[a] malt, natural flavoring (may contain malt), hydrolyzed vegetable protein,[a] chewing gum,[a] catsup,[a] mustard,[a] soy sauce,[a] curry powder,[a] horseradish, vegetable gum Emulsifiers and stabilizers[a] may be derived from or contain wheat, rye, oats, or barley Vinegar,[a] distilled vinegar, malt vinegar Pickles[a] Chili powder[a]

[a] Some may be used if checked with manufacturer and found to be gluten-free.

Appendix XI. ANTIBODIES REACTIVE TO HUMAN TISSUE USED IN MEDICAL DIAGNOSIS[a]

Antibody	Antigen	Interpretation
Acetylcholine receptor-binding antibody	Antibody directed to acetylcholine receptors at neuromuscular junctions of skeletal muscle	Elevated in myasthenia gravis
Acetylcholine receptor-blocking antibody	Antibody directed to acetylcholine receptors that block binding of ^{125}I alpha-bungarotoxin	Elevated in one-third of patients with myasthenia gravis. Indicated when acetylcholine receptor-binding antibodies are not elevated
Antiadrenal cortex antibody	Antibody directed to adrenal cortex cells	Elevated in 75% of patients with autoimmune hypoadrenal corticism
Anticardiolipin antibody	Antibody directed to cardiolipin	Present in systemic lupus erythematosus (SLE) associated with arterial and venous thromboses and in patients with placental infarcts in early pregnancy with or without SLE. Elevation may be predictive of risk of thrombosis or recurrent spontaneous abortions of early pregnancy
Anticentromere antibody	Antibody directed to chromosome centromeres	Elevated in the CREST syndrome; also elevated in 30% of patients with Raynaud disease
Antiglomerular basement membrane antibody	Antibody directed to renal glomerular basement membrane	Presence suggests Goodpasture syndrome and autoimmune glomerulonephritis

[a]Tests are used to support medical diagnosis. Sensitivity and specificity are variable. Method of detection and reference standards vary among laboratories. Interpretation should be confirmed with the laboratory performing the test.
CREST, calcinosis, Raynaud phenomenon, esophageal involvement, sclerodactyly, and telangiectasia syndrome.

Appendix XII. **MANUFACTURERS OF ALLERGENIC EXTRACTS FOR DIAGNOSIS AND TREATMENT**

ALK-Abello, 800-325-7354, 1700 Royston Lane, Round Rock, TX 78644

Allergy Laboratories, Inc., 405-235-1451, 1005 Southwest 2nd Street, Oklahoma City, OK 73109

Allermed Laboratories, Inc., 800-221-2748, 7203 Convoy Court, San Diego, CA 92111

Greer Laboratories, Inc., 800-438-0088, P.O. Box 800, Lenoir, NC 28645

Hollister-Stier Laboratories, 800-992-1120, 3525 North Regal Street, Spokane, WA 99207

Nelco Laboratories, 631-242-3662, 154 Brook Ave., Deer Park, NY 11729

Appendix XIII. **COMMERCIAL SOURCES FOR ENVIRONMENTAL CONTROL PRODUCTS**

Allergy Clean Environments, 800-882-4110

Allergy Control Products, 800-442-DUST

Allergy-Products.Net, 877-437-2247

Allergy Shop, 800-211-5549

Allergy Supply Company, 800-323-7644

Allerx Allergy Products, 972-635-2580

ComfortLiving.com, 877-378-4411

Home Care America, 877-SHOP-HCA

National Allergy Supply, Inc., 800-522-1448

**Allergy and Asthma Network/
Mothers of Asthmatics, Inc.**
2751 Prosperity Avenue
Suite 1501
Fairfax, VA 22030
800-878-4403
www.aanma.org

**Asthma & Allergy Foundation
of America**
125 Fifteenth Street, N.W.
Suite 502
Washington, DC 20005
800-7-ASTHMA
www.aafa.org

Allergy Foundation of Canada
P.O. Box 1904
Saskatoon, S7K 3S
Canada
306-652-1608

Asthma Society of Canada
5130 Bridgeland Avenue
Suite 425
Toronto, Ontario M6A 1Z4
800-787-3880
416-787-4050 Toronto residents
Fax: 416-787-5807

**American Academy of Allergy,
Asthma & Immunology**
611 East Wells Street
Milwaukee, WI 53202
800-822-ASMA or 414-272-6071
www.aaaai.org

**Centers for Disease Control
and Prevention**
1600 Clifton Road
Atlanta, GA 30333
800-311-3435
www.cdc.gov

**American College of Allergy,
Asthma & Immunology**
84 West Algonquin Road
Suite 550
Arlington Heights, IL 60005
800-842-7777 or 847-427-1200
www.acaai.org

The Food Allergy Network
10400 Eaton Pl., Suite 107
Fairfax, VA 22030
800-929-4040
www.foodallergy.org

The American Lung Association
For the affiliate nearest you,
Call 800-LUNG-USA
www.lungusa.org

Immune Deficiency Foundation
25 W. Chesapeake Avenue
Suite 206
Towson, MD 21204
800-296-4433
www.primaryimmune.org

The American Thoracic Society
1740 Broadway
New York, NY 10019-4315
212-315-8700

**National Heart, Lung
& Blood Institute**
(National Asthma Education
& Prevention Program)
P.O. Box 30105
Bethesda, MD 20824
301-251-1222
www.nhbli.nih.org

**National Institute of Allergy
& Infectious Diseases**
Building 31, Room 7A-50
National Institutes of Health
Bethesda, MD 20892
301-496-5717
www.niaid.nih.gov

**U.S. Environmental
Protection Agency**
Indoor Environments Division
401 M Street, S.W. (6604J)
Washington, DC 20460
202-233-9370

**Indoor Air Quality Information
Clearinghouse**
800-438-4318
www.epa.gov/iaq

* Resources are provided as information only and not as endorsements.

SUBJECT INDEX

Note: Page numbers followed by "f" indicate figures; those followed by "t" indicate tabular material.